GERIATRIC NUTRITION

NUTRITION AND DISEASE PREVENTION

1. Genomics and Proteomics in Nutrition, *edited by Carolyn D. Berdanier and Naima Moustaid-Moussa*

2. Perinatal Nutrition: Optimizing Infant Health and Development, *edited by Jatinder Bhatia*

3. Soy in Health and Disease Prevention, *edited by Michihiro Sugano*

4. Nutrition and Cancer Prevention, *edited by Atif B. Awad and Peter G. Bradford*

5. Cancer Prevention and Management through Exercise and Weight Control, *edited by Anne McTiernan*

6. Nutritional Strategies for the Diabetic/Prediabetic Patient, *edited by Jeffrey I. Mechanick and Elise M. Brett*

7. Nutrient–Drug Interactions, *edited by Kelly Anne Meckling*

8. Geriatric Nutrition, *edited by John E. Morley and David R. Thomas*

Related Volumes

Introduction to Clinical Nutrition: Second Edition, Revised and Expanded, *edited by V. Sardesai*

Pediatric Gastroenterology and Nutrition in Clinical Practice, *edited by Carlos Lifschitz*

Nutrients and Cell Signaling, *edited by Janos Zempleni and K. Dakshinamurti*

Mitochondria in Health and Disease, *edited by Carolyn D. Berdanier*

Thiamine, *edited by Frank Jordan and Mulchand Patel*

Phytochemicals in Health and Disease, *edited by Yongping Bao and Roger Fenwick*

Handbook of Obesity: Etiology and Pathophysiology, Second Edition, *edited by George Bray and Claude Bouchard*

Handbook of Obesity: Clinical Applications, Second Edition, *edited by George Bray and Claude Bouchard*

GERIATRIC NUTRITION

Edited by

John E. Morley
David R. Thomas

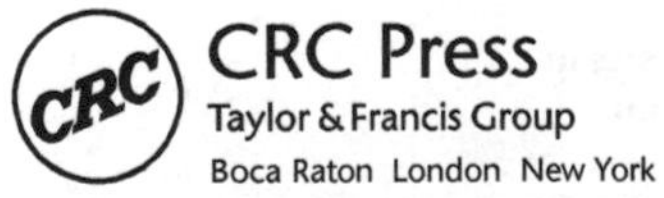

CRC Press is an imprint of the
Taylor & Francis Group, an informa business

CRC Press
Taylor & Francis Group
6000 Broken Sound Parkway NW, Suite 300
Boca Raton, FL 33487-2742

First issued in paperback 2019

ISBN-13: 978-0-8493-3815-1 (hbk)
ISBN-13: 978-0-367-38907-9 (pbk)

Library of Congress Cataloging-in-Publication Data

Geriatric nutrition / editors, John E. Morley and David R. Thomas.
p. ; cm. -- (Nutrition and disease prevention ; 8)
"A CRC title."
Includes bibliographical references and index.
ISBN-13: 978-0-8493-3815-1 (alk. paper)
ISBN-10: 0-8493-3815-8 (alk. paper)
1. Nutrition disorders in old age. 2. Older people--Nutrition. I. Morley, John E. II. Thomas, D. R. (David R.) III. Series.
[DNLM: 1. Nutrition Physiology. 2. Aged--physiology. WT 115 G3689 2007]

RC620.6.G38 2007
618.97--dc22 2006038911

Visit the Taylor & Francis Web site at
http://www.taylorandfrancis.com

and the CRC Press Web site at
http://www.crcpress.com

Contents

Preface

Food is essential to life. Absent adequate nutrition, depletion in both fat and fat-free mass leads to detrimental effects on an individual's health, ultimately progressing to death. Moreover, coexisting disease causes catastrophic effects on nutritional health, and poor nutritional health leads to acute and chronic disease. The magnitude of nutritional depletion from any cause depends to a large extent on the nutrient reservoir accumulated over time in each individual. In our increasingly older population, nutritional health is more marginal and the magnitude of the effect on nutritional health is amplified.

In this comprehensive text, normal nutrition, pathological nutrition, and optimal nutrition are carefully examined by a group of outstanding experts in the field. From these experts, a substantial difference in nutritional health in older individuals compared to younger persons emerges. The strategies to improve nutritional health in older individuals require unique approaches, are often frustrating, and require sensitivity to each individual's needs and belief system.

We commend to you the work of the authors of this book. We believe that you will both find basic knowledge and explore exciting new ideas in this volume, just as we did in reading the chapters. The text and chapters have been expanded and clarified with the aim to produce a state-of-the-art review of current nutritional thinking. To all of those who deal with nutritional health, whether as family, nutritional educators, dietitians, gerontologists, or geriatricians, we anticipate that this book will be useful in furthering our understanding of nutrition in older persons.

David R. Thomas
John E. Morley

The Editors

David R. Thomas is professor of internal medicine and geriatric medicine in the Division of Geriatric Medicine at Saint Louis University Health Sciences Center. Dr. Thomas serves as director of clinical research for the Division of Geriatric Medicine. He is medical director for two teaching nursing homes.

Dr. Thomas is certified in both internal medicine and the subspecialty of geriatric medicine by the American Board of Internal Medicine. He has been elected fellow of the American College of Physicians, the American Geriatrics Society, and the Gerontological Society of America. Dr. Thomas is a certified medical director in long-term care by the American Medical Directors Association. He has received the Sir William Osler Award for Excellence in Clinical Teaching at the Saint Louis University Department of Medicine.

Dr. Thomas currently serves as associate editor for the *Journal of the American Medical Directors Association* and on the editorial advisory board for the *Annals of Long Term Care*. He is a past associate editor of the *Journals of Gerontology: Medical Sciences*.

He has previously served on the board of directors of the National Pressure Ulcer Advisory Panel and as an associate editor of *Advances in Wound Care*. He serves on the American College of Physicians, Professional Information and Education Resource (PIER) Consultant Board, Pressure Ulcer Module, and on the Wound Healing Society Guideline Development Committee for pressure ulcers and venous stasis ulcers. Dr. Thomas is a member of the National Council for Nutritional Strategies in Long-Term Care. He serves on the Clinical Practice Committee of the American Medical Directors Association.

He has been honored with a John A. Hartford Faculty Fellow Award in Geriatrics and, by inclusion, in the Marquis *Who's Who in America* and is listed in *The Best Doctors in America* and *Top Doctors in Saint Louis*. He is a frequent invited educational speaker both nationally and internationally. Dr. Thomas is active in the American Geriatrics Society, the Gerontological Society of America, the American College of Physicians, the American Federation for Clinical Research, the American Medical Directors Association, the American Society of Parenteral and Enteral Nutrition, and the Wound Healing Society. He has authored over 120 publications and clinical investigations as well as 31 books or book chapters. His research interests include wound healing and clinical nutrition.

John Edward Morley completed his medical degree at the University of Witwatersrand in Johannesburg, South Africa in 1972. After completing his internal medicine residency in South Africa, he held a fellowship in endocrinology at UCLA. He was subsequently a staff endocrinologist at the Minneapolis VA Medical Center and the University of Minnesota. In January 1985, he moved to California to become director of the Geriatric Research, Education, and Clinical Center, Sepulveda, VA Medical Center, and a professor of medicine, University of California, Los Angeles. He is board certified in internal medicine, endocrinology, and geriatric medicine.

Dr. Morley has edited 21 books, including *Medical Care in the Nursing Home*, *Geriatric Nutrition*, *Endocrinology of Aging*, and *Principles and Practice of Geriatric Medicine*. He has published over 1000 papers, with a major research emphasis on the role of neuropeptides in the modulation of hormonal responses and behavior, as well as nutrition and hormones in older persons. For his work in appetite regulation, he received the Mead Johnson Award of the American Institution of Nutrition in 1985. His work has been cited over 20,000 times.

He has served on the editorial boards of nine journals. He was the associate editor of the *Journal of American Geriatrics Society.* He edits the geriatrics section of *Cyberounds*. He served as editor for the *Journal of Gerontology: Medical Sciences* from January 2000 through December 2005. He is the editor of the *Journal of the American Medical Director's Association.* He has been an invited speaker at numerous national and international meetings.

He was the Medical Director of the Year for Life Care Centers of America in 1998. In 1999, he was awarded the IPSEN Foundation Longevity Prize, which is one of the most prestigious European awards for research in gerontology. In 2001, he received the Gayle and Richard Olson Prize for Most Outstanding Behavioral Paper Published the Previous Year in the journal *Peptides*, as well as receiving the Circle Award from the American Dietetic Association. In 2002, he was chosen to receive the American Geriatrics Society's Nascher/Manning Award for his lifelong achievements in clinical geriatrics. In November 2004, he was awarded the Joseph T. Freeman Award by the Gerontological Society of America for his work in geriatrics in both research and practice. In June 2005, he was honored as the recipient of the Marsha Goodwin-Beck Interdisciplinary Award for Excellence in Geriatric Leadership by the Department of Veterans Affairs National Leadership Board.

In July 1989, Dr. Morley moved to St. Louis, Missouri to become the Dammert Professor of Gerontology and director of the Division of Geriatric Medicine at Saint Louis University Medical Center and director of the Geriatric Research, Education, and Clinical Center at the St. Louis Veterans Affairs Medical Center. He is the medical director of two nursing homes.

Contributors

Wasseem Aneed
Saint Louis University Medical Center
St. Louis, Missouri

H.J. Armbrecht
St. Louis VA Medical Center
and
Saint Louis University Medical Center
St. Louis, Missouri

Connie W. Bales
Durham VA Medical Center
and
Duke University Medical Center
Durham, North Carolina

Gwendolen T. Buhr
Duke University Medical Center
Durham, North Carolina

Linda S. Evanko
Durham VA Medical Center
Durham, North Carolina

Julie K. Gammack
Saint Louis University Medical Center
and
St. Louis VA Medical Center
St. Louis, Missouri

Nathalia Garcia
Saint Louis University Medical Center
St. Louis, Missouri

Mehret Gebretsadik
Saint Louis University Medical Center
St. Louis, Missouri

George T. Grossberg
Saint Louis University Medical Center
St. Louis, Missouri

Ramzi R. Hajjar
St. Louis VA Medical Center
and
Saint Louis University Medical Center
St. Louis, Missouri

Victoria H. Hawk
Duke University Medical Center
Durham, North Carolina

Matthew T. Haren
St. Louis VA Medical Center
and
Saint Louis University Medical Center
St. Louis, Missouri

Aminah Jatoi
Mayo Clinic
Rochester, Minnesota

Seema Joshi
Saint Louis University Medical Center
St. Louis, Missouri

Rafi Kevorkian
St. Louis VA Medical Center
and
Saint Louis University Medical Center
St. Louis, Missouri

Juergen Martin Bauer
Friedrich Alexander Universitat
Erlangen Nurnberg
Nurnberg, Germany

Angela Mazza
Saint Louis University Medical Center
St. Louis, Missouri

Heidi McKean
Mayo Clinic
Rochester, Minnesota

D. Douglas Miley
Saint Louis University Medical Center
St. Louis, Missouri

John E. Morley
Saint Louis University Medical Center
and
St. Louis VA Medical Center
St. Louis, Missouri

Devaraj Munikrishnappa
Saint Louis University Medical Center
St. Louis, Missouri

Zeina Nahhas
Industry Representative
Beirut, Lebanon

M. Louay Omran
Saint Louis University Medical Center
St. Louis, Missouri

Shailaja Pulisetty
Saint Louis University Medical Center
St. Louis, Missouri

Neelavathi Senkottaiyan
Saint Louis University Medical Center
St. Louis, Missouri

Zareen Syed
Saint Louis University Medical Center
St. Louis, Missouri

Syed H. Tariq
Saint Louis University Medical Center
St. Louis, Missouri

David R. Thomas
Saint Louis University Medical Center
St. Louis, Missouri

Chantri Trinh
Saint Louis University Medical Center
St. Louis, Missouri

Nina Tumosa
St. Louis VA Medical Center
and
Saint Louis University Medical Center
St. Louis, Missouri

Dorothee Volkert
Rheinische Friedrich Wilhelms
Universität Bonn
Bonn, Germany

Kent R. Wehmeier
Saint Louis University Medical Center
St. Louis, Missouri

Heidi K. White
Durham VA Medical Center
and
Duke University Medical Center
Durham, North Carolina

Gary A. Wittert
University of Adelaide
Adelaide, South Australia

1 The Aging Society and Nutrition Epidemiology

Shailaja Pulisetty, M.D.
John E. Morley, M.B., B.Ch.

CONTENTS

Both the number and proportion of older persons are growing in all countries; the trends worldwide are likely to continue unabated. Issues in geriatric nutrition are inextricably linked to broader issues facing the aging population. This chapter sets the stage for this volume's discussion of geriatric nutrition by providing an overview of some of these broader issues facing the aging population.

There are 380 million people aged 65 years and above, and by the year 2020, the over-65 population is projected to increase to more than 690 million.[1] The number of persons aged 60 years or older is projected to grow to almost 2 billion by 2050.[2] For the first time in human history, the population of older persons will be larger than the population of children (0 to 14 years).[2] This trend has been amplified by fall in mortality and increased life expectancy. The increasing demands on national health budgets and other resources are a matter of considerable future concern. The oldest old (80+) make up 12% of the population aged 60 years or older. Table 1.1 depicts the percentage of population aged 60 years and older in selected countries.

In 2000, approximately 10% of world's population was 60 years old or older. This figure is expected to rise to 20% by 2050. This means that 400 million older people will be living in the developed countries and over 1.5 billion in the less developed world.[3]

The demographic transition from predominantly young to predominantly middle-aged or old populations is taking place, and this epidemiological transition is changing the pattern of morbidity dominated by infectious diseases to chronic diseases and disabilities. Many of the diseases suffered by older persons are a result of dietary factors operating from infancy and physiological changes occurring with the aging process.[4,5] The leading cause of death in older people worldwide is vascular disease and associated chronic conditions.[6] There exists a great potential

TABLE 1.1
Percentage of Population Aged 60+ Years (2004)

Country	Percentage
Japan	25.6
San Marino, Italy	25.3
Germany	24.8
Sweden	23.0
Greece	22.9
U.K., Spain, Switzerland	21.0
Canada	17.5
U.S.	16.5
Ireland	15.0
Chile	11.3
China	10.8
Jamaica	10.1
India	7.8
Pakistan	5.8
Kuwait	3.0

Source: Abstracted from World Health Organization, *The World Health Report 2006*, Geneva, 2006.

for prevention of these diseases through exercise, nutritious diet, and avoidance of smoking. Nutrition intervention holds the promise of mitigating the growing burden of chronic disease and disability and improving the quality of life of the rapidly growing older population.

Table 1.2 and Table 1.3 depict life expectancies at birth for males and females in various countries. For both men and women the Japanese have the longest-lived population. For reasons that are not entirely agreed upon, women have an advantage of higher life expectancy at birth and at older ages in both developed and most developing countries. This pattern has significant consequences for the health of these older women. The longer life span of women, combined with the fact that men marry younger women and that widowed men remarry more often than widowed women, means that there are more widows in the world than widowers. Women in many countries rely on men for economic resources, making them at risk for dependency, isolation, neglect, and poverty.[3]

Table 1.4 shows that of the total 182 million men over 65 years, 9 million are 85+. Numbers for women over 65 are 237 million, of which 19 million are 85+. Table 1.5 shows that Japan has the longest life expectancy at age 60 for both men and women.

Whether the increase in life expectancy means more health or more years of sickness is one of the most difficult questions for health planners and politicians trying to allocate funds.

TABLE 1.2
Life Expectancy at Birth in Years for Males

Country	Age (years)
Japan, Iceland	79
Australia, Canada, Israel, Italy, Monaco	78
Andorra, Greece, Norway, New Zealand	77
Netherlands, Spain, Singapore	77
Austria, France, Germany, U.K.	76
Belgium, Cuba, Denmark, U.S., Finland	75
Chile	74
Mexico	72
China, Bosnia	70
Philippines	65
India, Nepal, Mongolia	61

Source: Abstracted from World Health Organization, *The World Health Report 2006*, Geneva, 2006.

TABLE 1.3
Life Expectancy at Birth in Years for Females

Country	Age (years)
Japan	86
Monaco	85
Italy, San Marino	84
Andorra, Australia, France, Spain	83
Austria, Germany, Greece, Israel, Norway	82
Cuba, Denmark	80
Mexico, Bosnia	77
U.K., Romania, Bulgaria	76
U.S., Equador, Mauritius, Sri Lanka	75
China, Brazil, Jamaica, Saudi Arabia	74
India, Pakistan, Bangladesh	63
Nepal	61

Source: Abstracted from World Health Organization, *The World Health Report 2006*, Geneva, 2006.

The percentage of the population aged 60 or above is currently much higher in more developed countries, but the pace of aging is more rapid in the developing regions.[2] In 1975 about 52% of all persons aged 60 and over lived in developing countries, and this proportion is expected to reach nearly 72% by 2005 (http://www.un.org/esa/socdev/ageing/ageipaal.htm).

TABLE 1.4
Number of Men and Women 65 and Older Worldwide by Age Group, 2000 (in millions)

Age (years)	85+	75–84	65–74
Male	9	48	125
Female	19	72	146

Source: World Health Organization, *Gender, Health and Ageing*, http://www.int/gender/documents/en/gender_ageing.pdf.

TABLE 1.5
Life Expectancy at Age 60 in Selected Countries (2000–2005)

Country	Women (years)	Men (years)
Japan	27	22
Switzerland	26	21
France	26	20
Italy, Canada, Australia	25	21
Iceland	25	22
Spain	25	20
Germany, Netherlands	24	19
U.S., Chile	24	20
U.K.	23	20
China	20	17
India	18	16
South Africa	18	14
Nepal	17	15

Source: http://unstats.un.org/unsd/demographic/products/indwm/ww2005/tab3a.htm.

An older person's energy requirement per kilogram of body weight is reduced due to decline in lean body mass and basal metabolic rate with aging. Although total energy intake declines with age, nutrient requirements go up to maintain organ systems with declining functionality. Moreso, the nutritional requirements in the older population are not very well defined. The elderly in tropical regions of the third world may have greater or lesser nutrient requirements than their peers in Europe and North America, as lifestyle, lifelong environmental and dietary exposures, parasites, and foods can condition the uptake or utilization of nutrients.[7]

The operation of the multiple risk factors is modified by the country of origin, beginning with genetic and ethnic makeup of the population and extending to cultural assumptions about aging and the access of individuals to health care resources.[8] The ability to purchase, prepare, consume, and absorb food is dependent on multiple factors, as listed in Table 1.6. With aging there is reduced absorption of iron and some micronutrients. Visual impairments associated with aging impede self-feeding and food preparation. Poor dentition and difficulty with chewing can cause inadequate nutritional intake. As chewing becomes difficult, older persons often choose soft foods that are high in sugars and carbohydrates over fresh vegetables and meats. People with dementia are at risk for malnutrition because they often forget to eat, cannot make proper judgments about type of foods to eat, or become too impaired to feed themselves.

In the developing world, the percentage of gross domestic product expended on health is often lower than in developed countries and health ministries are

TABLE 1.6
Risk Factors for Undernutrition in Elderly

Physiological
Declining absorption
Reduced visual, olfactory, taste acuity
Food intolerance
Anorexia
Physical
Poor dentition
Chewing difficulty
Impaired mobility
Psychological
Depression
Loneliness
Dementia
Food likes/dislikes
Social and Economical
Poverty
Transportation availability
Lack of knowledge of nutrition
Inadequate cooking knowledge (men)
Cultural beliefs
Availability of familiar foods
Availability of transportation
Others
Prescribed diets
Medication side effects
Alcoholism

underfinanced.[8] It will not take much of an increase in the older population to make the funding for health even more precarious.[8] Whereas statistics show that most of the world's elderly live in the developing world, most of the research pertaining to nutrition in older persons has been carried out in developed countries. The results of studies on developed countries are not transferable to developing countries, as the older people in these countries are old at a chronologically younger age and are likely to have reached their old age after a lifetime of suboptimal nutrition and poor health.[9] There exists a significant need for geriatric nutrition research in the developing world. Additionally, the systems of home care nurses, geriatric specialists, nursing homes, senior nutrition programs, and senior centers do not exist in most of developing countries.[10]

Table 1.7 illustrates per capita food consumption globally and regionally. Patterns of increasing dietary excess are seen in higher-income Central and South America and most of the Caribbean, where intake of animal products and fat has increased, with a decline in intake of fruits and vegetables.[11] Asian nations showed a decline in the availability of complex carbohydrates and an increase in total fats.[12] In Brazil, obesity is prevalent among even the least-income sector.[13] The per capita energy supply has declined from both animal and vegetable sources in the countries in economic transition, while it has increased in the developing and developed countries. The per capita supply of animal protein is three times higher in developed countries and the supply of vegetable protein is higher in developing countries. The highest consumption of fat is in parts of North America and Europe, and the least consumption is in Africa.

Fish consumption is highest in Japan, Iceland, and some small island states. Fish consumption is associated with a decrease in atherosclerotic cardiovascular disease.[14] A recent study based on data from 36 countries reported that fish consumption leads to reduced risk of death from all causes as well as cardiovascular deaths.[15] The lowest fat consumption is recorded in Africa, and the highest consumption occurs in North America and Europe. In South Africa, there has been increased consumption of fat and reduction in carbohydrate intake.[16] In China, there is a greater fat intake from both animal and vegetable sources.[17] Similarly, in India a large community-based survey showed higher intake of fat in higher socioeconomic groups than in lower-income groups and the prevalence of heart disease was higher in high-income groups than in lower-income groups. The dietary changes combined with growth of the aging population suggest an escalating epidemic of diabetes, obesity, and heart disease in the developing countries.

Obesity also makes direct contributions to risk of chronic disease, and in parallel with dietary changes, there is rapidly increasing prevalence of obesity worldwide. Latin America and the Caribbean have a high prevalence of obesity currently. In the developing countries, factors associated with obesity are urbanization, increased life expectancy, mechanization and lower-energy-expending labor, television and other sedentary activities, and consumption of a higher-energy

TABLE 1.7
Global and Regional Per Capita Food Consumption

Region	Calories (kcal/day), 1997–1999	Meat (kg/year)	Milk (kg/year)	Vegetables (kg/year)	Fat (g/day), 1997–1999
World	2803	36.4	78.1	101.9	73.0
Developing countries	2681	25.5	44.6	98.8	—
Sub-Sahara Africa	3006	13.4	29.1	52.1	45.0
Near East, North Africa	2195	21.2	72.3	—	—
Latin America	2824	76.6	110.2	—	79.0
East Asia	2921	58.5	10.0	—	52.0
South Asia	2403	11.7	67.5	116.2	52.0
Industrialized countries	3380	100.1	212.2	112.8	100.1
Transition countries	2906	60.7	159.1	—	60.7

Source: Abstracted from World Health Organization, *Global and Regional Food Consumption Patterns and Trends*, Geneva, 2003; FAOSTAT, 2003.

dense diet.[18] In Chile, from 1988 to 1997, prevalence of obesity increased by 9% in women and by 10% in men.[19] In China, obesity is associated with higher income in both rural and urban regions.[20]

There are considerable challenges to research on the nutritional status of the elderly in developing countries. Due to incomplete information in nutrient databases, particularly in regard to the nutrients of concern in the elderly, such as vitamins B6, B12, D, and E, folate, and carotenoids, dietary intake remains difficult to assess in many regions.[21] Micronutrient deficiencies are very common among the elderly population in the developing world, and they have been linked to chronic diseases. Vitamin B12 has been associated with neurologic and cognitive function.[22] Vitamins B6 and B12 and folate are required to prevent elevation of homocysteine, which in turn is linked with risk of vascular disease.[23] Calcium and Vitamin D are also important nutrients in the elderly, as the requirements increase with aging. The low calcium and vitamin D intake in developing countries suggests osteoporosis risk is an increasingly major problem. The requirements for vitamin A are lower in the elderly due to reduced hepatic clearance.

Some countries have taken initiatives in improving the nutritional status of the aging population. In Chile, individuals over 70 who are registered at primary health clinics receive a powdered mixture (2 kg/month) providing 400 kcal/100 g as well as array of micronutrients.[9]

More research is needed to assess the nutritional status of the aging population in developing nations. Additionally, international dietary guidelines for older individuals are needed to guide community awareness and interventions.

REFERENCES

1. http://www.who.int/whr/1997/media_centre/50facts.
2. United Nations, *Population Aging, 2002*, http://unstats.un.org/unsd/demographic/products/indwm/ww2005/tab39.htm.
3. World Health Organization, *Gender, Health and Ageing,* http://www.int/gender/documents/en/gender_ageing.pdf.
4. World Health Organization, *Programming of Chronic Disease by Impaired Fetal Nutrition: Evidence and Implications for Policy and Intervention Strategies*, Geneva, 2002.
5. Godfrey, K.M. and Barker, D.J., Fetal nutrition and adult disease, *Am. J. Clin. Nutr.*, 71, 1344S, 2000.
6. Murray, C.J. and Lopez, A.D., Mortality by cause for eight regions of the world: global burden of disease study, *Lancet*, 349, 1269, 1997.
7. Solomons, N.W., Nutrition and aging: potentials and problems for research in developing countries, *Nutr. Rev.*, 50, 224, 1992.
8. Solomons, N.W., Demographic and nutritional trends among the elderly in developed and developing regions, *Eur. J. Clin. Nutr.*, 54, S2, 2000.
9. Dangour, A.D. and Ismail, S.J., Tropical medicine and international health, *Trop. Med. Int. Health*, 8, 287, 2003.
10. World Health Organization, *Ageing and Nutrition: A Growing Global Challenge*, Geneva, 2001.
11. Popkin, B.M., The nutrition transition in low-income countries: an emerging crisis, *Nutr. Rev.*, 52, 285, 1994.
12. Drewnowski, A. and Popkin, B.M., The nutrition transition: new trends in global diet, *Nutr. Rev.*, 55, 31, 1997.
13. Monteiro, C.A., Mondini, L., deSouza, A.L., et al., The nutrition transition in Brazil, *Eur. J. Clin. Nutr.*, 49, 105, 1995.
14. Kromhout, D., Bosschieter, E.B., and deLezenne, C.C., The inverse relation between fish consumption and 20-year mortality from coronary heart disease, *N. Engl. J. Med.*, 312, 1205, 1985.
15. Zhang, J., Sasaki, S., Amano, K., et al., Fish consumption and mortality from all causes, ischemic heart disease, and stroke: an ecological study, *Prev. Med.*, 28, 520, 1999.
16. Bourne, L.T., Langenhoven, M.L., Steyn, K., et al., Nutrient intake in the urban African population of the Cape Peninsula, South Africa. The Brisk Study, *Cent. Afr. J. Med.*, 39, 238, 1993.
17. Popkin, B.M., Keyou, G., Zhai, F., et al., The nutrition transition in China: a cross sectional analysis, *Eur. J. Clin. Nutr.*, 47, 333, 1993.
18. Caballero, B., Introduction. Symposium: obesity in developing countries: biological and ecological factors, *J. Nutr.*, 131, 855S, 2001.
19. Vio, F. and Albala, C., Nutrition policy in the Chilean transition, *Public Health Nutr.*, 3, 49, 2000.
20. Du, S., Lu, B., Zhai, F., et al., The new stage of the nutrition transition in China, *Public Health Nutr.*, 5, 169, 2002.
21. Tucker, K.L. and Buranapin, S., Nutrition and aging in developing countries, *J. Nutr.*, 131, 21417S, 2001.
22. Russell, R.M., Micronutrient requirements of the elderly, *Nutr. Rev.*, 50, 463, 1992.

23. Hattersley, A.T. and Tooke, J.E., The fetal insulin hypothesis: an alternative explanation of the association of low birthweight with diabetes and vascular disease, *Lancet*, 353, 1789, 1999.

2 Molecular Theories of Aging and Nutritional Interventions

H.J. Armbrecht, Ph.D.

CONTENTS

Gerontological research has made great strides in recent years in understanding how we age.[1] Aging is a biological process that occurs at the molecular, cellular, and systems levels. These levels are both interdependent and independent. As molecules, cells, and systems change with age, the capacity of an organism to regulate itself declines. One of the hallmarks of the aging process is this decreased regulatory capacity in the face of external stressors.[2] It ultimately leads to death. This research has provided new support for some theories of aging. Other theories now seem less useful or have been merged with others.

Nutritional research has also made great strides in understanding the beneficial effects of food components at the molecular level. Some food components have the capacity to increase mean life span (vitamin E). Some food manipulations (dietary restriction) have the capacity to increase maximal life span in animal studies. Other food components (polyphenols) may have beneficial effects on specific tissues, such as the brain. We can now study these food components and food manipulations in light of biological aging to better understand their beneficial effects.

The purpose of this chapter is to briefly present theories of aging and their interaction at the molecular, cellular, and systems levels. At each level we will discuss some nutritional interventions suggested by these theories. In general, these will be interventions with the significant experimental support in model systems. Most of the experimental studies will involve rodent models of aging, although there will be a few references to roundworms and flies. Where they exist, studies in tissues and isolated cells will also be cited. Hopefully, this review will provide a basis for understanding current human studies and for proposing new human interventions.

2.1 AGING AT THE MOLECULAR LEVEL: FREE RADICALS

2.1.1 The Free Radical Theory of Aging

The major biochemical components of cells are proteins, nucleic acids (DNA and RNA), and lipids. There is experimental evidence, particularly in animal models of aging, that these components become altered with time to the point that their molecular function is compromised. The main driving force behind these molecular alterations is thought to be free radicals in the form of highly reactive oxygen and nitrogen compounds. The free radicals themselves are generated by such things as energy production by the cell and the activity of certain cellular enzymes. These molecular alterations lead to alterations in cell function, which in turn lead to alterations in tissue function. Altered tissue function ultimately leads to aging and death of the whole organism.[3] In its broadest form, this has come to be known as the free radical theory of aging. This concept dominates much of the present thinking about the biology of aging.

A number of experimental correlations in animals support the free radical theory.[4] First, oxidative damage to DNA, protein, and membrane lipids increases with age. Second, species longevity is directly related to the efficiency of its repair mechanisms. Third, a high metabolic rate generates more free radicals and is associated with a shorter life span. Finally, organisms such as roundworms, fruit flies, and mice that are engineered to have higher antioxidant defenses live longer.

2.1.1.1 Scope of the Free Radical Theory

Because of these correlations, the free radical theory has gradually expanded to include previous theories of aging. The rate of living theory, proposed years ago,[5] states that a high metabolic rate is associated with a shorter life span. Since a higher metabolic rate would be expected to produce more free radicals, this is now interpreted in terms of increased free radical damage.

The error catastrophe theory predicted that as proteins became damaged with age they would produce more damaged proteins.[6] The protein machinery that made proteins from messenger RNA would itself become dysfunctional, leading to even more errors in protein synthesis. However, there do not appear to be large changes in the numbers or amounts of proteins in a given tissue with age. Rather, the changes in proteins tend to be more subtle, with proteins being oxidized or nitrosylated with age. This, in itself, can have dramatic effects. It can lead to decreased protein degradation and to proteins aggregating in unhealthy ways (i.e., beta-amyloid). Another theory involving the modification of existing proteins is the glycation theory. Glycation is the progressive attachment of sugar groups to certain proteins with the passage of time. Since glycation is speeded up by free radicals, this too has become a component of the free radical theory.

The DNA damage theory of aging has focused on the chemical modifications that take place in the individual bases that make up the DNA double helix.[7] Most of the DNA damage is the result of free radical reactions. If not repaired, these modifications can lead to DNA strand breaks, chromosomal rearrangement, aberrant DNA replication, and altered transcription of genes. At the cellular level, this can lead to cell death or uncontrolled cell growth.

Finally, the membrane theory of aging stresses the importance of the lipid membranes that compartmentalize the cell.[8] The cellular plasma membrane encloses the cell and is involved in the transport of nutrients and in cell-to-cell recognition. The mitochondrial and nuclear membranes delineate their respective subcellular organelles and regulate transport. The endoplasmic reticulum/golgi membranes are involved in protein synthesis and export. There is evidence that the elasticity (fluidity) of these membranes may change with age, affecting their function as part of the cell. These elasticity changes are due to lipid oxidation, which is a result of free radical generation.

2.1.1.2 Predictions of the Free Radical Theory

In addition to the experimental correlations listed previously, the free radical theory also makes testable predictions. It predicts positive effects from (1) slowing down the rate of radical formation, (2) increasing protection against free radicals, or (3) repairing free radical damage. These effects may be in delaying the start of aging or in slowing down the rate of aging. This results in an increase in maximal life span or at least an increase in functional life span. In this regard, the free radical theory has been the inspiration for many nutritional interventions in the aging process (see below).

One cellular location where many components of the free radical theory come together and perhaps synergize is in the mitochondria. Mitochondria generate the energy for the cell adenosine triphosphate (ATP) via the process of oxidative phosphorylation. Oxidative phosphorylation, although critical to cell function, itself generates free radicals. The mitochondria contain attractive targets for free radical attack—an outer and inner lipid membrane, circular DNA, and proteins, including those proteins involved in oxidative phosphorylation. Because of all these potential interactions, it has been proposed that age-related changes in mitochondria may account for many of the features of cell and tissue aging—the mitochondrial theory of aging.[9] Because mitochondria are attractive targets for nutritional intervention, we will consider mitochondrial aging separately (see below).

2.1.2 Nutritional Interventions Based on the Free Radical Theory

As mentioned above, the free radical theory predicts that slowing down the rate of radical formation, or increasing protection against free radicals, or repairing free radical damage should have positive effects on functionality and longevity. From a nutritional standpoint, this has most often been attempted by (1) feeding vitamins with antioxidant properties, (2) feeding foods rich in phytochemicals such as carotenoids, flavonoids, and polyphenols, or (3) feeding natural foods high in antioxidant activity. We will discuss examples of each of these strategies. These examples and their actions are summarized in Table 2.1.

TABLE 2.1
Interventions Based on the Free Radical Theory

Action	Experimental System	Reference
Vitamin E		
Blocked oxidative stress due to hypoxia or inflammation	Young rats	11, 12
Blocked lipid peroxidation and inflammation (with ascorbate)	Old rats	13
Maintained long-term potentiation and reversed oxidative stress	Old rats	14
Reversed sensitivity to oxidative stress	Brain slices from old rats	15
Blocked toxicity and oxidative stress from amyloid	Cultured rat neuronal cells	16
Enhanced immune function	Old mice	17, 18
Ginkgo biloba		
Increased survival time under hypoxia	Young mice	22
Reduced lipid peroxidation and increased antioxidant pathways in brain	Young rats	23
Increased cell survival after oxidative stress	Cultured rat neuronal cells	24, 25
Blocked toxicity of amyloid peptide	Cultured rat neuronal cells	26, 27
Fruit Polyphenols		
Retarded age-related cognitive decline	Aging rats	29
Reversed behavioral deficits and improved neuronal function	Old rats	30
Prevented memory deficits in Alzheimer's disease model	Mice overproducing amyloid	31

2.1.2.1 Antioxidant Vitamins: Vitamin E

The antioxidant vitamins include vitamins E, C, and A. Vitamin E (alpha-tocopherol) is lipid soluble and protects membrane lipids by functioning as an antioxidant. It functions to break the chain of free radical reactions that result in lipid peroxidation. Vitamin C (ascorbate) is a water-soluble free radical scavenger that may help to inhibit lipid peroxidation. Vitamin A (carotinoids) has many diverse actions on systems, such as the immune system, in addition to being an antioxidant.

Vitamin E has been one of the most studied of the antioxidant vitamins. There is evidence from animal studies that it extends mean (average) life span, but there is controversy as to whether it extends maximal life span.[10] However, it does have beneficial effects in a number of experimental models relevant to aging. One of these models is the simulation of hypoxia and the resulting oxidative damage in young rats.[11] Organs such as the brain and kidneys with a high oxygen requirement may be particularly susceptible to hypoxia with age. In this rat model of hypoxia, vitamin E supplementation prevented the oxidative damage seen with inadequate oxygen availability.

In another model of oxidative stress, lipopolysaccharide (LPS) was used to induce an inflammatory response that resulted in oxidative stress in young rats.[12] Many age-related diseases, such as Alzheimer's disease, are thought to have an inflammatory component. Vitamin E administration prior to LPS injection reduced a number of biochemical parameters related to oxidative stress.

With regard to aging itself, the protective effects of vitamin E have been studied in the brain tissue of aging rats. One study compared several biochemical markers in the brain cortex from young and old rats.[13] It found that markers for lipid peroxidation and inflammation were higher in the old rats. These elevated markers were not observed in old animals fed a diet of vitamin E and ascorbate for 12 weeks.

The capacity of rats to sustain long-term potentiation (LTP) is impaired in old rats.[14] LTP is a biochemical process in the brain that may be related to long-term memory. There are also increases in lipid peroxidation and inflammation in old animals that may be related to increased oxidative stress. Feeding the aged rats vitamin E reversed the markers for oxidative stress and restored the ability of the animals to sustain LTP.

The effects of vitamin E have also been studied in isolated brain preparations. Brain striatal slices from young and old rats were studied directly in perfusion chambers.[15] Neurotransmitter release from these slices is sensitive to agents that produce oxidative stress. Slices from old animals were more sensitive to oxidative stress than slices from young animals. However, preincubation with vitamin E reversed the sensitivity to oxidative stress. This suggests that the old striatum has decreased antioxidant capacity compared to the young, but that this capacity can be boosted by exogenous antioxidants.

One factor in the pathogenesis of Alzheimer's disease in humans may be increased oxidative stress with age. The peptide molecule that may play a major role in Alzheimer's disease, amyloid beta-protein, may also contribute to this oxidative stress. There is evidence for this from cell culture studies. For example, culturing primary rat embryonic hippocampal neurons with the full-length peptide (Abeta(1-42)) results in increased protein oxidation, oxygen radical formation, and neurotoxicity.[16] These effects of Abeta(1-42) were blocked by the presence of vitamin E.

In addition to possible protective effects in the brain, dietary vitamin E has been shown to be beneficial to the immune system. Feeding vitamin E for 6 weeks boosted the immune response of aged mice to that seen in young mice.[17] This action of vitamin E may be mediated by suppression of prostaglandin synthesis. In a direct test of immune function, old mice were challenged with influenza virus.[18] Those mice fed a diet containing vitamin E for 6 months prior to the challenge had significantly lower viral titers and were able to maintain their body weight compared to control animals. These effects of vitamin E may be independent of its antioxidant properties, since other antioxidants had no effect in the same study.

2.1.2.2 Phytochemical Supplements: *Ginkgo biloba*

Phytochemicals are a group of natural substances with variable phenolic structures. Flavonoids are the most widely occurring group.[19] Some common flavonoids are quercetin (found in onions, apples, broccoli, and berries), the flavanones (found in citrus fruit), the catechins (found in green and black tea and red wine), and the anthocyanins (found in strawberries, grapes, wine, and tea).[20] Curcumin, a yellow curry spice used in India, is another well-known flavonoid. Traditionally, the beneficial effects of the flavonoids have been attributed to their ability to act as antioxidants by neutralizing free radical compounds. However, recent studies have indicated that flavonoids can also modulate cell signaling pathways independent of their antioxidant properties.[21]

The most well studied of the phytochemical-rich supplements is *Ginkgo biloba* extract. The standardized *Ginkgo* extract preparation, EGb761, contains 24% flavonoids. In intact mouse studies, this preparation was found to considerably prolong the survival time of mice undergoing lethal hypoxia.[22] This parallels the effect of vitamin E in the hypoxia model discussed previously.[11] Interestingly, the nonflavone fraction of the *Ginkgo* preparation was reported to be the source of the antihypoxia activity in this study. In a study in normal rats, treatment with EGb761 was found to reduce lipid peroxidation but also to increase the activity of some antioxidant enzymes in the brain.[23] This is evidence that EGb761 has biochemical effects in addition to its antioxidant properties.

The actions of *Ginkgo* have also been studied in cell culture models. In one study using rat cerebellar neurons, pretreatment with *Ginkgo* extract increased the survival of cells subsequently challenged by oxidative stress induced by hydrogen peroxide.[24] In a similar experiment, two different *Ginkgo* extracts increased the survival of cultured neurons challenged by oxidative stress from hydrogen peroxide and iron.[25] Likewise, EGb761 blocked the toxicity of Abeta(1-42) in primary hippocampal cells in part by blocking the accumulation of free radicals.[26] A similar effect was demonstrated in a rat nerve cell line, perhaps by interacting with Abeta itself.[27] This action is similar to the ability of vitamin E to block the toxicity of Abeta fragments, discussed earlier.

2.1.2.3 Natural Foods: Fruit Polyphenols

A number of epidemiological studies have suggested that diets rich in fruits and vegetables have positive effects in older persons. This has led to the study of the possible benefits of fruit and vegetable polyphenolic compounds. Extracts of fruits and vegetables have been studied extensively by Joseph et al.[28] In initial studies, the ability of extracts to retard age-related cognitive changes was studied. Rats were fed diets containing 1 to 2% extracts of strawberry or spinach from 6 to 14 months of age.[29] These diets were successful in retarding the age-related declines in learning and memory seen in these animals. These behavioral changes correlated with retardation of age-related changes in brain biochemical function. The spinach extract had the most beneficial effect, but the strawberry extract was also effective. These results prompted the question of whether fruit extracts could reverse already existing deficits. The effects of strawberry, spinach, and blueberry extracts were studied in old rats with behavioral deficits.[30] When these extracts were fed for 8 weeks, they reversed these behavioral deficits along with improving biochemical parameters related to neuronal function.

Blueberry supplementation has also been studied in an Alzheimer's disease model.[31] Mice engineered to overproduce beta-amyloid and develop amyloid plaques show memory deficits by 12 months. Blueberry supplementation started at 4 months prevented these deficits. Interestingly, it did so without reducing the beta-amyloid burden. However, the blueberry diet stimulated hippocampal signaling pathways in ways associated with improved memory. This suggests that fruit polyphenols may have specific effects in the brain not related to their antioxidant properties. These effects may include increasing receptor sensitivity, improving ion buffering, and reducing premature death of neuronal cells.[28]

2.2 AGING AT THE CELLULAR LEVEL: MITOCHONDRIA

The mitochondria are subcellular organelles delineated by an inner and outer membrane. The inner membrane is the site of the proteins involved in the electron transport that generates ATP. Mitochondria also contain circular DNA that codes for specific proteins not coded for by the nuclear chromosomal DNA. Some of these proteins are components of the mitochondrial electron transport chain. Mitochondria perform many other functions in the cell in addition to generating energy, such as regulating intracellular calcium and participating in apoptotic pathways. As a byproduct of their ATP generation via electron transport, they also generate free radical compounds. To counteract this, they have their own antioxidant defenses, such as mitochondrial superoxide dismutase (SOD).

2.2.1 Mitochondrial Aging

Mitochondria show a number of changes with age that may be related to free radical generation and oxidative damage. These include an increase in oxidized lipids and alteration in membrane fluidity.[8] There is also an increase in mitochondrial DNA mutations and oxidized proteins with age.[32,33] This leads to functional changes such as decreased mitochondrial membrane potential, decreased ATP production, and increased free radical production with age.[34,35]

2.2.2 Nutritional Interventions Based on Mitochondrial Aging

The concept of improving mitochondrial function by nutritional means has been extensively explored by Liu and Ames.[36] Their idea has been to reduce age-related "mitochondrial decay" and thereby ameliorate cognitive dysfunction, Alzheimer's disease, and Parkinson's disease. This group proposes several ways by which nutrients may have a positive effect on mitochondrial function: (1) protecting and enhancing mitochondrial enzymes, (2) increasing antioxidant defenses, (3) reducing oxidant stress by reducing free radical production, and (4) repairing mitochondrial structural damage. Three dietary compounds that may have one or more of these effects are L-carnitine, lipoic acid, and coenzyme Q. Their actions are summarized in Table 2.2.

2.2.2.1 L-Carnitine

L-Carnitine is needed to transport fatty acids into and out of mitochondria as part of their ATP synthesizing function.[36] The derivative acetyl-L-carnitine (ALCAR) is used in nutritional studies because it enters cells and crosses membranes more easily. Its benefits include antioxidant activity, improved mitochondrial energy production, and stabilization of intracellular membranes.[37] ALCAR has been used to treat a number of neurological disorders and to prevent ischemic damage. Liu and coworkers showed

TABLE 2.2
Interventions Based on Mitochondrial Aging

Action	Experimental System	Reference
L-Carnitine		
Reduced mitochondrial oxidative damage and partially reversed memory loss	Old rats	9, 38
Reduced toxicity of amyloid peptide	Cultured neuronal cells	39
Lipoic Acid		
Reduced mitochondrial oxidative damage and partially reversed memory loss	Old rats	9, 38
Reduced age-related oxidative stress in heart	Aging mice	41
Improved age-related memory loss in mouse model	SAMP8 mice	42
Reduced toxicity of amyloid peptide	Cultured neuronal cells	43
Coenzyme Q		
Improved tolerance to pacing stress in myocardium	Old rats	45
Reduced age-related oxidative stress in heart	Aging mice	41
Neuroprotective effect	Mouse model of ALS	46

that feeding ALCAR to old rats for 7 weeks ameliorated mitochondrial oxidative damage and dysfunction.[9] In addition, the same feeding schedule partially reversed memory loss in old rats.[38]

The effects of ALCAR have also been studied *in vitro* in neuronal cell cultures.[39] When Abeta(1-42), the peptide associated with Alzheimer's disease, is added to neuronal cells, it causes oxidative damage and cell death. However, pretreatment of cells with ALCAR reduced the oxidative damage and toxicity of Abeta(1-42) exposure. In these studies, ALCAR increased levels of glutathione, an endogenous antioxidant, and heat shock proteins, which are important stress response proteins. This suggests that ALCAR may directly increase cellular antioxidant defenses in addition to its effect on mitochondria.

2.2.2.2 Lipoic Acid

R-Alpha-Lipoic acid (LA) is a coenzyme involved in mitochondrial metabolism and is a mitochondrial antioxidant.[36] It has been proposed as a therapy for diseases involving oxidative stress and has proven effective in the treatment of diabetic neuropathy.[40] Liu and coworkers showed that feeding LA to old rats for 7 weeks ameliorated mitochondrial oxidative damage and dysfunction.[9] These were the same feeding experiments that showed a similar effect of ALCAR. In the parallel studies of memory loss in old animals, LA partially reversed memory, as did ALCAR.[38] In general, the effects of LA were similar to those of ALCAR, although in some cases feeding LA and ALCAR together had an even greater effect on some of the parameters measured. In a study of LA effects in the heart, feeding LA starting at 14 months in mice produced alterations in gene expression consistent with reduced oxidative stress.[41] LA had no effect on longevity in these studies. Finally, in a mouse model of age-related memory loss, giving LA for 4 weeks improved the cognition of 12-month-old SAMP8 mice.[42] LA also reversed indices of oxidative stress in the brain.

As with ALCAR, the effects of LA have been studied in neuronal cell cultures.[43] In these studies, primary hippocampal cells were challenged with Abeta(25-35) and iron/hydrogen peroxide. Pretreatment with LA significantly increased survival in the face of this oxidative challenge. Interestingly, when LA was added simultaneously with the oxidants, it potentiated cell death and increased free radical production. The authors interpreted this in terms of the fact that LA can also serve as a pro-oxidant. In this case it may be interacting with the iron to increase oxidative stress.

2.2.2.3 Coenzyme Q10

Coenzyme Q10 (CoQ10), or ubiquinone, performs at least three functions in mitochondria. It serves as a mitochondrial antioxidant, it carries electrons as part of the electron transport chain generating ATP, and (somewhat paradoxically) it is a major source of oxygen radical generation.[44] Coenzyme Q10 has been reported to improve stress tolerance in the myocardium of senescent rats.[45] Senescent rats who were given CoQ10 daily for 6 weeks showed the same positive cardiac response to pacing stress as young rats. This is consistent with a more recent report in mice that feeding CoQ10 produced gene alterations consistent with reduced oxidative stress in the heart.[41] Likewise, CoQ10 has been reported to have neuroprotective effects in a mouse model of amyotropic lateral sclerosis (ALS).[46]

However, a long-term feeding study of CoQ10 started at 3.5 months in mice found no effect on life span.[44] This is consistent with a study that found no effect of CoQ10 started at 14 months on life span.[41] More difficult to interpret, however, was the fact that the long-term feeding study found no detectable effect of CoQ10 on antioxidant defenses or pro-oxidant generation (since it can also generate free radicals) in old animals.[44] There was no difference despite the fact that dietary supplementation did boost endogenous CoQ10 levels in mitochondria. It may be that the effects of CoQ10 are more evident when older animals are stressed rather than in longitudinal aging studies.

2.3 AGING AT THE SYSTEMS LEVEL: CALORIC RESTRICTION

Free radicals are generated at the molecular level and cause damage to proteins, lipids, and nucleic acids. At the cellular level, the mitochondria are both a source and a target for free radicals. This results in decreased energy production for the cell. In addition, the fate of the cell itself may lie in part with mitochondria, since they play a role in cell death, cell senescence, and apoptosis. As cellular function and cell cycles change with age, the regulatory systems of which they are a part also change. This results in the decreased capacity of an organism to regulate itself in the face of external stressors.[2]

2.3.1 Aging at the Systems Level

There are several homeostatic systems that are especially important with regard to aging and nutrition. These include the glucose/insulin system, the growth hormone/insulin-like growth factor (IGF) system, the neuroendocrine stress response system, and the immune system.[1]

2.3.1.1 The Glucose/Insulin System

Interest in the glucose/insulin system has been stimulated by studies in mice showing that inactivating the insulin receptor in fat tissue leads to an increase in longevity.[47] These animals have normal food intake and reduced fat mass. In addition, increased longevity is associated with low insulin and glucose levels and increased sensitivity to insulin, such as in dwarf mice.[48]

2.3.1.2 The Growth Hormone/IGF System

Related to the glucose/insulin system is the growth hormone/IGF system. Dwarf mice, which lack growth hormone and therefore have low levels of IGF-1, have increased longevity.[48] Support for the importance of this pathway in aging also comes from gene inactivation studies. When the gene for the growth hormone receptor/binding protein is disrupted in mice, they live significantly longer.[49] Likewise, partially inactivating the IGF-1 receptor has been reported to increase maximal life span in male and female mice, although the increase was not significant in the males.[50] Inactivating the insulin-like signaling systems in roundworms and fruit flies also increases life span, suggesting that this is a fundamental regulatory pathway.

2.3.1.3 The Neuroendocrine/Stress Response System

The neuroendocrine stress response system has long been implicated in the aging process.[51] Glucocorticoids, which are the adrenal steroids secreted in response to stress, can be beneficial in the acute response to stress. However, long-term exposure to high glucocorticoid levels may have negative effects on the nervous system, including neuronal degeneration.[52] Glucocorticoid levels have been shown to rise with age in rats, making them suspects in the aging of the nervous system.[53]

2.3.1.4 The Immune System

Changes in the immune system with age have been well documented.[54] These changes include the involution of the thymus gland, lower numbers of T cells, a decrease in cell-mediated immunity, and decreased response to vaccines.[55] An age-related decline in spleen cell proliferation has been seen in rats,[56] and a decline in antibody production in response to influenza has been seen in mice.[57] Both of these findings were linked to a decrease in naïve T cells with age. It has been argued that the aging of the immune system may be due in part to chronic stress and elevated glucocorticoids.[55]

2.3.2 Caloric Restriction

Dietary restriction is the experimental manipulation of feeding animals significantly less than they would eat on their own (*ad libitum*). It has been known for many years that this significantly increases mean and maximal life span in rodents.[58] A number of studies have shown that the key component that needs to be restricted in order to extend longevity is total calories. Hence, this experimental manipulation, the only one that consistently increases longevity in mammals, is referred to as caloric restriction (CR). In addition to increasing longevity, CR retards the onset of many age-related diseases, as well as many of the physiological manifestations of aging. CR also works in lower animals, such as roundworms and fruit flies. In lower organisms, the effect of CR is even more pronounced than in rodents, indicating that some basic biological mechanism may be at work.

2.3.3 Possible Mechanisms of Caloric Restriction

Since its effects are triggered by withholding calories, CR is an important nutritional phenomenon. It has been proposed that CR occurs when "an organism's perception of a reduced energy supply elicits a coordinated set of transcriptional regulatory events leading to increased protection against a variety of stressors and the damage they cause as well as the maintenance of reserve capacity."[59] In general, it has been thought that CR works by modifying the rate of aging rather than just delaying the time at which aging begins.[58] However, this interpretation has sometimes been called into question.[60] Although CR is a relatively simple experimental maneuver, it causes profound effects at the molecular, cellular (mitochondrial), and systems levels. Historically, almost every theory of aging has been invoked to explain the mechanism of CR.[58]

2.3.3.1 Free Radical Mechanisms

At the molecular level, there is much evidence that CR slows the increase in oxidative damage to molecules with age.[4] This could be due to (1) decreased generation of free radicals, (2) increased free radical defenses, or (3) increased repair of oxidative damage. The effect of CR on free radical defenses has been unclear. Some studies show an increase in enzymatic activity associated with free radical defenses in some tissues. Other studies show no effect or even a decrease. With regard to repair of oxidative damage, there are studies indicating a positive effect of CR on DNA repair.

2.3.3.2 Mitochondrial Mechanisms

The effect of CR on the generation of free radicals has focused on mitochondria, the major site of free radical production. Most studies, but not all, have reported that CR decreases free radical production by isolated mitochondria.[60] However, care must be taken in extrapolating this finding to intact tissue due to the possibility of artifacts in mitochondrial isolation. It has been more difficult to see an effect of CR on free radical generation at the cellular level. The decreased oxidative damage that is generally seen in CR animals may be due to a combination of decreased free radical production and increased antioxidant defenses. This combination may vary with tissue and species.

2.3.3.3 Systems Mechanisms

Finally, the effects of CR have been explained as alterations in homeostatic systems.[58] CR reduced plasma insulin and glucose levels when measured over the whole life span of the rat.[61] The authors proposed that these results could be explained in part by increased sensitivity to insulin. These changes in the glucose/insulin system are similar to those seen in long-lived dwarf mice.[48]

CR also markedly lowered levels of IGF-1, suggesting an effect on the growth hormone/IGF-1 system.[62] However, arguing against this is the fact that the life span of long-lived dwarf mice, which have low levels of growth hormone and IGF-1, can be further extended by CR.[63] This suggests separate mechanisms for the life extension effects of dwarfism and CR.

The effects of CR on the neuroendocrine/stress response system are paradoxical. CR increases stress in rodents,[53] and yet they live longer.[64] These findings may be related to the concept of hormesis (see below).

Finally, the effects of CR have also been interpreted in terms of the immune system. The age-related decline in naïve T cell levels were blunted by CR in both rats[56] and mice.[57] This leads to improved immune function in old CR animals.

2.3.4 Nutritional Interventions Based on Caloric Restriction

2.3.4.1 Caloric Restriction Mimetics

As summarized above, CR is the most reproducible manipulation that extends life span in mammals. It has beneficial effects at the molecular, cellular, and homeostatic systems levels in rodents. Ongoing studies in nonhuman primates have suggested that CR has similar beneficial effects at the systems level in monkeys.[65] These primate studies have been too brief to see an effect on longevity. All of this makes CR a potentially attractive nutritional intervention for humans. However, the restrictedness of the diet and its composition would make it impractical as a general intervention in a food-conscious Western society. This has led to the search for CR mimetics, dietary or pharmacological compounds that mimic the biological effects of CR without restricting diet itself.[66]

Information on many CR mimetic studies is minimal due to the proprietary nature of the work. However, there have been some reviews of noncommercial strategies.[59] The first candidate mimetics have targeted energy metabolism, since this appears to be a fundamental trigger of the CR response. The first compound to be tested was 2-deoxyglucose, a glycolytic inhibitor. In one study, the effects of feeding 2-deoxyglucose were compared to the effects of intermittent feeding, a type of dietary restriction, over a 6-month period in young rats.[67] Feeding 2-deoxyglucose decreased blood pressure, heart rate, and serum and insulin levels in a manner similar to intermittent feeding. Both treatments also raised stress hormone levels.

In addition to glucose metabolism, lipid metabolism may also be a target for CR mimetics.[59] The compounds alpha-lipoic acid and carnitine have been discussed previously in the context of antioxidants (see above). However, in addition to being antioxidants, they also have effects on fatty acid oxidation in mitochondria. Ultimately, a combination of compounds may be required to mimic the many effects of CR. Feeding a diet composed of vitamins, minerals, herbs, and antioxidants has been reported to extend longevity in mice.[68]

2.3.4.2 Hormesis

Masoro defines hormesis in the context of aging research as "the beneficial action resulting from the response of an organism to a low-intensity stressor."[58] Masoro has argued that CR is a low-intensity stressor. It increases stress hormone levels even as it increases life span and improves physiological functioning. In the context of brain aging, this has been referred to as the glucocorticoid paradox of CR. In their review of the literature, Patel and Finch[64] concluded that the positive neuroprotective effects of CR outweighed the increase in glucocorticoids that it also produced. However, Masoro proposes that the increase in glucocorticoids itself may be beneficial, perhaps by reducing inflammation.[58]

In addition to CR, other stressors that may work through hormesis include pro-oxidants, irradiation, heat shock, and exercise.[69] From a nutritional standpoint, the most interesting of these is dietary pro-oxidants. As an example, curcumin, an antioxidant derived from turmeric, a curry spice, also induces heat shock proteins, a stress response.[70] This compound has been cited as contributing to the reduced incidence of Alzheimer's disease in India. This raises the interesting possibility that dietary intake of small amounts of compounds normally considered harmful may induce antioxidant defenses and have long-term beneficial effects.

2.4 SUMMARY

This review has highlighted our knowledge of aging at the molecular level and its interaction with nutrition. Recent studies suggest why certain nutrients may be beneficial and also suggest new strategies. Some of the nutritional interventions are very familiar, such as the antioxidant vitamins. However, even here there are some surprises, as antioxidants such as vitamin E seem to have specific actions in cells that go far beyond their antioxidant properties. These multiple actions are also seen in studies of the *Ginkgo* preparation EGb761. In recent years, it has become clearer how fruit polyphenols may have beneficial effects at the molecular level. These studies are exciting because this class of compounds is found in fruits such as strawberries, spinach, and blueberries.

Studies of mitochondrial aging have suggested new nutritional interventions such as L-carnitine and lipoic acid. These compounds appear to have specific effects on mitochondrial energy production and antioxidant capability. They have not yet been demonstrated to have an effect on longevity, but they do have an effect on cognitive function in old animals. This would have important implications if they were found to have the same effects in humans.

Finally, recent studies suggest that a mechanism exists in rodents, probably in nonhuman primates and possibly in humans, that responds to caloric stress. This provides a new target for nutritional intervention. This target is particularly attractive since the response to caloric stress is so robust. It may be that true caloric mimetics will be found given the great commercial interest. On the other hand, caloric stress may be just one of broader classes of stress responses. Activating these by nutritional means could potentially give the benefits of an enhanced stress response while minimizing the unpleasant side effects (i.e., hunger) of the stressor itself.

REFERENCES

1. Armbrecht HJ. The biology of aging. *J Lab Clin Med* 138: 220–225, 2001.
2. Miller RA. The biology of aging and longevity. In *Principles of Geriatric Medicine and Gerontology*, Hazzard WR, Blass JP, Ettinger WH, Halter JB, and Ouslander JG, Eds. New York: McGraw-Hill, 1998, pp. 3–19.
3. Harmon D. Aging: a theory based on free radical and radiation chemistry. *J Gerontol* 2: 298–300, 1956.
4. Sohal RS and Weindruch R. Oxidative stress, caloric restriction, and aging. *Science* 273: 59–63, 1996.
5. Pearl R. *The Rate of Living*. London: University of London Press, 1928.
6. Gallant J, Kurland C, Parker J, Holliday R, and Rosenberger R. The error catastrophe theory of aging. Point counterpoint. *Exp Gerontol* 32: 333–346, 1997.
7. Vijg J and Gossen JA. Somatic mutations and cellular aging. *Comp Biochem Physiol* 104B: 429–437, 1993.

8. Yu BP. Membrane alteration as a basis of aging and the protective effects of calorie restriction. *Mech Ageing Dev* 126: 1003–1010, 2005.
9. Liu J, Killilea DW, and Ames BN. Age-associated mitochondrial oxidative decay: improvement of carnitine acetyltransferase substrate-binding affinity and activity in brain by feeding old rats acetyl-L-carnitine and/or R-alpha-lipoic acid. *Proc Natl Acad Sci USA* 99: 1876–1881, 2002.
10. Meydani M. Nutrition interventions in aging and age-associated disease. *Ann NY Acad Sci* 928: 226–235, 2001.
11. Ilavazhagan G, Bansal A, Prasad D, Thomas P, Sharma SK, Kain AK, Kumar D, and Selvamurthy W. Effect of vitamin E supplementation on hypoxia-induced oxidative damage in male albino rats. *Aviat Space Environ Med* 72: 899–903, 2001.
12. Kheir-Eldin AA, Motawi TK, Gad MZ, and Abd-ElGawad HM. Protective effect of vitamin E, beta-carotene and N-acetylcysteine from the brain oxidative stress induced in rats by lipopolysaccharide. *Int J Biochem Cell Biol* 33: 475–482, 2001.
13. O'Donnell E and Lynch MA. Dietary antioxidant supplementation reverses age-related neuronal changes. *Neurobiol Aging* 19: 461–467, 1998.
14. Murray CA and Lynch MA. Dietary supplementation with vitamin E reverses the age-related deficit in long term potentiation in dentate gyrus. *J Biol Chem* 273: 12161–12168, 1998.
15. Joseph JA, Villalobos-Molina R, Denisova N, Erat S, Cutler R, and Strain J. Age differences in sensitivity to H2O2- or NO-induced reductions in K(+)-evoked dapamine release from superfused striatal slices: reversals by PBN or Trolox. *Free Radic Biol Med* 20: 821–830, 1996.
16. Yatin SM, Varadarajan S, and Butterfield DA. Vitamin E prevents Alzheimer's amyloid beta-peptide (1-42)-induced neuronal protein oxidation and reactive oxygen species production. *J Alzheimers Dis* 2: 123–131, 2000.
17. Meydani SN, Meydani M, Verdon CP, Shapiro AA, Blumberg JB, and Hayes KC. Vitamin E supplementation suppresses prostaglandin E1(2) synthesis and enhances the immune response of aged mice. *Mech Ageing Dev* 34: 191–201, 1986.
18. Han SN, Meydani M, Wu D, Bender BS, Smith DE, Vina J, Cao G, Prior RL, and Meydani SN. Effect of long-term dietary antioxidant supplementation on influenza virus infection. *J Gerontol A Biol Sci Med Sci* 55: B496–B503, 2000.
19. Rice-Evans C. Flavonoid antioxidants. *Curr Med Chem* 8: 797–807, 2001.
20. Esposito E, Rotilio D, Di MV, Di GC, Cacchio M, and Algeri S. A review of specific dietary antioxidants and the effects on biochemical mechanisms related to neurodegenerative processes. *Neurobiol Aging* 23: 719–735, 2002.
21. Williams RJ, Spencer JP, and Rice-Evans C. Flavonoids: antioxidants or signalling molecules? *Free Radic Biol Med* 36: 838–849, 2004.
22. Oberpichler H, Beck T, Abdel-Rahman MM, Bielenberg GW, and Krieglstein J. Effects of *Ginkgo biloba* constituents related to protection against brain damage caused by hypoxia. *Pharmacol Res Commun* 20: 349–368, 1988.
23. Bridi R, Crossetti FP, Steffen VM, and Henriques AT. The antioxidant activity of standardized extract of *Ginkgo biloba* (EGb 761) in rats. *Phytother Res* 15: 449–451, 2001.
24. Oyama Y, Chikahisa L, Ueha T, Kanemaru K, and Noda K. *Ginkgo biloba* extract protects brain neurons against oxidative stress induced by hydrogen peroxide. *Brain Res* 712: 349–352, 1996.
25. Guidetti C, Paracchini S, Lucchini S, Cambieri M, and Marzatico F. Prevention of neuronal cell damage induced by oxidative stress *in-vitro*: effect of different *Ginkgo biloba* extracts. *J Pharm Pharmacol* 53: 387–392, 2001.

26. Bastianetto S, Ramassamy C, Dore S, Christen Y, Poirier J, and Quirion R. The *Ginkgo biloba* extract (EGb 761) protects hippocampal neurons against cell death induced by beta-amyloid. *Eur J Neurosci* 12: 1882–1890, 2000.
27. Yao Z, Drieu K, and Papadopoulos V. The *Ginkgo biloba* extract EGb 761 rescues the PC12 neuronal cells from beta-amyloid-induced cell death by inhibiting the formation of beta-amyloid-derived diffusible neurotoxic ligands. *Brain Res* 889: 181–190, 2001.
28. Joseph JA, Shukitt-Hale B, and Casadesus G. Reversing the deleterious effects of aging on neuronal communication and behavior: beneficial properties of fruit polyphenolic compounds. *Am J Clin Nutr* 81: 313S–316S, 2005.
29. Joseph JA, Shukitt-Hale B, Denisova NA, Prior RL, Cao G, Martin A, Taglialatela G, and Bickford PC. Long-term dietary strawberry, spinach, or vitamin E supplementation retards the onset of age-related neuronal signal-transduction and cognitive behavioral deficits. *J Neurosci* 18: 8047–8055, 1998.
30. Joseph JA, Shukitt-Hale B, Denisova NA, Bielinski D, Martin A, McEwen JJ, and Bickford PC. Reversals of age-related declines in neuronal signal transduction, cognitive, and motor behavioral deficits with blueberry, spinach, or strawberry dietary supplementation. *J Neurosci* 19: 8114–8121, 1999.
31. Joseph JA, Denisova NA, Arendash G, Gordon M, Diamond D, Shukitt-Hale B, and Morgan D. Blueberry supplementation enhances signaling and prevents behavioral deficits in an Alzheimer disease model. *Nutr Neurosci* 6: 153–162, 2003.
32. Gredilla R and Barja G. Minireview: the role of oxidative stress in relation to caloric restriction and longevity. *Endocrinology* 146: 3713–3717, 2005.
33. Lambert AJ, Portero-Otin M, Pamplona R, and Merry BJ. Effect of ageing and caloric restriction on specific markers of protein oxidative damage and membrane peroxidizability in rat liver mitochondria. *Mech Ageing Dev* 125: 529–538, 2004.
34. Hagen TM, Yowe DL, Bartholomew JC, Wehr CM, Do KL, Park JY, and Ames BN. Mitochondrial decay in hepatocytes from old rats: membrane potential declines, heterogeneity and oxidants increase. *Proc Natl Acad Sci USA* 94: 3064–3069, 1997.
35. Harper ME, Monemdjou S, Ramsey JJ, and Weindruch R. Age-related increase in mitochondrial proton leak and decrease in ATP turnover reactions in mouse hepatocytes. *Am J Physiol* 275: E197–E206, 1998.
36. Liu J and Ames BN. Reducing mitochondrial decay with mitochondrial nutrients to delay and treat cognitive dysfunction, Alzheimer's disease, and Parkinson's disease. *Nutr Neurosci* 8: 67–89, 2005.
37. Calabrese V, Giuffrida Stella AM, Calvani M, and Butterfield DA. Acetylcarnitine and cellular stress response: roles in nutritional redox homeostasis and regulation of longevity genes. *J Nutr Biochem* 17: 73–88, 2006.
38. Liu J, Head E, Gharib AM, Yuan W, Ingersoll RT, Hagen TM, Cotman CW, and Ames BN. Memory loss in old rats is associated with brain mitochondrial decay and RNA/DNA oxidation: partial reversal by feeding acetyl-L-carnitine and/or R-alpha-lipoic acid. *Proc Natl Acad Sci USA* 99: 2356–2361, 2002.
39. Abdul HM, Calabrese V, Calvani M, and Butterfield DA. Acetyl-L-carnitine-induced up-regulation of heat shock proteins protects cortical neurons against amyloid-beta peptide 1-42-mediated oxidative stress and neurotoxicity: implications for Alzheimer's disease. *J Neurosci Res* 84: 398–408, 2006.
40. Smith AR, Shenvi SV, Widlansky M, Suh JH, and Hagen TM. Lipoic acid as a potential therapy for chronic diseases associated with oxidative stress. *Curr Med Chem* 11: 1135–1146, 2004.

41. Lee CK, Pugh TD, Klopp RG, Edwards J, Allison DB, Weindruch R, and Prolla TA. The impact of alpha-lipoic acid, coenzyme Q10 and caloric restriction on life span and gene expression patterns in mice. *Free Radic Biol Med* 36: 1043–1057, 2004.
42. Farr SA, Poon HF, Dogrukol-Ak D, Drake J, Banks WA, Eyerman E, Butterfield DA, and Morley JE. The antioxidants alpha-lipoic acid and N-acetylcysteine reverse memory impairment and brain oxidative stress in aged SAMP8 mice. *J Neurochem* 84: 1173–1183, 2003.
43. Lovell MA, Xie C, Xiong S, and Markesbery WR. Protection against amyloid beta peptide and iron/hydrogen peroxide toxicity by alpha lipoic acid. *J Alzheimers Dis* 5: 229–239, 2003.
44. Sohal RS, Kamzalov S, Sumien N, Ferguson M, Rebrin I, Heinrich KR, and Forster MJ. Effect of coenzyme Q10 intake on endogenous coenzyme Q content, mitochondrial electron transport chain, antioxidative defenses, and life span of mice. *Free Radic Biol Med* 40: 480–487, 2006.
45. Rowland MA, Nagley P, Linnane AW, and Rosenfeldt FL. Coenzyme Q10 treatment improves the tolerance of the senescent myocardium to pacing stress in the rat. *Cardiovasc Res* 40: 165–173, 1998.
46. Matthews RT, Yang L, Browne S, Baik M, and Beal MF. Coenzyme Q10 administration increases brain mitochondrial concentrations and exerts neuroprotective effects. *Proc Natl Acad Sci USA* 95: 8892–8897, 1998.
47. Bluher M, Kahn BB, and Kahn CR. Extended longevity in mice lacking the insulin receptor in adipose tissue. *Science* 299: 572–574, 2003.
48. Bartke A and Brown-Borg H. Life extension in the dwarf mouse. *Curr Top Dev Biol* 63: 189–225, 2004.
49. Coschigano KT, Clemmons D, Bellush LL, and Kopchick JJ. Assessment of growth parameters and life span of GHR/BP gene-disrupted mice. *Endocrinology* 141: 2608–2613, 2000.
50. Holzenberger M, Dupont J, Ducos B, Leneuve P, Geloen A, Even PC, Cervera P, and Le BY. IGF-1 receptor regulates lifespan and resistance to oxidative stress in mice. *Nature* 421: 182–187, 2003.
51. Landfield PW. Nathan Shock Memorial Lecture 1990. The role of glucocorticoids in brain aging and Alzheimer's disease: an integrative physiological hypothesis. *Exp Gerontol* 29: 3–11, 1994.
52. Sapolsky RM. Glucocorticoids, stress, and their adverse neurological effects: relevance to aging. *Exp Gerontol* 34: 721–732, 1999.
53. Sabatino F, Masoro EJ, McMahan CA, and Kuhn RW. Assessment of the role of the glucocorticoid system in aging processes and in the action of food restriction. *J Gerontol* 46: B171–B179, 1991.
54. Ernst DN and Hobbs MV. Age-related changes in cytokine expression by T cells. In *The Science of Geriatrics*, Morley JE, Armbrecht HJ, Coe RM, and Vellas B, Eds. Paris: Serdi Publisher, 2000, pp. 541–554.
55. Bauer ME. Stress, glucocorticoids and ageing of the immune system. *Stress* 8: 69–83, 2005.
56. Fernandes G, Venkatraman JT, Turturro A, Attwood VG, and Hart RW. Effect of food restriction on life span and immune functions in long-lived Fischer-344 × Brown Norway F1 rats. *J Clin Immunol* 17: 85–95, 1997.
57. Effros RB, Walford RL, Weindruch R, and Mitcheltree C. Influences of dietary restriction on immunity to influenza in aged mice. *J Gerontol* 46: B142–B147, 1991.
58. Masoro EJ. Overview of caloric restriction and ageing. *Mech Ageing Dev* 126: 913–922, 2005.

59. Roth GS, Lane MA, and Ingram DK. Caloric restriction mimetics: the next phase. *Ann NY Acad Sci* 1057: 365–371, 2005.
60. Merry BJ. Dietary restriction in rodents: delayed or retarded ageing? *Mech Ageing Dev* 126: 951–959, 2005.
61. Masoro EJ, McCarter RJ, Katz MS, and McMahan CA. Dietary restriction alters characteristics of glucose fuel use. *J Gerontol* 47: B202–B208, 1992.
62. Breese CR, Ingram RL, and Sonntag WE. Influence of age and long-term dietary restriction on plasma insulin-like growth factor-1 (IGF-1), IGF-1 gene expression, and IGF-1 binding proteins. *J Gerontol* 46: B180–B187, 1991.
63. Tsuchiya T, Dhahbi JM, Cui X, Mote PL, Bartke A, and Spindler SR. Additive regulation of hepatic gene expression by dwarfism and caloric restriction. *Physiol Genomics* 17: 307–315, 2004.
64. Patel NV and Finch CE. The glucocorticoid paradox of caloric restriction in slowing brain aging. *Neurobiol Aging* 23: 707–717, 2002.
65. Roth GS, Mattison JA, Ottinger MA, Chachich ME, Lane MA, and Ingram DK. Aging in rhesus monkeys: relevance to human health interventions. *Science* 305: 1423–1426, 2004.
66. Weindruch R, Keenan KP, Carney JM, Fernandes G, Feuers RJ, Floyd RA, Halter JB, Ramsey JJ, Richardson A, Roth GS, and Spindler SR. Caloric restriction mimetics: metabolic interventions. *J Gerontol A Biol Sci Med Sci* 56: 20–33, 2001.
67. Wan R, Camandola S, and Mattson MP. Intermittent fasting and dietary supplementation with 2-deoxy-D-glucose improve functional and metabolic cardiovascular risk factors in rats. *FASEB J* 17: 1133–1134, 2003.
68. Lemon JA, Boreham DR, and Rollo CD. A complex dietary supplement extends longevity of mice. *J Gerontol A Biol Sci Med Sci* 60: 275–279, 2005.
69. Rattan SI. Aging intervention, prevention, and therapy through hormesis. *J Gerontol A Biol Sci Med Sci* 59: 705–709, 2004.
70. Calabrese V, Scapagnini G, Colombrita C, Ravagna A, Pennisi G, Giuffrida Stella AM, Galli F, and Butterfield DA. Redox regulation of heat shock protein expression in aging and neurodegenerative disorders associated with oxidative stress: a nutritional approach. *Amino Acids* 25: 437–444, 2003.

3 The Role of Nutrition in the Prevention of Age-Associated Diseases

John E. Morley, M.B., B.Ch.

CONTENTS

Disease prevention can be divided into primary, secondary, and tertiary prevention. Primary prevention occurs when steps are taken before the disease has developed to prevent its occurrence, e.g., the use of influenza vaccine to prevent influenza epidemics or the institution of good sanitary practices in food handling to prevent food poisoning. Secondary prevention is the early detection of a disease that may remain occult for a period of time before manifesting itself. Secondary prevention can also be included in aggressive early treatment of disease, e.g., treating influenza with rimantidine or oseltamivir to ameliorate the development of serious complications. Under tertiary prevention is included the rehabilitation process, such as when an elderly patient is admitted to a geriatric evaluation unit for a period of physical therapy and nutritional support before being discharged home.

Nutritional interventions can clearly be applied at the primary, secondary, and tertiary levels of disease prevention. However, in developing an understanding of the role of nutrition in the prevention of age-associated diseases, it is important to realize that these interventions are unlikely to make major changes in life expectancy.

In the U.S., since the beginning of the 20th century, life expectancy has risen from 45 to 77.4 years. From 1970 to 2001, life expectancy in persons over 65 years of age increased by 2.9 years, or 0.1 year of age for each calendar year. This has occurred during a period when food intake has increased and the U.S. has become the most obese nation in the world. Some of this can be explained by the effects of protein and micronutrients on fetal development. For example, large babies at birth have stronger grip strength at 70 years of age, and higher weight at 10 years of age is inversely related to ischemic heart disease, systolic blood pressure, and glucose intolerance. Poor nutrition during phases of accelerated growth may also have an effect, as suggested by a Japanese study showing that those age 5 to 20 years during World War II, when there were multiple nutritional shortages, have an increased mortality from diabetes mellitus and ischemic heart disease. Other factors associated with the decline in atherosclerosis have been the improvement in food processing, i.e., elimination of animal infections and thermal processing of food, which leads to decreased infections for the initiation of atherosclerosis. Improvement in water quality has resulted in a decrease in peptic ulcers and gastric cancer. Increased food intake is related to decreased risk of atherosclerotic heart disease. This may be due to increased ingestion of antioxidants in food. Poor food intake may be related to borderline immune deficiency and decreased ability to inhibit the development of cancers.

For these reasons, it becomes increasingly important to measure the impact of nutritional intervention programs on morbidity. Small changes in morbidity can have a major impact on the quality of life. For example, as shown in Figure 3.1, the world record for the 1-mile run has improved by 1% every 7 years. In real terms, this is a 1% improvement in an international-class athlete that would put him or her 7 years ahead of other competitors. This would almost certainly guarantee an Olympic gold medal, or in the case of a professional football player, could represent the difference between being a millionaire or a street person. The impact on quality of life of a 95-year-old who does not fracture a hip when falling because of nutritional (calcium and vitamin D) and exercise interventions is immeasurable. Interventions that prevented the development of a nonfatal stroke would likewise have a major effect in compressing morbidity and improving quality of life.

Thus, it is reasonable to explore the available evidence that nutritional intervention can modulate either life expectancy or morbidity. The focus of this chapter is on the effect of nutritional manipulation in late life, that is, in humans over the age of 70 years. It should be stressed that there is no nutritional manipulation that comes close to abstaining from cigarette smoking in its power to ameliorate disease. Thus, it makes no sense to accede to requests for a dietary change in patients who persist in smoking.

3.1 PRIMARY PREVENTION

3.1.1 Nutrition and Hypertension

Hypertension is an extremely common problem in older individuals, with the National Health and Nutrition Examination Survey (NHANES) finding that 44% of whites and 60% of blacks aged 65 to 74 years have a blood pressure in excess of

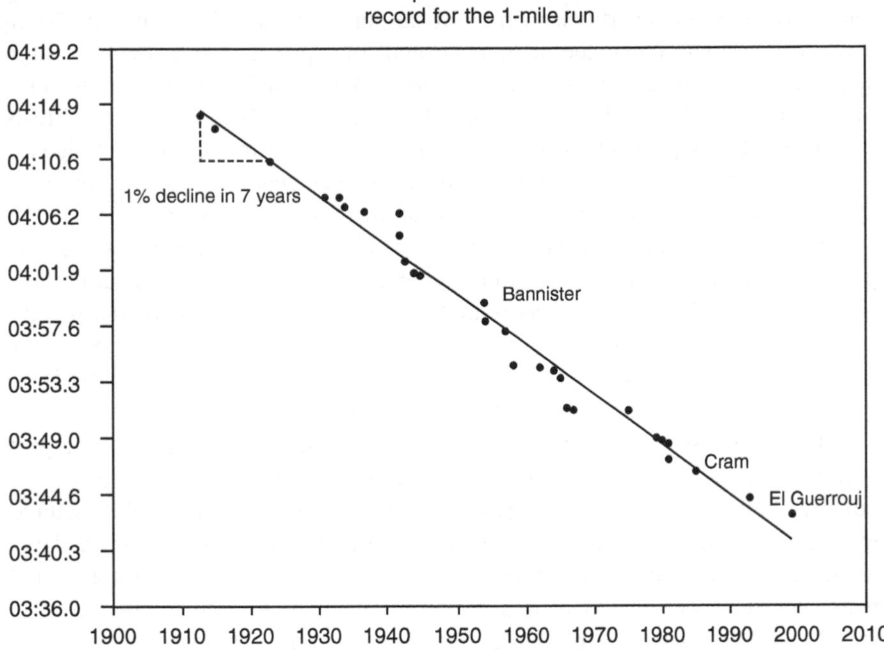

FIGURE 3.1 Pictorial representation of the world record for the 1-mile run.

160/95 mmHg.[1] The prevalence of hypertension is increasing with the increasing prevalence of obesity, and this increase was particularly noticeable from 1990 to 2000.[2] Both the Framingham Study and the Chicago Stroke Study have shown that untreated hypertension in older individuals is strongly associated with an increased risk of stroke and cardiovascular disorders.[3] Studies such as the Systolic Hypertension in the Elderly Program (SHEP) have shown that lowering blood pressure has decreased the occurrence of stroke.[4] Thus, nutritional interventions that would lower the prevalence of hypertension in older individuals could have a major impact on the health status of this group.

In younger patients, being overweight has been linked to hypertension, and with age there is an increase in body fat. Malnourished patients in nursing homes often display a marked amelioration of preexisting hypertension. These findings suggest that excess weight could contribute to hypertension in older individuals.

Epidemiologic studies have long suggested a relationship between hypertension and salt intake. Luft et al.[5] suggested that 25 to 30% of individuals over 40 years of age may display sodium-sensitive blood pressure responses. A difference of 100 meq/day in sodium intake is associated with a 3- to 6-mm difference in systolic blood pressure.[6] It has been suggested that older individuals (mean age, 85 years) are especially sensitive to the effects of a high-salt diet on blood pressure.[7] This increased sensitivity may be secondary to the reduced rate of urinary sodium excretion in older individuals. It would appear prudent to suggest that most elderly should avoid adding table salt to their food and should not use excessive salt for cooking. Some drinking water is particularly high in salt; tap water should not exceed 20 mg of sodium per liter. When the sodium content of tap water is particularly high, consideration should be given to drinking and cooking with bottled water. However, severe sodium restriction should be avoided wherever possible in older individuals, as it can result in unpalatable food and the development of malnutrition. It also can lead to severe postural hypotension.[8] There is some evidence that long-term use of very low sodium diets may actually lead to an increased mortality.[9]

Low calcium intake has been associated with increased arterial pressure,[10] and high calcium intakes ameliorate systolic hypertension.[11] A meta-analysis found that many older individuals have a suboptimal calcium intake. In view of the putative protective effects of high calcium intake on bone (*vide infra*), it seems reasonable to liberalize calcium intake to 1 to 1.5 g in subjects 50 years of age or older in the hope that it will also result in a lower blood pressure.

Both low potassium and magnesium are associated with increased blood pressure, and administration of these ions produces a small decrease in blood pressure.[12,13] Insulin resistance is associated with hypertension, and persons with insulin resistance have increased salt sensitivity.[14] Consuming one or two alcoholic drinks a day is associated with a lower blood pressure than seen in persons who do not drink.[15] Greater consumption of alcohol is associated with hypertension. A meta-analysis showed that 3.7 g of fish oil produced a small reduction in blood pressure.[16]

Overall, geriatric hypertension appears to have a relatively strong relationship to diet; a lifetime of moderate salt and caloric intake, as well as an adequate calcium intake, appears to be a prudent preventive medicine approach. The Trial of Non-Pharmacologic Intervention in the Elderly (TONE) showed that over a 4-year period of sodium reduction and weight loss, 23% of patients did not need medications to control their blood pressure compared to 7% in the usual-care group.[17] In view of the high cost of antihypertensive medications, careful dietary intervention in older subjects (mild salt restriction or added calcium intake) may represent the most prudent approach to the management of borderline elevations in blood pressure. This approach is particularly relevant in the "stroke belt" of the southern U.S., where NHANES III showed this region to have the highest salt and lowest potassium, calcium, and magnesium intakes.[18]

3.1.2 Osteopenia

The development of osteoporosis and subsequent fractures is a major cause of morbidity in postmenopausal Caucasian females. Clearly, the first approach to prevention is measurement of bone mineral density and appropriate bisphosphonate therapy in severely osteopenic persons. In addition, there is reasonable epidemiologic evidence linking the development of type II (age-related) osteopenia to lifetime calcium intake.[19] Studies in Hong Kong have suggested that subjects with a calcium intake below 400 mg/day are particularly at risk for the development of osteoporosis and hip fractures.[20] Osteoporosis is more prevalent in subjects with lactose intolerance, which leads to poor intake of dairy products and thus calcium, and in subjects with malabsorption syndromes, again suggesting a role for dietary calcium in bone protection. For these reasons, it seems appropriate to suggest a total calcium intake of the order of 1 to 1.5 g/day.

The role of vitamin D deficiency in the pathogenesis of hip fractures in individuals over 70 years of age is rapidly emerging.[21] A number of factors make older individuals at risk for developing vitamin D deficiency. These include decreased dietary intake, decreased sun exposure, the use of sunscreen to prevent recurrent skin cancer, impairment of the ability of ultraviolet light to produce cholecalciferol in older skin, decreased conversion of 25(OH) vitamin D to 1,25(OH) vitamin D by the kidney, and decreased intestinal reception for vitamin D. Studies from Israel have suggested that even elderly subjects living in high-sun-exposure areas can develop vitamin D deficiency.[22] A longitudinal study over 14 years showed that even very healthy older persons living in New Mexico had declines in their 25(OH) vitamin D levels.[23] Elderly in institutions appear to be particularly vulnerable to developing vitamin D deficiency, which increases their chances of having a hip fracture. For this reason, all institutionalized older subjects should receive 800 IU of vitamin D daily. If this is given, calcium levels need to be checked regularly to avoid the development of unrecognized hypercalcemia. A placebo controlled study of 3270 healthy ambulatory women aged 84 ± 6 years who were supplemented with 1.2 g of elemental calcium and 800 IU of vitamin D daily for 18 months produced a 43% decrease in hip fracture.[24] Recent studies have supported the need to have vitamin D levels of at least 30 mg/dl.

3.1.3 Cholesterol

Is it rational to have embarked on a national campaign to lower cholesterol? McCormick and Skrabanek[25] have argued that future generations will look back at the era of population interventions to reduce coronary artery disease with disbelief and contempt for the epidemiologic analysis that supported these political actions. Alternatively, Fries et al.,[26] although accepting that cholesterol reduction is unlikely to reduce mortality, have cogently argued that, at least in some populations, reduction in cholesterol may compress morbidity by reducing morbid cardiovascular events. Thus, in the Helsinki Heart Study trial, for example, there was a 37% reduction in nonfatal coronaries.[26] In addition, it is possible but not proven that such prevention may reduce medical expenditures. Thus, it would appear still reasonable to pursue cholesterol reduction vigorously in high-risk groups, such as those with a previous myocardial infarction or those subjects with a strong family history of atherosclerotic heart disease. The cholesterol level at which intervention should begin is uncertain, although values above 300 mg/dl would certainly warrant attention. For the best overall mortality target, levels of cholesterol should probably be in the range of 200 to 220 mg/dl in subjects under 65 years of age. One study suggested that, even in subjects with a mean age of 82 years, a total cholesterol greater than 250 mg/dl and a high-density lipoprotein cholesterol less than <35 mg/dl remain indicators of subsequent coronary events.[27] However, in other studies a high total cholesterol was associated with longevity,[28] and in a study of 3572 men aged 71 to 93 years, persons with the lowest quartile had a higher all-cause mortality than those in the highest quartile.[29] However, there is no evidence that routine intervention in subjects over

65 years of age has any benefit on mortality or mental or function status.[30] In addition, the Women's Health Initiative could show no major health benefits of a low-fat diet.[31–33] It is now recognized that small, dense low-density lipoprotein (LDL) is easily absorbed and oxidized by blood vessels. This is in contrast to large, foamy LDL, which is not atherogenic and found in high amounts in many centenarians. Treatment of elevated cholesterol levels in older persons requires understanding that all LDL is not bad. In view of these facts—that major interventions in diet in older subjects may result in malnutrition—it seems reckless to attempt to alter the cholesterol content of diets in the populations over 70 years of age. In addition, animal and human studies have suggested that lowering cholesterol may result in cognitive impairment.[34,35]

3.1.4 Fish and Fish Oils

Greenland Eskimos, despite their high fat intake, have a low prevalence of atherosclerosis and develop acute myocardial infarction at 10% the rate of Danes or North Americans. The difference is explained by the quality of fats ingested, with the Eskimos ingesting high qualities of omega-3 fatty acids derived mainly from seals and whales, whereas the other populations eat more saturated fats and omega-6 fatty acids.

These epidemiologic findings have led to the suggestion that polyunsaturated fatty acids, such as eicosopentanoic and docoscipentanoic acid, may decrease coronary artery disease both by decreasing platelet adhesiveness and by lowering triglycerides and, to a lesser extent, low-density lipoprotein cholesterol.[36] As these fatty acids are the predominant fat in fish, eating a high-fish diet may also prove protective against heart disease. Population studies have suggested that eating fish regularly may reduce atherosclerotic disease.[37] Mortality from coronary artery disease was 50% lower among those who consumed fish than among those who did not. At present, no large population trials showing the efficacy of raw fish oils over a prolonged period have been published. Because of the increased bleeding tendency produced by fish oil ingestion, intake of excess fish oil should be avoided in older subjects. However, there would appear to be minimal risk and potentially some benefit of increasing fish consumption to three or four times per week. Other polyunsaturated fatty acids, as seen in the Mediterranean diet, may be equally effective.

3.1.5 Cancer

Approximately half of all the new cancers in the U.S. can occur in individuals over the age of 65 years. Gastrointestinal, prostate, and breast cancer are responsible for over half the cancers in patients over 60 years of age. Although the cancer incidence rises with age, it begins to decrease in those 85 to 90 years of age. The concept that diet can modulate the prevalence of cancer is not a new one. In 1933, Morison and Orr[38] suggested that cancer in betel nut chewers was less prevalent in those with high vitamin A intake. In the same year, Stocks and Karn[39] found that high intake of whole-meal bread, vegetables, and fresh milk was associated with a decrease in cancer incidence at multiple sites.

Animal studies have suggested that food restriction reduces the cancer rate.[40] Further, feeding high-fat diets to animals induces breast and colon cancers. Human epidemiologic studies support the increased occurrence of carcinoma of the colon and breast in subjects on high-fat diets.[41] However, recent large prospective studies have considerably weakened the support for a major role of fat intake independent of calories as a major pathogenic factor in breast and colon cancer.[42] There is stronger evidence to support a relationship between aggressive prostate cancer and fat intake.[43] There is a 15% increase in colon cancer for each 100-g increase in red meat[44] and a 30% increase in prostate cancer in high-red-meat eaters.[45] This may be due to N-nitrose compounds formed from nitrogenous residues in red meat. Vegetarian groups, such as the Seventh Day Adventists, have a low occurrence of carcinoma of the colon, which could be related to low fat intake, the effect of lack of meat, or, most likely, the increased fiber in the diet. Numerous animal and human studies have supported the protective effect of dietary fiber against the development of colon cancer.

Iron deficiency has been associated with hypopharyngeal cancers in women.[46] Iodine deficiency predisposes to thyroid cancer.[47] Aflatoxin, from *Aspergillus flavus*, is a contaminant of peanuts and cereals in some situations and has been associated with hepatoma.[48] In Japan, eating bracken fern is associated with a five-fold increase in esophageal cancer.[49]

Epidemiologic studies have suggested a decrease in lung cancer in subjects with high intakes or serum levels of beta-carotene or vitamin A.[50] Vitamin A ingestion can lead to hypercalcemia by cathespin D activation and release of parathormone. For this reason, supplementation with vitamin A is never recommended. In the Alpha-Tocopherol Beta-Carotene (ATBC) trial, there was no association with lung cancer but a 34% lower incidence of prostate cancer in heavy smokers.[51] Long-term use of folate supplementation reduced the risk of colon cancer by approximately 40%.[52]

Low selenium levels in the blood have been associated with an increase in cancer incidence.[53] The combination of low selenium and low vitamin E levels seems to be highly predictive of increased risk, especially for gastrointestinal cancers.[54] Countries with high selenium levels in the soil, such as Venezuela, have much lower colon carcinoma rates than do those with lower selenium levels in the soil, such as the U.S. Overall, there is mounting evidence that selenium deficiency may predispose to the development of cancer.

Unfortunately, diets that protect against some cancers are associated with an increase in prevalence of cancers at other sites. For example, cereal cultures, such as those of Japan and Southeast Asia, have a high prevalence of stomach and esophageal cancer, whereas the incidence of breast, colon, and prostate cancers is decreased. Meat-eating cultures, such as the U.S., show exactly the opposite cancer pattern. Table 3.1 summarizes some of the known dietary influences on cancer.

3.1.6 Exercise

There is mounting evidence that moderate exercise can prolong the life span.[55] Exercise is associated with salutary effects on the cardiovascular system, bone, and muscle. The strengthening of muscle and bone may decrease the incidence of hip fracture. In addition, evidence in both animal[56] and human[57] studies suggests that

TABLE 3.1
Potential Dietary Influences on Cancer

Cancer	Effects of Nutrients
Lung	Decreased prevalence with increased beta-carotene, vitamin A, carrots, and green leafy vegetable intake
Esophageal	Increased rates with high bread or bracken from consumption
Stomach	Increased risk with dried salty fish consumption; decreased risk with vegetable and fruit consumption
Pancreas	Increased risk with butter, fried and grilled meal; decreased risk with raw fruits, vegetables, and vitamin C
Colon	Increased risk with pasta, rice, and cereals; decreased risk with vegetables, fiber, selenium, and vitamin C
Hypopharyngeal skin cancers	Increased risk with iron deficiency; decreased risk with selenium consumption

exercise is associated with a decrease in cancer. Recent studies have shown that exercise produces an acute increase in nature killer (NK) cell activity, most probably secondary to the release of beta-endorphin from the pituitary gland.[58] NK cells are responsible for scavenging circulating tumor cells. Thus, there is now a biochemical basis for the cancer-protective effect of moderate exercise.

Overall, it would seem that mild to moderate exercise can produce myriad beneficial effects when introduced at almost any age. This includes decreased brain atrophy, improved memory, and decreased depression. In older individuals, the exercise program should be tailored to the individual's capacity. All exercise programs should consist of endurance, resistance, balance, flexibility, and posture elements.

3.1.7 Life Extension

Since Ponce de Leon set out from Puerto Rico in search of the fountain of youth, only to discover Florida instead (in view of the senior migration to Florida, he might be considered to have been at least partially successful in his quest), many humans have craved a magic potion that would prolong their life span. Books and magazines on life extension have proved to be particularly successful with the lay public. Although clearly this author joins with Fries[59] in feeling that we should spend more time searching for ways to compress morbidity, it is nevertheless appropriate to review briefly dietary studies on life extension.

Numerous animal studies in many species from *Drosophila* to rodents have demonstrated that dietary restriction leads to a prolongation of life span.[60] Dietary restriction seems to be most effective when calories are restricted by approximately 25%. However, dietary restriction is not capable of extending life in rotifers.[61] No single macronutrient appears to be specifically responsible for the life span extension. The mechanism by which mild caloric deprivation enhances life span is uncertain, with theories ranging from a reduction in free radical generation or tissue glycation to a delay in thymic involution. There is relatively strong support for the growth hormone/insulin-like growth factor 1 (IGF-1) hypothesis. Caloric restriction appears to work by increasing the silent information regulator 2 (SIR2) or its mammalian ortholog (Sirt).[62] SIR2 is an NAD-dependent deacetylase. Besides altering histone deacetylation, Sirt also suppresses p53 and Foxo medicated apoptons and inactivates the proapoptotic factor, BAX. Sirt1 also decreases insulin, growth hormone/IGF-1, and leptin and increases adiponectin. It should be realized that such studies as these can be interpreted as demonstrating that overnutrition is not good for an animal, rather than demonstrating an effect of undernutrition per se. There is an attempt to develop caloric restriction mimetics, such as 2-dioxyglucose, to produce the beneficial effects of caloric restriction.[63]

Attempts to prove that the spartan existence increases life span led to searches for long-lived human populations. Three such populations were putatively identified—the Georgians in Russia, the Afghans in the Khyber Pass, and the people of Villacabamba in Ecuador. After much excitement concerning the ability of these individuals to live high-quality lives on a frugal diet, it rapidly becomes obvious that the great ages attained by these individuals were more closely linked to their inability to count correctly, rather than to their dietary and exercise habits. The longest-documented human life span is 122 years in a French woman. The most long lived population in the U.S. is in Hawaii, hardly a group of people who follow a spartan nutritional existence. Caloric restriction in rhesus monkeys lowers body temperature and energy expenditure, but also causes an increased loss of bone from the hip.[64–66] Attempts at caloric restriction in humans show a decrease in body temperature, oxidative stress, cholesterol, triglycerides, fasting glucose and insulin, c-reactive protein, and carotid artery intema media thickness.[67–69]

One theory of aging proposes that the generation of free radicals causes tissue damage and ultimately death. If this is true, then one would expect that intake of free radical scavengers, such as selenium or vitamin E, or antioxidants would result in a prolongation of life span. It is important to recognize that in these situations vitamins are used as pharmacological agents and not as nutritional supplements. Unfortunately, this question has been addressed in very few animal studies, and the paucity of data makes it impossible to make any conclusive comments on this issue. In one retrospective analysis, vitamin C ingestion slightly prolonged life in males but not in females.[70] There is some evidence in rodents that alpha-lipoic acid reduces oxidative metabolism and extends life.

Overall, it would appear that at present there is no dietary fountain of youth and that the best advice is to partake of a balanced diet that maintains weight around that of the population average.

3.2 SECONDARY PREVENTION

Much of the approach to the early detection and treatment of nutritional diseases is reviewed in detail in other sections of this book. For this reason, approaches to secondary prevention are reviewed only briefly here. The development of classical nutrient deficiencies, such as pellagra or scurvy, is extremely rare in the older populations of developed countries. More commonly, some older individuals who are suffering from intercurrent illnesses may develop borderline deficiency states.

For example, an older patient with type II diabetes mellitus may be losing zinc in the urine. He then develops a leg ulcer and has recurrent urinary tract infections, resulting in anorexia and decreased intake. His leg ulcer heals slowly because he has now developed a zinc deficiency that impairs wound healing. Zinc replacement eventually allows the full healing of his ulcer. Many patients in nursing homes are at particular risk for the development of borderline vitamin and tract mineral deficiencies and, as such, should be carefully monitored for signs and symptoms of these deficiencies.

Numerous drugs that are commonly used in older individuals interfere with nutrient bioavailability. Diuretics can cause magnesium, potassium, and zinc deficiency. Tuberculosis therapy with isoniazid can lead to vitamin B_6 deficiency. Epileptic treatment with phenytoin or phenobarbitone can result in folate deficiency. Laxative abuse with mineral oil can result in deficiency of vitamins A, D, and K. For these reasons, it is important for older patients receiving medications to be monitored carefully for nutrient deficiencies. In addition, the older person's need for the variety of drugs he is receiving should be assessed carefully. Not only does polypharmacy increase the likelihood of drug interactions, but it also increases the possibility of nutrient deficiencies. For the elderly, it is just as important that they learn to "just say no to drugs" when they are inappropriate as it is for our younger population.

Protein-energy malnutrition (PEM) is reaching endemic proportions among older Americans. In the prevention of this disease, primary prevention programs, such as meals at senior citizen centers and Meals on Wheels, can play an important role. In addition, the development of bereavement squads who visit an older person a week after a spouse dies and bring food with them may reduce the protein-energy malnuturition commonly associated with a spouse's death. In the long-term care setting, ensuring sufficient money to prepare attractive food and hire a dietitian is the major primary prevention need.

Because the onset of PEM is often insidious, early detection is of paramount importance. Many older subjects present with a marasmic picture, with weight loss rather than hypoalbuminemia dominating the situation. Weight loss needs to be pursued vigorously in older individuals and treatable causes, such as occult depression, carefully excluded. Patients at risk for malnutrition include those who are unable to shop for themselves. In a diagnosis-related group (DRG)-driven world, the physician needs to be particularly aware that many older patients admitted with infection have occult malnutrition. If the patient is discharged home too quickly, he may be too weak to prepare meals, resulting in a vicious cycle of worsening malnutrition, further impairment of the immune system, and subsequent hospital readmissions for infection. It is important to realize that, in many cases, the best result that can be obtained from tube feeding is a maintenance of body weight at the level prevailing at the time of tube insertion. For this reason, if successful secondary prevention of PEM is to occur, it is necessary that tube feedings are begun earlier, rather than later, with the expectation that the tube may be removed as soon as weight stabilization occurs.

Diabetes mellitus is an extremely common disease, occurring in up to 18% of individuals over 65 years of age.[71] Yet in approximately half of these individuals, the diagnosis is not made. Regular screening programs for diabetes mellitus in seniors should be undertaken using glucose or fructosamine levels. Not only does diabetes mellitus cause retinopathy, neuropathy, and nephropathy, but there is also increasing evidence that it may result in premature aging and accelerated atherosclerosis.

3.3 TERTIARY PREVENTION

Exercise therapy and aggressive nutritional therapy are the cornerstones of the ability of the frail elderly person to return to the community.

Patients with well-established PEM often require prolonged hospitalization or admission to a skilled nursing facility. Carefully designed swallowing therapy programs may be necessary to allow the patient to eat again. When the patient fails to respond to routine measures, heroic therapy, such as the use of the anabolic growth hormone, may be indicated. Restoration of the severely malnourished patient requires a maximum effort by all the members of the interdisciplinary team. The ability of handicapped or frail elderly to eat can be greatly improved by the use of specialized eating utensils that have been developed to aid patients with strokes or amputations (Figure 3.2).

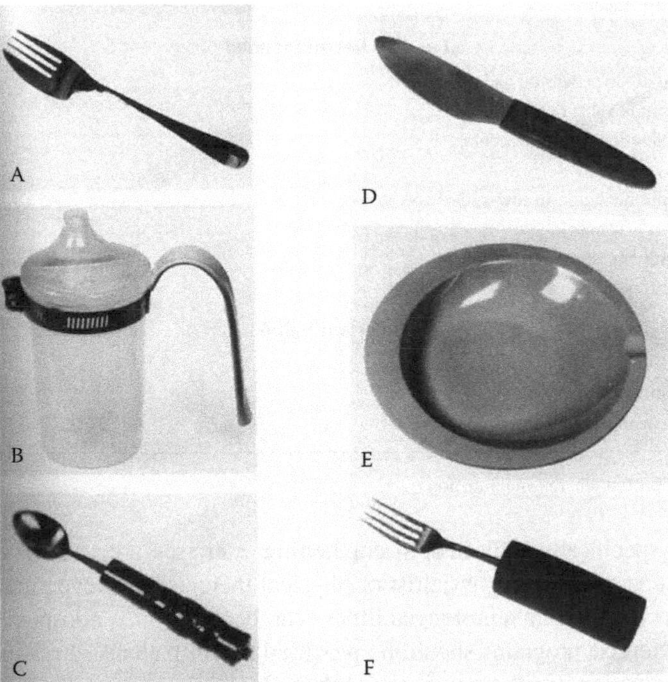

FIGURE 3.2 Examples of utensils used to improve food intake in handicapped elderly: (A) Side-cutter fork with sharpened edge, which allows cutting and eating with one hand. (B) Flow-restricted cup in a cup holder. Cup can be used with or without a straw. Spout is large enough for thick soups. (C) Weighted spoon for use by patients with Parkinson's disease or other tremors. (D) Rocker-bottom knife allows for meat cutting with one hand by rocking back and forth. (E) Scoop dish. One side is elevated, allowing for easier scooping by moving food against the edge. (F) Soft built-up fork used by a person with limited grip.

TABLE 3.2
Nutritional Approaches to Prevention of Age-Associated Diseases

Primary Prevention	Secondary Prevention	Tertiary Prevention
Highly Recommended		
No added salt—hypertension	Screening for weight loss	Exercise
Calcium supplementation—bone and hypertension	Screening for diabetes mellitus	Vigorous treatment of PEM—early tube feeding
Increased fish intake—cardiovascular disease	No megavitamin use—hypercalcemia	Specialized eating utensils
Avoidance of very high fat diets—cancer	Use of indicated drugs only—decrease drug–nutrient interactions	PEM
Moderate exercise—cancer, cardiovascular disease, bone		
Meals at senior citizen centers		
Meals on Wheels—PEM		
Vitamin D—hip fracture		
Possibly Recommended		
Weight reduction—hypertension and diabetes mellitus; uncertain value over 60 years		
Cholesterol reduction—cardiovascular morbidity		
Selenium supplementation in low-soil-selenium areas—cancer		
Vitamin and mineral supplementation to prevent infection attack rates		
Uncertain Value		
Cholesterol reduction—total mortality		
Dietary restriction—life extension		
Free radical scavengers—life extension		

Note: PEM = protein-energy malnutrition.

Where specifically indicated, strengthening exercises are usually carried out under the supervision of a physiatrist or physical therapist. However, many patients who are recovering from a prolonged illness can benefit from a nonspecific exercise program. Exercise programs should be provided for all patients in rehabilitation or geriatric evaluation wards, as well as for those in nursing homes. Special attention should be paid to strengthening leg muscles in the hope of preventing future falls.

3.4 CONCLUSION

Our knowledge concerning nutritional prevention of age-associated diseases is similar to that of the two blind men, one at the trunk and one at the tail of the elephant.

We have made an excellent start in understanding the nutritional bases of some of these diseases, but the lack of a full understanding makes it difficult to be absolutely certain that any recommendation will be proven to be correct. Table 3.2 summarizes the potential nutritional approaches to prevention. As we embark on the exciting field of health promotion and disease prevention in older individuals, we need to be exquisitely sensitive that the programs we institute do no harm. It should be remembered that, in many healthy older individuals, the less we intervene, the more likely they are to survive.

REFERENCES

1. National Center for Health Statistics. *Plan and Operation of the National Health and Nutrition Examination Survey. United States 1971–1973. Vital and Health Statistics*, Series 1, No. 10a and b. Washington, DC: U.S. Government Printing Office, 1973, pp. 1–16 (DHEW Publication 73-1310).
2. Perry, H.M., Jr., Davis, B.R., Price, T.R., et al. Effect of treating isolated systolic hypertension on the risk of developing various types and subtypes of stroke: the Systolic Hypertension in the Elderly Program (SHEP). *JAMA*, 284, 465, 2000.
3. Tuck, M.L., Griffiths, R.F., Johnson, L.E., et al. UCLA geriatric grand rounds. Hypertension in the elderly. *J. Am. Geriatr. Soc.*, 36, 630, 1988.
4. Bhatt, D.L., Steg, P.G., Ohman, E.M., et al. International prevalence, recognition, and treatment of cardiovascular risk factors in outpatients with atherothrombosis. *JAMA*, 295, 180, 2006.
5. Luft, F.C., Weinberger, M.H., Fineberg, N.S., et al. Effects of age on renal sodium homeostatis and its relevance to sodium sensitivity. *Am. J. Med.*, 82, 9, 1987.
6. Dickinson, H.O., Mason, J.M., Nicolson, D.J., et al. Lifestyle interventions to reduce raised blood pressure: a systematic review of randomized controlled trials. *Hypertension*, 24, 215, 2006.
7. Lustig, G., Palmer, R., Stern, N., et al. The effect of dietary salt ingestion on blood pressure of old-old subjects. *Clin Res.*, 36, 177A, 1988.
8. Morley, J.E. Is low pressure dangerous? *J. Am. Geriatr. Soc.*, 39, 1239, 1991.
9. Alderman, M.H., Cohen, H., and Madhavan, S. Dietary sodium intake and mortality: the National Health and Nutrition Examination Survey (NHANES 1). *Lancet*, 351, 781, 1998.
10. Bucker, H.C., Cook, R.J., Guyatt, G.H., et al. Effects of dietary calcium supplementation on blood pressure. A meta-analysis of randomized controlled trials. *JAMA*, 275, 1016, 1996.
11. Cappuccio, F.P., Elliott, P., Allender, P.S., et al. Epidemiologic association between dietary calcium intake and blood pressure: a meta-analysis of published data. *Am. J. Epidemiol.*, 142, 935, 1995.
12. Whelton, P.K. and He, J. Potassium in preventing and treating high blood pressure. *Semin. Nephrol.*, 19, 494, 1999.
13. Jee, S.H., Miller, E.R., Guallar, E., et al. The effect of magnesium supplementation on blood pressure: a meta-analysis of randomized clinical trials. *Am. J. Hypertens.*, 15, 691, 2002.
14. Kotchen, T.A., Kotchen, J.M., and O'Shaughnessy, I.M. Insulin and hypertensive cardiovascular disease. *Curr. Opin. Cardiol.*, 11, 483, 1996.

15. Victor, R.G. and Hansen, J. Alcohol and blood pressure: a drink a day. *N. Engl. J. Med.*, 332, 1782, 1995.
16. Morris, M.C., Sacks, F., and Rosner, B. Does fish oil lower blood pressure? A meta-analysis of controlled trials. *Circulation*, 88, 523, 1993.
17. Kostis, J.B., Wilson, A.C., Shindler, D.M., et al. Persistence of normotension after discontinuation of lifestyle intervention in the trial of TONE. Trial of Nonpharmacologic Interventions in the Elderly. *Am. J. Hypertens.*, 15, 732, 2002.
18. Hajjar, I. and Kotchen, T.A. Regional variations of blood pressure in the United States are associated with regional variations in dietary intakes: the NHANES-III data. *J. Nutr.*, 133, 211, 2003.
19. Morley, J.E., Gorbien, M.J., Mooradian, A.D., et al. UCLA geriatric grand rounds: osteoporosis. *J. Am. Geriatr. Soc.*, 36, 845, 1988.
20. Lau, E., Donnan, S., Barker, D.J., et al. Physical activity and calcium intake in fracture of the proximal femur in Hong Kong. *Br. Med. J.*, 297, 1441, 1988.
21. Pierron, R.L., Perry, H.M., 3rd, Grossberg, G., et al. *J. Am Geriatr. Soc.*, 38, 1339, 1990.
22. Goldray, D., Mizrahi-Sasson, E., Merdler, C., et al. Vitamin D deficiency in elderly patients in a general hospital. *J. Am. Geriatr. Soc.*, 37, 589, 1989.
23. Perry, H.M., 3rd, Horowitz, M., Morley, J.E., et al. Longitudinal changes in serum 25-hydroxyvitamin D in older people. *Metabolism*, 48, 1028, 1999.
24. Chapuy, M.C., Arlot, M.E., Delmas, P.D., et al. Effect of calcium and cholecalciferol treatment for three years on hip fractures in elderly women. *Br. Med. J.*, 308, 1081, 1994.
25. McCormick, J. and Skrabanek, P. Coronary artery disease is not preventable by population interventions. *Lancet*, 2, 839, 1988.
26. Fries, J.F., Green, L.W., and Levine, S. Health promotion and the compression of morbidity. *Lancet*, 1, 481, 1989.
27. Aronow, W.S., Herzig, A.H., Etienne, F., et al. 41-month follow-up of risk factors correlated with new coronary events in 708 elderly patients. *J. Am. Geriatr. Soc.*, 37, 501, 1989.
28. Weverling-Rijnsburger, A.W., Blauw, G.J., Lagaay, A.M., et al. Total cholesterol and risk of mortality in the oldest old. *Lancet*, 350, 1119, 1997.
29. Schatz, I.J. Masaki, K., Yano, K., et al. Cholesterol and all-cause mortality in elderly people from the Honolulu Heart Program: a cohort study. *Lancet*, 358, 351, 2001.
30. Shepherd, J., Blauw, G.J., Murphy, M.B., et al. Pravastatin in elderly individuals at risk of vascular disease (PROSPER): a randomized controlled trial. *Lancet*, 360, 1623, 2002.
31. Prentice, R.L., Caan, B., Chlebowski, R.T., et al. Low-fat dietary pattern and risk of invasive breast cancer: the Women's Health Initiative Randomized Controlled Dietary Modification Trial. *JAMA*, 295, 629, 2006.
32. Beresford, S.A., Johnson, K.C., Ritenbaugh, C., et al. Low-fat dietary pattern and risk of colorectal cancer: the Women's Health Initiative Randomized Controlled Dietary Modification Trial. *JAMA*, 295, 643, 2006.
33. Howard, B.V., Manson, J.E., Stefanick, M.L., et al. Low-fat dietary pattern and weight change over 7 years: the Women's Health Initiative Dietary Modification Trial. *JAMA*, 295, 39, 2006.
34. Swan, G.E., LaRue, A., Carmelli, D., et al. Decline in cognitive performance in aging twins. Heritability and biobehavioral predictors from the National Heart, Lung, and Blood Institute Twin Study. *Arch. Neurol.*, 49, 476, 1992.
35. Kessler, A.R., Kessler, B., and Yehuda, S. *In vivo* modulation of brain cholesterol level and learning performance by a novel plant lipid: indications for interactions between hippocampal-cortical cholesterol and learning. *Life Sci.*, 38, 1185, 1986.

36. Leaf, A. and Weber, P.C. Cardiovascular effects of n-3 fatty acids. *N. Engl. J. Med.*, 318, 549, 1988.
37. Kromhout, D., Bosschieter, E.B., and de Lezenne Coulander, C. The inverse relation between fish consumption and 20-year mortality from coronary heart disease. *N. Engl. J. Med.*, 312, 1205, 1985.
38. Morison, I. and Orr, M.B. Oral cancer in betel nut chewers in travancore. *Lancet*, 2, 575, 1933.
39. Stocks, P. and Karn, M.N. A co-operative study of the habits, home life, dietary and family histories of 450 cancer patients and of an equal number of control patients. *Ann. Eugenics*, 5, 237, 1933.
40. Fanestil, D.D. and Barrows, C.M., Jr. Aging in rotifer. *J. Gerontol.*, 20, 462, 1965.
41. Linn, B.S. and Linn, M.S. Dietary patterns and practices which affect the incidence of cancer in the elderly. In *Handbook of Nutrition in the Aged,* Watson, R.W., Ed. CRC Press, Boca Raton, FL, 1986, p. 299.
42. Macrae, F.A. Fat and calories in colon and breast cancer: from animal studies to controlled clinical trials. *Prev. Med.*, 22, 750, 1993.
43. Fair, W.R., Fleshner, N.E., and Heston, W. Cancer of the prostate: a nutritional disease? *Urology*, 50, 840, 1997.
44. Biesalski, H.K. Meat and cancer: meat as a component of a healthy diet. *Eur. J. Clin. Nutr.*, 56, S2, 2002.
45. Shirai, T., Asamoto, M., Takahashi, S., et al. Diet and prostate cancer. *Toxicology*, 181/182, 89, 2002.
46. Larsson, L.G, Sandstrom, A., and Westling, P. Relationship of Plummer-Vinson disease to cancer of the upper alimentary tract in Sweden. *Cancer Res.*, 35, 3308, 1975.
47. Cowdry, E.V. Malignant neoplasms of thyroid gland. In *Etiology and Prevention of Cancer in Man*, Cowdry, E.V., Ed. Appleton, New York, 1968, p. 277.
48. Linsell, C.A. and Peers, F.G. Field studies on liver cell cancer. In *Origin of Human Cancer*, Hiatt, H.H., Watson, J.D., and Winsten, J.A., Eds. Cold Spring Harbor Lab, New York, 1977, p. 549.
49. Pamukcu, A.M., Erturk, E., Yalciner, S., et al. Carcinogenic and mutagenic activities of milk from cows fed bracken fern (*Pteridium aquilinum*). *Cancer Res.*, 38, 1556, 1978.
50. Menkes, M.S., Comstock, G.W., Vuilleumier, J.P., et al. Serum beta-carotene, vitamins A and E, selenium, and the risk of lung cancer. *N. Engl. J. Med.*, 315, 1250, 1986.
51. Virtamo, J., Pietinen, P., Huttunen, J.K., et al. Incidence of cancer and mortality following alpha-tocopheral and beta-carotene supplementation: a post intervention follow-up. *JAMA*, 2980, 476, 2003.
52. Martinez, M.E. Primary prevention of colorectal cancer: lifestyle, nutrition, exercise. *Recent Results Cancer Res.*, 166, 177, 2005.
53. Morley, J.E., Mooradian, A.D., Silver, A.S., et al. Nutrition in the elderly. *Ann. Intern. Med.*, 109, 890, 1988.
54. Salonen, J.T., Salonen, R., Lappetelainen, R., et al. Risk of cancer in relation to serum concentrations of selenium and vitamins A and E: matched case-control analysis of prospective data. *Br. Med. J.*, 290, 417, 1985.
55. Paffenbarger, R.S., Jr., Hyde, R.T., Wing, A.S., et al. Physical activity, all-cause mortality, and longevity of college alumni. *N. Engl. J. Med.*, 314, 605, 1986.
56. Hoffman, S.A., Paschkis, K.E., and DeBias, D.A. The influence of exercise on the growth of transplanted rat tumors. *Cancer Res.*, 22, 597, 1962.
57. Gerhardsson, M., Norell, S.E., Kiviranta, H., et al. Sedentary jobs and colon cancer. *Am. J. Epidemiol.*, 123, 775, 1986.

58. Fiatarone, M.A., Morley, J.E., Bloom, E.T., et al. Endogenous opioids and the exercise-induced augmentation of natural killer cell activity. *J. Lab. Clin. Med.*, 112, 544, 1988.
59. Fries, J.F. Aging, natural death, and the compression of morbidity. *N. Engl. J. Med.*, 303, 130, 1980.
60. Masoro, E.J. Overview of caloric restriction and ageing. *Mech. Ageing Dev.*, 126, 913, 2005.
61. Shanley, D.P. and Kirkwood, T.B.L. Caloric restriction does not enhance longevity in all species and is unlikely to do so in humans. *Biogerontology*, 7, 165, 2006.
62. Guarente, L. and Picard, F. Calorie restriction: the SIR2 connection. *Cell*, 120, 473, 2005.
63. Roth, G.S., Lane, M.A., and Ingram, D.K. Caloric restriction mimetics: the next phase. *Ann. N.Y. Acad. Sci.*, 1057, 365, 2005.
64. Lane, M.A., Baer, D.J., Rumpler, W.V., et al. Calorie restriction lowers body temperature in rhesus monkeys, consistent with a postulated anti-aging mechanism in rodents. *Proc. Natl. Acad. Sci. U.S.A.*, 93, 4159, 1996.
65. Raman, A., Ramsey, J.J., Kemnitz, J.W., et al. Influences of calorie restriction and age on energy expenditure in the rhesus monkeys. *Am. J. Physiol. Endocrinol. Metab.*, Epub, August 8, 2006.
66. DeLany, J.P., Hansen, B.C., Bodkin, N.L., et al. Long-term caloric restriction reduces energy expenditure in aging monkeys. *J. Gerontol. A Biol. Sci. Med. Sci.*, 54, B5, 1999.
67. Racette, S.B., Weiss, E.P., Villareal, D.T., et al. One year of caloric restriction in humans: feasibility and effects on body composition and abdominal adipose tissue. *J. Gerontol. A Biol. Sci. Med. Sci.*, 61, 943, 2006.
68. Fontana, L., Meyer, T.E., Klein, S., et al. Long-term calorie restriction is highly effective in reducing the risk for atherosclerosis in humans. *Proc. Natl. Acad. Sci. U.S.A.*, 101, 6659, 2004.
69. Heilbronn, L.K., deJonge, L., Frisard, M.I., et al. Effect of 6-month calorie restriction on biomarkers of longevity, metabolic adaptation, and oxidative stress in overweight individuals: a randomized controlled trial. *JAMA*, 295, 1539, 2006.
70. Enstrom, J.E., Kanim, L.E., and Klein, M.A. Vitamin C intake and mortality among a sample of the United States population. *Epidemiology*, 3, 194, 1992.
71. Morley, J.E., Mooradian, A.D., Rosenthal, M.J., et al. Diabetes mellitus in elderly patients. Is it different? *Am. J. Med.*, 83, 533, 1987.

4 Obesity in Older Adults

Gary A. Wittert, M.B.B.S.

CONTENTS

4.1 SUMMARY

Increased body fat, redistribution of body fat to the abdomen, and loss of muscle mass (sarcopenia) are all problems in old age, which are increasing in frequency. Decreased physical activity and decreased energy expenditure with aging predispose to fat accumulation and fat redistribution. The risks of obesity in old age are dependent on the distribution of the fat, increasing with a predominant visceral distribution; prior weight history; and associated sarcopenia. The use of the body mass index (BMI; kg/m^2) to assess obesity in the elderly may be misleading. An increased BMI has a smaller effect on overall and cardiovascular mortality in the elderly, although it is associated with decreased mobility. Overall mortality is more likely to increase when the BMI decreases. Waist circumference is a more useful measure since intra-abdominal fat is clearly related to increased morbidity and mortality. Increased physical activity is a preferable management strategy to diet-induced weight loss, other than in those with predominantly obesity-related mobility disorders, and also has beneficial effects on muscle strength, endurance, and overall well-being. Those exercise regimens that include strength training have benefits over and above those focusing on endurance training alone. An active lifestyle should be promoted early and maintained through adulthood to prevent substantial weight gain and obesity with age.

4.2 AGE-RELATED CHANGES IN BODY COMPOSITION

On average, body weight increases until approximately age 60 to 65 and decreases in approximately 60% of the population thereafter. The contribution of fat mass to the weight loss that occurs in the elderly is small and seen predominantly in women over the age of 70 years.[1,2] In general, fat mass increases with increasing age[3] and tends to be redistributed viscerally, in both genders.[4] Muscle mass and strength decrease by approximately 15 and 30%, respectively, between the second and seventh decades.[3]

In the SENECA study (Survey in Europe on Nutrition and the Elderly; a Concerted Action), a longitudinal assessment of changes in body composition that occurred between the ages of 65 to 70 and 80 to 85 in Europeans from nine towns, stature decreased by 1.5 to 2 cm and average body weight increased by 5 kg in 13% of men and women and decreased by 5 kg in 23% of men and 27% of women. In contrast, waist circumference increased by 3 to 4 cm.[5] A U.S. study followed a group of men and women age over 60 at enrollment. In men, overall body weight did not change significantly, fat mass increased by approximately 1.2 kg, and total appendicular skeletal muscle decreased by approximately 0.8 kg. In women, both body weight and fat mass were reduced by about 0.8 kg and appendicular skeletal muscle mass decreased by about 0.4 kg.[6] In another study, the oldest subjects had a thinner body frame and malnutrition was present in 5% of both genders. Waist circumference and waist:hip ratio values were higher for the youngest men than for the oldest men, whereas in women the waist:hip ratio values were higher in the oldest women, suggesting that visceral redistribution in old age predominantly affects females.[7]

4.3 MECHANISMS RESPONSIBLE FOR THE CHANGES IN BODY COMPOSITION WITH AGING

4.3.1 Changes in Energy Expenditure

Energy expenditure decreases by around 165 kcal/decade in men and 103 kcal/decade in women, primarily due to changes in voluntary physical activity and, to a lesser extent, a decrease in resting metabolic rate (RMR).[8] In a population-based cohort of 33,466 men age 45 to 79 years in central Sweden, total daily physical activity was found to decrease by approximately 4% between ages 45 and 79. Obese men reported 2.6% lower physical activity than normal-weight men. Men with self-rated poor health had –11.3% lower levels of physical activity than those reporting very good health.[9] Data from cross-sectional studies show that after the age of 40 there is a progressive decline is resting metabolic rate, which is explained by both a loss of fat-free mass and a decrease in physical activity. Up to 30% of community-dwelling older persons have diets deficient in at least one major nutrient.[10]

4.3.2 Changes in Nutrient Intake

In a cross-sectional study of 15,266 healthy men age 55 to 79 years, total energy and energy from fat, but not from other nutrients, increased linearly with increasing BMI. BMI increased by 0.53 and 0.14 kg/m^2 for every 500 kcal of fat and total energy consumed, respectively.[11] While many elderly people consume adequate amounts of protein, many older people have a reduced appetite and consume less than the protein Recommended Dietary Allowance (RDA), likely resulting in an accelerated rate of sarcopenia. In very old men and women, the use of a protein-calorie supplement was associated with greater strength and muscle mass gains, and an increased protein intake enhances the response of muscle to resistance exercise in the elderly.[12]

4.3.3 Changes in Fat Metabolism

Changes that occur with aging that increase the propensity to the accumulation of fat include a decrease in whole body fat oxidation (0.5 g/year from age 30 to 70) associated with the decrease in fat-free mass, a diminished ability to use fat as a fuel during exercise,[13] reduced adipose tissue lipoprotein lipase activity,[14] and catecholamine[13] and leptin[14] resistance. In women, both aging and the menopause transition are associated with a number of changes in fat metabolism, which may contribute to the accumulation of body fat after menopause.[15]

4.3.4 Changes in Muscle Metabolism

In muscle there is a disproportionate atrophy of type II (fast-twitch) muscle fibers and a decrease in the number of functional motor units accompanied by irregularity of motor unit firing. There is also a decrease in muscle protein synthesis, mitochondrial oxidative enzyme activity, muscle capillarization, myosin heavy-chain synthesis, and a decline in mitochondrial function.[16] Factors that may be responsible for, or are at least associated with, these changes are decreased physical activity, inadequate nutrition, vascular disease, increased activity of inflammatory cytokines, and decreased levels of anabolic hormones.[17,18]

4.4 ASSESSMENT OF OBESITY IN THE ELDERLY

Body mass index (BMI) calculated as kg/m^2, which is used as an approximation of fat mass in adults, reaches a maximum in the fifth decade in both males and females. The 75th year of age is a turning point for BMI.[7] At different ages, however, the same levels of BMI correspond to different amounts of fat and fat-free mass. Some individuals with low BMI have as much fat as those with high BMI.[19] BMI is therefore of limited use to evaluate the prevalence of overweight and obesity in the elderly unless very high.[20] Waist circumference is a good index of visceral fat mass at all ages[19,20] and relates well to obesity-related health risks in the elderly.[21]

The accurate identification of a combination of low muscle mass with increased fat mass (sarcopenic obesity) requires precise methods of simultaneously measuring fat and lean components, such as dual-energy X-ray absorptiometry.[20] The measurement of the waist:hip ratio may serve clinical purposes; it relates particularly well to the risk of diabetes mellitus and cardiovascular disease (CVD).[22,23]

4.5 PREVALENCE OF OBESITY IN THE ELDERLY

Studies of the prevalence of obesity in the elderly have most frequently been based on standard BMI criteria. In elderly Italians age 65 to 95, the prevalence of obesity in 1985, which was 28% in women and 13% in men, increased to 16% in men in a little over a decade, while remaining unchanged in the women.[7] In a more recent analysis (2004), 38.8% of Italian women were overweight and 13.8% obese. Age- and sex-standardized prevalence of overweight or obesity was 36.0% for more educated subjects and 54.0% for less educated ones.[24] Among 4009 community-living men and women over the age of 60 in Spain, the prevalence of overweight and obesity in men was 49 and 31.5%, respectively. The corresponding percentages in women were 39.8 and 40.8%. The prevalence of central obesity was 48.4% in men and 78.4% in women. The prevalence of obesity was highest in the uneducated, particularly among women, where the prevalence of central obesity was 80.9% in those with no education.[25] In urban Mexican women (mean age, 71.6), the proportions of overweight and obese women were 60.7, 36.2, and 76.5% in urban, rural, and marginal areas, respectively.[26] In a representative sample of elderly Mexicans from five Southwestern states in the U.S., 23% of men and 35% of women were obese.[27] In elderly Taiwanese subjects, the prevalence of overweight was 27.3% in men and 34.9% in women, and that of obesity was 3.2% in men and 6.4% in women.[28] The Dutch nutrition survey of 539 apparently healthy, independently living elderly age 65 to 79 years found an overall prevalence of obesity of 13%.[29]

Among residents over 50 years in a defined area in Jerusalem, the prevalence of obesity standardized by age and sex was 21% in 1970 and 25% in 1986, although the increase was statistically significant only in men.[30] Analysis of data from the Longitudinal Study of Aging and the Assets and Health Dynamics of the Oldest Old Survey showed that the prevalence of obesity, over time, increased among those 70 and older.[31] Data from male participants of the Normative Aging Study showed that new cases of obesity, defined on the basis of BMI, increased over time, while the numbers of subjects classified as lean and intermediate decreased. Among oldest subjects, both the lean and obese had slight but significant decreases in mean BMI. Among the lean, only the young showed consistent increments.[32]

4.6 CONSEQUENCES OF OBESITY IN THE ELDERLY

4.6.1 Overall Mortality

The relative contribution of increased fat mass to mortality may be less pronounced in elderly people. There is some variability between studies. In 2032 subjects (999 men, 1033 women; mean age, 80 years) recruited by random sampling of the Old Age and Disability Allowance Schemes in Hong Kong, stratified by sex and 5-year age groups from 70 years onward, overall mortality was negatively associated with body mass index and participation in physical activity, after adjusting for age and sex.[33] In another study, older men and women at a BMI range of 25 to less than 32 kg/m^2 were shown to have no excess mortality.[34] The BMI range of 25 to 27 has also been reported not to be risk factor for all-cause and cardiovascular mortality among elderly persons, whereas overweight (BMI ≥ 27) was a significant prognostic factor for all-cause and cardiovascular mortality among 65- to 74-year-olds, and there was also a significant positive association between overweight and all-cause mortality among those 75 years or older. Overall, it is clear that higher BMI values are associated with a smaller relative mortality risk in elderly persons than in young and middle-aged populations. The standardized mortality rate increases with increasing BMI, but within each BMI group, the standardized mortality rate decreases with age.[35]

A high waist circumference (in nonsmoking men) may be a better predictor of all-cause mortality than high BMI.[19] In a prospective cohort study of 31,702 healthy Iowa women age 55 to 69 years, the waist:hip ratio was the best anthropometric predictor of total mortality.[36] In men and women age 67 to 78, the waist circumference and supine sagittal abdominal diameter are most closely related to CVD risk factors.[37]

In 1996, a health survey was mailed to all surviving participants 65 years or older from the Chicago Heart Association Detection Project in Industry Study (1967 to 1973). The response rate was 60%, and the sample included 3981 male and 3099 female respondents. Compared with normal-weight people, both underweight and obese older adults reported impaired quality of life, particularly worse physical functioning and physical well-being. These results reinforce the importance of normal body weight in older age.[38]

The elderly at greatest risk are those who are simultaneously sarcopenic and obese.[17] Low BMI and weight loss in the elderly are both strong and independent predictors of subsequent mortality, and low BMI better predicts mortality than low waist circumference.[19] Prior weight history has also been shown to be important in predicting risk. Older heavier people who gained more than 10% of mid-life body weight or thinner older people who had lost 10% or more of body weight show high risk compared with thinner people with stable weight.[39] Using data from a large, population-based California cohort study, the Leisure World Cohort Study, it has been shown that in the elderly obesity has been associated with increased mortality only among persons under age 75 years and among never or past smokers. In addition, being overweight or obese in young adulthood and underweight or obese in later life increases the risk of premature mortality in the elderly.[40]

4.6.2 General Health and Well-Being

In the elderly, as in younger individuals, although there have been health improvements in a number of areas, chronic and obesity-related diseases are increasing. For example, in Manitoba, Canada, the prevalence of diabetes, hypertension, and dementia increased substantially over a 14-year period in approximately 50,000 individuals over the age of 65.[41]

4.6.3 Disease-Specific Risks

4.6.3.1 Mobility-Related Disability

Among 2714 women and 2095 men, 65 to 100 years, there was a positive association between fat mass and disability at baseline. Moreover, fat mass was predictive of disability 3 years later, independent of low fat-free mass, age, physical activity, or chronic disease.[42] Data from the U.S. National Health and Nutrition Examination Survey (NHANES) I (1971 through 1987) showed that high BMI is a strong predictor of long-term risk for mobility disability in older women and that this risk persists even to very old age. In the English Longitudinal Study of Ageing, a national population sample of 1030 women and 888 men age 55 to 74 years, body mass and shape were major determinants of disability. Increased waist circumference was the best predictor for most disability outcomes.[21] Sarcopenic obesity at baseline is particularly predictive of independent activities of daily living (IADL) disability at follow-up after 8 years.[43]

Large population-based studies have shown that obesity is a significant independent predictor for older persons being homebound[44] or losing independence, particularly when associated with an unhealthy diet and physical inactivity.[45] A paradoxical increase in risk in disability has been associated with weight loss in very elderly women.[46] Moreover, the Women's Health Initiative Observational Study undertaken in 40 U.S. clinical centers and involving 40,657 women age 65 to 79 at baseline and 3 years of follow-up showed that both obesity and underweight were strongly associated with the development of frailty.[47]

4.6.3.2 Impaired Glucose Tolerance and Type 2 Diabetes Mellitus

The prevalence of type 2 diabetes increases progressively with age, peaking at 16.5% in men and 12.8% in women age 75 to 84 years. Over age 65, diabetes or glucose intolerance was present in 30 to 40% of Framingham Study subjects.[48] Among 1972 male participants in the Department of Veterans Affairs Normative Aging Study cohort, there was a prospective relation between abdominal adiposity and the risk of diabetes.[49] An age-associated increase in total adiposity is a major contributor to impaired glucose tolerance in middle-aged and older men. Increased body fatness and increased abdominal obesity, rather than aging per se, are thought to be directly linked to the greatly increased incidence of type 2 diabetes mellitus among the elderly.[50] Nevertheless, there is evidence that insulin secretion decreases with age even after adjustments for differences in adiposity, fat distribution, and physical activity.[51]

4.6.3.3 Hypertension and Cardiovascular Disease

Data from the Honolulu Heart Program show that obesity and high blood pressure continue to be highly correlated even in old age.[52] Furthermore, the Veterans Administration Normative Aging Study showed that abdominal accumulation of body fat, apart from overall level of adiposity, was associated with both increased blood pressure and an increased risk of hypertension.[53]

Fat and distribution in the middle appear to be the dominant predictor of cardiovascular risk in the elderly. Body mass index has been shown to be an important risk factor for fatal coronary heart disease (CHD), and its prognostic significance remains after up to 30 years of follow-up.[54] Moreover, for individuals with no cardiovascular risk factors, as well as for those with one or more risk factors, those who are obese in middle age have a higher risk of hospitalization and mortality from CHD, cardiovascular disease, and diabetes in older age than those who are normal weight.[55]

4.6.3.4 Fatty Liver

The prevalence of fatty liver has been reported to be 3.3% in male and 3.8% in female nonobese and 21.6% in male and 18.8% in female obese elderly individuals, and was shown to be an independent correlate of coronary risk factors.[56]

4.6.3.5 Pulmonary Function

Among 1094 men and 540 women from the Baltimore Longitudinal Study of Aging there was a strong inverse association of waist/hip ratio (WHR) with FEV(1) and FVC in men but not women.[57] In a cross-sectional evaluation, the effects of fat distribution and body composition on lung function were determined in 2744 men age 60 to 79 years from towns in Britain. All men were free of cardiovascular disease and cancer. Total body fat and central adiposity were found to be inversely associated with lung function. Increased fat free mass (FFM) reflecting increased muscle mass was associated with better lung function and lower odds of low FEV1:FVC with aging.[58] Weight loss has been shown to improve static lung volume, not dynamic pulmonary function, in moderately obese, sedentary men.[59]

4.6.3.6 Autonomic Nervous System Dysfunction

Abdominal-to-peripheral fat distribution explains a significant portion of the variance in a number of autonomic-circulatory functions attributable to aging.[60]

4.6.3.7 Cognitive Function

Obesity is defined by BMI and waist circumference is associated with poorer cognition in the elderly.[61] Moreover, obesity at midlife is associated with an increased risk of dementia and Alzheimer's disease (AD) later in life, and clustering of vascular risk factors increases the risk in an additive manner.[62] A larger WHR may be related to neurodegenerative, vascular, or metabolic processes that affect brain structures underlying cognitive decline and dementia.[63]

4.6.3.8 Other Adverse Effects of Obesity in the Elderly

Obesity is independently associated with the presence and severity of urinary incontinence[64] and lower limb joint pain.[65] Obesity also increases the risk of overall cancer, non-Hodgkin's lymphoma, leukemia, multiple myeloma, and cancers of the kidney, colon, rectum, breast (in postmenopausal women), pancreas, ovary, and prostate.[66]

4.7 MANAGEMENT OF OBESITY IN THE ELDERLY

4.7.1 Benefits and Risks of Weight Loss

For overweight individuals in good health, there is no good evidence to show that mortality rates are reduced with weight loss. Even among overweight persons with one or more obesity-related health conditions, specific weight loss recommendations may be unnecessary.[67] Modifiable behavioral factors (physical activity, smoking, and obesity) and cardiovascular risk factors (diabetes, HDL cholesterol, and blood pressure) are associated with maintenance of good health in older adults.[68] Many obesity-related health conditions (e.g., hypertension, dyslipidemia, insulin resistance, glucose intolerance) can be ameliorated independently of weight loss.[67] While the benefits of weight loss in the elderly have been the subject of considerable uncertainty, it has been shown that it is feasible for self-selected obese older women to achieve a moderate weight loss and increase in physical activity resulting in short-term improvements in laboratory, physical performance, self-reported function, vitality, and life quality outcomes.[69] Nevertheless, in well-functioning elderly people, the functional consequences of past weight change depended on the type of weight change, intentionality, and current measured body weight. For example, unintentional weight loss in the previous year has been associated with increased risk for mobility limitation regardless of weight status, and in the overweight (but not obese) elderly, intentional weight and weight fluctuation with any intention increased the risk for mobility limitation.[70] Similarly, data from another cohort have also shown that change in weight is associated with worse health-related quality of life among the older adults, principally women, and therefore it is desirable to prevent weight gain, especially among the obese, and weight loss, especially among the nonobese.[71]

The North American Society of the Study of Obesity has taken the position that weight loss therapy improves physical function, quality of life, and the medical complications associated with obesity in older persons. Therefore, weight loss therapy that minimizes muscle and bone losses is recommended for older persons who are obese and who have functional impairments or medical complications that can benefit from weight loss.[72]

4.7.2 Specific Modalities for Inducing Weight Loss

4.7.2.1 Calorie Restriction

Thinness and weight loss (regardless of initial BMI) are associated with increased mortality rates in humans, independent of smoking or weight loss resulting from subclinical disease. In general, it is not appropriate to advise caloric restriction in the elderly as the primary modality to induce weight loss, although it may be appropriate where the major problem is mobility or when part of a balanced eating plan, of modest degree, of adequate protein content and combined with appropriate physical activity. It is generally appropriate, however, to advise a reduction in saturated fat intake, to increase fiber, and to ensure that the diet contains sufficient micronutrients.

4.7.2.2 Physical Activity

Regular exercise is the best predictor of successful weight maintenance. An increase in physical activity leads to an improved insulin sensitivity and glucose tolerance,[73] and a reduction in all-cause and cardiovascular mortality.[67] Endurance training increases fatty acid oxidation, leads to a reduction in visceral fat, and increases, or attenuates, the decline in RMR.[74] Beginning moderately vigorous sports activity, quitting cigarette smoking, maintaining normal blood pressure, and avoiding obesity were separately associated with lower rates of death from all causes and from coronary heart disease among middle-aged and older men.[75] Resistive training has particular benefits and improves quality and function of skeletal muscle, decreases total and intra-abdominal fat, improves insulin action, and lowers blood pressure.[76,77] Improvements in fitness have been shown to attenuate age-related increases in adiposity. People who exercise regularly have a lower risk of cardiovascular disease[75] and appear to accumulate less adipose tissue in upper, central body regions as they get older, potentially reducing the risk for the metabolic disorders associated with upper-body obesity.[78]

4.7.2.3 Pharmacotherapy

Most clinical trials exclude older patients, and little is known about benefits of diets or drugs inducing weight loss in these age groups.

4.7.2.4 Bariatric Surgery

Bariatric surgery can be safely performed in patients above age 70 with the same benefits as for younger subjects. Laparoscopically performed Roux-en-Y gastric bypass (LRYGBP) in patients >60 years of age is associated with significant weight loss, resolution of obesity-associated comorbidities,[79–81] reduction of medication needs, and very large cost savings.[80] Although there is a higher morbidity and mortality, the risk–benefit ratio is considered acceptable.

REFERENCES

1. Mott JW, Wang J, Thornton JC, Allison DB, Heymsfield SB, Pierson RN, Jr. Relation between body fat and age in 4 ethnic groups. *Am J Clin Nutr* 69:1007–1013, 1999.
2. Perry HM, 3rd, Morley JE, Horowitz M, Kaiser FE, Miller DK, Wittert G. Body composition and age in African-American and Caucasian women: relationship to plasma leptin levels. *Metabolism* 46:1399–1405, 1997.
3. Hughes VA, Frontera WR, Roubenoff R, Evans WJ, Singh MA. Longitudinal changes in body composition in older men and women: role of body weight change and physical activity. *Am J Clin Nutr* 76:473–481, 2002.
4. Beaufrere B, Morio B. Fat and protein redistribution with aging: metabolic considerations. *Eur J Clin Nutr* 54 (Suppl 3):S48–S53, 2000.
5. de Groot CP, Enzi G, Matthys C, Moreiras O, Roszkowski W, Schroll M. Ten-year changes in anthropometric characteristics of elderly Europeans. *J Nutr Health Aging* 6:4–8, 2002.
6. Gallagher D, Ruts E, Visser M, Heshka S, Baumgartner RN, Wang J, Pierson RN, Pi-Sunyer FX, Heymsfield SB. Weight stability masks sarcopenia in elderly men and women. *Am J Physiol Endocrinol Metab* 279:E366–375, 2000.
7. Perissinotto E, Pisent C, Sergi G, Grigoletto F. Anthropometric measurements in the elderly: age and gender differences. *Br J Nutr* 87:177–186, 2002.
8. Elia M. Obesity in the elderly. *Obes Res* 9 (Suppl 4):244S–248S, 2001.
9. Norman A, Bellocco R, Vaida F, Wolk A. Total physical activity in relation to age, body mass, health and other factors in a cohort of Swedish men. *Int J Obes Relat Metab Disord* 26:670–675, 2002.
10. Morley JE. Nutritional status of the elderly. *Am J Med* 81:679–695, 1986.
11. Satia-Abouta J, Patterson RE, Schiller RN, Kristal AR. Energy from fat is associated with obesity in U.S. men: results from the Prostate Cancer Prevention Trial. *Prev Med* 34:493–501, 2002.
12. Evans WJ. Protein nutrition, exercise and aging. *J Am Coll Nutr* 23:601S–609S, 2004.
13. Blaak EE. Adrenergically stimulated fat utilization and ageing. *Ann Med* 32:380–382, 2000.
14. Berman DM, Rogus EM, Busby-Whitehead MJ, Katzel LI, Goldberg AP. Predictors of adipose tissue lipoprotein lipase in middle-aged and older men: relationship to leptin and obesity, but not cardiovascular fitness. *Metabolism* 48:183–189, 1999.
15. Misso ML, Jang C, Adams J, Tran J, Murata Y, Bell R, Boon WC, Simpson ER, Davis SR. Differential expression of factors involved in fat metabolism with age and the menopause transition. *Maturitas* 51:299–306, 2005.
16. Waters DL, Brooks WM, Qualls CR, Baumgartner RN. Skeletal muscle mitochondrial function and lean body mass in healthy exercising elderly. *Mech Ageing Dev* 124:301–309, 2003.
17. Morley JE, Baumgartner RN, Roubenoff R, Mayer J, Nair KS. Sarcopenia. *J Lab Clin Med* 137:231–243, 2001.
18. Nikolic M, Bajek S, Bobinac D, Vranic TS, Jerkovic R. Aging of human skeletal muscles. *Coll Antropol* 29:67–70, 2005.
19. Seidell JC, Visscher TL. Body weight and weight change and their health implications for the elderly. *Eur J Clin Nutr* 54 (Suppl 3):S33–S39, 2000.
20. Baumgartner RN, Heymsfield SB, Roche AF. Human body composition and the epidemiology of chronic disease. *Obes Res* 3:73–95, 1995.
21. Angleman SB, Harris TB, Melzer D. The role of waist circumference in predicting disability in periretirement age adults. *Int J Obes* (Lond) 30:364–373, 2006.

22. Canoy D, Luben R, Welch A, Bingham S, Wareham N, Day N, Khaw KT. Fat distribution, body mass index and blood pressure in 22,090 men and women in the Norfolk cohort of the European Prospective Investigation into Cancer and Nutrition (EPIC-Norfolk) study. *J Hypertens* 22:2067–2074, 2004.
23. Dalton M, Cameron AJ, Zimmet PZ, Shaw JE, Jolley D, Dunstan DW, Welborn TA. Waist circumference, waist-hip ratio and body mass index and their correlation with cardiovascular disease risk factors in Australian adults. *J Intern Med* 254:555–563, 2003.
24. Gallus S, Colombo P, Scarpino V, Zuccaro P, Negri E, Apolone G, Vecchia CL. Overweight and obesity in Italian adults 2004, and an overview of trends since 1983. *Eur J Clin Nutr* 60: 1174–1179, 2006.
25. Gutierrez-Fisac JL, Lopez E, Banegas JR, Graciani A, Rodriguez-Artalejo F. Prevalence of overweight and obesity in elderly people in Spain. *Obes Res* 12:710–715, 2004.
26. Gutierrez LM, Llaca MC, Cervantes L, Velasquez Alva MC, Irigoyen ME, Zepeda M. Overweight in elderly Mexican women of a marginal community. *J Nutr Health Aging* 5:256–258, 2001.
27. Ostir GV, Markides KS, Freeman DH, Jr., Goodwin JS. Obesity and health conditions in elderly Mexican Americans: the Hispanic EPESE. Established Population for Epidemiologic Studies of the Elderly. *Ethn Dis* 10:31–38, 2000.
28. Chiu HC, Chang HY, Mau LW, Lee TK, Liu HW. Height, weight, and body mass index of elderly persons in Taiwan. *J Gerontol A Biol Sci Med Sci* 55:M684–690, 2000.
29. Lowik MR, Schrijver J, Odink J, van den Berg H, Wedel M, Hermus RJ. Nutrition and aging: nutritional status of "apparently healthy" elderly (Dutch nutrition surveillance system). *J Am Coll Nutr* 9:18–27, 1990.
30. Gofin J, Abramson JH, Kark JD, Epstein L. The prevalence of obesity and its changes over time in middle-aged and elderly men and women in Jerusalem. *Int J Obes Relat Metab Disord* 20:260–266, 1996.
31. Himes CL. Obesity, disease, and functional limitation in later life. *Demography* 37:73–82, 2000.
32. Grinker JA, Tucker K, Vokonas PS, Rush D. Overweight and leanness in adulthood: prospective study of male participants in the Normative Aging Study. *Int J Obes Relat Metab Disord* 20:561–569, 1996.
33. Woo J, Ho SC, Yuen YK, Yu LM, Lau J. Cardiovascular risk factors and 18-month mortality and morbidity in an elderly Chinese population aged 70 years and over. *Gerontology* 44:51–55, 1998.
34. Bender R, Jockel KH, Trautner C, Spraul M, Berger M. Effect of age on excess mortality in obesity. *JAMA* 281:1498–1504, 1999.
35. Heiat A, Vaccarino V, Krumholz HM. An evidence-based assessment of federal guidelines for overweight and obesity as they apply to elderly persons. *Arch Intern Med* 161:1194–1203, 2001.
36. Folsom AR, French SA, Zheng W, Baxter JE, Jeffery RW. Weight variability and mortality: the Iowa Women's Health Study. *Int J Obes Relat Metab Disord* 20:704–709, 1996.
37. Turcato E, Bosello O, Di Francesco V, Harris TB, Zoico E, Bissoli L, Fracassi E, Zamboni M. Waist circumference and abdominal sagittal diameter as surrogates of body fat distribution in the elderly: their relation with cardiovascular risk factors. *Int J Obes Relat Metab Disord* 24:1005–1010, 2000.
38. Yan LL, Daviglus ML, Liu K, Pirzada A, Garside DB, Schiffer L, Dyer AR, Greenland P. BMI and health-related quality of life in adults 65 years and older. *Obes Res* 12:69–76, 2004.

39. Harris TB, Launer LJ, Madans J, Feldman JJ. Cohort study of effect of being overweight and change in weight on risk of coronary heart disease in old age. *BMJ* 314:1791–1794, 1997.
40. Corrada MM, Kawas CH, Mozaffar F, Paganini-Hill A. Association of body mass index and weight change with all-cause mortality in the elderly. *Am J Epidemiol* 163:938–949, 2006.
41. Menec VH, Lix L, Macwilliam L. Trends in the health status of older Manitobans, 1985 to 1999. *Can J Aging* 24 (Suppl 1):s5–s14, 2005.
42. Visser M, Langlois J, Guralnik JM, Cauley JA, Kronmal RA, Robbins J, Williamson JD, Harris TB. High body fatness, but not low fat-free mass, predicts disability in older men and women: the Cardiovascular Health Study. *Am J Clin Nutr* 68:584–590, 1998.
43. Baumgartner RN, Wayne SJ, Waters DL, Janssen I, Gallagher D, Morley JE. Sarcopenic obesity predicts instrumental activities of daily living disability in the elderly. *Obes Res* 12:1995–2004, 2004.
44. Jensen GL, Silver HJ, Roy MA, Callahan E, Still C, Dupont W. Obesity is a risk factor for reporting homebound status among community-dwelling older persons. *Obesity* (Silver Spring) 14:509–517, 2006.
45. Sulander T, Martelin T, Rahkonen O, Nissinen A, Uutela A. Associations of functional ability with health-related behavior and body mass index among the elderly. *Arch Gerontol Geriatr* 40:185–199, 2005.
46. Launer LJ, Harris T, Rumpel C, Madans J. Body mass index, weight change, and risk of mobility disability in middle-aged and older women. The epidemiologic follow-up study of NHANES I. *JAMA* 271:1093–1098, 1994.
47. Woods NF, LaCroix AZ, Gray SL, Aragaki A, Cochrane BB, Brunner RL, Masaki K, Murray A, Newman AB. Frailty: emergence and consequences in women aged 65 and older in the Women's Health Initiative Observational Study. *J Am Geriatr Soc* 53:1321–1330, 2005.
48. Wilson PW, Kannel WB. Obesity, diabetes, and risk of cardiovascular disease in the elderly. *Am J Geriatr Cardiol* 11:119–123, 125, 2002.
49. Cassano PA, Rosner B, Vokonas PS, Weiss ST. Obesity and body fat distribution in relation to the incidence of non-insulin-dependent diabetes mellitus. A prospective cohort study of men in the normative aging study. *Am J Epidemiol* 136:1474–1486, 1992.
50. Colman E, Katzel LI, Sorkin J, Coon PJ, Engelhardt S, Rogus E, Goldberg AP. The role of obesity and cardiovascular fitness in the impaired glucose tolerance of aging. *Exp Gerontol* 30:571–580, 1995.
51. Muller DC, Elahi D, Tobin JD, Andres R. The effect of age on insulin resistance and secretion: a review. *Semin Nephrol* 16:289–298, 1996.
52. Masaki KH, Curb JD, Chiu D, Petrovitch H, Rodriguez BL. Association of body mass index with blood pressure in elderly Japanese American men. The Honolulu Heart Program. *Hypertension* 29:673–677, 1997.
53. Cassano PA, Segal MR, Vokonas PS, Weiss ST. Body fat distribution, blood pressure, and hypertension. A prospective cohort study of men in the normative aging study. *Ann Epidemiol* 1:33–48, 1990.
54. Kim J, Meade T, Haines A. Skinfold thickness, body mass index, and fatal coronary heart disease: 30 year follow up of the Northwick Park Heart Study. *J Epidemiol Community Health* 60:275–279, 2006.
55. Yan LL, Daviglus ML, Liu K, Stamler J, Wang R, Pirzada A, Garside DB, Dyer AR, Van Horn L, Liao Y, Fries JF, Greenland P. Midlife body mass index and hospitalization and mortality in older age. *JAMA* 295:190–198, 2006.

56. Akahoshi M, Amasaki Y, Soda M, Tominaga T, Ichimaru S, Nakashima E, Seto S, Yano K. Correlation between fatty liver and coronary risk factors: a population study of elderly men and women in Nagasaki, Japan. *Hypertens Res* 24:337–343, 2001.
57. Harik-Khan RI, Wise RA, Fleg JL. The effect of gender on the relationship between body fat distribution and lung function. *J Clin Epidemiol* 54:399–406, 2001.
58. Wannamethee SG, Shaper AG, Whincup PH. Body fat distribution, body composition, and respiratory function in elderly men. *Am J Clin Nutr* 82:996–1003, 2005.
59. Womack CJ, Harris DL, Katzel LI, Hagberg JM, Bleecker ER, Goldberg AP. Weight loss, not aerobic exercise, improves pulmonary function in older obese men. *J Gerontol A Biol Sci Med Sci* 55:M453–M457, 2000.
60. Christou DD, Jones PP, Pimentel AE, Seals DR. Increased abdominal-to-peripheral fat distribution contributes to altered autonomic-circulatory control with human aging. *Am J Physiol Heart Circ Physiol* 287:H1530–H1537, 2004.
61. Jeong SK, Nam HS, Son MH, Son EJ, Cho KH. Interactive effect of obesity indexes on cognition. *Dement Geriatr Cogn Disord* 19:91–96, 2005.
62. Kivipelto M, Ngandu T, Fratiglioni L, Viitanen M, Kareholt I, Winblad B, Helkala EL, Tuomilehto J, Soininen H, Nissinen A. Obesity and vascular risk factors at midlife and the risk of dementia and Alzheimer disease. *Arch Neurol* 62:1556–1560, 2005.
63. Jagust W, Harvey D, Mungas D, Haan M. Central obesity and the aging brain. *Arch Neurol* 62:1545–1548, 2005.
64. Melville JL, Katon W, Delaney K, Newton K. Urinary incontinence in US women: a population-based study. *Arch Intern Med* 165:537–542, 2005.
65. Adamson J, Ebrahim S, Dieppe P, Hunt K. Prevalence and risk factors for joint pain among men and women in the West of Scotland Twenty-07 study. *Ann Rheum Dis* 65:520–524, 2006.
66. Pan SY, Johnson KC, Ugnat AM, Wen SW, Mao Y. Association of obesity and cancer risk in Canada. *Am J Epidemiol* 159:259–268, 2004.
67. Gaesser GA. Thinness and weight loss: beneficial or detrimental to longevity? *Med Sci Sports Exerc* 31:1118–1128, 1999.
68. Burke GL, Arnold AM, Bild DE, Cushman M, Fried LP, Newman A, Nunn C, Robbins J. Factors associated with healthy aging: the cardiovascular health study. *J Am Geriatr Soc* 49:254–262, 2001.
69. Jensen GL, Roy MA, Buchanan AE, Berg MB. Weight loss intervention for obese older women: improvements in performance and function. *Obes Res* 12:1814–1820, 2004.
70. Lee JS, Kritchevsky SB, Tylavsky F, Harris T, Simonsick EM, Rubin SM, Newman AB. Weight change, weight change intention, and the incidence of mobility limitation in well-functioning community-dwelling older adults. *J Gerontol A Biol Sci Med Sci* 60:1007–1012, 2005.
71. Leon-Munoz LM, Guallar-Castillon P, Banegas JR, Gutierrez-Fisac JL, Lopez-Garcia E, Jimenez FJ, Rodriguez-Artalejo F. Changes in body weight and health-related quality-of-life in the older adult population. *Int J Obes* (Lond) 29:1385–1391, 2005.
72. Villareal DT, Apovian CM, Kushner RF, Klein S. Obesity in older adults: technical review and position statement of the American Society for Nutrition and NAASO, The Obesity Society. *Obes Res* 13:1849–1863, 2005.
73. Laws A, Reaven GM. Effect of physical activity on age-related glucose intolerance. *Clin Geriatr Med* 6:849–863, 1990.
74. Kim HJ, Lee JS, Kim CK. Effect of exercise training on muscle glucose transporter 4 protein and intramuscular lipid content in elderly men with impaired glucose tolerance. *Eur J Appl Physiol* 93:353–358, 2004.

75. Paffenbarger RS, Jr., Hyde RT, Wing AL, Lee IM, Jung DL, Kampert JB. The association of changes in physical-activity level and other lifestyle characteristics with mortality among men. *N Engl J Med* 328:538–545, 1993.
76. Ryan AS, Hurlbut DE, Lott ME, Ivey FM, Fleg J, Hurley BF, Goldberg AP. Insulin action after resistive training in insulin resistant older men and women. *J Am Geriatr Soc* 49:247–253, 2001.
77. Hurley BF, Roth SM. Strength training in the elderly: effects on risk factors for age-related diseases. *Sports Med* 30:249–268, 2000.
78. Kohrt WM, Malley MT, Dalsky GP, Holloszy JO. Body composition of healthy sedentary and trained, young and older men and women. *Med Sci Sports Exerc* 24:832–837, 1992.
79. Sosa JL, Pombo H, Pallavicini H, Ruiz-Rodriguez M. Laparoscopic gastric bypass beyond age 60. *Obes Surg* 14:1398–1401, 2004.
80. Snow LL, Weinstein LS, Hannon JK, Lane DR, Ringold FG, Hansen PA, Pointer MD. The effect of Roux-en-Y gastric bypass on prescription drug costs. *Obes Surg* 14:1031–1035, 2004.
81. Papasavas PK, Gagne DJ, Kelly J, Caushaj PF. Laparoscopic Roux-En-Y gastric bypass is a safe and effective operation for the treatment of morbid obesity in patients older than 55 years. *Obes Surg* 14:1056–1061, 2004.

5 Sarcopenia and Cachexia

John E. Morley, M.B., B.Ch.
Matthew T. Haren, Ph.D.

CONTENTS

> ...for wasting which represents old age (sarcopenia) and wasting that is secondary to fever (cachexia) and wasting that is called doalgashi (starvation).
>
> **—Maimonides (1135–1204)**

Sarcopenia can be defined as severe loss of muscle mass that is related to aging. Cachexia, on the other hand, is excessive weight loss associated with disease. The other major causes of weight loss in older persons are anorexia and dehydration. All causes of weight loss can lead to frailty and a decline in muscle strength.

5.1 SARCOPENIA

The age-related loss of muscle mass commonly occurs in older persons. In addition to the loss of muscle mass, aging is associated with increase in intramuscular fat. This has been called myosteatosis. Sarcopenia has been defined as a decline in muscle mass that is two standard deviations less than the muscle mass of young individuals age 20 to 40 years. Overall, the prevalence of sarcopenia is approximately 13% of 60-year-olds and about half of 80-year-olds.[1] Sarcopenic individuals have a marked increase in having disability, and the increased cost of sarcopenia among older persons has been estimated in the order of $18.4 billion in the U.S.[2,3]

An important subset of sarcopenic persons are those who are obese but have lost excessive muscle mass. These older persons have been characterized as the "fat frail" or having sarcopenic obesity. In the New Mexico Aging Process Study sarcopenic obesity was found to be longitudinally the best predictor of future disability and mortality.[4] In distinction from these obese, persons who have an appropriate muscle mass have better outcomes than normal-weight older persons.

The causes of sarcopenia are multifactorial (Table 5.1). In the Hertfordshire Cohort Study grip strength was shown to correlate with birth weight but not weight

TABLE 5.1
The Putative Factors Involved in the Pathogenesis of Sarcopenia

1. Genetic, e.g., angiotensin-converting enzyme polymorphism
2. Congenital—low birth weight
3. Testosterone
4. Vitamin D
5. DHEA
6. Growth hormone
7. ICG-1
8. Mechanogrowth factor
9. Ghrelin
10. Creatine
11. Myostatin
12. Cytokines
13. Insulin resistance
14. Anorexia
15. Lack of physical activity
16. Motor neuron activity
17. Atherosclerotic vascular disease

at 1 year of age, suggesting that *in utero* factors or genetics play a role in the subsequent development of sarcopenia.[5] There is emerging evidence that genetic factors, such as the different alleles of the angiotensin-converting enzyme, may play a role in late-life sarcopenia.

To understand the pathogensis of sarcopenia it is important to realize that muscle is a dynamic tissue that is in a continuous state of both anabolism and catabolism (Figure 5.1). Whenever a muscle contracts, muscle injury is created (Figure 5.2). Mechanoreceptors (such as titin and dystroglycan) recognize, then stimulate, the production of muscle growth factors, which lead to muscle repair through satellite cells and protein synthesis. This results in muscle regeneration and improved function. With aging, this system is impaired, resulting over time in an impaired fiber number (especially type II fibers), leading to a decline in strength and power. Muscle anabolism involves both hypertrophy and regeneration, whereas catabolism involves atrophy and apoptosis. Besides age, predictors of the decline in muscle mass and strength with aging include energy intake, physical activity, insulin-like growth factor 1 (IGF-1), and testosterone.[6] It is important to recognize that muscle mass gain is not always associated with enhanced muscle strength and power in older persons.

Testosterone levels in males decline with aging at the rate of 1% per annum beyond 30 years of age.[7] Testosterone replacement therapy in older males increased muscle mass and strength.[8–10] Testosterone stimulates mesenchymal stem cells to produce satellite cells and inhibits the production of pre-adipocytes. The satellite cells are responsible for repair of muscle tissue during regeneration. In addition, testosterone stimulates muscle protein synthesis and inhibits muscle protein turnover by direct effects on the cellular death chamber, i.e., the ubiquitin–proteasome pathway. These effects of testosterone appear to involve the Wnt pathway indirectly by stimulating beta-catenin,

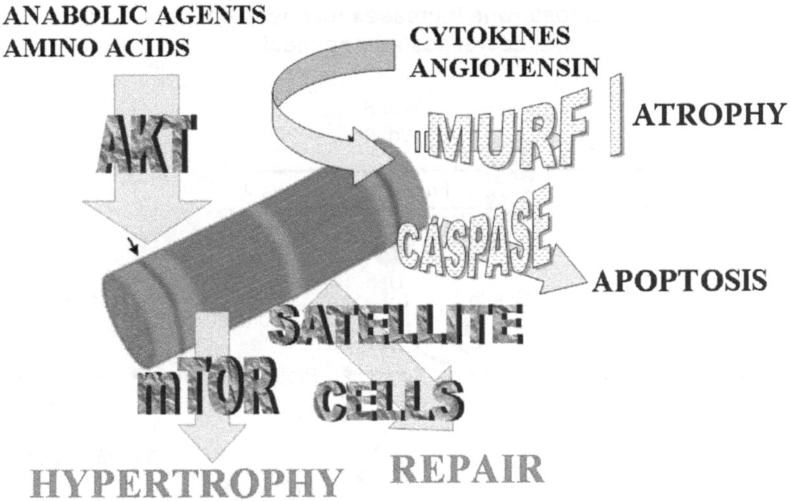

FIGURE 5.1 The ying and yang of muscle survival. Muscle mass and strength is a balance between anabolism and catabolism.

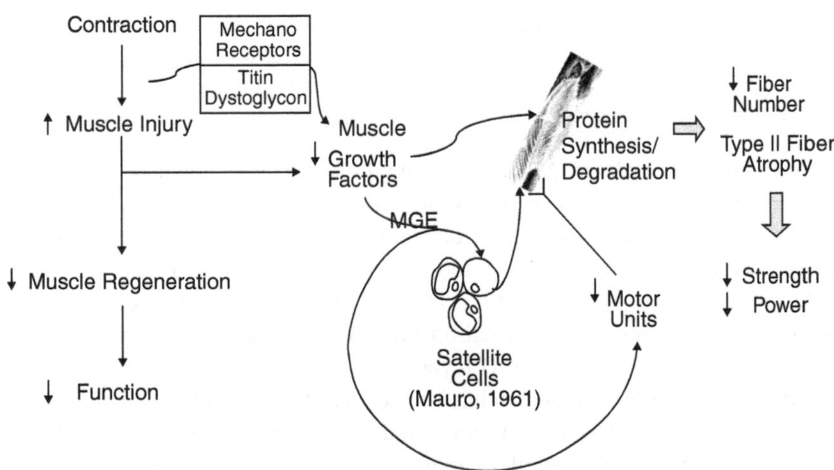

FIGURE 5.2 The effects of aging on the exercise muscle injury and repair cycle. MGF = mechanogrowth factor; = increased with aging; = decreased with aging.

which results in decreased adipogenesis and increased cell cycling and myogenesis (Figure 5.3). Because androgens have effects that may be considered less desirable in older men, e.g., effects on prostate and libido, there have been and are being developed a number of selective androgen receptor molecules (SARMs). Available steroid SARMs include nandrolone, oxandrolone, and oxymethalone. Under development are nonsteroidal SARMs related to 2-quinolones, coumarins, and bicalutamide. There are very preliminary data suggesting that testosterone will also increase strength in older women.

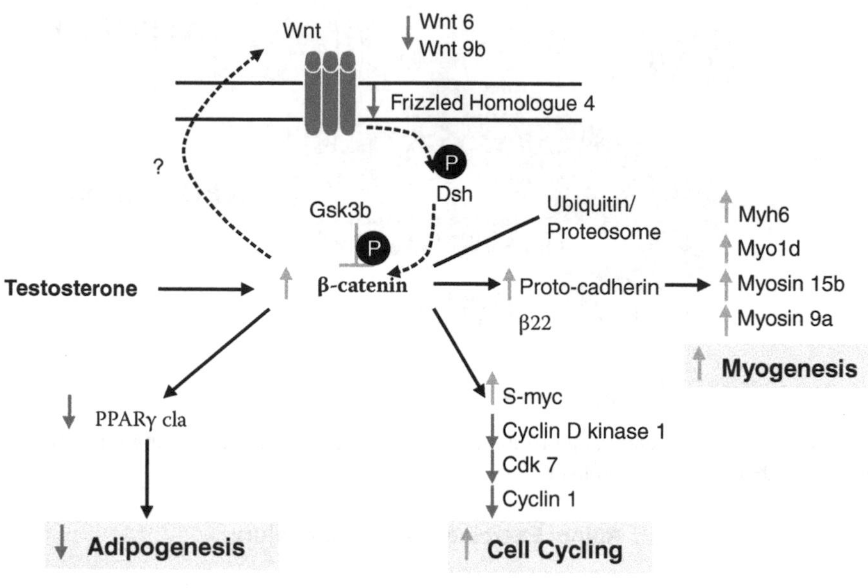

FIGURE 5.3 The putative molecular mechanism by which testosterone regulates muscle mass and strength in older persons.

A longitudinal study of 25(OH) vitamin D levels has shown that they fall in older persons even when the persons are highly healthy and living in a sunny climate.[11] Hypovitaminosis D is associated with declines in muscle strength and reported disability.[12] Low vitamin D and high parathyroid hormone levels are associated with sarcopenia.[13] Low vitamin D levels are an independent predictor of falls.[14] Vitamin D and calcium supplementation improves strength and performance only in older persons with low vitamin D levels.[15]

DHEA is a steroid hormone that has been called the mother hormone. A yearlong study of DHEA at 50 mg daily in males and females age 60 to 70 years failed to show an effect on muscle strength or muscle and fat cross-sectional areas.[16]

Growth hormone and ICG-1 levels decline with aging.[17] Growth hormone increases nitrogen retention, produces weight gain, and increases muscle mass but fails to increase muscle strength. ICF-1, which is predominantly produced in the liver, is under growth hormone regulation. IGF-1 increases protein synthesis but has no effect on satellite cells and muscle repair.

Mechanogrowth factor (MGF) is an alternative splicing variant of IGF-1 that is produced in muscle. MGF levels are increased during mechanical overload, and this increase declines over the life span. In older persons, MGF levels increase with resistance training and growth hormone has no effect on basal levels. However, growth hormone will synergize with resistance training to further increase MGF levels. MGF enhances satellite cell proliferation. Localized MGF transgenic expression sustains hypertrophy and regeneration in senescent skeletal muscle.[18]

Creatine is an amino acid supplement that is essential for muscle function. Creatine is found mainly in meat in the diet. Chrusch et al.[19] demonstrated that in older men creatine supplementation increased lean mass and knee extension/flexion power.

Myostatin is a powerful inhibitor of satellite cells and muscle regeneration. Myostatin gene deletion in a human was associated with a marked increase in muscle mass.[20] Animal studies using antibodies to myostatin have shown muscle hypertrophy. Antibodies that inhibit myostatin have been developed and are entering clinical trials for the treatment of sarcopenia.

Cytokins, such as interleukin-1, interleukin-6, and tumor necrosis factor (TNF) alpha, have been shown to potentially increase the turnover of the atrogin–ubiquitin–proteasome pathway, resulting in loss of muscle mass. Excess cytokines are associated with a decline in handgrip strength, physical performance scores, disability, and death.[21]

The metabolic or insulin resistance syndrome is associated with an increased accumulation of fat in muscle and decreased muscle function. Accumulation of triglycerides in muscle attenuates the orderly phosphorylation of the insulin receptor sulstrate, and thus the ability of the muscle cell to appropriately respond to insulin. With aging there is an increase in mitochondrial deletions, which can lead to an intracellular increase in triglycerides, as the mitochondria can no longer adequately utilize lipids as their energy source.[22] This explains, in part, the decrease in muscle function and increased falls in older diabetics.[23]

Motor neuron nerve units deteriorate with aging. Lack of continuous neuronal electrical impulses results in loss of muscle mass as well as poorly coordinated muscle contraction. There is some evidence that the ciliary neurotrophic factor, which declines with aging, may be responsible for the decreased motor neuron activity associated with aging.

Peripheral vascular disease is a common concomitant of aging. Decreased blood flow to muscles and decreased tissue oxygenation can result in marked muscle atrophy.

Finally, while obvious, it needs to be stressed that the major factor involved in the development of sarcopenia with aging is the lack of physical exercise. Resistance exercise is the centerpiece of the management of sarcopenia. Increasing spontaneous physical activity by getting an older person to leave the house on a daily basis is an important component of the prevention of frailty.

5.2 CACHEXIA

Cachexia involves severe loss of muscle and adipose tissue mass. Cachexia was named from the Greek *Kakos*, meaning bad, and *kexis*, a condition. Cachexia is very common, with over 5 million persons in the U.S. alone suffering from this condition. It is usually associated with anorexia and is associated with illness. It is most commonly, if not universally, associated with a marked excess production of cytokines. Suggested criteria for the diagnosis of cachexia are listed in Table 5.2.

Excessive productions of cytokines, such as TNF alpha and interleukin-6, have multiple effects that lead to the cachexia syndrome[23] (Table 5.3). Cytokines have direct effects on muscle, activating NF-kappa beta, resulting in decreased protein syn-

TABLE 5.2
Suggested Diagnostic Criteria for Cachexia

1. Loss of weight (at least 5%)
2. Body mass index
   <20 in those under 65 years
   <22 in those older than 65 years
3. Albumin < 35 g/l (3.5 g/dl)
4. Low fat-free mass (lowest, 10%)
5. Evidence of cytokine excess, e.g., C-reactive protein

TABLE 5.3
The Role of Cytokines in the Pathogenesis of Cachexia

I. Muscle
   Decreased protein synthesis
   Increased activity of the ubiquitin–proteasome system
   Catabolism
   Decrease NF-kappa beta
II. Liver
   Decreased albumin synthesis
   Decreased lipoprotein lipase activity
   Hyperlipidemia
   Increased acute phase—proteins, e.g., CRP and serum amyloid protein
III. Fat
   Increased lipolysis
   Hypertriglyceridemia
   Increased circulating free fatty acids
IV. Gastrointestinal tract
   Decreased gastric emptying
   Decreased intestinal motility
V. Central nervous system
   Anorexia
   Cognitive dysfunction
   Sickness behavior
VI. Adrenal
   Increased epinephrine
   Increased cortisol

thesis and activation of the ubiquitin–proteasome system leading to muscle catabolism. The available amino acids then are transported to the liver and used to produce acute phase reactants, such as CRP and serum amyloid protein. Cytokines also lead to insulin resistance, thus making increased glucose available for vital organs, such as the brain. Cytokines decrease protein synthesis in the liver and also cause third spacing of albumin into the extravascular space. The latter is the reason for the rapid decline in albumin in sick persons admitted to the hospital. Cytokines produce lipolysis, leading to increased circulating triglycerides and free fatty acids. In the liver, cytokines decrease the activity of lipoprotein lipase, resulting in hyperlipidemia. Cytokines decrease gastric emptying and intestinal motility. Effects of cytokines on the central nervous system include anorexia, memory disturbance, and sickness behavior. Sickness behavior leads to decreased voluntary energy utilization. Cytokine activation of the adrenal medulla leads to increased epinephrine release into the circulation, resulting in an increased resting metabolic rate. The cytokine effect to increase cortisol by activating the hypothalamic (CRF)–pituitary (ACTH)–adrenal axis leads to further muscle protein wasting.

Cachexia occurs in all diseases of major organs, e.g., heart (cardiac cachexia), kidney, chronic obstructive pulmonary disease, multiple infections, and cancer. In these conditions cachexia appears to be an independent predictor of poor outcome. Anker et al.[24] demonstrated that cardiac cachexia (defined as a weight loss of greater than 7.5%) predicted survival independently of peak VO_2, left ventricular ejection fraction, New York Heart Association class, sodium, and age.

In cancer, other factors besides cytokines have been implicated in the pathogenesis of cachexia. These include lipid-mobilizing factor (a zinc $alpha_2$ glycoprotein), proteolysis-inhibiting factor, lactate, increased circulating tryptophan, which leads to anorexia by increasing central nervous system serotonin, ciliary neurotrophic factor, prostaglandins, and zinc deficiency. In addition, depression can play a major role in producing anorexia in these patients; as demonstrated in Figure 5.4, there are numerous possible treatment options for the cancer–anorexia syndrome.

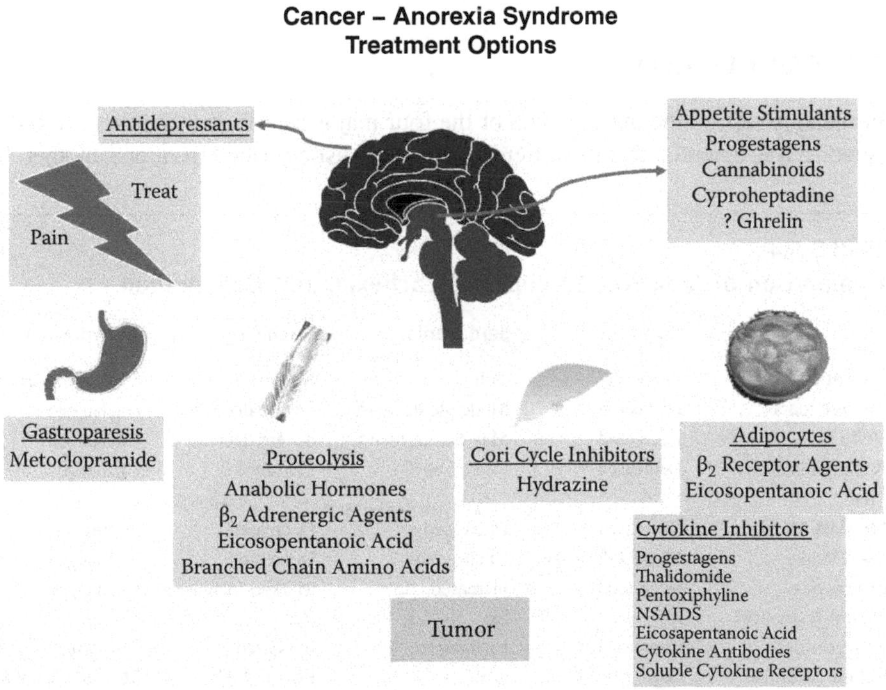

FIGURE 5.4 Treatment options for the cancer–anorexia syndrome.

In renal failure, malnutrition has been divided into two types: type I, or starvation type, which is reversed by adequate dialysis and nutritional support, and type II, which is considered a cachectic type associated with elevated resting energy metabolism and an increased oxidation stress and is resistant to increased dialysis and nutritional support.[25] Type II malnutrition in renal failure is associated with the MIA syndrome. In this syndrome, malnutrition is associated with inflammation and accelerated atherosclerosis. Besides cytokines, causes of malnutrition in renal failure patients include inadequate dialysis, dietary restrictions, depression, zinc deficiency, medications, metabolic acidosis, insulin resistance, and nutrient losses during peritoneal dialysis.

AIDS is the classical cachexia syndrome of the modern age.[23] Wasting syndrome in AIDS is highly predictive of death. In seniors, there has been a marked increase in AIDS in the U.S. from 1981–1987, when only 1413 older persons had AIDS, to 2000, when 8373 persons had AIDS. In older persons the most common presentations of AIDS are wasting syndrome and pneumocystes pneumonia. In AIDS wasting, besides cytokine malabsorption and diarrhea, testosterone deficiency and hyperlactemia associated with nucleoside analog reverse transcrystase inhibitors play a role in its pathogenesis.

At present the drugs most utilized to treat cachexia include megestrol acetate, dronabinol, eicosapentanoic acid, thalidomide and its newer derivatives, and corticosteroids. The nanocrystal form of megestrol acetate can be absorbed better in the absence of food, making it an atheoretically useful drug for cachectic/anorectic patients. Megestrol is a "bastard" drug with a combination of progestational, corticosteroid, and anabolic properties. It is more effective in females.

5.3 CONCLUSION

In the approach to the management of the four major causes of weight loss in older persons, it is essential that the different forms are distinguished from one another. In

TABLE 5.4
Comparison of Anorexia, Sarcopenia, Cachexia, and Dehydration

	Anorexia	Sarcopenia	Cachexia	Dehydration
Weight loss	Moderate	Mild	Severe	Mild to moderate
Fat-free mass	Decreased	Moderate decrease	Severe decrease	Unchanged
Body fat	Decreased	May be increased	Severe decrease	Unchanged
Resting metabolic rate	Decreased	Decreased	Increased	Unchanged
Physical activity	Decreased	Decreased	Decreased	Decreased
Food intake	Marked decrease	Unchanged	Decreased	Unchanged
Proteolysis	Decreased	Increased	Marked increase	Unchanged
Insulin resistance	No	No	Yes	No
Triglycerides	Decreased	Unchanged	Increased	Decreased
Serum creatinine	Low	Low	Low to high	May be increased
Blood urea nitrogen	Low	Low	Low to high	Elevated
Cytokines	Minimal change	Mild increase	Marked increase	Unchanged

this chapter, two of these causes—sarcopenia and cachexia—have been discussed in detail. Table 5.4 compares the major features of the four common causes of weight loss in older persons. Other causes for weight loss in older persons include malabsorption and increased metabolism, e.g., hyperthyroidism and pheochromocytoma.

REFERENCES

1. Morley, J.E., Baumgarter, R.N., Roubenoff, R., et al., Sarcopenia, *J. Lab. Clin. Med.*, 137, 231, 2001.
2. Janssen, I., Baumgartner, R.N., Ross, R., et al., Skeletal muscle cutpoints associated with elevated physical disability risk in older men and women, *Am. J. Epidemiol.*, 159, 413, 2004.
3. Janssen, I., Influence of sarcopenia on the development of physical disability: the Cardiovascular Health Study, *J. Am. Geriatr. Soc.*, 54, 56, 2006.
4. Baumgartner, R.N., Wayne, S.J., Waters, D.L., et al., Sarcopenic obesity predicts instrumental activities of daily living disability in the elderly, *Obes. Res.*, 12, 1995, 2004.
5. Sayer, A.A., Syddall, H.E., Gilbody, H.J., et al., Does sarcopenia originate in early life? Findings from the Hertfordshire Cohort Study, *J. Gerontol. A Biol. Sci. Med. Sci.*, 59, M930, 2004.
6. Baumgartner, R.N., Waters, D.L., Gallagher, D., et al., Predictors of skeletal muscle mass in elderly men and women, *Mech. Ageing Dev.*, 107, 123, 1999.
7. Morley, J.E., Kaiser, F.E., Perry, H.M., 3rd, et al., Longitudinal changes in testosterone, luteinizing hormone, and follicle-stimulating hormone in healthy older men, *Metabolism*, 46, 410, 1997.
8. Sih, R., Morley, J.E., Kaiser, F.E., et al., Testosterone replacement in older hypogonadal men: a 12-month randomized controlled trial, *J. Clin. Endocrinol. Metab.*, 82, 1661, 1997.
9. Wittert, G.A., Chapman, I.M., Haren, M.T., et al., Oral testosterone supplementation increases muscle and decreases fat mass in healthy elderly males with low-normal gonadal status, *J. Gerontol. A Biol. Sci. Med. Sci.*, 58, 618, 2003.
10. Bhassin, S., Woodhouse, L., Casaburi, R., et al., Older men are as responsive as young men to the anabolic effects of graded doses of testosterone on the skeletal muscle, *J. Clin. Endocrinol. Metab.*, 90, 678, 2005.
11. Perry, H.M., 3rd, Horowitz, M., Morley, J.E., et al., Longitudinal changes in serum 25-hydroxyvitamin D in older people, *Metabolism*, 48, 1028, 1999.
12. Zamboni, M., Zoico, E., Tosoni, P., et al., Relation between vitamin D, physical performance, and disability in elderly persons, *J. Gerontol. A Biol. Sci. Med. Sci.*, 57, M7, 2002.
13. Visser, M., Deeg, D.J., and Lips, P., Low vitamin D and high parathyroid hormone levels as determinants of loss of muscle strength and muscle mass (sarcopenia): the Longitudinal Aging Study Amsterdam, *Clin. Endocrinol. Metab.*, 88, 5766, 2003.
14. Flicker, L., Mead, K., MacInnis, R.J., et al., Serum vitamin D and falls in older women in residential care in Australia, *J. Am. Geriatr. Soc.*, 51, 1533, 2003.
15. Latham, N.K., Anderson, C.S., and Reid, I.R., Effects of vitamin D supplementation on strength, physical performance, and falls in older persons: a systematic review, *J. Am Geriatr. Soc.*, 51, 1219, 2003.
16. Percheron, G., Hogrel, J.Y., Denot-Ledunois, S., et al., Effect of 1-year oral administration of dehydroepiandrosterone to 60- to 80-year-old individuals on muscle function and cross-sectional area: a double-blind placebo-controlled trial, *Arch. Int. Med.*, 133, 720, 2003.

17. Morley, J., Hormones and the aging process, *J. Am. Geriatr. Soc.*, 51, S333, 2003.
18. Musaro, A., McCullagh, K., Paul, A., et al., Localized Igf-1 transgene expression sustains hypertrophy and regeneration in senescent skeletal muscle, *Nat Genet.*, 27, 195, 2001.
19. Chrusch, M.J., Chilibeck, P.D., Chad, K.E., et al., Creatine supplementation combined with resistance training in older men, *Med. Sci. Sports Exerc.*, 33, 2111, 2001.
20. McNally, E.M., Powerful genes: myostatin regulation of human muscle mass, *N. Engl. J. Med.*, 360, 2642, 2004.
21. Morley, J.E. and Baumgartner, R.N., Cytokine-related aging process, *J. Gerontol. A Biol. Sci. Med. Sci.*, 59, M924, 2004.
22. Petersen, K.F., Befroy, D., Dufour, S., et al., Mitochondrial dysfunction in the elderly: possible role in insulin resistance, *Science*, 300, 1140, 2003.
23. Morley, J.E., Thomas, D.R., and Wilson, M.M., Cachexia: pathophysiology and clinical relevance, *Am. J. Clin. Nutr.*, 83, 735, 2006.
24. Anker, S.D., Ponikowski, P., Varney, S., et al., Wasting as independent risk factor for mortality in chronic heart failure, *Lancet*, 349, 1050, 1997.
25. Dombros, N.V., Pathogenesis and management of malnutrition in chronic peritoneal dialysis patients, *Nephrol. Dial. Transplant*, 16, 111, 2001.

6 Immunity and Nutrition

Chantri Trinh, M.D.

CONTENTS

According to the U.S. Census Bureau, there were 31 million of the population age 65 and older in 1990, and by the year 2050, there will be about 80 million of this population. For the oldest old population (>85 years), that would be a five-fold increase. Parallel to this drastic rise in the elderly population is the significant increase in health care expenses due to the increased risk of infection, cancer, and other diseases in the aged group. This population is also at greater risk of contracting more severe and longer-lasting infections, particularly respiratory infections. Moreover, they are more prone to develop invasive *Staphylococcus aureus* infections[1] and waning immunity to tetanus,[2] thereby increasing their susceptibility to diphtheria.[3] Furthermore, the aged population is known to have poor responses to influenza vaccination[4,5] and also has a higher incidence of infections and sepsis after a traumatic injury than their younger counterparts.[6] Despite increased health care expenses spent in research development and clinical intervention, death due to cancer and infection remains significant. In the population 65 years and older, death due to cancer is the second most common, while that due to influenza or pneumonia stays the fifth most common cause (Table 6.1). An age-related decline in immunity has been implicated as the cause for these clinical cases. This has been extensively studied over the past few decades with the common conclusion of dysfunction of the cell-mediated immunity and impaired delayed hypersensitivity reaction to antigens.

Dietary intake plays a major role in a person's health and disease. Elderly persons are particularly at risk of inadequate intake due to various factors, i.e., medical diseases, poor taste, physical disability, chewing and swallowing problems, living condition, polypharmacy, and limited income. Based on the National Health and Nutrition Examination Survey (NHANES) III data evaluating the impact of diet on health and diseases, elderly people were found to have total energy intake below the recommended level. Older age and lower energy intake have been shown to be independent risk factors for nosocomial infections.[7] Furthermore, nutrition, measured by serum albumin, has been known to be a major contributing factor in mortality and morbidity outcomes in hospitalized elderly,[8–10] in recovering patients after discharge,[9]

TABLE 6.1
Leading Causes of Death among Those Age 65 and Older (Year 2002)

Leading Causes	Number	Percentage of Total Deaths
1. Diseases of the heart	576,301	31.8
2. Malignant neoplasms	391,001	21.6
3. Cerebrovascular diseases	143,293	7.9
4. Chronic lower respiratory diseases	108,313	6.0
5. Influenza and pneumonia	58,826	3.2
6. Alzheimer's disease	58,289	3.2
7. Diabetes	54,715	3.0

Source: U.S. National Center for Health Statistics, *Vital Statistics of the United States*, annual; *National Vital Statistics Report*, Vol. 53, No. 17, March 7, 2005.

as well as in apparently healthy community-dwelling elderly.[11,12] Evident in different parts of the world where areas were ravaged by famine, the mortality rate rises significantly in the very young and old age groups due mainly to dysentery/diarrheal diseases (Ireland's Great Famine, 1840s), malaria (famine in tropical countries), and AIDS (areas of famine in Africa). This provides additional evidence of the important impact of nutritional status on the body's immune defense. Due to multiple medical comorbidities, poor nutritional status, frailty, and a weakened immune system, the elderly are more likely to harbor frequent infections with higher degree of severity than the younger population. These infections are common and include pneumonia, influenza, urinary tract infections, skin and soft tissue infections, diverticulitis, and zoster (shingles).[13]

This chapter will first provide a general review of the immune system and its components. Then it will address the changes in the immune system associated with the aging body, common features of the immune components in healthy elderly vs. frail and undernutrition individuals, and the possible mechanisms, and will examine the clinical evidence of nutritional intervention and supplementation to improve immune response.

6.1 OVERVIEW OF THE IMMUNE SYSTEM

The immune system is designed to protect the body from foreign organisms. It discriminates self from nonself and eliminates foreign invasion. It is crucial for survival of the host body. Not only does the immune system protect its host from external factors, but it also fends against internal aberrations that give rise to cancer and autoimmune diseases. There are two levels of response against external threat, an **innate system (natural immunity)** and an **adaptive system (acquired immunity)**. Innate immunity starts at birth and is **nonspecific**. This includes the natural barrier of the body, the skin, and the alternative complement system, acute-phase proteins, natural killer cells, and cytokines. Cells of the innate system recognize pathogen molecular motifs that are highly conserved among many microbes (i.e., bacterial endotoxin) and kill the pathogens directly or trigger a series of events and activate the adaptive system. The adaptive system involves an intricate network of exposure to foreign material (immunologic priming), immunologic memory specific for the antigen, activation of lymphocytes, and elimination of the antigen. There are two arms of the adaptive immune system: clearance of foreign particles via direct killing by cytotoxic T lymphocytes **(cellular immunity)** and removal of antigens via the chain of events mediated by antibodies produced by B lymphocytes **(humoral immunity)**.

6.2 ORGANS AND CELLS OF THE IMMUNE SYSTEM

The **bone marrow** gives rise to almost all cells of the immune system through differentiation of pluripotent stem cells into lymphocytes, granulocytes, monocytes, erythrocytes, and megakaryocytes. B lymphocytes undergo early maturation in the bone marrow, whereas T lymphocytes are produced and differentiate in the **thymus**.

The bone marrow and the thymus are primary lymphoid organs. Secondary lymphoid organs include the lymph nodes, spleen, and gut-associated lymphoid tissue. These organs are interconnected by blood and lymphatic vessels. **Lymph nodes** form an intricate network to defend the body against infection locally and prevent spread of infection and contain mostly B and T lymphocytes. The spleen is but a giant lymph node. It filters and processes the antigens. **Gut-associated lymphoid tissues** include the tonsils, Peyer's patches of the small intestine, and appendix. They function like the spleen and the lymph nodes.

Monocytes and **macrophages** are derived from blood monocytes. They function to phagocytize the antigen, then process and present the antigen to T lymphocytes. Activated macrophages secrete proteolytic enzymes, oxygen radicals, cytokines (interleukin (IL) 1, IL-6, IL-8), tumor necrosis factor (TNF), and others.

Dendritic cells are bone-marrow-derived antigen-presenting cells (APCs) such as Langerhans' cells and oligodendrocytes. These cells defend the body's integrity at the skin, respiratory, and gastrointestinal (GI) levels and transport the antigen to regional lymphoid tissues. When bound to antigens, the dendritic cells release cytokines to recruit other cells of the innate system and T and B cells of the adaptive system.

Lymphocytes play a major role in the adaptive immunity. Their function is specific. They recognize specific antigen and process that for immunologic memory. About 75% of the circulating blood lymphocytes are T lymphocytes (Table 6.2) and 10 to 15% are B lymphocytes. The remaining lymphocytes are referred to as null cells. B and T lymphocytes are distinguishable only by flow cytometry and immunophenotyping through recognition of cell surface markers and clusters of differentiation (CD markers).

Null cells include different cell types, one of which is the **natural killer (NK) cells**. They have a membrane receptor for the immunoglobulin G (IgG) molecule and act to destroy the antibody-coated foreign organism or cell **(antibody-dependent**

TABLE 6.2
T Cell Classes and Functions

CD8+ T cells	Cytotoxic; lysis of virus-infected or foreign cells
CD4+ T cells	Primary regulatory cells of T and B cells and monocyte function by producing cytokines and by direct cell contact
T_H1-type (helper T cells)	Subclass of CD4 cells; secrete IL-2, IFN-*r*, IL-3, TNF-α, GM-CSF, and TNF-β; promote production of opsonizing antibodies and induction of cytotoxic T cells and macrophage activation; mediate delayed hypersensitivity responses (HIV or *M. tuberculosis*)
T_H2-type (helper T cells)	Subclass of CD4 cells; secrete IL-3, IL-4, IL-5, IL-6, IL-10, and IL-13; help to regulate humoral immunity and isotype switching; help B cell with specific Ig production; help to regulate proinflammatory responses mediated by T_H1 cells
CD4+ and CD8+ T regulatory cells	Control immune responses; produce large amount of IL-10; can suppress T and B cell responses; loss of these cells gives rise to organ-specific autoimmune disease in mice

Notes: IFN-*r*: interferon gamma; GM-CSF: granulocyte-macrophage colony stimulating factor; HIV: human immunodeficiency virus; Ig: immunoglobulin; T_H1: T-helper 1 subset.

cell-mediated cytotoxicity). Alternatively, NK cells can destroy virus-infected cells, transplanted foreign cells, or tumor cells without antibody coating. Other functions include nonspecific recognition of antigens without immunologic memory and regulation of cytokines.

Polymorphonuclear leukocytes (neutrophils) are granulocytes derived from the bone marrow. They contain cytoplasmic granules filled with degradative enzymes and superoxide radicals in acidic medium. They clear the foreign particles and organisms by phagocytosis and process them through the reticuloendothelial system.

Eosinophils share many functions with neutrophils but are much less efficient at phagocytosis. They often respond to inflammation and are key cytotoxic effector cells in the defense against parasites. However, they can cause potential damage and exacerbate a hyperresponsiveness of the immune system, as in the hypereosinophilic syndromes, causing major organ system dysfunction of the heart, central nervous system, kidneys, lungs, gastrointestinal tract, and skin.

Basophils and **mast cells** are central to both immediate and late-phase allergic responses. They release many potent mediators (e.g., IL-4) that affect the vasculature and mediate hypersensitivity responses.

6.3 INFLAMMATORY MEDIATORS

Inflammatory mediators include histamine, leukotrienes, prostaglandins, platelet-activating factor, complement proteins, and cytokines, among others. They act to modulate, mediate, or activate a chain of immunologic response that results in elimination of the foreign particle or organism. In addition to activating cells of the immune system, some **cytokines** function as growth factors and induce immunoglobulin synthesis and acute-phase reactants. A subset of T cells was classified based on the function of cytokines secreted by these T cells into the T_H2 (humoral immune response) or T_H1 (cell-mediated immune response) class (Table 6.3).

6.4 HYPERSENSITIVITY IMMUNE RESPONSES

Type I is an anaphylactic or immediate hypersensitivity reaction that happens after the binding of a previously exposed antigen to its specific IgE antibodies, and this combination, once bound to the surface of a mast cell or basophil, triggers the release of inflammatory mediators. The clinical manifestations are usually seen within 12 hours of exposure. Examples include anaphylactic shock, allergic rhinitis, allergic asthma, and allergic drug reactions.

Type II hypersensitivity reactions are cytotoxic and involve IgG or IgM recognition of antigen bound to the cell membrane. Upon antibody–antigen binding, the complement cascade is activated, resulting in destruction of the antigen-labeled cell. Examples of this type are immune hemolytic anemia and Rh hemolytic disease of the newborn.

Type III reactions are immune complex mediated. Immune complexes (ICs) are formed from antibody–antigen binding. These are then cleared from the circulation by the phagocytic system. Deposition of ICs in the vascular endothelium can cause

TABLE 6.3
Cytokines and Functions

Cytokine	Cell Source	Biologic Activity	Clinical Applications
IL-1α, IL-1β	Monocytes/macrophages, B cells, fibroblasts, thymic epithelium, endothelial and epithelial cells	Upregulates adhesion molecule expression and hepatic acute-phase protein production; chemotactic for neutrophil and macrophage; modulates shock/fever reaction and hematopoiesis	Pyrogenic; anticytokine therapy with NSAIDS; COX-I or COX-II inhibitors, steroids, and acetaminophen are used to treat fever; inflammatory arthritis; IL-1 receptor antagonist is used to treat rheumatoid arthritis (RA)
IL-2	T cells	Regulates T cell and NK cell activation and proliferation and B cell growth; enhances monocyte/macrophage cytotoxicity	Recombinant IL-2 used to treat renal cell cancer and melanoma; IL-2 receptor antibody is used as immunosuppressant therapy after renal transplant to prevent acute rejection
IL-3	T cells, NK cells, mast cells	Stimulates hematopoetic progenitors	
IL-4	T cells, mast cells, basophils, bone marrow	Stimulates T_H2 helper T cell differentiation and proliferation; induces B cells to produce IgG4 and IgE; modulates the inflammatory response	
IL-5	T cells, eosinophils, mast cells	Stimulates eosinophil functions and proliferation; activates eosinophils and B cell differentiation; chemoattractant for eosinophils	
IL-6	Similar source as IL-1	Proinflammatory and anti-inflammatory; induction of acute-phase protein production; growth factor for T and B cells, myeloma cells, and osteoclast growth and activation	Pyrogenic (proinflammatory function); IL-6 antagonist may have additional benefit in combination with methotrexate for treatment of RA
IL-7	Bone marrow, thymic epithelial cells	Differentiation and activation of T and NK cells	
IL-8	Similar source as IL-1	Chemoattractant for T cells, neutrophils, and monocytes; stimulates angiogenesis	

IL-10	T and B cells, monocytes, and macrophages	Inhibits cytokine synthesis in activated T_H1 helper T cells, monocytes, and NK cells; inhibits NK cell function; inhibits differentiation of T_H1 helper T cells; stimulates mast cell and B cell activation and differentiation	IL-10 agonists developed to treat RA but no significant clinical benefit
IFN-α, IFN-β	All cells	Antiviral activity; stimulate T cell, macrophage, and NK cells; direct antitumor effects; upregulate MHC class I antigen expression; have therapeutic use in viral and autoimmune diseases	Treatment of chronic hepatitis B, C, and D by IFN-α alone or in combination with ribavirin; IFN-β in treatment of chronic hepatitis C and in combination with ribavirin
IFN-γ	T cells, NK cells	Activates macrophages and others (fibroblasts, endothelial cells, parenchymal cells); induces differentiation of CD4+ T cells into T_H1 helper T cells; inhibits TH2 cell proliferation[14]	Prophylactic use in patients with chronic granulomatous disease; adjunctive therapy for visceral and cutaneous leishmaniasis; disseminated *Mycobacterium avium* complex infection and leprosy
TNF-α	Macrophages, mast cells, NK cells	Mediates sepsis/fever/shock, capillary leak syndrome, acute-phase protein synthesis, and proinflammatory cytokine production	Induces anorexia and wasting effects; pyrogenic; anti-TNF is used to treat Crohn's, ulcerative colitis, and rheumatoid arthritis
G-CSF	Monocytes/macrophages, endothelial cells, and fibroblasts	Stimulates myelopoiesis; increases number of cell divisions and shortens bone marrow transit time; enhances function and life span of mature neutrophils; immunomodulatory for macrophages and lymphocytes[15,16]	Human recombinant G-CSF used during chemotherapy or to treat prophylax neutropenia in patients receiving chemotherapy; used in stem cell transplant, HIV, diabetes, trauma and sepsis, and fungal infections
GM-CSF	T cells, monocytes, macrophages, fibroblasts, endothelial cells, and smooth muscle cells	Stimulates progenitor cells to differentiate into neutrophils, eosinophils, and monocytes; decreases neutrophil apoptosis and enhances neutrophil function[15,17]	Human recombinant GM-CSF used for patients on myeloablative chemotherapy, patients with AML, Hodgkin's and non-Hodgkin's lymphomas, and HIV, and patients undergoing stem cell transplantation

tissue injury by IC-mediated immune response involving complement activation, mobilization of leukocytes, phagocytosis, and tissue injury. Clinical examples are serum sickness and lupus nephritis.

Type IV reactions are also called delayed hypersensitivity reactions. Cellular response to antigen is seen 48 to 72 hours after exposure. This reaction is similar to type I, but the time to clinical response is delayed. It is mediated by T cells, interferon (IFN)-*r*, IL-2, TNF-α-secreting T_H1-type T cells, and macrophages. With exposure to the antigen, local immune response causes an upregulation of endothelial cell adhesion molecules to promote lymphocyte migration to the site. The antigen is processed by dendritic cells and then presented to CD4+ T cells. Cytokines are released by the APCs and induce a T_H1 response. T_H1 cells promote production of opsonizing antibodies and induce cytotoxic T cells and macrophage activation. Activated macrophages fuse to form multinucleated giant cell infiltrate called granulomatous inflammation. Examples of this type of reaction are fungal infections (histoplasmosis), mycobacterial infections (tuberculosis (TB), leprosy), and chlamydial infections (lymphogranuloma venereum).

6.5 IMMUNOSENESCENCE: THE AGING IMMUNE RESPONSE

Older age has been associated with an increase in infection rate and mortality due to infections, particularly influenza, pneumonia, urinary tract infections, skin infections, tetanus, and reactivation of latent infections such as herpes zoster and tuberculosis. For patients suffering from influenza, the mortality rate showed little change among those age 65 to 84 years but increased among those 85 years and older in the state of Wisconsin from 1980 to 2003.[18] During flu seasons, a mortality rate as high as 90% can occur in the elderly,[19] and nursing home patients are at increased risk of contracting the disease and have a high mortality rate from pneumonia despite appropriate interventions of vaccination, amantadine administration, and infection control measures.[20] Aging is also associated with an increase in the prevalence of diseases related to impaired or dysregulated immune systems, for example, increased incidence of cancer with age, increased monoclonal immunoglobulins with age and suboptimal health status,[21] and increased autoantibody levels in an apparent healthy study group age 95 and older.[22] While some level of immune component decreases with aging, others increase with aging, such as IL-6.[23] This leads to a concept of age-related immune dysfunction. However, some other causes of immune deficiency in the elderly other than immunosenescence include comorbid illness, medication use, depression, malnutrition, and sedentary lifestyle.[24]

Immunosenescence has been a topic of investigation for many decades and has gathered much interest in recent years since nutrition was examined for a possible link to decline in immune response in the elderly. It is well noted that older patients do not manifest as vigorous an immune response as their younger counterparts, especially in the setting of infections and sepsis. Many cardinal signs of immune response were absent in the infected elderly, for example, fever and leukocytosis. Many studies have based their data from apparently healthy elderly using the

TABLE 6.4
Criteria for Very Healthy Elderly

SENIEUR criteria[25] (apparently healthy)	1.	In good health
	2.	No ongoing, developing, or degenerative diseases
	3.	Normal adult values for laboratory variables (leukocytes with differentials, blood glucose, SGOT, SGPT, urinalysis for protein, glucose sediment)
	4.	No drugs acting on the immune system
Additional criteria for the very healthy[26]	1.	No disease in the past 5 years
	2.	No motor skill difficulties
	3.	Normal physical activity: >4-km walk/day
	4.	No drug treatment for cardiac, neurological, or psychotropic diseases (including depression)
	5.	Normal mental status (mini mental status of Folstein ≥ 28/30)
	6.	Serum albumin ≥ 3.9 g/dl
	7.	No low values for trace elements (Zn and Se) or vitamins (B_6, folate, B_{12}, A, and C)

SENIEUR protocol of the European Community's Concerted Action Program on Ageing (EURAGE). This protocol gives the selection criteria for study subjects who fit the apparently healthy elderly[25] (Table 6.4) and designates young as 25 to 34 years old and aged as 65 years and above. Other investigators considered that the SENIEUR protocol was not precise enough to exclude underlying infection or inflammatory diseases and clinically hidden nutritional deficiencies. Lesourd et al. added new exclusion criteria to select for the very healthy elderly[26] (Table 6.4). With that in mind, the findings discussed below are from the very healthy and the apparently healthy elderly.

6.5.1 Cell-Mediated Immunity: Changes with Aging

Cell-mediated immunity responses seem to be impaired with aging. This is evident in impaired primary immunization with T-cell-dependent antigens such as tetanus toxoid and delayed hypersensitivity responses to tuberculin skin test. As discussed earlier, findings of immune impairment with aging may have contradicting results due to uncertainties of study subjects' underlying micronutrient deficiencies and underlying inflammatory diseases not yet identifiable. Below are discussions of general concensus on immune aging. Whenever strict criteria were applied to select a very healthy elderly population, the results could be subject to selection bias of choosing the best cohort with the possible best genetic pool.

6.5.1.1 Decrease in New T Lymphocyte Generation

Stem cells give rise to many cells of the immune system. The ability of stem cells to undergo clonal differentiation decreases with age. T cells are generated from hematopoietic stem cells in the bone marrow. These precursor T cells then migrate to the thymus for differentiation and maturation. Mature T cells (CD3+) then migrate from the thymus to the periphery. Only about 5% of the mature T cells make it to the periphery under optimal conditions.[27] Thymus involution starts early in life and by age 60 it is completed. This is a process where the thymus undergoes a progressive reduction in size, resulting in loss of thymic epithelial cells and decrease in new T cell production. And by age 60, new T lymphocyte generation is almost absent.[26] Thymus tissue becomes atrophic and is then replaced by fat. This involution results in decreased numbers of circulating naive T cells, impaired cell-mediated immunity, and a higher number of immature T cells (CD2+CD4–CD8–). It has been suggested by Lesourd et al.[28] that these immature T cells are not produced in the thymus but in another primary immune organ, probably the liver, where it has been shown in aged mice as another lymphoid organ.

6.5.1.2 Changes in Peripheral Blood Lymphocytes

Total lymphocyte number in peripheral blood decreases with age.[29] This change is observed in the apparent healthy elderly 65 years and older (SENIEUR criteria) and in the oldest old (85 years and older) of the very carefully selected healthy elderly without any micronutrient deficiency (SENIEUR criteria with strict exclusions).[28,30–32] Furthermore, there is a shift in the B cell subset from antibody production (B2 cells) in response to foreign antigen to increase in autoantibody production (B1 cells). This age-associated increase in B1 lymphocyte number and activity contributes to the increased serum concentration of autobodies seen in the aging population.[33]

6.5.1.3 Changes in T Cell Subsets and Functions

Aged individuals are found to have reversal shifts of number and function in T cell subsets. There are fewer mature T cells (CD3+) and more immature T cells (CD2+CD3–)[29] due to atrophic thymus. There is a decrease in the CD8+ subset, but the CD4+ subset remains unchanged in the very healthy elderly. The observed changes are minor and may not be able to explain any clinical state of immunodeficiency. Natural killer cells (CD57+) also seem to increase with age and may have decreased cytotoxicity and decreased response to IL-2 stimulation.[34,35] The changes in NK cell activity may have contributed to longer-lasting infections and lower defense against tumor cells by the elderly.

Another important change in T cell subset involves the switching of naïve (CD45RA) T cells (before antigen recognition) to memory (CD45RO) lymphocytes (after antigen contact). This change is more pronounced early in life until age 30 and continues into later years but with a much lower rate.[36] This is of immunologic importance since memory T cells are poor IL-2 secretors and have poor proliferative capacity.[37]

In addition, aging has been associated with an imbalance of $T_H1:T_H2$ function (decreased or unchanged in T_H1 function and an enhanced T_H2 function). T cell helper functions are assessed by the change in quantity of cytokines produced. T_H1 cells produce IL-2, IL-12, and IFN-γ, resulting in T cell proliferation and macrophage activation, features of cell-mediated immunity. In contrast, T_H2 cells produce IL-4, IL-5, IL-6, and IL-10, cytokines that augment antibody responses. Previous studies have shown that interleukin-2 secretion, a T_H1 function, is decreased in the apparent healthy elderly, but recent studies show that such decline is not significant in the very healthy group except the oldest olds.[26,38–40] Other cytokines studied to assess T_H1 function include interferon and IL-12. Interferon was reported as decreased or unchanged in the very healthy elderly,[41,42] and IL-12 release was found to be similar to young adult values.[43] These findings suggest that T_H1 function does not decline with age in the very healthy elderly, only in the very old population. And the observed decreased T_H1 function in the apparent healthy elderly reported in earlier studies might in fact be due to diseases or nutritional deficiencies.

Interleukin-6 secretion, a function of T_H2 subset, was found to be increased in both the apparent healthy[23,44,45] and the very healthy elderly.[32] The increase in IL-6 starts in the middle age (36 to 59 years) and is more pronounced in the very old (>85 years) than in the young old (75 to 84 years) and has been linked to an increased mortality rate in the elderly.[46] From the contradicting findings in the population study based on the SENIEUR protocol and the strict SENIEUR criteria, it can be concluded that most of what had been regarded as age-related immune changes may in fact be the consequence of subclinical diseases or nutritional deficiencies that have been previously overlooked. It also suggests the importance of micro- and macronutrients on function of the immune system when more selective criteria were used to exclude vitamin and mineral deficiencies in the study subjects. The decline in T_H1 function occurs only in the oldest olds but not in the healthy young elderly. The borderline disequilibrium in T_H1:T_H2 function results in decreased CD8+ cytotoxic T cell maturation and activation (T_H1 function). However, CD4+ subset seems to be unchanged in the elderly.[47,32]

Aging is also associated with an increase in CD28– T cells. The CD28 molecule is expressed constitutively on T cells and its signal transduction results in IL-2 production. This molecule is expressed on more than 99% of human T cells at birth (CD28+ T cells). With aging, the CD28– T cells progressively increase, particularly within the CD8 T cell subset. This deficiency manifests as poor proliferative capacity to signaling, shorter telomeres, and resistance to superantigen apoptosis. The increase in CD28– T cells correlates with reduced antibody response to vaccination, increased mortality in elderly person 80 years and older, and increased osteoporotic fractures in the elderly.[48,49]

6.5.2 Anergy and Delayed Cutaneous Hypersensitivity Reaction

Type IV hypersensitivity reaction measured by skin reaction to antigens was found to be reduced in the independent-living healthy elderly compared to young controls[50] when a multitest was performed with seven antigens. Anergy, defined as a lack of response greater than 5 mm of induration when read at 48 hours to standard antigens, is found more frequently in healthy elderly than in younger controls.[51] The delayed cutaneous hypersensitivity (DCH) reaction is mediated by T_H1 response. T cells sensitized by prior infection are recruited to the skin site where the antigen was deposited and release cytokines. These cytokines induce induration by local inflammatory reaction, including vasodilatation, edema, fibrin deposition, and further recruitment of other inflammatory cells to the area.[52] Anergy or decreased response of the DCH reaction is due to impairment in cell-mediated immune system, namely, changes in the T_H1 subset and functions, cytokines produced, and changes in inflammatory cells as described. It was believed that anergy to skin test is common in the elderly, but was found unlikely when five or more antigens were used.[53]

6.5.3 Humoral Immunity: Changes with Aging

6.5.3.1 B Lymphocytes

There is impaired production of naïve B cells in the bone marrow, but B cell number does not decrease with aging. This is due to peripheral production and self-renewal at the lymph nodes and spleen. However, this production is under strict regulation and is compromised by other processes, for example, medications, infections, and chronic illnesses. Aging is associated with changes in B cell subsets with a shift from antibody production specific to antigens from foreign to autologous (decreased antibody response to vaccines but higher level of autoantibodies found in aged individuals). Aging is also associated with increased B clonal expressions, giving rise to monoclonal immunoglobulins and B cell neoplasms (multiple myeloma, monoclonal gammopathy).[33,54]

6.5.3.2 Immunoglobulin (Ig) Levels

Although some study reported no difference in the Ig level when comparing the very old and centenarians to young normal people,[55,56] the general concensus was that immunoglobulin serum levels in aged individuals seem to rise with age. The increase was due mainly to serum IgG and IgA. The IgA increase in both serum and secretions of elderly individuals is due to the IgA1 subclass, while IgA2 is significantly decreased.[57] Since IgA2 antibodies are produced in the mucosal defense against pathogens, the decrease in production of IgA2 may contribute to the high susceptibility and incidence of pulmonary infection in this age group. Among the IgG subclasses, there is a significant increase in IgG 1, 2, and 3 subclasses and no change in IgG4.[58,59] Oligoclonal Ig was also found in the healthy centenarian subpopulation.[58,60]

6.5.3.3 Antibody Response

Antibody production in response to antigen or vaccination is reduced. The affinity and specificity of the secreted antibody are also impaired, leading to less adapted antibody responses.[26] B cells from older individuals show impaired activation and proliferation that may also be related to changes in stimulatory molecules. Both the primary and secondary antibody responses to vaccination are impaired, and to a greater extent, especially when the responses involve T cell activation. Based on the data in the NHANES III study, immunity to tetanus declines starting at age 40 and continues until only 20% of those age 80 and over are immune to tetanus.[3] A quantitative and qualitative study of primary antibody response to tetanus toxoid was done in healthy aged subjects who had not been vaccinated. There was a lack of antibody response in general, and in those that mounted an antibody response, the level was lower than in young healthy volunteers, even after a booster dose. Response rate significantly improved only in those receiving the booster dose enhanced with thymostimulin administration.[61] Baseline diphtheria antibody levels were found to be significantly lower in older adults than in younger individuals, and among the elderly with detectable diphtheria antibodies, the higher the level, the higher the response to conjugated pneumococcal polysaccharide vaccine.[62] A quantitative review of antibody response to influenza vaccine in groups of elderly vs. younger adults shows a considerably lower antibody response in the elderly group (Centers of Disease Control and Prevention (CDC) estimates of clinical efficacy of 70 to 90% in young adults vs. 17 to 53% in the elderly).[63,64] When healthy elderly subjects who were vaccinated yearly with influenza vaccine were compared to young subjects without previous history of vaccination, the seroconversion rate was significantly higher in the younger group and much less in the elderly group, even after booster immunization.[65] The reason could be due to a defect in antigen presentation or defective T–B cell interaction, as demonstrated by defective IL-2 production by helper T cells in response to antigenic stimulation (influenza vaccine)[66] and an increase in CD28– T cells with aging, resulting in decreased IL-2 production.[48,49]

6.5.4 Increased Autoantibody Production

As mentioned earlier, autoimmunity was presumed to arise from changes in B cell repertoire with age, i.e., an increase in the B1 lymphocyte subset, resulting in an increased level of autoantibodies in the elderly,[33] for example, pernicious anemia. Another theory suggests that memory B cells accumulated over time and reactivated later in life (recall memory) when reexposed to an antigen. This induces an autoimmune memory response through molecular mimicry, leading to production of autoantibodies. This concept is known as immune risk phenotype and is influenced by changes in T cell subset and functions, the type of cytokines produced, defective immune surveillance, and self-regulation and tolerance.[67,68]

6.5.5 Innate Immune Cells

The number of blood monocytes is similar in both elderly and young subjects, but there is evidence of a significant decrease of macrophage precursors as well as a number of macrophages in the bone marrow of elderly subjects.[19] Toll-like receptors (TLRs) on macrophages recognize pathogen-associated molecular patterns and respond by activating the cascade of production and release of proinflammatory cytokines such as TNF- and IL-6 to initiate the response to eliminate the invading organism. There seems to be a defect at the TLR expression and function with the aged population.[69] This reduced cytokine activation due to impaired TLRs may also contribute to low cytokine response in the setting of infection. This may explain the reason why elderly often fail to manifest classic signs and symptoms of infection and fail to mount an adequate response to infection.

Macrophages play an important role in wound repair, in the initial inflammatory stages, and also in the growth phase by secreting angiogenic and fibrogenic growth factors. A review of macrophage function on wound repair shows qualitative changes that include enhanced platelet aggregation, delayed reepithelialization, delayed angiogenesis, delayed collagen deposition, turnover and remodeling, delayed healing strength, decreased wound strength, and delayed infiltration and function of macrophages; and often, complete wound healing is suboptimal.[19]

The production of reactive oxygen species and nitrogen species is significantly impaired in neutrophils and macrophages. Studies on polymorphonuclear (PMN) leukocytes yielded conflicting results, but generally, aging seems to be associated with impairment of microbactericidal and killing activity of PMNs (oxidative burst,) but has little influence on other PMN functions (adhesion, chemotaxis, migration, phagocytosis, etc.).[40,70] Natural killer cells are also affected by the aging process. For studies following the SENIEUR protocol, NK cells increase in number and have more mature phenotype with advancing age. Yet they may have less cytolytic ability and are unable to properly proliferate following IL-2 stimulation. NK cells are also less able to destroy tumor cells,[70] and the incidence of cancer increases in the subpopulation with lower NK cytotoxic activity.[71] The NK cell proliferative response to IL-2 is decreased by 40 to 60% among the elderly.[70,34]

6.5.6 Cytokines

Aging is also linked to a low baseline increase in proinflammatory cytokines and acute-phase proteins (TNF-, IL-6, soluble TNF receptors, C-reactive protein [CRP]). A review on cytokines and their association with diseases and mortality finds that TNF- and IL-6 elevation in the elderly was associated with increased risk of mortality independent of comorbidities.[72] Furthermore, TNF- was found to be an independent prognostic marker for mortality in the very old (100 years and over).[73] Cytokines are generally classified based on the type of cells that produce them. Type 1 cytokines are produced by the T_H1 (T helper 1) and Tc1 (T cytotoxic 1) cells and are represented by IFN- and TNF-. Type 2 cytokines are characterized by IL-4 production from T helper 2 (T_H2) and cytotoxic 2 (Tc2) T cells. Aging has been associated with a shift toward dominance of type 2 cytokines and a diminished role of type 1 cytokines.[74,75] Much literature suggested that circulating levels of proinflammatory cytokines are increased in the aged, and macrophages are presumed to be the primary producers of these cytokines. Other studies have demonstrated that the low baseline elevation in these cytokines is due to underlying inflammatory diseases and poor nutrition rather than the natural aging process.[70]

In contrast to decreased IL-2 production in response to antigenic stimulation in aged individuals, IL-10, a T_H2 cytokine, has been reported to be increased. This interleukin has suppressive effects on cell-mediated immunity by inhibiting IFN- production and downregulates antigen-presenting cells' function by inhibiting T_H1 cytokine production, particularly IL-12, the cytokine responsible for initiation of cell-mediated immunity (CMI).[76]

Cytokine production in the elderly is generally decreased in response to immune challenge, for example, vaccination. Decreased or impaired pro- and anti-inflammatory cytokine secretion and a lesser increase in the acute-phase protein were observed.[59,77] This was shown to be predictive of frailty in old age and could be associated with a genetic predisposition with the IL-10 promoter gene.[78] In summary, age-associated alterations in immune function may be linked to an imbalance in production of several cytokines, rather than due to any particular cytokine derangement. And this shift in cytokine balance likely accounts for the observed changes in cellular differentiation and cell-to-cell signaling of the immune system.

6.6 IMMUNITY IN THE MALNOURISHED

While caloric restriction has been shown to prolong survival, as first demonstrated in 1935,[79] the same conclusion cannot be substantiated in humans. Much evidence and many observations link the importance of nutrition and its effects on immunity. In the hospitals of the Warsaw ghetto in 1942, Jewish physicians noted that tuberculosis was much more severe in the malnourished, the tuberculin skin test was impaired in malnourished patients with TB, and allergic diseases improved spontaneously as malnutrition worsened. In the two groups of British and Russian prisoners of war who had similar food rations and living and working conditions, the British group received daily food supplements from the Red Cross. There was a marked difference in the incidence of tuberculosis in the two groups, with a lower incidence in the British group, indicating the importance of nutrition on the immune response.[80,81]

Malnutrition is a common clinical entity found with increased prevalence in the elderly population. Malnutrition can be caused by many different etiologies: physical disability, medication-induced anorexia, anorexia of aging, restrictive diets, poor dentition, chronic medical conditions, living situations, psychosocial issues, and depression. All these factors lead to a common endpoint of malnutrition, worsening function, and frailty.

6.6.1 Cell-Mediated Immunity in the Malnourished

In patients with impaired nutritional status, either lower serum albumin (3.0 to 3.9 g/dl) or normal albumin but lower micronutrient status, the changes in T cell subsets (CD3+, CD8+, and CD4+) and function (decreased IL-2, IL-6 release) were marked compared to the discussed changes with aging in the healthy aged population.[28,32] In addition, the immune responses of the elderly are very sensitive to nutritional influences, for example, folic acid deficiency. Even in the very healthy elderly group, minor changes in folic acid level were found to result in decreased T cell subsets and lower cell-mediated immune (CMI) responses, while young adults with low folic acid levels do not exhibit a lower immune response.[40] In ambulatory elderly individuals with serum albumin less than 3 g/dl, the peripheral lymphocyte count was shown to be suboptimal and CD4 T cells lower than 400/mm^3, a level comparable to acute acquired immune deficiency syndrome in human immunodeficiency virus infection.[82]

In general, poor nutritional status exacerbates the already impaired function of the aging immune system and resembles the same pattern as those discussed in the immunosenescence section, but the degree of impairment is more marked.

Delayed cutaneous hypersensitivity (DCH) reaction declines significantly in the elderly population at risk for nutritional deficiencies of vitamins,[82] and when replaced with nutritional supplement, the DCH reaction seems to improve.[83] In hospitalized elderly at risk for malnutrition[84,85] and in idiopathic senile anorectic elderly,[86] the DCH reaction is significantly depressed. Anergy is also found to be more prevalent in nursing home residents than in geriatric clinic patients (community dwellers).[87] Although elderly subjects with chronic diseases have a significantly lower DCH reaction than young controls, only a small subpopulation show some anergy to the common antigens.[53] Deficiency of essential omega-3 fatty acids may also contribute to cutaneous anergy in the malnourished elderly.[88]

6.6.2 Macrophage–T Cell Interactions: Cytokine Production

Undernutrition also affects cytokine production. Macrophages release cytokines in response to stress. The decreased T cell functions in the frail elderly result in decreased cytokine release from macrophages. These cytokines modify metabolic functions and induce utilization of body reserves of nutrients, resulting in hypercatabolic syndrome (proteolysis, osteolysis, changes in protein synthesis in the liver, decrease in insulin).[40] The vicious cycle continues with further body reserve depletion under longer stress reaction, and the elderly undergo accelerated aging when under prolonged stress. The elderly recover in a more frail state and lower body reserve (lower muscle mass), and thus exemplify the importance of nutrition on frailty progression and accelerated aging. In idiopathic senile anorexia, there is increased production of several cytokines, such as TNF-α, IL-1β, IL-6, and IFN-γ,[86] and this increase in proinflammatory cytokines may contribute to protein-energy malnutrition (PEM), frequently found in chronic nonmalignant disorders.[89]

When undernutrition reaches the PEM state, all immune responses are decreased, including macrophage cytokine synthesis. This leads to lower nutritional utilization and impaired lymphocyte activation and results in longer duration of disease and longer inflammatory response, leading to more decreases in body nutritional reserves, a more profound malnourished state,[40] and eventually to death.

6.6.3 Mucosal Immune System in Aging and Malnutrition

Mucosal immunity is primed after birth and develops throughout life via the interaction of microflora with the gut immune system (gastrointestinal-associated lymphoid tissue, or GALT). Any changes in the gut with aging affect the microenvironment, and therefore the mucosal immune system. Mucosal defense utilizes innate and adaptive immune cells. The innate immune cells, namely, monocytes, macrophages, NK cells, and dendritic cells, recognize the specific pathogen motif and mount an immediate immune reaction. Available studies show mucosal immune deficits in the differentiation and migration of immunoglobulin A cells to the intestinal lamina propria, and the initiation or regulation of local antibody production with aging.[90,91] This results in impaired secretory IgA responses, induction of anergy, and suppression or tolerance to oral antigen in the elderly. Furthermore, GALT-mediated responses are more susceptible to aging than are lymphoid tissues elsewhere in the body. These changes may be due to the reduced size of Peyer's patches and decreased cytokine production and response.[92]

Nutritional deficiencies of vitamins and minerals pose different influences on the immune system as a whole and play an important role in growth and diseases. Microflora of the gut, respiratory tract, perineum, vagina, and distal urethra control the homeostasis of the mucosal immune system. Malnutrition can shift the balance of normal flora and result in increased susceptibility to infections and other derangements, for example, coagulopathy and *Clostridium difficile* colitis. Studies have found some benefits of probiotic bacteria effective against antibiotic-associated diarrhea, such as *C. difficile* colitis. Probiotic lactobacilli can decrease tumor risk by neutralizing carcinogens and producing antitumor factors and by replacing microflora that produce carcinogens and tumor promoters.[93–97] Moreover, lactobacilli can be used to increase a weak systemic immune response, even in an HIV-positive host.[93,98]

The route of nutrition delivery may greatly affect the mucosal immunity of the intestine, liver, and lungs. It has been hypothesized that there is an immunologic link between the gastrointestinal tract and respiratory tract via a common mucosal immune system. Results from experimental and clinical studies in animals and humans support the hypothesis that immune cells sensitized in the Peyer's patches of the intestine can migrate to other intestinal and extraintestinal sites and induce specific mucosal immune responses at these sites. In animal models, mice fed parenterally were found to have marked reduction of B and T lymphocytes in the intestinal lamina propria and a significant shift of the CD4:CD8, ratio resulting in decreased cytokines, specifically IL-4 and IL-10, which are important for B cell switching to sIgA-producing plasma cells, and decreased IgA production. When mice immunized with a respiratory virus were then fed parenterally, 50% of the animals lost protection against the virus and had continued viral shedding 40 hours after rechallenge; all animals fed via the gastrointestinal tract cleared the virus. However, immunologic memory was restored with enteral refeeding.[99,100] In human trials, patients postoperatively were randomized to start enteral feeding vs. parenteral nutrition; the enteral group was found to have significantly lower incidence of pneumonia and trending to lower incidence of intra-abdominal abscess.[101–103]

Glutamine is an amino acid recognized for its role in modulating the immune changes with parenteral nutrition. Adding glutamine to the parenteral preparation improves intestinal lymphocyte number, preserves IL-4 function, increases intestinal and respiratory tract IgA levels, and may partially reverse the impaired antiviral and antibacterial immune response due to parenteral feeding.[100]

6.7 IMMUNE RECONSTITUTION AND ENHANCEMENT

6.7.1 VACCINES

Faced with the deleterious consequences of declining immunity in the aged, vaccinations offer an effective intervention combating mortality and morbidity risks in the elderly (Table 6.5). Vaccines are effective in preventing and reducing mortality and morbidity associated with influenza A and B and pneumococcal pneumonia, tetanus, and diphtheria. Although elderly patients have lower antibody titers to vaccination, most healthy elderly achieve titers that are generally protective and proven to be effective in reducing hospitalization rate due to influenza by at least 30%,[104] as well as a 38% relative risk reduction for patients vaccinated with pneumococcal vaccine.[105] For the frail, chronically ill patients, instutionalized and malnourished, it has been suggested that an additional booster dose may be required to mount an adequate immune response.[106] However, with influenza and bacterial pneumonia among the top leading causes of death in the elderly, the percentage vaccinated was disappointing, with the highest vaccination rate in Caucasians (66.6%), African Americans (43.3%), and Hispanics (52.5%) among the Medicare beneficiaries.[107]

6.7.2 NUTRIENT DEFICIENCIES AND INTERVENTION

Before the introduction of the SENIEUR protocol to standardize selection criteria for a healthy population for the study of immunity in the aged, outcomes from these earlier studies could be flawed due to selection bias. Study subjects were not tested for micro- or macronutrient deficiency, and thus the findings from these earlier studies might actually be due to nutritional deficiency. Animal and human studies have shown that dietary modifications and supplements can be used to improve and reverse the immune dysfunction caused by malnutrition. Clinical reviews on the outcomes of these studies show improvement in CD4 T cell numbers, NK cell activity, mitogenic responses, IL-2 release and expression, and enhanced DCH responses, and clinically reduce the number of infectious illness days and antibiotic use.[24,43,108,109] However, caution must be taken with oversupplementation due to potential risk of toxicity and increased mortality of some vitamins and minerals (i.e., vitamin A, vitamin E, zinc). Recent meta-analysis of vitamin E has shown that high-dose supplementation with vitamin E daily may increase all-cause mortality[110] and impaired immune responses.[111]

TABLE 6.5
Available Therapies for Immune Enhancement in the Elderly

1. Vaccines
2. Intravenous immunoglobulin (only for special cases of immunodeficiency; quite costly)
3. Nutritional interventions
4. Exercise
5. Mental and social well-being

6.7.2.1 Iron Deficiency

This is the single most common nutrient deficiency in the world. Its impact on the immune system includes reduced intracellular killing of bacteria by phagocytes, decreased T cell numbers, and proliferation *before* anemia develops. This dysfunction is due to decreased activity of ribonucleotide reductase and myeloperoxidase.[112] Uncorrected, iron deficiency is associated with low IL-2 production, leading to impaired cell-mediated immunity.

6.7.2.2 Zinc

Zinc deficiency results in atrophy of the lymphoid organs that could have a prolonged lasting effect when it occurs in the fetus. Zinc acts as a cofactor in many activation sequences for cell proliferation and plays an important role in cell-mediated immunity through its interaction with thymulin, a hormone produced by the thymus that regulates T cell differentiation. Thymulin has a higher affinity for zinc than for other metals. When zinc intake is deficient, serum thymulin activity decreases as well as IL-2 production and response, CD8 T cell cytotoxicity is diminished,[112] and lymphopenia is moderate.[84] Supplemention with zinc significantly improves the above biochemical parameters, increases DCH reaction, and increases CMI responses.[83] Yet, oversupplementation with zinc may cause a decreased benefit in a dose–response pattern.[113]

6.7.2.3 Vitamin E

Vitamin E is an antioxidant important in prostaglandin E2 production (PGE2) and has been found to be deficient in a significant percentage of the healthy elderly population. PGE2 has been found to be elevated in human and animal models and is associated with decreased proliferative capacity and IL-2 production and increased IL-10 production. Vitamin E acts to inhibit PGE2 production. Supplementation improves DCH response and IL-2 release, increases proliferative response, and decreases PGE2 production. Higher dose supplementation, 200 to 800 mg/day, is needed to boost antibody response to vaccines and decreases the self-reported infection rate.[114–117] However, a recent trial tested the effect of a high-dose (200 mg/day) supplement of vitamin E, 17 to 20 times the Recommended Dietary Allowance (RDA), and showed no effect on incidence of infection, but rather increased several markers of illness severity, namely, duration, number of symptoms, fever, and activity restriction.[118] A more recent double-blind, placebo-controlled trial confirms the significant reduction of common colds and decreased incidence of respiratory infection among elderly nursing home patients with a daily vitamin E supplement of 200 i.u.[119] However, long-term antioxidant treatment with vitamins E and C in healthy elder men has no effects on inflammatory markers TNF-α, IL-6, and CRP.[120]

6.7.3 Nutritional Supplementation and Cancer Prevention

With increased awareness that supplementation of dietary nutrients improves immune function, the role of each nutrient supplementation remains to be investigated.

Observational study on high-vitamin C diets suggests protection of some cancers,[121] and a low level of ascorbate was linked to increased all-cause mortality in older people.[122] In a large corhort of elderly age 67 to 105 years, reported use of vitamins E and C was associated with decreased risk of all-cause mortality up to 42%, yet reported use of vitamin C alone had no effect on mortality.[123] Several studies were conducted to investigate the possible cancer prevention role of antioxidants, but so far scant evidence has been found for a beneficial effect. A recent review and meta-analysis evaluating vitamins C and E on treatment and cancer prevention concluded that were no benefits from the doses tested in the population studied.[124]

Other studies addressed the possible association of diets rich in beta-carotene and reduced incidence of cancer. Due to their antioxidant properties, the carotenoids (beta-carotene, lutein, and lycopene) seem to protect against DNA damage[125] in healthy elderly. Although their role in cancer prevention is unproven, common findings in these trials show a beneficial effect of enhanced cell-mediated immune responses.[126] In another prospective cohort study, a relationship was established between dietary intake of tocopherols and increased risk of gastric cardia cancer, while dietary intake of fruits, vitamin C, tocopherols, and lycopene seemed to be protective for gastric noncardia cancer.[127] While some trials may show positive effects, others fail to replicate the immune enhancement of beta-carotene and lycopene in healthy study subjects.[128,129]

Dietary folate, a water-soluble B vitamin found in a variety of fruits and vegetables, has garnered much interest due to its role in DNA methylation and DNA synthesis and repair. Various observational studies have been conducted to study the role of folate in cancer prevention and have found that high dietary folate intake is associated with decreased risk of bladder cancer,[130] and may modify and inhibit colorectal cancer development.[131] There is an increased risk of breast cancer with increasing alcohol consumption, but no association could be made with dietary intake of folate and breast cancer.[132] Furthermore, high folate intake was associated with decreased lung cancer risk by 40% with an inverse dose–response relationship.[133]

Selenium and cadmium may also have important roles in prostate cancer risk and modulation. While cadmium is carcinogenic for prostate epithelials by promoting growth and malignant transformation, selenium in a randomized controlled trial has been shown to be protective in prostate cancer risk.[134] Another randomized trial testing supplementation of antioxidants, selenium, and zinc showed significant reduction in prostate cancer incidence only in men with normal prostate specific antigen (PSA) values.[135] In the cancer prevention study, vitamin E use has no significant reduction on prostate cancer risk and incidence of bladder cancer.[136]

In summary, there are many observational and epidemiologic studies that suggest a beneficial role of dietary supplements, such as antioxidants, vitamins, and minerals, for cancer reduction benefits, and more randomized controlled trials in progress or planned to further assess the actual risk reduction of these supplements in cancer prevention. One must not overlook the potential toxicity of these in high doses and interactions between the supplements themselves. It is prudent to emphasize the importance of a healthy and balanced diet consisting of a wide variety of plant-based foods and fish, avoiding a high-fat diet or diet rich in advanced glycation end products (fried, browned, baked, cooked, barbecued). A Mediterranean-type diet was proposed (higher intake of fruits, vegetables, fish, and olive oil, and a lower intake of sugar, starch, and dairy products). Adherence to this diet has been shown to significantly decrease all-cause mortality and death due to coronary heart disease and cancer.[137] Results from observational studies at times are not concordant with those obtained from randomized clinical trials; therefore, vitamin supplements are appropriate for recognized deficiencies. However, evidence to support their benefits in cancer protection remains to be investigated.

6.7.4 Role of Probiotics or Prebiotics?

Future prospectives to treatment and modification of impaired immune systems hold great promise. Is there a role of probiotics or prebiotics as an adjunct or alternative to treatment of certain clinical conditions to reduce mortality and morbidity? Probiotics are live microorganisms, usually components of the normal human intestinal flora, that when given in adequate dosage can promote health and prevent and cure diseases. Probiotics given to patients on antibiotic therapy have been shown to reduce the incidence of antibiotic-associated diarrhea in two large meta-analyses[138,139] in children and in adults and have been recommended for use in gastroenterology as level 1A evidence.[140] Recent reviews on probiotics found that specific strains of lactic acid bacteria, such as *Lactobacillus* or *Bifidobacterium* species, have been

TABLE 6.6
Probiotics in Evidence-Based Medicine[140]

Grade A Recommendation (Level 1A Evidence)
Prevention of antibiotic-associated diarrhea
Treatment of lactose malabsorption
Grade A Recommendation (Level 1B Evidence)
Prevention of pouchitis and maintenance of remission
Prevention of postoperative infections
Grade B Recommendation (Level 2B Evidence)
Prevention of travelers' diarrhea
Maintenance of remission of ulcerative colitis

Note: Grade A recommendations: Evidence with clinically proven benefits.

Grade B recommendations: Therapeutic option supported by level 2 evidence; recommendations could change in the future.

Level 1A evidence: Evidence from high-quality randomized controlled trials with statistically significant results and few limitations on the design, or by conclusions of systematic reviews of the trials.

Level 1B evidence: Evidence comes from single high-quality clinical trials with narrow intervals of confidence and clear positive or negative results.

Level 2 evidence: Randomized controlled trials with some limitations or results and wide confidence intervals.

shown to increase phagocytic activity and receptor expression in granulocytes, increase NK number and function, enhance antibody response to vaccines, and may have an anticarcinogenic property.[140] Furthermore, the immunomodulatory effect of lactic acid bacteria differs with each strain of bacteria, is dose dependent, and exhibits greater improvements in people older than 70 years than those younger.[140] These changes in T cell numbers and functions of CD4+ and activated T and NK cells are more marked, especially in patients with poor pretreatment immune responses.[141] However, other studies failed to show any modulatory effect of probiotics on phagocytic function.[142,143] Commonly, probiotics are found in yogurt, drinks such as cow milk, goat milk, and fruit juices, and commercially prepared supplement capsules, tablets, or powders. Probiotics can be used in clinical conditions of malnourishment, lactose intolerance, constipation, and antibiotic-associated diarrhea.

Prebiotics are a more recent concept developed in the past decade. They are chemical compounds, usually oligosaccharides, that act as substrates for the probiotics and potentiate the growth of gut normal flora. Prebiotics are found naturally in breast milk and certain vegetables, such as Jerusalem artichokes, onions, and chicory, and are nondigestible. Synthetic prebiotics are oligosaccharides based on fructose or galactose that can be added to foods or combined with a probiotic to make a *synbiotic*. Other prebiotics, such as lactulose and inulin, act as dietary fiber and can be used to treat constipation by acting as substrates for lactic acid bacteria and bifidobacteria for catabolism and inducing an osmotic effect. Increased calcium bioavailability was shown in two trials of prebiotics.[144,145] This raises a possible role of prebiotics in increasing calcium absorption and osteoporosis treatment or prevention in the future. More research in the field of probiotics and prebiotics is warranted to find new immunoadjuvants in the quest for modulating immune response in aging.

6.7.5 Exercise

Exercise has been frequently recommended to modulate diseases and improve function and physical and mental wellness at all ages, including the elderly. Exercise was shown to be an immune inducer, but much of the underlying interaction requires further investigation. Previous evidence demonstrated clinical benefits with moderate aerobic exercise, but strenuous exercise proved to be deleterious to the aging immunity in the elderly. This is termed the inverted J hypothesis. The visually inverted J delineates improvement of immune function with increasing intensity of exercise until a threshold is reached, after which immune function starts to decline precipitously.[146] Furthermore, strenuous exercise induces a state of exhaustion and immunosuppression in the host (Table 6.7) that usually lasts from 3 to 72 hours postexertion, but may manifest clinical symptoms of upper respiratory tract infection in 1 to 2 weeks after heavy periods of training.[147] Even though data from human and animal studies imply a possible enhancement of immunity with exercise, lifelong continuation of physical activity and positive lifestyle changes may be needed to achieve a physical fitness before any benefit in the immune system can be expected in the aged body.[147]

TABLE 6.7
Immunocompromised Host after Prolonged Strenuous Exertion[147]

1. Neutrophilia and lymphopenia induced by high plasma catecholamines, growth hormones, and cortisol
2. Increased inflammatory markers from granulocytes and monocytes
3. Decreased granulocyte oxidative burst activity
4. Decreased nasal neutrophil phagocytosis
5. Decreased NK cytotoxic activity
6. Decreased nasal mucociliary clearance
7. Decreased nasal neutrophil phagocytosis
8. Decreased mitogen-induced lymphocyte proliferation
9. Decreased DCH response
10. Increased pro- and anti-inflammatory cytokines

Are nutritional supplements effective immune modulators in exercise-induced inflammation and immunosuppression? Several studies have addressed the influence of nutritional supplements, primarily zinc, dietary fat, vitamin C, glutamine, and carbohydrate, on immune response after intense and prolonged exercise. None of the nutrients or vitamin has proven beneficial except carbohydrate administration during strenuous exercise. During exercise, the blood glucose level was found to be reduced, and this was thought to be due to activation of the hypothalamic–pituitary–adrenal axis, leading to increased catecholamine release, increased cortisol and growth hormone, and decreased insulin level. Several studies have tested the hypothesis that carbohydrate ingestion during exercise would maintain blood glucose level, attenuate stress hormone release, and therefore lessen the changes in the immune system. Results have shown that subjects that ingest carbohydrate drink during exercise have higher blood glucose level, lower plasma cortisol and growth hormone, decreased inflammatory markers IL-1 and IL-6, and less changes in peripheral leukocyte counts and other immune response parameters.[147]

So, how do these findings translate to clinical outcomes in our elderly population? A recent review on the clinical significance of exercise to modulate immune changes with aging has concluded that long-term exercise seems to have the most benefit to improve changes in immunosenescence, such as antibody response to vaccines and novel antigens, T cell functions and subsets, and cytokine production.[148,149] Yet for a population of frail elderly nursing home patients, endurance and resistance exercise intervention for 8 months showed no difference in immune parameters and incidence of infections[150] compared to placebo. In another population of frail independent living elderly, a 4-month intervention of enriched food showed no effect on the cellular immunity measured by the DCH reaction to seven antigens, but exercise seemed to slow the decline in DCH response compare to the placebo group.[151] The immune modulatory effect of moderate exercise in the elderly population may have to be lifelong to show clinical benefit. Nevertheless, moderate exercise is an important recommendation to help improve other aspects of life, such as fall risk reduction, cardiovascular fitness, physical and mental wellness, and preservation of function in the elderly, both frail and healthy.

6.7.6 Psychosocial Wellness

Social isolation, depression, and mental stress have been linked to poor outcomes in the elderly. A recent study showed peak antibody response to influenza vaccine at 1 month in patients with bereavement in the year prior to vaccination, and also in married couples and those with higher marital satisfaction. The response was more evident in the younger half of the married sample.[152] In the elderly depressed patients, lymphocyte stimulation and T cell growth factor production, when stimulated with phytohemagglutinin, are decreased, and the DCH reaction was also decreased.[153] Moreover, the levels of proinflammatory cytokines TNF and IL-6 were found to be increased and there was a decrease in suppressive IL-10 cells.[154] In the elderly caregiver wives of demented patients, levels of stress and depression showed a strong association with impaired T cell proliferation, change in T cell subpopulation to increased CD8+ T cells, and significant reduction in NK cells and CD56+T cells, a subset important in MHC-unrestricted cytotoxicity found increased in healthy centenarians.[155] However, a similar study was done on younger caregivers with the same morbidity, and there was no significant change found in immune parameters measured, indicating no degree of impairment with stress and depression.[156] This difference in immune response in the elder caregivers compared to the younger caregivers, when subjected to stress and depression, could be due to immunosenescence already in place in the elderly. However, improvement in physical activity and modifications of psychosocial factors may help to modulate and improve immune response in the elderly,[148] leading to a better outcome.

Despite efforts at boosting immune responses by various methods, the best proven, with significant reduction in all endpoints, is a healthy lifestyle. This includes physical exercise and mental wellness, stress control, limited exposure to tobacco and alcohol, and healthy nutrition to minimize risk and maximize successful aging. A large study with a 10-year follow-up for patients adhering to the Mediterranean diet, moderate alcohol consumption and physical activity, and no smoking was found to be associated with significant risk reduction in all-cause mortality and mortality from cardiovascular diseases, coronary heart diseases, and cancer.[157,158]

6.8 OVERNUTRITION AND IMMUNITY

Overnutrition also has its effects on the immune system. Obesity correlates with higher respiratory morbidity and impairment of cell-mediated immunity, as well as reduced NK cells and phagocytic activity. Studies that examined the effects of high fatty acids in the diet on T-cell-mediated responses revealed reduced cytotoxic T cell activity and reduced antibody responses to T-cell-dependent antigens. Macrophage functions are also affected by high-fat diets. This includes reduced phagocytosis, impaired activity against tumor cells, and decreased cytotoxic activity.[159]

The role of lipids in the age-related changes in immune responses involves membrane fluidity. Variation in the fatty acid composition of membranes poses an important influence on lipid peroxidation, and consequently on the rate of aging and life span determination. The products of lipid peroxidation are reactive molecules that can cause damage to cellular structures and shorten life span. It is possible that the reduced oxidative stress by caloric restriction changes fatty acid composition of the membrane, making it more resistant to lipid peroxidation and explaining the longer life span in some species.[160] In humans, membrane lipid composition changes during T cell proliferation induced by mitogens, and this change in aged individuals correlates with a decrease in mitogenic response.[161] It was observed that peripheral lymphocytes of aged individuals have a higher membrane viscosity, and this change is associated with a lower mitogenic response, i.e., lower proliferative ability of lymphocytes.[162] Changes in membrane viscosity are observed to be more pronounced in the frail than in the healthy elderly. When treated *in vivo* with lipid-lowering drug or dietary modification (low-fat diet), membrane viscosity was reduced and mitogenic activity increased.[161] This suggests that part of the altered lymphocyte proliferative capacity in the elderly is due to increased membrane viscosity caused by increased dietary lipid intake.

Leptin is a protein hormone produced by fat cells and functions to decrease food intake and increase metabolic rate. Leptin levels correlate closely with fat mass and decrease with decline in body fat as one ages. Leptin resistance has been implicated in abnormal lipid metabolism and insulin resistance of the metabolic syndrome in the elderly. Leptin also has a direct effect on T-cell-mediated immunity and promotes lymphocyte survival in T and B cells. In a diet-induced obese mouse model of obesity and leptin resistance, leptin receptor-mediated signaling in T cell is reduced.[163] Peroxisome proliferator-activated receptor (PPAR)-alpha, a member of the nuclear receptor family that regulates the expression of genes associated with lipid metabolism and adipocyte differentiation, is upregulated by hyperleptinemia. PPAR-alpha activators (i.e., the fibric acid derivatives, thiazolidinediones) have been shown to improve glucose utilization, insulin resistance, and lipid metabolism. Furthermore, treatment with PPAR agonist results in decreased levels of spontaneous inflammatory cytokines[164,165] and induces a shift in cytokine secretion of human T cells by inhibiting IFN-γ and promoting IL-4 secretion.[166] Are the PPARs the next antiaging agents? Much remains to be investigated.

6.9 CONCLUSION

As presented earlier, the immune system functions to defend its host from extrinsic (bacteria, carcinogens) and intrinsic (self-repair, growth, tumor control) pathogenic agents. As thc immune system ages, its function is compromised, leaving the host vulnerable to harm and diseases. Nutrition plays an important role in maintaining the vigor of the immune system, since nutritional deficits and malnutrition further aggravate the already weakened immune system in the elderly. Dietary supplements have been studied over the years and have been found to improve immune responses in malnourished individuals. However, extra supplements as means of antiaging or cancer prevention in healthy individuals have no proven clinical benefits but can potentially cause harm in high doses. Vessels to healthy and successful aging are therefore a balanced diet and healthy lifestyle habits that include moderate exercise, limited intake of alcohol, no tobacco, and being happy. For chronically ill or institutionalized individuals, special attention should be directed to ensure proper nutrition and supplements, yearly vaccination, and social interaction.

REFERENCES

1. Laupland, K.B., Church, D.L., Mucenski, M., et al., Population-based study on the epidemiology of and the risk factors for invasive *Staphylococcus aureus* infections, *J. Infect. Dis.*, 187, 1452, 2003.
2. Pascual, F.B., McGinley, E.L., Zanardi, L.R., et al., Tetanus surveillance: United States, 1998–2000, *Morb. Mortal Wkly. Rep. Surveill. Summ.*, 52, 1, 2003.
3. Marwick, C., NHANES III health data relevant for aging nation, *JAMA*, 227, 100, 1997.
4. Bridges, C.B., Fukuda, K., Uyeki, T.M., et al., Advisory Committee on Immunization Practices. Prevention and control of influenza. Recommendations of the Advisory Committee on Immunization Practices (ACIP), *Morb. Mortal Wkly. Rep. Recomm. Rep.*, 51, 1, 2003.
5. Potter, J.M., O'Donnel, B., Carman, W.F., et al., Serological response to influenza vaccination and nutritional and functional status of patients in geriatric medical long-term care, *Age Ageing*, 28, 141, 1999.
6. Linn, B.S., Age differences in the severity and outcomes of burns, *J. Am. Geriatr. Soc.*, 28, 118, 1980.
7. Paillaud, E., Herbaud, S., Caillet, P., et al., Relations between undernutrition and nosocomial infections in elderly patients, *Age Ageing*, 34, 619, 2005.
8. Sullivan, D.H., Patch, G.A., Walls, R.C., et al., Impact of nutritional status on morbidity and mortality in a select population of geriatric rehabilitation patients, *Am. J. Clin. Nutr.*, 51, 749, 1990.
9. Sullivan, D.H., Walls, R.C., and Bopp, M.M. Protein-energy undernutrition and the risk of mortality within one year of hospital discharge: a follow-up study, *J. Am. Geriatr. Soc.*, 43, 507, 1995.
10. Kagansky, N., Berner, Y., Koren-Morag, N., et al., Poor nutritional habits are predictors of poor outcome in very old hospitalized patients, *Am. J. Clin. Nutr.*, 82, 784, 2005.
11. Klonoff-Cohen, H., Barrett-Connor, E.L., and Edelstein, S.L., Albumin levels as a predictor of mortality in the healthy elderly, *J. Clin. Epidemiol.*, 45, 207, 1992.
12. Corti, M.C., Guralnik, J.M., Salive, M.E., et al., Serum albumin level and physical disability as predictors of mortality in older persons, *JAMA*, 272, 1036, 1994.
13. Bender, B.S., Infectious disease risk in the elderly, *Immunol. Allergy Clin. N. Am.*, 23, 57, 2003.
14. Murray, H.W., Interferon-gamma and host antimicrobial defense: current and future clinical applications, *Am. J. Med.*, 97, 459, 1994.
15. Lieschke, G.J., and Burgess, A.W., Granulocyte colony-stimulating factor and granulocyte-macrophage colony-stimulating factor (2), *N. Engl. J. Med.*, 327, 99, 1992.
16. Dale, D.C., Liles, W.C., Summer, W.R., et al., Review: granulocyte colony-stimulating factor: role and relationships in infectious diseases, *J. Infect. Dis.*, 172, 1061, 1995.
17. Root, R.K. and Dale, D.C., Granulocyte colony-stimulating factor and granulocyte-macrophage colony-stimulating factor: comparisons and potential for use in the treatment of infections in nonneutropenic patients, *J. Infect. Dis.*, 179, S342, 1999.

18. Schumann, C.L., Hoxie, N.J., and Vergeront, J.M., Wisconsin trends in pneumonia and influenza mortality, 1980–2003, *WMJ.*, 105, 40 2006.
19. Plowden, J., Renshaw-Hoelscher, M., Engleman, C., et al., Innate immunity in aging: impact on macrophage function, *Aging Cell*, 3, 161, 2004.
20. Morens, D.M. and Rash, V.M., Lessons from a nursing home outbreak of influenza A, *Infect. Control Hosp. Epidemiol.*, 16, 275,1995.
21. Ligthart, G.J., Radl, J., Corberand, J.X., et al., Monoclonal gammopathies in human aging increased occurrence with age and correlation with health status, *Mech. Ageing Dev.*, 52, 235, 1990.
22. Hijmans, W., Radl, J., Bottazzo, G.F., et al., Autoantibodies in highly aged humans, *Mech. Ageing Dev.*, 26, 83, 1984.
23. Ershler, W.B., Sun, W.H., Binkley, N., et al., Interleukin-6 and aging: blood levels and mononuclear cell production increase with advancing age and *in vitro* production modifiable by dietary restriction, *Lymphokine Cytokine Res.*, 12, 225, 1993.
24. Salvador, J., Adams, E.J., Ershler, R., et al., Future challenges in analysis and treatment of human immune senescence, *Immunol. Allergy Clin. N. Am.*, 23, 133, 2003.
25. Ligthart, G.J., Corberand, J.X., Fournier, C., et al., Admission criteria for immunogerontological studies in man: the SENIEUR protocol, *Mech. Ageing Dev.*, 28, 47, 1984.
26. Lesourd, B. and Mazari, L., Nutrition and immunity in the elderly, *Proc. Nutr. Soc.*, 58, 685, 1999.
27. Dominguez-Gerp, L. and Rey-Mendez, M., Evolution of the thymus size in response to physiological and random events throughout life, *Microsc. Res. Tech.*, 62, 464, 2003.
28. Lesourd, B. et al., Decreased maturation of T cell population factors on the appearance of double negative CD4–, CD8–, CD2+ cells, *Arch. Gerontol. Geriatr.*, 4, 139, 1994.
29. Kawakami, K., Kadota, J., Iida, K., et al., Reduced immune function and malnutrition in the elderly, *Tohoku J. Exp. Med.*, 187, 157, 1999.
30. Lesourd, B.M. and Meaume, S., Cell-mediated immunity changes in aging: relative importance of cell subpopulation switches and of nutritional factors, *Immunol. Lett.*, 40, 235, 1994.
31. Huppert, F.A., Solomou, W., O'Connor, S., et al., Aging and lymphocyte subpopulations: whole-blood analysis of immune markers in a large population sample of healthy elderly individuals, *Exp. Gerontol.*, 33, 593, 1998.
32. Mazari, L. and Lesourd, B., Nutritional influences on immune response in healthy aged persons, *Mech. Ageing Dev.*, 104, 25, 1998.
33. Weksler, M.E., Changes in the B-cell repertoire with age, *Vaccine*, 18, 1624, 2000.
34. Borrego, F., Alonso, M.C., Galiani, M.D., et al., NK phenotypic markers and IL-2 response in NK cells from elderly people, *Exp. Gerontol.*, 34, 253, 1999.
35. Albright, J.W. and Albright, J.F., Impaired natural killer cell function as a consequence of aging, *Exp. Gerontol.*, 33, 13, 1998.
36. Cossarizza, A. et al., Age-related imbalance of virgin (CD45RA+) and memory (CD45RO+) cells between CD4+ and CD8+ T lymphocytes in humans: study from newborns to centenarians, *J. Immunol. Res.*, 4, 117, 1992.
37. Hobbs, M.V. and Ernst, D.N., T cell differentiation and cytokine expression in late life, *Dev. Comp. Immunol.*, 21, 464, 1997.
38. Ahluwalia, N., Mastro, A.M., Ball, R., et al., Cytokine production by stimulated mononuclear cells did not change with aging in apparently healthy, well-nourished women, *Mech. Ageing Dev.*, 122, 1269, 2001.
39. Krause, D., Mastro, A.M., Handte, G., et al., Immune function did not decline with aging in apparently healthy, well-nourished women, *Mech. Ageing Dev.*, 112, 43, 1999.

40. Lesourd, B.M., Nutrition: a major factor influencing immunity in the elderly, *J. Nutr. Health Aging*, 8, 28, 2004.
41. Chen, W.F., Liu, S.L., Gao, X.M., et al., The capacity of lymphokine production by peripheral blood lymphocytes from aged human, *Immunol. Invest.*, 15, 575, 1987.
42. Sinderman, J., Kruse, A., Frercks, H.J., et al., Investigations of the lymphokine system in elderly individuals, *Mech. Ageing Dev.*, 70, 149, 1993.
43. Castle, S., Uyemura, K., Wong, W., et al., Evidence of enhanced type 2 immune responses and impaired upregulation of a type 1 response in frail elderly nursing home residents, *Mech. Ageing Dev.*, 94, 7, 1997.
44. Daynes, R.A., Araneo, B.A., Ershler, W.B., et al., Altered regulation of IL-6 production with normal aging, *J. Immunol.*, 150, 5219, 1993.
45. James, K., Premchand, N., Skibinska, A., et al., IL-6, DHEA and the ageing process, *Mech. Ageing Dev.*, 93, 15, 1997.
46. Harris, T.B., Ferrucci, L., Tracy, R.P., et al., Associations of elevated interleukin-6 and C-reactive protein levels with mortality in the elderly, *Am. J. Med.*, 106, 506, 1999.
47. Grossmann, A., Ledbetter, J.A., and Rabinovitch, P.S., Reduced proliferation in T lymphocytes in aged humans is predominantly in the CD8+ subset, and is unrelated to defects in transmembrane signaling which are predominantly in the CD4+ subset, *Exp. Cell Res.*, 180, 367, 1989.
48. Effros, R.B., Replicative senescence of CD8 T cells: effect on human ageing, *Exp. Gerontol.*, 39, 517, 2004.
49. Effros, R.B., Problems and solutions to the development of vaccines in the elderly, *Immun. Allergy Clin. N. Am.*, 23, 41, 2003.
50. Blackburn, E., Mur, P., Jofre, B., et al., Immunosenescence: delayed cutaneous hypersensitivity tests in independently-living Chilean elderly individuals, *Rev. Med. Chile*, 128, 397, 2000.
51. Fietta, A., Merlini, C., Dos Santos, C., et al., Influence of aging on some specific and nonspecific mechanisms of the host defense system in 146 healthy subjects, *Gerontology*, 40, 237, 1994.
52. Colvin, R.B., Mosesson, M.W., and Dvorak, H.F., Delayed-type hypersensitivity skin reactions in congenital afibinogenemia: lack of fibrin deposition and induration, *J. Clin. Invest.*, 63, 1302, 1979.
53. Delafuente, J.C., Meuleman, J.R., and Nelson, R.C., Anergy testing in nursing home residents, *J. Am. Geriatr. Soc.*, 36, 733, 1988.
54. Weksler, M.E. and Szabo, P., The effect of age on the B-cell repertoire, *J. Clin. Immunol.*, 20, 240, 2000.
55. Dworsky, R., Paganini-Hill, A., Arthur, M., et al., Immune responses of healthy humans 83–104 years of age, *J. Natl. Cancer Inst.*, 71, 265, 1983.
56. Thompson, J.S., Wekstein, D.R., Rhoades, J.L., et al., The immune status of healthy centenarians, *J. Am. Geriatr. Soc.*, 32, 274, 1984.
57. Ventura, M.T., Evaluation of IgA1-IgA2 levels in serum and saliva of young and elderly people, *Immunol. Clin.*, 7, 135, 1988.
58. Paganelli, R., Quinti, I., Fagiolo, U., et al., Changes in circulating B cells and immunoglobulin classes and subclasses in a healthy aged population, *Clin. Exp. Immunol.*, 90, 351, 1990.
59. Paganelli, R., Scala, E., Quinti, I., et al., Humoral immunity in aging, *Aging Clin. Exp. Res.*, 6, 143, 1994.
60. Radl, J., Sepers, J.M., Skvaril, F., et al., Immunoglobulin patterns in humans over 95 years of age, *Clin. Exp. Immunol.*, 22, 84, 1975.

61. Fagiolo, U., Amadori, A., Biselli, R., et al., Quantitative and qualitative analysis of anti-taetanus toxoid antibody response in the elderly. Humoral immune response enhancement by thymostimulin, *Vaccine*, 11, 1336, 1993.
62. Shelly, M.A., Pichichero, M.E., and Treanor, J.J., Low baseline antibody level to diphtheria is associated with poor response to conjugated pneumococcal vaccine in adults, *Scand. J. Infect. Dis.*, 33, 542, 2001.
63. Goodwin, K., Viboud, C., and Simonsen, L., Antibody response to influenza vaccination in the elderly: a quantitative review, *Vaccine*, 24, 1159, 2006.
64. Powers, D.C., Murphy, B.R., Fries, L.F., et al., Reduced infectivity of cold-adapted influenza A H1N1 viruses in the elderly: correlation with serum and local antibodies, *J. Am. Geriatr. Soc.*, 40, 163, 1992.
65. Fagiolo, U., Amadori, A., Cozzi, E., et al., Humoral and cellular immune response to influenza virus vaccination in aged humans, *Aging Clin. Exp. Res.*, 5, 451, 1993.
66. McElhaney, J.E., Beattie, B.L., Devine, R., et al., Age-related decline in interleukin 2 production in response to influenza vaccine, *J. Am. Geriatr. Soc.*, 38, 652, 1990.
67. Boren, E. and Gershwin, M.E., Inflamm-aging: autoimmunity, and the immune-risk phenotype, *Autoimmun. Rev.*, 3, 401, 2004.
68. Stacy, S., Krolick, K.A., Infante, A.J., et al., Immunological memory and late onset autoimmunity, *Mech. Ageing Dev.*, 123, 975, 2002.
69. Renshaw, M., Rockwell, J., Engleman, C., et al., Cutting edge: impaired toll-like receptor expression and function in aging, *J. Immunol.*, 169, 4697, 2002.
70. Plackett, T.P., Boehmer, E.D., Faunce, D.E., et al., Aging and innate immune cells, *J. Leukoc. Biol.*, 76, 291, 2004.
71. Imai, K., Matsuyama, S., Miyake, S., et al., Natural cytotoxic activity of peripheral-blood lymphocytes and cancer incidence: an 11-year follow-up study of a general population, *Lancet*, 356, 1795, 2000.
72. Bruunsgaard, H. and Pedersen, B.K., Age-related inflammatory cytokines and disease, *Immunol. Allergy Clin. N. Am.*, 23, 15, 2003.
73. Bruunsgaard, H., Andersen-Ranberg, K., Hjelmborg, J.B., et al., Elevated levels of tumor necrosis factor alpha and mortality in centenarians, *Am. J. Med.*, 115, 278, 2003.
74. Alberti, S., Cevenini, E., Ostan, R., et al., Age-dependent modifications of type 1 and type 2 cytokines within virgin and memory CD4+ T cells in humans, *Mech. Ageing Dev.*, 127, 560, 2006.
75. Sandmand, M., Bruunsgaard, H., Kemp, K., et al., Is ageing associated with a shift in the balance between type 1 and type 2 cytokines in humans? *Clin. Exp. Immunol.*, 127, 107, 2002.
76. Koichi, U., Castle, S.C., and Takashi, M., The frail elderly: role of dendritic cells in the susceptibility of infection, *Mech. Ageing Dev.*, 123, 955, 2002.
77. Yousfi, M.E., Mercier, S., Breuille, D., et al., The inflammatory response to vaccination is altered in the elderly, *Mech. Ageing Dev.*, 126, 874, 2005.
78. van den Biggelaar, A.H., Huizinga, T.W., de Craen, A.J., et al., Impaired innate immunity predicts frailty in old age. The Leiden 85-plus study, *Exp. Gerontol.*, 39, 1407, 2004.
79. McCay, C.M., Cromwell, M.F., and Maynard LA., The effect of retarded growth upon the length of the lifespan and ultimate body size, *J. Nutr.*, 10, 63, 1935.
80. Martin, D.R., The relationship between malnutrition and lung infections, *Clin. Chest Med.*, 8, 359, 1987.
81. Winick M, Ed., *Hunger Disease: Studies by the Jewish Physicians in the Warsaw Ghetto*, Wiley, New York, 1979.

82. Lesourd, B., Protein undernutrition as the major cause of decreased immune function in the elderly: clinical and functional implications, *Nutr. Rev.*, 53, S86, 1995.
83. Buzina-Soboticanec, K., Buzina, R., Stavijenic, A., et al., Ageing, nutritional status and immune response, *Int. J. Vitamin Nutr. Res.*, 68, 133, 1998.
84. Congy, F., Clavel, J.P., Devillechabrolle, A., et al., Plasma zinc levels in elderly hospitalized subjects. Correlation with other nutritional and immunological markers and survival, *Semaine Hopitaux*, 59, 3105, 1983.
85. Cederholm, T., Lindgren, J.A., and Palmblad, J., Impaired leukotriene C4 generation in granulocytes from protein-energy malnourished chronically ill elderly, *J. Intern. Med.*, 247, 715, 2000.
86. Analich, F. et al., Cell-mediated immune response and cytokine production in idiopathic senile anorexia, *Mech. Ageing Dev.*, 77, 67, 1994.
87. Rodysill, K.J., Hansen, L., and O'Leary, J.J., Cutaneous-delayed hypersensitivity in nursing home and geriatric clinic patients. Implications for the tuberculin test, *J. Am. Geriatr. Soc.*, 37, 435, 1989.
88. Cederholm, T.E., Berg, A.B., Johansson, E.K., et al., Low levels of essential fatty acids are related to impaired delayed skin hypersensitivity in malnourished chronically ill elderly people, *Eur. J. Clin. Invest.*, 24, 615, 1994.
89. Cederholm, T., Wretlind, B., Hellstrom, K., et al., Enhanced generation of interleukins 1 beta and 6 may contribute to the cachexia of chronic disease, *Am. J. Clin. Nutr.*, 65, 876, 1997.
90. Schmucker, D.L., Heyworth, M.F., Owen, R.L., et al., Impact of aging on gastrointestinal mucosal immunity, *Dig. Dis. Sci.*, 41, 1183, 1996.
91. Cunningham-Rundles, S., The effect of aging on mucosal host defense, *J. Nutr. Health Aging*, 8, 20, 2004.
92. Fujihashi, K. and McGhee, J.R., Mucosal immunity and tolerance in the elderly, *Mech. Ageing Dev.*, 125, 889, 2004.
93. Bergogne-Berezin, E., Treatment and prevention of antibiotic associated diarrhea, *Int. J. Antimicrob. Agents*, 521, 2000.
94. Majamaa, H., Isolauri, E., Saxelin, M., et al., Lactic acid bacteria in the treatment of acute rotavirus gastroenteritis, *J. Pediatr. Gastroenterol. Nutr.*, 20, 333, 1995.
95. Hirayama, K. and Rafter, J., The role of lactic acid bacteria in colon cancer prevention: mechanistic considerations, *Antonie Van Leeuwenhoek*, 76, 391, 1999.
96. Kirjavainen, P.V., Apostolou, E., Salminen, S.J., et al., New aspects of probiotics: novel approach in the management of food allergy, *Allergy*, 54, 909, 1999.
97. Hove, H., Norgaard, H., and Mortensen, P.B., Lactic acid bacteria and the human gastrointestinal tract, *Eur. J. Clin. Nutr.*, 53, 339, 1999.
98. Cunningham-Rundles, S., Ahrne, S., Bengmark, S., et al., Probiotics and immune response, *Am. J. Gastroenterol.*, 95, S22, 2000.
99. Kudsk, K.A., Current aspects of mucosal immunology and its influence by nutrition, *Am. J. Surg.*, 183, 390, 2002.
100. Kudsk, K.A., Effect of route and type of nutrition on intestine-derived inflammatory responses, *Am. J. Surg.*, 185, 16, 2003.
101. Kudsk, K.A., Croce, M.A., Fabian, T.C., et al., Enteral versus parenteral feeding. Effects on septic morbidity after blunt and penetrating abdominal trauma, *Ann. Surg.*, 215, 503, 1992.
102. Moore, F.A., Moore, E.E., Jones, T.N., et al., TEN versus TPN following major abdominal trauma: reduced septic morbidity, *J. Trauma*, 29, 916, 1989.

103. Moore, F.A., Feliciano, D.V., Andrassy, R.J., et al., Early enteral feeding, compared with parenteral, reduces postoperative septic complications, the results of a meta-analysis, *Ann. Surg.*, 216, 172, 1992.
104. Yoo, B.K. and Frick, K.D., The instrumental variable method to study self-selection mechanism: a case of influenza vaccination, *Value Health*, 9, 114, 2006.
105. Ansaldi, F., Turello, V., Lai, P., et al., Effectiveness of a 23-valent polysaccharide vaccine in preventing pneumonia and non-invasive pneumococcal infection in elderly people: a large-scale retrospective cohort study, *J. Intern. Med. Res.*, 33, 490, 2005.
106. Peters, N.J., Meiklejohn, G., and Jahnigen, D.W., Antibody response of an elderly population to a supplemental dose of influenza B vaccine, *J. Am. Geriatr. Soc.*, 36, 593, 1988.
107. Hebert, P.L., Frick, K.D., Kane, R.L., et al., The causes of racial and ethnic differences in influenza vaccination rates among elderly Medicare beneficiaries, *Health Serv. Res.*, 40, 517, 2005.
108. Girodon, F., Lombard, M., Galan, P., et al., Effect of micronutrient supplementation on infection in institutionalized elderly subjects: a controlled trial, *Ann. Nutr. Metab.*, 41, 98, 1997.
109. Chandra, R.K., Nutrition and the immune system from birth to old age, *Eur. J. Clin. Nutr.*, 56, S73, 2002.
110. Miller, E.R., 3rd, Pastor-Barriuiso, R., Dalal, D., et al., Meta-analysis: high dosage vitamin E supplementation may increase all-cause mortality, *Ann. Intern. Med.*, 142, 37, 2005.
111. Chandra, R.K., Graying of immune system. Can nutrient supplements improve immunity in the elderly? *JAMA*, 227, 1398, 1997.
112. Bradley, J. and Xu, X., Diet, age, and the immune system, *Nutr. Rev.*, 54, S43, 1996.
113. Bogden, J.D., Oleske, J.M., Lavenhar, M.A., et al., Effect of one year of supplementation with zinc and other micronutrients on cellular immunity in the elderly, *J. Am. Coll. Nutr.*, 9, 214, 1990.
114. Castle, S.C., Impact of age-related immune dysfunction on risk of infections, *Z. Gerontol. Geriatr.*, 33, 341, 2000.
115. Meyandi, S.N., Vitamin E enhancement of T cell-mediated function in healthy elderly: mechanisms of action, *Nutr. Rev.*, 53, S52, 1995.
116. Meyandi, S.N. and Beharka, A.A., Recent developments in vitamin E and immune response, *Nutr. Rev.*, 56, S49, 1996.
117. Meyandi, S.N. et al., Vitamin E supplementation and *in vivo* immune response in healthy elderly subjects: a randomized controlled trial, *JAMA*, 227, 1380, 1997.
118. Graat, J.M., Schouten, E.G., and Kok, F.J., Effect of daily vitamin E and multivitamin-mineral supplementation on acute respiratory tract infections in elderly persons: a randomized controlled trial, *JAMA*, 288, 715, 2002.
119. Meydani, S.N., Han, S.N., and Hamer, D.H., Vitamin E and respiratory infection in the elderly, *Ann. N.Y. Acad. Sci.*, 1031, 214, 2004.
120. Bruunsgaard, H., Poulsen, H.E., Pedersen, B.K., et al., Long-term combined supplementations with alpha-tocopherol and vitamin C have no detectable anti-inflammatory effects in healthy men, *J. Nutr.*, 133, 1170, 2003.
121. Fairfield, K.M. and Fletcher, R.H., Vitamins for chronic disease prevention in adults: scientific review, *JAMA*, 287, 3116, 2002.
122. Fletcher, A.E., Breeze, E., and Shetty, P.S., Antioxidant vitamins and mortality in older persons: findings from the nutrition add-on study to the Medical Research Council Trial of Assessment and Management of Older People in the Community, *Am. J. Clin. Nutr.*, 78, 999, 2003.

123. Losonczy, K.G., Harris, T.B., and Havlik, R.J., Vitamin E and vitamin C supplement use and risk of all-cause and coronary heart disease mortality in older persons: the Established Populations for Epidemiologic Studies of the Elderly, *Am. J. Clin. Nutr.*, 64, 190, 1996.
124. Coulter, I.D., Hardy, M.L., Morton, S.C., et al., Antioxidants vitamin C and vitamin E for the prevention and treatment of cancer, *J. Gen. Intern. Med.*, 21, 735, 2006.
125. Zhao, X., Aldini, G., Johnson, E.J., et al., Modification of lymphocyte DNA damage by carotenoid supplementation in postmenopausal women, *Am. J. Clin. Nutr.*, 83, 163, 2006.
126. Hughes, D.A., Effects of carotenoids on human immune function, *Proc. Nutr. Soc.*, 58, 713, 1999.
127. Nouraie, M., Pietinen, P., Kamangar, F., et al., Fruits, vegetables, and antioxidants and risk of gastric cancer among male smokers, *Cancer Epidemiol. Biomarkers Prev.*, 14, 2087, 2005.
128. Corridan, B.M., Low-dose supplementation with lycopene or beta-carotene does not enhance cell-mediated immunity in healthy free-living elderly humans, *Eur. J. Clin. Nutr.*, 55, 627, 2001.
129. Watzl, B., Bub, A., Blockhaus, M., et al., Prolonged tomato juice consumption has no effect on cell-medicated immunity of well-nourished elderly men and women, *J. Nutr.*, 130, 1719, 2000.
130. Schabath, M.B., Spitz, M.R., Lerner, S.P., et al., Case-control analysis of dietary folate and risk of bladder cancer, *Nutr. Cancer*, 53, 144, 2005.
131. Strohle, A., Wolters, M., and Hahn, A., Folic acid and colorectal cancer prevention: molecular mechanisms and epidemiological evidence, *Int. J. Oncology*, 26, 1449, 2005.
132. Feigelson, H.S., Jonas, C.R., Robertson, A.S., et al., Alcohol, folate, methionine, and risk of incident breast cancer in the American Cancer Society Cancer Prevention Study II Nutrition Cohort, *Cancer Epidemiol. Biomarkers Prev.*, 12, 161, 2003.
133. Shen, H., Wei, Q., Pillow P.C., et al., Dietary folate intake and lung cancer risk in former smokers: a case-control analysis, *Cancer Epidemiol. Biomarkers Prev.*, 12, 980, 2003.
134. Drasch, G., Schopfer, J., and Schrauzer, G.N., Selenium/cadmium ratios in human prostates: indicators of prostate cancer risk of smokers and nonsmokers, and relevance to the cancer protective effects of selenium, *Biol. Trace Elem. Res.*, 103, 103, 2005.
135. Meyer, F., Falan, P., Douville, P., et al., Antioxidant vitamin and mineral supplementation and prostate cancer prevention in the SU.VI.MAX trial, *Int. J. Cancer*, 116, 182, 2005.
136. Rodriguez, C., Jacobs, E.J., Mondul, A.M., et al., Vitamin E supplements and risk of prostate cancer in U.S. men, *Cancer Epidemiol. Biomarkers Prev.*, 13, 378, 2004.
137. Trichopoulou, A., Costacou, T., Bamia, C., et al., Adherence to a Mediterranean diet and survival in a Greek population, *N. Engl. J. Med.*, 348, 2599, 2003.
138. D'Souza, A.L., Rajkumar, C., Cooke, J., et al., Probiotics in prevention of antibiotic associated diarrhoea: metaanalysis, *Br. Med. J.*, 324, 1361, 2002.
139. Cremonini, F., DeCaro, S., Nista, E.C., et al., Meta-analysis: the effect of probiotic administration on antibiotic-associated diarrhea, *Aliment Pharmacol. Ther.*, 16, 1461, 2002.
140. Gill, H.S. and Guarner, F., Probiotics and human health: a clinical perspective [review], *Postgrad. Med. J.*, 80, 516, 2004.
141. Gill, H.S., Rutherfurd, K.J., Cross, M.L., et al., Enhancement of immunity in the elderly by dietary supplementation with the probiotic *Bifidobacterium lactis* HN019, *Am. J. Clin. Nutr.*, 74, 833, 2001.

142. Spanhaak, S., Havenaar, R., and Schaafsma, G., The effect of consumption of milk fermented by *Lactobacillus casei* strain Shirota on the intestinal microflora and immune parameters in humans, *Eur. J. Clin. Nutr.*, 52, 899, 1998.
143. Yoon, H. et al., New insights in the validation of specific biomarkers for the evaluation of the immunoregulatory properties of milk fermented with yogurt culture *Lactobacillus casei* (ACTIMEL): a prospective trial, *Int. J. Immunother.*, 15, 79, 1999.
144. van den Heuvel, E.G., Schoterman, M.H., and Muijs, T., Transgalactooligosaccharides stimulate calcium absorption in post-menopausal women, *J. Nutr.*, 130, 2938, 2000.
145. Cashman, K., Prebiotics and calcium bioavailability, in *Probiotics and Prebiotics: Where Are We Going?* Tannock, G.W., Ed., Caister Academic Press, Wymondham, 2002, p. 149.
146. Woods, J.A., Lowder, T.W., and Keylock, K.T., Can exercise training improve immune function in the aged? *Ann. N.Y. Acad. Sci.*, 959, 117, 2002.
147. Nieman, D.C., Exercise immunology: future directions for research related to athletes, nutrition, and the elderly, *Int. J. Sports Med.*, 21, S61, 2000.
148. Kohut, M.L., Marian, L., Cooper, M.M., et al., Exercise and psychosocial factors modulate immunity to influenza vaccine in elderly individuals, *J. Gerontol. A. Biol. Sci. Med. Sci.*, 57, M557, 2002.
149. Kohut, M.L. and Senchina, D.S., Reversing age-associated immunosenescence via exercise, *Exerc. Immunol. Rev.*, 10, 6, 2004.
150. Kapasi, Z.F., Ouslander, J.G., Schnelle, J.F., et al., Effects of an exercise intervention on immunologic parameters in frail elderly nursing home residents, *J. Gerontol. A Biol. Sci. Med. Sci.*, 58, 636, 2003.
151. Chin, A., Paw, M.J., deJong, N., et al., Immunity in frail elderly: a randomized controlled trial of exercise and enriched foods, *Med. Sci. Sports Exerc.*, 32, 2005, 2000.
152. Phillips, A.C., Carroll, D., Burns, V.E., et al., Bereavement and marriage are associated with antibody response to influenza vaccination in the elderly, *Brain Behav. Immun.*, 20, 279, 2006.
153. Bartoloni, C., Guidi, L., Antico, L., et al., Psychological status and immunological parameters of institutionalized aged, *Panminerva Med.*, 33, 164, 1991.
154. Trzonkowski, P., Mysliwska, J., Godlewska, B., et al., Immune consequences of the spontaneous pro-inflammatory status in depressed elderly patients, *Brain Behav. Immun.*, 18, 135, 2004.
155. Castle, S., Wilkins, S., Heck, E., et al., Depression in caregivers of demented patients is associated with altered immunity: impaired proliferative capacity, increased CD8+, and a decline in lymphocytes with surface signal transduction molecules (CD38+) and a cytotoxicity marker (CD56+ CD8+), *Clin. Exp. Immunol.*, 101, 487, 1995.
156. Vedhara, K., McDermott, M.P., Evans, T.G., et al., Chronic stress in nonelderly caregivers: psychological, endocrine and immune implications, *J. Psychosomatic Res.* 53, 1153, 2002.
157. Knoops, K.T., deGroot, L.C., Kromhout, D., et al., Mediterranean diet, lifestyle factors and 10 year mortality in elderly European men and women, *JAMA*, 292, 1433, 2004.
158. Rimm, E.B. and Stampfer, M.J., Diet, lifestyle and longevity: the next steps? *JAMA*, 292, 1490, 2004.
159. Chandra, R.K., Effects of nutrition on the immune system, *Nutrition*, 10, 207, 1994.
160. Hubert, A.J., On the importance of fatty acid composition of membranes for aging, *J. Theor. Biol.*, 234, 277, 2005.
161. Wick, G., Huber, L.A., Xu, Q.B., et al., The decline of the immune response during aging: the role of an altered lipid metabolism, *Ann. N.Y. Acad. Sci.*, 621, 277, 1991.

162. Wick, G. and Grubeck-Lowenstein, B., Primary and secondary alterations of immune reactivity in the elderly: impact of dietary factors and disease, *Immunol. Rev.*, 160, 171, 1997.
163. Papathanassoglou, E., El-Haschimi, K., Li, XC, et al., Leptin receptor expression and signaling in lymphocytes: kinetics during lymphocyte activation, role in lymphocyte survival, and response to high fat diet in mice, *J. Immunol.*, 176, 7745, 2006.
164. Erol, A., PPARalpha activators may be good candidates as antiaging agents, *Med. Hypotheses*, 65, 35, 2005.
165. Israelian-Konaraki, A. and Reaven, P.D., Peroxisome proliferator-activated receptor-alpha and atherosclerosis: from basic mechanisms to clinical implications, *Cardiol. Rev.*, 13, 240, 2005.
166. Lovett-Racke, A.E., Hussain, R.Z., Northrop, S., et al., Peroxisome proliferator-activated receptor alpha agonists as therapy for autoimmune disease, *J. Immunol.*, 172, 5790, 2004.

7 Nutritional Requirements in Older Adults

David R. Thomas, M.D.

CONTENTS

7.1 INTRODUCTION

Food is essential to survival and health. Our ability to expend energy depends on adequate intake of protein and calories. Aging itself is associated with a lower energy intake. Hallfrisch et al.[1] have shown a decline in total daily energy requirements after age 40. Energy intake of older men (40 to 74 years old) is nearly a third less (2100 to 2300 calories/day) than that of men age 24 to 34 years old (2700 calories/day). On average, persons over the age of 70 years consume one third less calories than younger persons.[2] Sixteen to eighteen percent of community-dwelling elderly persons consume less than 1000 kcal daily.[3]

By the seventh decade, total energy intake decreases by 1000 to 1200 kcal in men and by 600 to 800 kcal in women. This results in concomitant decline in most nutrient intakes. Ten percent of men and twenty percent of women have intakes of protein below the Recommended Dietary Allowance (RDA); one third consume less calories than the RDA. Lower food intake among the elderly has been associated with lower intakes of calcium, iron, zinc, B vitamins, and vitamin E.[4] Fifty percent of older adults have a vitamin and mineral intake less than the RDA, while 10 to 30% have subnormal levels of vitamins and minerals.[5]

Older adults tend to consume less energy-dense sweets and fast foods, and consume more energy-dilute grains, vegetables, and fruits. The daily volume of foods and beverages also declines as a function of age. Physiological changes associated with age, including slower gastric emptying, altered hormonal responses, decreased basal metabolic rate, and altered taste and smell, may also contribute to lowered energy intake. Other factors, such as marital status, income, education, socioeconomic status, diet-related attitudes and beliefs, and convenience, likely play a role as well. Many age-related nutritional problems may be remedied to some extent by providing nutrient-dense meals through home delivery or meal congregate programs.[6] However, this low energy intake or low nutrient density of the diet may increase the risk of diet-related illnesses. Thus, even when adequate calories are available, nutritional deficiency diseases can occur.

Populations at high risk for inadequate vitamin intake include older persons, vegans, alcohol-dependent individuals, and patients with malabsorption syndromes.

7.2 RECOMMENDED DIETARY ALLOWANCES

The U.S. (and other governments) has established minimum levels of nutrient intakes. These levels are typically referred to as Recommended Dietary Allowances. The Recommended Dietary Allowances program was begun in 1941 by the Food and Nutrition Board. Nutrient requirements were expressed as a Recommended Dietary Allowance (RDA). The Recommended Dietary Allowances were based on the minimal requirement for 95% of the population based on a reference male, age 25, 5 feet 10 inches tall, 150 pounds, with a normal body composition.[7] No differential recommendations were made for persons older than 70 years due to higher prevalence of chronic disease, insufficient data, and heterogeneity of the population. Lower energy requirements were assumed for older persons, and adjustments for differences in sex after age 51 years were made.[10] The guidelines are revised every 10 years by the National Academy of Sciences as new evidence becomes available. It is important to realize that the RDA is not intended to be regarded as a daily requirement of a specific nutrient, since the body is able to store most nutrients.

The definition of a nutrient requirement depends to a great extent on the measured outcome. A level of a nutrient required to prevent a dietary deficiency does not imply that the level of intake is optimal. A minimum level aimed at preventing a deficiency may differ from a level aimed at preventing a specific disease. Additionally, the question of whether a supratherapeutic level of a nutrient may be beneficial is highly controversial.

Recently, there has been a shift in emphasis from the individual to the population group. As a result, the RDA has been replaced by Dietary Reference Intakes. The intent is to present dietary data aimed at preventing disease rather than simply preventing dietary deficiency. The Dietary Reference Intake (DRI) is based on four assumptions. First, the amount consumed is the minimal value that will meet the nutrient need of 50% of the population. Second, the level will prevent a deficiency of the nutrient in 98% of the population. Third, for those nutrients that do not have an RDA, an estimated Adequate Intake is presented. Finally, the Tolerable Upper Limit, which includes all sources of the nutrient, whether natural or supplemental, represents the estimated highest level of the nutrient that is likely to pose no risk to 98% of the population. Since the DRI is population based rather than individual based, these values do not represent a daily consumption goal.

As data have become available for older populations, the Dietary Reference Intakes have been updated to include older persons, and gender adjustments for persons older than 51 years have also been reported. Table 7.1 shows the contrast between the Recommended Daily Allowances for vitamins and minerals published in 1968 and the current Dietary Reference Intake (1997 to 2001) for the older population.

Considerable change in the recommendations has occurred with the availability of newer data. However, on the whole, the requirements for nearly all nutrients show little change with age compared to younger persons, despite a lower energy intake among older adults.[8]

7.3 MACRONUTRIENTS

7.3.1 CALORIES

Daily caloric requirements range from 25 kcal/kg/day for sedentary adults to 40 kcal/kg/day for elderly patients under moderate stress (see Table 7.2). Various formulas, including the Harris–Benedict equation, can be used to predict caloric requirements, but controversy exists over accuracy in obese or severely undernourished individuals.[9] Other formulas have been adjusted for severely stressed hospitalized subjects.[10]

TABLE 7.1
Comparison of Recommended Dietary Allowances and Daily Recommended Intakes for Vitamins and Minerals

Vitamin	RDA (1968)	DRI (1997–2001) Age 50–79	DRI (1997–2001) Age >70	Tolerable UL
Vitamin A	5000 IU	900 µg males; 700 µg females (3000 IU)	900 µg males; 700 µg females (3000 IU)	3000 µg (10,000 IU)
Vitamin C	60 mg	90 mg males; 75 mg females	90 mg males; 75 mg females	2000 mg
Vitamin D	400 IU	600 IU 10 µg/day	600 IU 15 µg/day	2000 IU
Vitamin E	20 mg	15 mg	15 mg	1000 mg
Vitamin K	80 mg	120 mg males; 90 mg females	120 mg males; 90 mg females	ND
Thiamine	1.5 mg	1.2 mg males; 1.1 mg females	1.2 mg males; 1.1 mg females	ND
Riboflavin	1.7 mg	1.3 mg males; 1.1 mg females	1.3 mg males; 1.1 mg females	ND
Niacin	20 mg	16 mg males; 14 mg females	16 mg males; 14 mg females	35 mg
Vitamin B6	2 mg	1.7 mg males; 1.5 mg females	1.7 mg males; 1.5 mg females	100 mg
Folate	400 mg	400 mg from food; 200 mg supplement	400 mg from food; 200 mg supplement	1000 mg synthetic
Vitamin B12	6 µg	2.4 µg	2.4 µg	ND
Biotin	300 mg	30 mg	30 mg	ND
Pantothenic acid	10 mg	5 mg	5 mg	ND
Choline	ND	550 mg males; 450 mg females	550 mg males; 450 mg females	3500 mg

Mineral				
Calcium	1000 mg	1200 mg	1200 mg	4000 mg
Iron	8 mg	8 mg	8 mg	45 mg
Phosphorous	1000 mg	700 mg	700 mg	3000 mg
Iodine	150 mg	150 mg	150 mg	1100 mg
Magnesium	400 mg	420 mg males; 350 mg females	420 mg males; 350 mg females	350 mg, supplement only
Zinc	15 mg	11 mg males; 8 mg females	11 mg males; 8 mg females	40 mg
Selenium	70 mg	55 mg	55 mg	400 mg
Copper	2 mg	2.3 mg	900 µg/day	10,000 µg/day
Chromium	120 mg	30 mg males; 20 mg females	30 mg males; 20 mg females	ND
Molybdenum	75 mg	45 mg	45 mg	2000 mg

Note: RDA = Recommended Daily Allowances, based on the highest 1968 RDA for nutrition labeling by the Food and Drug Administration; DRI = Dietary Reference Intake, based on the highest DRI by the Food and Nutrition Board, Institute of Medicine, 1997–2001; UL = Upper Limit, considered safe; ND = not determined, no adverse effects from higher intake.

Source: Adapted from *Dietary Reference Intakes for Calcium, Phosphorous, Magnesium, Vitamin D, and Fluoride* (1997); *Dietary Reference Intakes for Thiamin, Riboflavin, Niacin, Vitamin B6, Folate, Vitamin B12, Pantothenic Acid, Biotin, and Choline* (1998); *Dietary Reference Intakes for Vitamin C, Vitamin E, Selenium, and Carotenoids* (2000); and *Dietary Reference Intakes for Vitamin A, Vitamin K, Arsenic, Boron, Chromium, Copper, Iodine, Iron, Manganese, Molybdenum, Nickel, Silicon, Vanadium, and Zinc* (2001). Copyright 2001 by the National Academy of Sciences. Used with permission.

TABLE 7.2
Dietary Reference Intakes (DRIs): Recommended Intakes for Individuals, Macronutrients

	DRI (1997–2001) Age 50–79	DRI (1997–2001) Age >70
Total water	3.7 l males; 2.7 l females	3.7 l males; 2.7 l females
Carbohydrates	130 g	130 g
Fat	ND	ND
Protein[a]	56 g male; 46 g female	56 g male; 46 g female
Fiber	30 g male; 21 g female	30 g male; 21 g female

Note: DRI = Dietary Reference Intake, based on the highest DRI by the Food and Nutrition Board, Institute of Medicine, 1997–2001; ND = not determined, no adverse effects from higher intake.

[a] Based on 0.8 g/kg/day for adults.

Source: Adapted from *Dietary Reference Intakes for Energy, Carbohydrate, Fiber, Fat, Fatty Acids, Cholesterol, Protein, and Amino Acids* (2002). Copyright 2002 by the National Academy of Sciences. Used with permission.

7.3.2 Protein

Protein is the only nutrient containing nitrogen in addition to carbon, hydrogen, and oxygen. Some proteins also contains sulfur and phosphorus. These elements combine to form amino acids, the smallest molecular units of protein. Nine amino acids cannot be synthesized by humans and are therefore considered essential. These include histidine, leucine, isoleucine, lysine, methionine, phenylalanine, threonine, tryptophan, and valine. Protein is responsible for repair and synthesis of enzymes involved in cell multiplication, collagen and connective tissue synthesis, and wound healing. Protein is a component of antibodies needed for immune system function. Twenty to twenty-five percent of calories should be obtained from protein sources.

The current Dietary Reference Intake in adults for protein is 0.8 g/kg/day.[11] However, some older persons are not able to maintain a positive nitrogen balance at this level.[12] For older persons under moderate stress, the requirement is likely to be 1.0 to 1.2 g/day.

7.3.3 Carbohydrates

Carbohydrates provide energy and prevent gluconeogenesis from protein stores. Carbohydrate calories should comprise 50 to 60% of the patient's total caloric needs. An inadequate supply of carbohydrates results in muscle wasting (when the body is forced to convert protein stores for energy use) and loss of subcutaneous tissue. Complex carbohydrates are encouraged rather than simple sugars. Whole-grain breads, cereals, legumes, fruits, vegetables, and milk are good sources of carbohydrate.

7.3.4 Fat

Fat is the most concentrated source of energy and provides a reserve source of energy in the form of stored triglycerides in adipose tissue. Fat calories should comprise 20 to 25% of the total calories. The amount and composition of fat for optimum nutrition remain undefined and controversial. Lean meats, poultry, fish, low-fat dairy products, and vegetable oils are preferred sources of fat.

7.3.5 Fiber

Dietary fiber refers to nondigestible carbohydrates and ligin derived from plants. *Added fiber* consists of nondigestible carbohydrates incorporated into foods because they are thought to have a beneficial effect in humans. Total dietary fiber is the sum of dietary fiber and added fiber.

Dietary fiber has been proposed to have a beneficial effect on health, especially in prevention of heart disease, stroke, and some cancers. The evidence for this rests solely on epidemiological associations. An inverse association between whole-grain intake and risk of ischemic heart disease mortality was found in a survey of post-menopausal women. The relative risk was 0.70 in the highest quintile of whole cereal consumption (p for trend = 0.02).[13] A similar decrease in relative risk (RR) for coronary heart disease was observed in the Nurses Health Study for women, who reported a median fiber intake of 22.9 g/day, compared to women who reported a median intake of 11.5 g/day, but diminished when adjusted for risk factors (RR, 0.77; 95% confidence interval (CI), 0.57 to 1.04). Among different sources of dietary fiber (e.g., cereal, vegetables, fruit), only cereal fiber was strongly associated with a reduced risk of coronary heart disease (RR, 0.63; 95% CI, 0.49 to 0.81) for each 5 g/day increase in cereal fiber.[14]

The relationship of fiber from fruits and vegetables and heart disease has been inconsistent. In persons age 44 to 64 years, followed for 11 years, whole-grain intake was inversely associated with total mortality and incident CAD (p for trend = 0.02). An inverse association between fruit and vegetable intake and CAD was observed among African Americans, but not among whites. The risk of ischemic stroke was not significantly related to whole-grain, refined-grain, or fruit and vegetable consumption.[15]

No similar observation has been observed for the effect of fiber on colorectal cancer. In a pooled analysis of 13 prospective cohort studies, fiber intake from cereals, fruits, and vegetables was not associated with risk of colorectal cancer, after accounting for other dietary risk factors (RR, 0.94; 95% CI, 0.86 to 1.03).[16]Total dietary fiber for adults is 38 g/day for men and 25 g/day for women. After age 50, the dietary reference intake is decreased to 30 g/day for men and 21 g/day for women. This amount of fiber is often difficult for older adults to ingest.

7.4 VITAMINS

7.4.1 The Vitamin A and Carotenoid Family

The carotenoids are a diverse group of more than 600 naturally occurring pigments. Natural sources include yellow, orange, and red plant compounds, such as carrots and green leafy vegetables. Humans cannot synthesize carotenoids and depend on dietary intake exclusively for these micronutrients. Beta-carotene and lycopene are the major dietary carotenoids. Lycopene is a natural pigment synthesized by plants and microorganisms but not by animals. It occurs in the human diet predominantly in tomatoes and processed tomato products. It is a potent antioxidant and the most significant free radical scavenger in the carotenoid family. There is no known deficiency state for carotenoids themselves and no Recommended Daily Intake. Beta-carotene can be converted to vitamin A, whereas lycopene cannot. All of the carotenoids are antioxidants, and approximately 50 are considered vitamins because they have pro-vitamin A activity. Vitamin A refers to preformed retinol and the carotenoids that are converted to retinol. Preformed vitamin A is found only in animal products, including organ meats, fish, egg yolks, and fortified milk. More than 1500 synthetic retinoids, analogs of vitamin A, have been developed.

7.4.2 Vitamin C

Vitamin C (ascorbic acid) is a water-soluble vitamin widely found in citrus fruits and raw leafy vegetables, strawberries, melons, tomatoes, broccoli, and peppers. Humans cannot synthesize vitamin C and a deficiency results in scurvy.

7.4.3 Vitamin D

Vitamin D occurs naturally in animal foods as the provitamin cholecalciferol. This requires conversion in the kidney to the metabolically active form, calcitriol. Vitamin D is not a true vitamin, since humans are able to synthesize it with adequate sunlight exposure. By photoconversion, 7-dehydrocholesterol becomes previtamin D3, which is metabolized in the liver to 25-hydroxyvitamin D3, the major circulating form of vitamin D. In the kidney, this is converted to two metabolites, the more active one being 1,25-dihydroxyvitamin D3. Food sources include fortified milk, saltwater fish, and fish liver oil.

7.4.4 Vitamin E

Vitamin E occurs in eight natural forms as tocopherols (alpha, beta, gamma, and delta) and tocotrienols (alpha, beta, gamma, and delta), all of which possess potent antioxidant properties. Gamma-Tocopherol is the predominant form of vitamin E in the human diet, yet most studies have focused on alpha-tocopherol, which is the type found in most over-the-counter supplements. One reason for this is that alpha-tocopherol is biologically more active than gamma-tocopherol. Vitamin E deficiency is rare and is seen primarily in special situations resulting in fat malabsorption, including cystic fibrosis, chronic cholestatic liver disease, abetalipoproteinemia, and short bowel syndrome.

7.4.5 B Vitamins

The B-complex vitamins contain a number of different compounds. The B-complex vitamins are found in brewer's yeast, liver, whole-grain cereals, rice, nuts, milk, eggs, meats, fish, fruits, leafy green vegetables, and many other foods.

7.4.5.1 Thiamine (B1)

Deficiency of thiamine is associated with beriberi, a disease that is characterized by anemia, paralysis, muscular atrophy and weakness, and spasms in the muscles of the legs. Neurological effects of thiamine deficiency include Wernicke's encephelopathy, which causes lack of coordination, and Korsakoff's psychosis, which affects short-term memory. The mouth can also be affected by thiamine deficiency, increasing the sensitivity of the teeth, cheeks, and gums, as well as fissures in the lips. Thiamine deficiency is rare but often occurs in alcoholics, because alcohol interferes with the absorption of thiamine through the intestines.

7.4.5.2 Riboflavin (B2)

A deficiency of riboflavin can cause seborrheic dermatitis, angular cheilosis, and glossitis.

7.4.5.3 Niacin (B3)

Niacin, also known as nicotinic acid and nicotinamide, is needed for the metabolism of food and the maintenance of healthy skin, nerves, and the gastrointestinal tract. A deficiency of niacin causes pellagra. Historically, this disease was often associated with the very poor and was also a major cause of mental illness. The symptoms of pellagra are sometimes referred to as the three D's—diarrhea, dermatitis, and dementia—ultimately resulting in a fourth D, death. The mouth is also affected by pellagra, which can cause the inside of the cheeks and tongue to become red and painful.

7.4.5.4 Pyridoxine (B6)

Pyridoxine, also known as pyridoxal phosphate and pyridoxamine, is needed for the breakdown of carbohydrates, proteins, and fats, and is necessary for the production of red blood cells. Due to the abundance of pyridoxine in many foods, a deficiency is rare except in alcoholics. A pyridoxine deficiency causes dermatitis, glossitis, peripheral neuropathy, incoordination, confusion, and insomnia.

7.4.5.5 Folate (B9)

Folic acid, also known as folacin and pteroylglutamic acid, interacts with vitamin B12 for the synthesis of DNA and hemoglobin. Folic acid is essential to virtually all biochemical reactions that use a one-carbon transfer and is produced by bacteria in the stomach and intestines. A deficiency of folic acid causes anemia, poor growth, and glossitis—all of which are similar to symtoms suffered by those with B12 deficiency. Folic acid is present in nearly all natural foods but can be damaged during cooking. Deficiencies are found mainly in alcoholics and persons who are unable to absorb food due to topical sprue or gluten enteropathy.

7.4.5.6 Cyancobalimine (B12)

Vitamin B12 is necessary for processing carbohydrates, proteins, and fats, hemoglobin synthesis, and maintenance of nerve sheaths. Vitamin B12 acts as a coenzyme in the synthesis and repair of DNA. Vitamin B12 cannot be absorbed by the body until it is combined with a stomach mucoprotein called intrinsic factor. Once the B12 becomes bound to the intrinsic factor, it is able to pass into the small intestine to be absorbed and used by the body.

Food-cobalamin malabsorption is caused primarily by gastric atrophy. Over 40% of patients older than 80 years have gastric atrophy that may or may not be related to *Helicobacter pylori* infection. Other factors that contribute to food-cobalamin malabsorption in elderly people include antacids, including H2-receptor antagonists and proton pump inhibitors, surgery or gastric reconstruction (e.g., bypass surgery for obesity), intestinal bacterial overgrowth (which can be caused by antibiotic treatment), long-term ingestion of biguanides (metformin), chronic alcoholism, partial pancreatic exocrine failure, and Sjögren's syndrome.[17]

Vitamin B12 deficiency is sometimes seen in strict vegetarians who do not take vitamin supplements. Enough B12 is stored in the liver to sustain a person for about 3 years. A deficiency of B12 causes pernicious anemia. Pernicious anemia is an autoimmune disease characterized by the destruction of the gastric mucosa, especially fundal mucosa, by a primarily cell-mediated process. Gastric secretions are neutral to slightly acidic even in the presence of gastrin (which normally increases acidity) and contain little or no intrinsic factor. Pernicious anemia causes anemia, peripheral neuropathy, and glossitis. B12 deficiency can produce cognitive impairment.

Treatment of intake deficiency should include 1000 μg intramuscularly for 1 month, followed by 125 to 500 μg daily orally for dietary deficiency or 1000 μg daily orally for pernicious anemia.[18]

7.4.5.7 Pantothenic Acid (B5) and Biotin (B7)

Pantothenic acid is used in the breakdown of carbohydrates, lipids, and some amino acids, and also for the synthesis of coenzyme A. Biotin functions as a coenzyme in carboxylation reactions (–COOH). Intestinal bacteria produce both pantothenic acid and biotin. There is no known disorder associated with pantothenic acid deficiency. The vitamin is found in abundance in meats, legumes, and whole-grain cereals. Large doses of pantothenic acid can cause diarrhea.

A deficiency of biotin is rare but can cause a skin disorder called eczematous dermatitis. Biotin deficiency may be found in individuals who eat large quantities of egg whites. These contain avidin, which binds biotin. Biotin is found in beef liver, egg yolk, brewer's yeast, peanuts, cauliflower, and mushrooms.

7.5 MICRONUTRIENT MINERALS

Minerals are soil elements that cannot be made by living organisms. Plants obtain minerals from the soil, and most of the minerals in our diets come directly from plants. Animals provide minerals indirectly from plants. Minerals may also be present in a person's drinking water. The content of minerals in plants, animals, or water varies with geographic locale.

7.5.1 Iron

Iron is an integral part of many proteins and enzymes and is necessary for the synthesis of hemoblobin. Dietary iron exists in two forms: heme and nonheme. Heme iron is found in animal foods that originally contained hemoglobin, such as red meats, fish, and poultry. Iron in plant foods such as lentils and beans is arranged in a chemical structure called nonheme iron. Nonheme iron is the form added to iron-enriched and iron-fortified foods. Heme iron is absorbed better than nonheme iron, but most iron in a diet is nonheme iron. Absorption of heme iron ranges from 15 to 35% and is not significantly affected by diet. Only 2 to 20% of nonheme iron in plant foods such as rice, maize, black beans, soybeans, and wheat is absorbed.

The World Health Organization considers iron deficiency the number one nutritional disorder in the world. As many as 80% of the world's population may be iron deficient, while 30% may have iron deficiency anemia.[19] Iron deficiency anemia can be associated with low dietary intake of iron, inadequate absorption of iron, or excessive blood loss.

Supplemental iron is available in two forms: ferrous and ferric. Ferrous iron salts (ferrous fumarate, ferrous sulfate, and ferrous gluconate) are the best absorbed forms of iron supplements. The amount of iron absorbed decreases with increasing doses. For this reason, it is recommended that most people take their prescribed daily iron supplement in two or three equally spaced doses. For adults who are not pregnant, the Centers for Disease Control and Prevention (CDC) recommends taking 50 to 60 mg of oral elemental iron (the approximate amount of elemental iron in one 300-mg tablet of ferrous sulfate) twice daily for 3 months for the therapeutic treatment of iron deficiency anemia. Therapeutic doses of iron supplements, which are prescribed for iron deficiency anemia, may cause gastrointestinal side effects such as nausea, vomiting, constipation, diarrhea, dark-colored stools, and abdominal distress. Excess amounts of iron can result in toxicity and even death. Starting with half the recommended dose and gradually increasing to the full dose will help minimize these side effects. Taking the supplement in divided doses and with food also may help limit these symptoms. Iron from enteric-coated or delayed-release preparations may have fewer side effects, but is not as well absorbed and is not usually recommended.[20]

7.5.2 Calcium

Calcium is a major component of mineralized tissues and is required for normal growth and development of the skeleton and teeth. In men and women 65 years of age and older, calcium intake of less than 600 mg/day is common. Furthermore, intestinal calcium absorption is often reduced because of the effects of estrogen deficiency in women and the age-related reduction in renal 1,25-dihydroxy vitamin D production. Calcium insufficiency due to low calcium intake and reduced absorption can translate into an accelerated rate of age-related bone loss in older individuals. Vitamin D insufficiency is common among the homebound elderly and residents of long-term care facilities, and contributes to reduced calcium absorption. Calcium intake among women later in menopause, in the range of 1500 mg/day, may reduce the rates of bone loss in selected sites of the skeleton, such as the femoral neck.

The physiology of calcium homeostasis in aging men over 65 is similar to that of women with respect to the rate of bone loss, calcium absorption efficiency, declining vitamin D levels, and changes in markers of bone metabolism. It seems reasonable, therefore, to conclude that in aging men, as in aging women, prevailing calcium intakes are insufficient to prevent calcium-related erosion of bone mass. Thus, in women and men over 65, a calcium intake of 1500 mg/day seems prudent.[21]

Vitamin D metabolites enhance calcium absorption. 1,25-Dihydroxy vitamin D, the major metabolite, stimulates active transport of calcium in the small intestine and colon. Deficiency of 1,25-dihydroxy vitamin D, caused by inadequate dietary vitamin D, inadequate exposure to sunlight, impaired activation of vitamin D, or acquired resistance to vitamin D, results in reduced calcium absorption. In the absence of 1,25-dihydroxy vitamin D, less than 10% of dietary calcium may be absorbed. Vitamin D deficiency is associated with an increased risk of fractures. Elderly patients are at particular risk for vitamin D deficiency because of insufficient vitamin D intake from their diet, impaired renal synthesis of 1,25-dihydroxy vitamin D, and inadequate sunlight exposure, which is normally the major stimulus for endogenous vitamin D synthesis. This is especially evident in homebound or institutionalized individuals. Supplementation of vitamin D intake to provide 600 to 800 IU/day has been shown to improve calcium balance and reduce fracture risk in these individuals. Sufficient vitamin D intake should be ensured for all individuals, especially the elderly, who are at greater risk for development of a deficiency. Sources of vitamin D, besides supplements, include sunlight, vitamin D-fortified liquid dairy products, cod liver oil, and fatty fish. Calcium and vitamin D need not be taken together to be effective. Excessive doses of vitamin D may introduce risks such as hypercalciuria and hypercalcemia and should be avoided. Anticonvulsant medications may alter both vitamin D and bone mineral metabolism, particularly in certain disorders, in the institutionalized and the elderly. Although symptomatic skeletal disease is uncommon in noninstitutionalized settings, optimal calcium intake is advised for persons using anticonvulsants.

Immobilization has been shown to produce a rapid decrease in bone mass. This loss has been well documented in individuals placed on bed rest and in individuals with regional forms of immobilization, such as that seen in para- and quadriplegia. Under these circumstances, the rate of bone loss may be rapid, which is in part related to an increase in bone resorption accompanied by a decrease in bone formation. There is concern that increased calcium intake may increase the risk of hypercalcemia, ectopic calcification, ectopic ossification, and nephrolithiasis in these individuals. Thus, any recommendations for increasing calcium intake are tempered in these individuals by the potential for undesirable consequences.

Dairy products are the chief sources of dietary calcium (for example, approximately 250 to 300 mg/8 oz of milk). Individuals with lactose intolerance frequently limit or exclude liquid dairy foods, but adequate calcium intake can be achieved through low-lactose-containing solid dairy food or through milk rendered lactose deficient. Vegans who voluntarily limit their intake of dairy products can obtain dietary calcium through other sources. Other good food sources of calcium include some green vegetables (e.g., broccoli, kale, turnip greens, Chinese cabbage), calcium-set tofu, some legumes, canned fish, seeds, nuts, and certain fortified food products. Breads and cereals, while relatively low in calcium, contribute significantly to calcium intake because of their frequency of consumption.

A number of calcium-fortified food products are currently available, including fortified juices, fruit drinks, breads, and cereals. Although some of these foods provide multiple nutrients and may be frequently consumed, their quantitative contribution and role in the total diet are not currently defined.

7.5.3 Phosphorus

Phosphorus is essential for the process of bone mineralization. Approximately 85% of phosphorus in the adult body is in bone. Phospholipids are necessary for the structure of cellular membranes, nucleic acids, and nucleotides, including adenosine triphosphate. Sources of phosphorous, mainly in the form of phosphates, are widely distributed in the food supply, and phosphorus intake from the normal diet is usually sufficient. Milk and milk products are particularly rich sources of phosphorus, containing about 1000 mg of phosphorus per liter of milk. Deficiency of phosphorus occurs mainly in malabsorption syndromes, alcoholics and critically ill patients, diabetic ketoacidosis, and diseases resulting in renal tubular losses of phosphorus. The refeeding syndrome can cause hypophosphatemia, which may be life threatening. Hypophosphatemia may result in anorexia, impaired growth, osteomalacia, skeletal demineralization, proximal muscle atrophy and weakness, cardiac arrhythmias, respiratory insufficiency, increased erythrocyte and lymphocyte dysfunction, susceptibility to infectious rickets, nervous system disorders, and even death. Phosphate salts are used in the treatment of acute phosphorus deficiency. Supplements containing phosphorus are contraindicated in hyperphosphatemia and in severely impaired renal function (less than 30% of normal).

Calcium phosphate, which is mainly used as a delivery form of calcium, increases phosphate levels. Calcium phosphate is contraindicated in those with hypercalcemia. Potassium phosphate is contraindicated in persons with hyperkalemia. The most common adverse reaction with sodium or potassium phosphate is diarrhea. Diarrhea is less likely to occur in phosphorus-deficient individuals than in persons with normal phosphorus status. Nausea, vomiting, and abdominal pain may also occur. Hyperphosphatemia can result in ectopic calcification. Prolonged use of high doses of inorganic phosphate salts may result in hypocalcemia even in healthy individuals with normal renal function. Aluminum-containing antacids decrease the absorption of phosphates and can be used in the treatment of hyperphosphatemia. Concomitant intake of zinc and phosphate salts (sodium phosphate, potassium phosphate, calcium phosphate) may decrease the absorption of zinc.

7.5.4 Sodium and Potassium

Sodium is the primary electrolyte that regulates the extracellular fluid levels and hydration status. In addition to maintaining water balance, sodium is necessary for osmotic equilibrium, acid–base balance, and regulation of plasma volume, nerve impulses, and muscle contractions. The typical American diet contains between 3000 and 5000 mg daily, thus exceeding the requirement for health (500 mg/day). Some endurance training (exercising >2 hours in duration) may require increased sodium intake due to excessive sweat losses. Hypertensive individuals respond to limiting their sodium intake to less than 2400 mg daily (along with eating a low-fat diet rich in fruits, vegetables, whole grains, and low-fat dairy foods) for blood pressure management. Hypoatremia may also be due to excessive intake of fluid, especially in those experiencing renal insufficiency. Hypoatremia is characterized by lethargy, confusion, muscle twitching, seizures, and coma. Excessive consumption of sodium on a regular basis is often associated with hypertension and edema. High intakes of sodium can also lead to osteoporosis because sodium can increase urinary calcium losses.

Potassium plays a key role in cardiac, skeletal, and smooth muscle contraction, and in renal function. The best dietary sources of potassium are fresh unprocessed foods, including meats, fish, vegetables (especially potatoes), fruits (especially avocados, dried apricots, and bananas), citrus juices (such as orange juice), dairy products, and whole grains. Most potassium needs can be met by eating a varied diet with adequate intake of milk, meats, cereals, vegetables, and fruits. Potassium levels may be increased by a number of medications, including nonsteroidal anti-inflammatory drugs (NSAIDs; such as ibuprofen, piroxicam, and sulindac), angiotensinin-converting enzyme inhibitors (such as captopril, enalapril, and lisinopril, especially in conjunction with NSAIDs), potassium-sparing diuretics (such as spironolactone, triamterene, or amiloride), or salt substitutes, along with the ACE inhibitors, heparin, cyclosporine, trimethoprim, and beta-blockers (such as metoprolol and propranolol). Potassium levels may be decreased by other medications, including thiazide diuretics (such as hydrochlorothiazide), loop diuretics (such as furosemide and bumetanide), corticosteroids, amphotericin B, antacids, insulin, theophylline, and laxatives.

7.5.5 Magnesium

Magnesium is the fourth most abundant mineral in the body and approximately 50% of total body magnesium is found in bone. The other half is found predominantly inside cells of body tissues and organs. Only 1% of magnesium is found in serum. Magnesium is involved in more than 300 biochemical reactions in the body, including muscle and nerve function, cardiac rhythm, immune function, and bone formation. Magnesium also helps regulate blood sugar levels, blood pressure, and energy metabolism and protein synthesis. Dietary sources include green vegetables such as spinach, legumes (beans and peas), nuts and seeds, and whole, unrefined grains. Refined grains are generally low in magnesium. Drinking water can be a source of magnesium, but the amount varies according to the water supply. Water that naturally contains more minerals is described as hard. Hard water contains more magnesium than soft water.

Approximately one third to one half of dietary magnesium is absorbed into the body. Gastrointestinal disorders that impair absorption, such as Crohn's disease, can limit the body's ability to absorb magnesium. Chronic or excessive vomiting and diarrhea may also result in magnesium depletion. Excretion by the kidneys can limit urinary excretion of magnesium to compensate for low dietary intake. Excessive loss of magnesium in urine can occur in renal disease, as a side effect of some medications, in cases of poorly controlled diabetes, and in alcohol abuse. Early signs of magnesium deficiency include loss of appetite, nausea, vomiting, fatigue, and weakness. Late magnesium deficiency demonstrates hypocalcemia, hypokalemia, numbness, tingling, muscle contractions and cramps, seizures, personality changes, abnormal heart rhythms, and coronary spasms.

Magnesium may influence the release and activity of insulin.[13] Low blood levels of magnesium (hypomagnesemia) are frequently seen in individuals with type 2 diabetes. Hypomagnesemia may worsen insulin resistance, a condition that often precedes diabetes, or may be a consequence of insulin resistance. Individuals with insulin resistance do not use insulin efficiently and require greater amounts of insulin to maintain blood sugar within normal levels. The kidneys possibly lose their ability to retain magnesium during periods of severe hyperglycemia (significantly elevated blood glucose). The increased loss of magnesium in urine may then result in lower blood levels of magnesium. In older adults, correcting magnesium depletion may improve insulin response and action.[28]

Several clinical studies have examined the potential benefit of supplemental magnesium on metabolic control of type 2 diabetes. In one such study, 63 subjects with below-normal serum magnesium levels received either 2.5 g of oral magnesium chloride daily "in liquid form" (providing 300 mg of elemental magnesium per day) or a placebo. At the end of the 16-week study period, those who received the magnesium supplement had higher blood levels of magnesium and improved metabolic control of diabetes, as suggested by lower hemoglobin A1C levels, than those who received a placebo.[22]

In another study, 128 patients with poorly controlled type 2 diabetes were randomized to receive a placebo or a supplement with either 500 mg or 1000 mg of magnesium oxide (MgO) for 30 days. All patients were also treated with diet or diet plus oral medication to control blood glucose levels. Magnesium levels increased in the group receiving 1000 mg of magnesium oxide per day (equal to 600 mg of elemental magnesium per day) but did not significantly change in the placebo group or the group receiving 500 mg of magnesium oxide per day (equal to 300 mg of elemental magnesium per day). However, neither level of magnesium supplementation significantly improved blood glucose control.[23]

7.5.6 Zinc

Zinc is involved in the activity of approximately 100 enzymes, in the immune system, and in DNA synthesis, and maintains the sense of taste and smell. The cheif dietary source of zinc is red meat and poultry. Oysters contain more zinc per serving than any other food. Other good food sources include beans, nuts, certain seafood, whole grains, fortified breakfast cereals, and dairy products. Absorption of zinc is greater from animal protein sources than plant proteins. Phytates, which are found in whole-grain breads, cereals, legumes, and other products, can decrease zinc absorption. There is no single laboratory test that adequately measures zinc nutritional status.[24] Risk factors for zinc deficiency include inadequate caloric intake, alcoholism, gastrointestinal surgery, malabsorption (such as sprue, Crohn's disease, and short bowel syndrome), and chronic diarrhea. Zinc toxicity has been seen associated with low copper status, altered iron function, reduced immune function, and reduced levels of high-density lipoproteins.

7.5.7 Copper

Copper is required in the formation of hemoglobin, elastin, and collagen. Copper is necessary for the manufacture of the neurotransmitter noradrenaline as well as for the pigmentation of hair. Copper is available from a variety of foods, such as whole grain, liver, molasses, and nuts, but water from copper pipes is a source of copper, and copper cooking utensils will also increase copper ingestion. It can be stored in the body, and daily presence in the diet is therefore not necessary. Deficiency of copper is associated with iron deficiency and with excess zinc. Copper deficiency has been associated with anemia, increased likelihood for infections, osteoporosis, thyroid gland dysfunction, heart disease, and abnormal nervous system function. Toxic levels may lead to diarrhea, vomiting, liver damage, and discoloration of the skin and hair, while mild excesses may result in fatigue, irritability, depression, and loss of concentration and learning disabilities.

7.5.8 Chromium

Chromium stimulates fatty acid and cholesterol synthesis, is an activator of several enzymes, and is also thought to be important in insulin metabolism. Rats fed a torula yeast-based diet developed abnormal glucose tolerance that could be reversed by supplements of brewer's yeast. Trivalent chromium ($CrCl_3$) was found to be the active factor in brewer's yeast. Further, it was reported that chromium formed a complex with insulin that enhanced insulin's activity. However, the relevance of animal studies of chromium deficiency to the effects of chromium in humans remains controversial.

Dietary sources of chromium include beef, liver, eggs, chicken, oysters, wheat germ, green peppers, apples, bananas, and spinach. The best source of chromium is brewer's yeast, but many people do not use it because it causes abdominal distention (a bloated feeling) and nausea. Black pepper, butter, and molasses are also good sources of chromium, but they are normally consumed only in small amounts.

7.5.9 Selenium

Selenoproteins have antioxidant properties that help prevent cellular damage from free radicals. Free radicals may contribute to the development of chronic diseases such as cancer and heart disease. Other selenoproteins help regulate thyroid function and play a role in the immune system. The dietary content of selenium depends on the selenium content of the soil where plants are grown or animals are raised. However, food distribution patterns across the U.S. help prevent people living in low-selenium geographic areas from having low dietary selenium intakes. Results of the National Health and Nutrition Examination Survey (NHANES III, 1988–1994) indicated that diets of most Americans provide the recommended amounts of selenium.[25] In the U.S., most cases of selenium depletion or deficiency are associated with severe gastrointestinal problems, such as Crohn's disease, or with surgical removal of part of the stomach.

7.6 SUMMARY

Many older persons have intakes of protein and calories below the daily recommended intake. Lower food intake among the elderly has been associated with lower intakes of calcium, iron, zinc, B vitamins, and vitamin E. Fifty percent of older adults have a vitamin and mineral intake less than the daily recommended intake, while 10 to 30% have subnormal levels of vitamins and minerals.

Evidence of epidemiological associations of vitamins and disease states has been found for nine vitamins. Inadequate folate status is associated with neural tube defect and some cancers. Folate and vitamins B6 and B12 are required for homocysteine metabolism and are associated with coronary heart disease risk. Vitamin E and lycopene may decrease the risk of prostate cancer. Vitamin D is associated with decreased occurrence of fractures when taken with calcium.[26] Zinc, beta-carotene, and vitamin E appear to slow the progression of macular degeneration, but do not reduce the incidence.

In observational studies (case-control or cohort design), people with high intake of antioxidant vitamins by regular diet or as food supplements generally have a lower risk of myocardial infarction and stroke than people who are low consumers of antioxidant vitamins. The associations in observation studies have been shown for carotene, ascorbic acid, and tocopherol. In randomized controlled trials, however, antioxidant vitamins as food supplements have no beneficial effects in the primary prevention of myocardial infarction and stroke.[27]

Serious adverse events have been reported. Toxicity may result from excessive doses of vitamin A during early pregnancy and from fat-soluble vitamins taken anytime. After an initial enthusiasm for antioxidants in the secondary prevention of cardiovascular disease, recent reports from several large randomized trials have failed to show any beneficial effects. Thus, the apparent beneficial results of high intake of antioxidant vitamins reported in observational studies have not been confirmed in large randomized trials.[29]

The use of various dietary supplements, including vitamins, to prevent or delay disease or aging rests for the most part on epidemiological associations. It does appear from this data that a diet rich in vitamins is associated with a tendency to improved health. However, the results from controlled trials are dismal. The discrepancies between different types of studies are probably explained by the fact that dietary composition and supplement use are components in a cluster of healthy behavior. An alternative hypothesis is that there are as yet unknown essential organic compounds in certain foods.

The most prudent approach is to recommend a daily intake of fruits and vegetables as a likely source of essential nutrients. Failing compliance with a natural source of essential nutrients, and in populations at high risk of vitamin deficiency, vitamin supplements should be encouraged.

REFERENCES

1. Hallfrisch J, Muller D, Drinkwater D, Tobin J, Andres R. Continuing diet trends in men: the Baltimore Longitudinal Study of Aging (1961–1987). *J Gerontol* 1990;45:M186–M191.
2. McGandy RB, Barrows CH Jr, Spanias A, Meredity A, Stone JL, Norris AH. Nutrient intake and energy expenditure in men of different ages. *J Gerontol* 1966;21:581–587.
3. Abraham S, Carroll MD, Dresser CM, et al. *Dietary Intake of Persons 1–74 Years of Age in the United States*, Advance Data from Vital and Health Statistics of the National Center for Health Statistics No. G. Rockville, MD, Public Health Service, March 30, 1977.
4. Wakimoto P, Block G. Dietary intake, dietary patterns, and changes with age: an epidemiological perspective. *J Gerontol A Biol Sci Med Sci* 2001;56:65–80.
5. Ritchie CR, Thomas DR. Aging. In *Handbook of Clinical Nutrition*, 3rd ed., Heimburger DC, Weinsier RL, Eds. Mosby, St. Louis, 1997.
6. Drewnowski A, Shultz JM. Impact of aging on eating behaviors, food choices, nutrition, and health status. *J Nutr Health Aging* 2001;5:75–79.
7. Food and Nutrition Board, National Research Council. *Recommended Dietary Allowances*, 10th ed. National Academy Press, Washington, DC, 1990.
8. Munro HN, Suter PM, Russel RM. Nutritional requirements of the elderly. *Ann Rev Nutr* 1987;7:23–49.
9. Choban PS, et al. Nutrition support of obese hospitalized patients. *Nutr Clin Pract* 1997;12:14–154.
10. Ireton-Jones CS. Evaluation of energy expenditures in obese patients. *Nutr Clin Pract* 1989;4:127–129.
11. National Research Council. *Recommended Dietary Allowances*, 10th ed. National Academy Press, Washington, DC, 1989.
12. Campbell WW, Trappe TA, Wolfe RR, Evans WJ. The recommend dietary allowance for protein may not be adequate for older people to maintain skeletal muscle. *J Gerontol A Biol Sci Med Sci* 2001;56:M373–M380.
13. Jacobs DR Jr, Meyer KA, Kushi LH, Folsom AR. Whole-grain intake may reduce the risk of ischemic heart disease death in postmenopausal women: the Iowa Women's Health Study. *Am J Clin Nutr* 1998;68:248–257.
14. Wolk A, Manson JE, Stampfer MJ, Colditz GA, Hu FB, Speizer FE, Hennekens CH, Willett WC. Long-term intake of dietary fiber and decreased risk of coronary heart disease among women. *JAMA* 1999;281:1998–2004.
15. Steffen LM, Jacobs DR Jr, Stevens J, Shahar E, Carithers T, Folsom AR. Associations of whole-grain, refined-grain, and fruit and vegetable consumption with risks of all-cause mortality and incident coronary artery disease and ischemic stroke: the Atherosclerosis Risk in Communities (ARIC) Study. *Am J Clin Nutr* 2003;78:383–390.

16. Park Y, Hunter DJ, Spiegelman D, Bergkvist L, Berrino F, van den Brandt PA, Buring JE, Colditz GA, Freudenheim JL, Fuchs CS, Giovannucci E, Goldbohm RA, Graham S, Harnack L, Hartman AM, Jacobs DR Jr, Kato I, Krogh V, Leitzmann MF, McCullough ML, Miller AB, Pietinen P, Rohan TE, Schatzkin A, Willett WC, Wolk A, Zeleniuch-Jacquotte A, Zhang SM, Smith-Warner SA. Dietary fiber intake and risk of colorectal cancer: a pooled analysis of prospective cohort studies. *JAMA* 2005;294:2849–2857.
17. Andrès E, Loukili NH, Noel E, Kaltenbach G, Ben Abdelgheni M, Perrin AE, et al. Vitamin B12 (cobalamin) deficiency in elderly patients. *CMAJ* 2004;171:251–259.
18. Andrès E, Noel E, Kaltenbach G. Treatment of vitamin B12 deficiency anemia: oral versus parenteral therapy. *Ann Pharmacother* 2002;36:1810.
19. Stoltzfus RJ. Defining iron-deficiency anemia in public health terms: reexamining the nature and magnitude of the public health problem. *J Nutr* 2001;131:565S–567S.
20. Disorders of iron metabolism: iron deficiency and overload. In *Hematology: Basic Principles and Practice*, 3rd ed., Hoffman R, Benz E, Shattil S, Furie B, Cohen H, Silberstein L, McGlave P, Eds. Churchill Livingstone, Harcourt Brace & Co., New York, 2000, chap. 26.
21. *Optimal Calcium Intake*, NIH Consensus Statement. June 6–8, 1994, 12:1–31.
22. Rodriguez-Moran M, Guerrero-Romero F. Oral magnesium supplementation improves insulin sensitivity and metabolic control in type 2 diabetic subjects. *Diabetes Care* 2003;26:1147–1152.
23. De Lourdes Lima M, Cruz T, Pousada JC, Rodrigues LE, Barbosa K, Canguco V. The effect of magnesium supplementation in increasing doses on the control of type 2 diabetes. *Diabetes Care* 1998;21:682–686.
24. Van Wouwe JP. Clinical and laboratory assessment of zinc deficiency in Dutch children. A review. *Biol Trace Elem Res* 1995;49:211–225.
25. Bialostosky K, Wright JD, Kennedy-Stephenson J, McDowell M, Johnson CL. *Dietary Intake of Macronutrients, Micronutrients and Other Dietary Constituents: United States 1988–94, Vital Health Statistics 11*. National Center for Health Statistics, 2002.
26. Fairfield KM, Fletcher RH. Vitamins for chronic disease prevention in adults: scientific review. *JAMA* 2002;287:3116–3126.
27. Asplund K. Antioxidant vitamins in the prevention of cardiovascular disease: a systematic review. *J Intern Med* 2002;251:372–392.
28. Laires MJ, Moreira H, Monteiro CP, Sardinha L, Limao F, Veiga L, Conclaves A, Ferreira A, Bieho M. Magnesium, insulin resistance and body composition in healthy potmenopausal women. *J Amer Coll Nutr* 2004;23:510–513S.
29. Thomas DR. Vitamins in health and aging. *Clinics in Geriatric Med* 2004;20: 259–74.

8 Energy Balance

John E. Morley, M.B., B.Ch.

CONTENTS

Maintenance of energy balance is an extraordinarily complex process. In its simplest form it can be considered that body weight (BW) = food intake (FT) – total energy expenditure (TEE) (Figure 8.1). TEE consists of resting metabolic rate (RMR), activity-related energy expenditure (AEE) (a combination of exercise and spontaneous physical activity, or SPA), and thermic energy of eating. Food intake is modulated by malabsorption and excretion of calories. With aging there are physiological alterations in both food intake and total energy expenditure. To some extent these changes can be predicted due to the loss of muscle mass (sarcopenia) that occurs during aging. In older persons, nearly one half will have a chronic disease or physical disability, which will further modulate energy balance. Finally, dramatic changes in energy balance occur when an older person develops an acute illness. In this instance, cytokines produce "sickness behavior" with a reduction in SPA but an increase in RMR.

While caloric restriction has been suggested as a way to extend life span as encapsulated by the concept that one should eat to live, rather than live to eat, it has become clear that prolonged underfeeding is perhaps more dangerous than overfeeding in older persons. With aging, many normal-weight healthy older men and women reduce their energy intake below their energy expenditure and thus lose weight.[1]

FOOD INTAKE = TOTAL ENERGY EXPENDITURE
(RMR + Physical Activity + TEE)

AGE EFFECT % OF DAILY ENERGY EXPENDITURE ← ALL DECREASED →

60–70% + 15–30% + 8–12% + 2–3%

FIGURE 8.1 Effects of aging on energy balance. RMR = resting metabolic rate; TEE = thermic energy of eating.

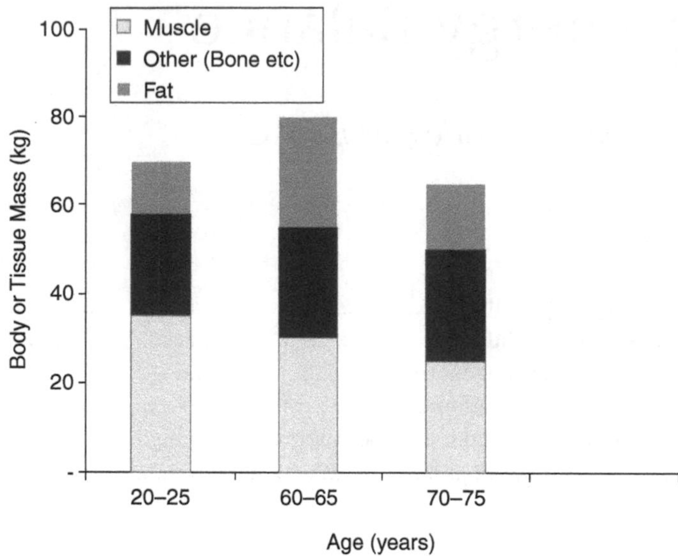

FIGURE 8.2 Changes in body mass with aging.

Loss of weight in older persons is associated with frailty, functional impairment, poor quality of life, and increased mortality. Overall, the physiological changes in body mass over the life span can be represented as a gain in weight from 30 to 60 years of age (mainly fat mass) and a loss of weight (due to loss of muscle, bone, and fat) after 70 years of age[2] (Figure 8.2).

8.1 TOTAL ENERGY EXPENDITURE

As might be expected, TEE deceases with aging.[3–5] In older persons, TEE is lower in women and in blacks.[6] This decrease was shown with double-labeled water, and thus we can be fairly confident that these findings apply to free-living persons and are not just confined to data for those living under experimental conditions in a metabolic chamber. A caveat to these findings is that these techniques have a large coefficient of variation. Because a 1% change in energy expenditure over a decade can result in major changes in body mass, it needs to be recognized that, with present techniques, data on TEE need to be interpreted with caution. While there is a high level of confidence that TEE declines with aging, present techniques do not allow us to determine if this is true in highly healthy groups of physically active elderly and the effect of long-term interventions on TEE.

8.2 RESTING METABOLIC RATE

The RMR is the energy cost of maintaining basal physiological functions. These include muscle tone, involuntary muscle activity, cardiopulmonary function, and the biochemical activities necessary to maintain homeostasis. The RMR is predominantly due to lean muscle mass basal activity. As such, it is higher in men than in women. However, this difference between the sexes cannot be completely explained by the difference in lean body mass.[6] In older males, but not females, blacks have a lower RMR, which again cannot be completely accounted for by the differences in free fat mass (FFM).

Basal metabolic rate (BMR) is the highly controlled RMR measure 12 to 14 hours after the last meal, at complete rest, while lying down and at a neutral environmental temperature. The BMR accounts for 60 to 65% of the TEE and is approximately 1500 kcal/day.

With aging there is a decline in the RMR.[6–9] This decrease is partly, but not completely, due to reduced free fatty mass. Intrinsic reduction of RMR is partly because of a decline in the N + K + ATPase activity, the decline in muscle protein turnover, and changes in mitochondrial membrane proton permeability.[10,11] Exercise results in an increase in RMR. The effects of disease in older persons with malnutrition have led to inconclusive results, with some suggesting that RMR may be elevated but the majority failing to show this.[1] In elderly nursing home patients, the RMR was 1174 kcal/day (29.3 kcal/kg FFM/day). This was lower than the overall range of 1131 to 1472 kcal/day reported in free-living elderly women.[12] Similarly, in patients with Alzheimer's disease there is a decline in RMR.[1] RMR increases in Parkinson's disease, but TEE drops because of the marked decrease in physical activity.[13] RMR did not increase in chronic obstructive pulmonary disease.[14] It is important to recognize that there is larger interindividual variation in RMR with aging.

A number of equations are available to predict RMR, such as the Harris–Benedict, WHO, or Schofield, and a standard calculation of 20 kcal/kg/day. The Harris–Benedict and Schofield tend to underpredict and the WHO equation overpredicts the RMR. Because of the large heterogeneity in older persons, these equations need to be used with caution. The ability of the equations to predict RMR can be improved by multiplying the derived RMR by 1.52 for persons of below-average physical activity, 1.67 for average physical activity, and 1.85 for persons of above-average physical activity.[6]

8.3 MEAL-INDUCED THERMOGENESIS

Following a meal, there is an increase in metabolic rate for about 6 hours. This increase is called meal-induced thermogenesis or the thermic effect of eating. Fat produces a lower effect on metabolic rate than does carbohydrate or protein. Meal-induced thermogenesis accounts for approximately 10% of energy utilization.

Overall, there appears to be a small decrease in the thermic effect of eating in older persons.[15] This decline in peak thermogenesis may be due to delayed gastric emptying in older persons when large meals are ingested. Other reasons for the change in adaptive thermogenesis in older persons are the decline in beta-adrenergic activity and insulin resistance.

8.4 PHYSICAL ENERGY EXPENDITURE

Functional status tends to predict energy expenditure in older persons. Overall, with aging there is a decrease in physical activity level. This appears to be due to both a decrease in exercise and a decrease in spontaneous physical activity. Recently it has been recognized that spontaneous physical activity plays an important role in maintaining body weight and physical fitness.

8.5 REGULATION OF FOOD INTAKE AND THE ANOREXIA OF AGING

The concept that there is a physiological decline in food intake over the ages of 20 to 80 years is now well accepted.[16,17] This has been termed the anorexia of aging and appears to be an appropriate response to the decline in physical activity that occurs over the life span.[18] This decline is due to both a reduction in intermeal snacking and early satiation that occurs in response to large meals.[19] Eating alone can further reduce the total amount of food ingested. While the overall change with aging is a decrease in food intake, Roberts et al.[20] have shown that the major change with food intake with aging is really a dysregulation (dysorexia). When older men and women are overfed, they are less capable of decreasing their food intake to return to their previous weight than are younger men and women. Similarly, older persons who were underfed continued to eat less and failed to regain their lost weight.

With aging there is an increase in taste threshold and a decline in the ability to detect odors.[21,22] The exact effect of these changes on food ingestion is controversial. Overall, it would appear that these changes account for about 100 kcal/day of the decline in food intake that occurs with aging, i.e., about 20% of the total decline in food intake.

Appetite regulation is a highly controlled process.[23] It is set so that the person will acquire slightly more food than needed so that there are sufficient energy stores to allow survival during time of famine. The major component of this system is the central feeding drive. The central feeding drive system is situated in the hypothalamus that receives input from the cortex, the amygdala, and other parts of the limbic system and a large number of inputs from the periphery. The multiple anatomical components of the hypothalamus interact with the midbrain to generate the feeding drive.

The central control of feeding is integrated by a number of orexigenic neurotransmitters, such as orexin neuropeptide Y, dynorphin, and norepinephrine. These orexigenic neurotransmitters are downregulated by large numbers of anorectic neurotransmitters such as serotonin, corticotrophin-releasing factor, and the melanocortins (alpha-MSH). The local cellular communication of these neurotransmitters appears to depend on nitric oxide.[24] While some animal studies have suggested small alternations in this system with aging, no data in humans confirm an important role for this hypothalamic system in the development of the anorexia of aging.

The central feeding drive system receives multiple inputs from the periphery providing information on the amount of food in the gastrointestinal tract, the state of adipose stores, and the availability of circulating nutrients. These messages are conveyed by ascending fibers of the autonomic nervous system, circulating hormones, and the availability of circulating nutrients. These systems are further modulated by endogenous steroid hormones. For example, increasing progesterone during pregnancy leads to an increase in food intake. A fall in testosterone during aging in males leads to an increase in the anorexic hormone, leptin, and a decrease in estrogen at menopause in females leads to an increase in food intake. Cytokines, produced in excess during illness, are potent anorexic agents.[25]

The gastrointestinal tract appears to be a major system involved in the pathogenesis of the physiological anorexia of aging.[26] Food entering the stomach releases nitric oxide from the wall of the fundus, resulting in smooth muscle relaxation to allow a large meal to be stored in the fundus. With aging there appears to be a decrease in the production of nitric oxide, and therefore a diminished capacity of the fundus to undergo adaptive relaxation. This results in food more rapidly entering the antrum of the stomach and producing antral stretch, leading to satiation signals being transmitted through ascending fibers of the vagus to the nucleus tractus solitarius, and from there to the hypothalamus.

Ghrelin is a peptide hormone produced by the fundus of the stomach. It crosses the blood–brain barrier and directly stimulates food intake and growth hormone release. The effect of aging on its level is controversial, and it does not appear to play a major role in the anorexia of aging.

There is evidence that slowed stomach emptying of large meals is important in producing the early satiety seen in many older persons.[27] When fatty or protein foods reach the duodenum, they release cholecystokinin (CCK), which plays an important role in satiation. CCK levels rise with aging, particularly after a high-fat meal, and CCK is a more potent anorectic agent in older persons.[28] Thus, CCK appears to play a central role in the anorexia of aging. Other anorectic peptides, such as glucagon-like peptide I, do not appear to be altered with aging.

Leptin is one of a number of peptide hormones produced from adipose cells. Leptin is a potent anorectic agent, and lack of leptin or its receptor in young children leads to obesity. Leptin resistance is present in middle-aged obese persons. This appears to be due to the fact that hypertriglyceridemia inhibits the ability of leptin to cross the blood–brain barrier into the central nervous system.[29] As alluded to, declining testosterone levels in males lead to increased leptin levels, and this is a convenient explanation for the greater degree of anorexia that occurs in males than in females with aging.[30]

While much has been written about the role of insulin as an appetite inhibitor in animals, in humans insulin infusion has no effect on appetite when glucose levels are maintained at a steady state.[31] Insulin given to humans in high doses invariably results in hyperphagia and weight gain.

To conclude, regulation of appetite is a complex process. The anorexia of aging appears to be an appropriate response to the decline in TEE that occurs with aging. Unfortunately, this dysregulation of the appetite process sets older persons up to develop severe anorexia when they become ill. Figure 8.3 summarizes the major factors involved in the anorexia of aging.

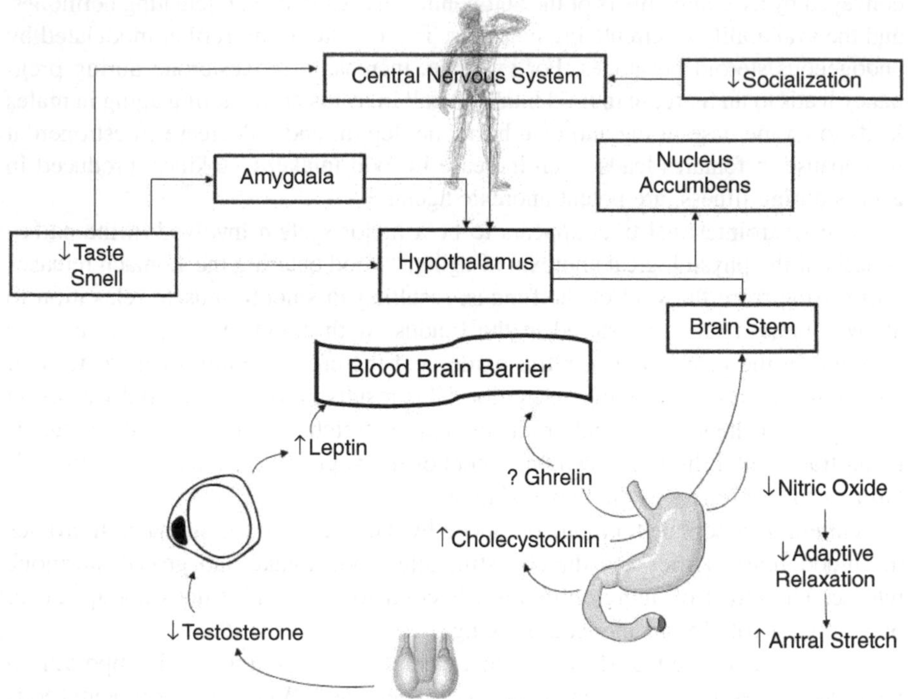

FIGURE 8.3 Factors involved in the anorexia of aging.

REFERENCES

1. Wilson, M.M. and Morley, J.E., Physiology of aging: invited review: aging and energy balance, *J. Appl. Physiol.*, 95, 1728, 2003.
2. Steen, B., Body composition and aging, *Nutr. Rev.*, 46, 45, 1988.
3. Delany, J.P. and Lovejoy, J.C., Energy expenditure, *Endocrinol. Metab. Clin. North Am.*, 25, 831, 1996.
4. Roberts, S.B., Use of the doubly labeled water method for measurement of total energy expenditure, total body water, and metabolizable energy intake in humans and small animals, *Can. J. Physiol. Pharmacol.*, 67, 1198, 1989.
5. Schoeller, D.A., Kushner, R.F., and Jones, P.J., Validation of doubly labeled water for measuring energy expenditure during parenteral nutrition, *Am. J. Clin. Nutr.*, 44, 291, 1986.
6. Blanc, S., Schoeller, D.A., Bauer, D., et al., Energy requirements in the eighth decade of life, *Am. J. Clin. Nutr.*, 79, 303, 2004.
7. Fukagawa, N.K., Bandini, L.G., and Young, J.B., Effect of age on body composition and resting metabolic rate, *Am. J. Physiol.*, 259, E233, 1990.
8. Visser, M., Deurenberg, P., vanStaveren, W.A., et al., Resting metabolic rate and diet-induced thermogenesis in young and elderly subjects: relationship with body composition, fat distribution, and physical activity level, *Am. J. Clin. Nutr.*, 61, 772, 1995.
9. Vaughan, L., Zurlo, F., and Ravussin, E., Aging and energy expenditure, *Am. J. Clin. Nutr.*, 53, 821, 1991.

10. Glick, Z., Energy balance, in *Geriatric Nutrition*, 2nd ed., Morley, J.E., Glick, Z., and Rubenstein, L.Z., Eds., Raven Press, New York, 1995, p. 15.
11. Simat, B.M., Morley, J.E., Frome, A.H., et al., Variables affecting measurements of human red cells Na+, K+, ATPase activity: technical factors, feeding, aging, *Am. J. Clin. Nutr.*, 40, 339, 1984.
12. Lammes, E. and Akner, G., Resting metabolic rate in elderly nursing home patients with multiple diagnoses, *J. Nutr. Health Aging*, 10, 263, 2006.
13. Toth, M.J., Fishman, P.S., and Poehlman, E.T., Free living daily energy expenditure in patients with Parkinson's disease, *Neurology*, 48, 88, 1997.
14. Tang, N.L., Chung, M.L., Elia, M., et al., Total daily energy expenditure in wasted chronic obstructive pulmonary disease patients, *Eur. J. Clin. Nutr.*, 56, 282, 2002.
15. Melanson, K.J., Saltzman, E., Vinken, A.G., et al., The effects of age on postprandial thermogenesis at four graded energetic challenges: findings in young and older women, *J. Gerontol. A Biol. Sci. Med. Sci.*, 53, B409, 1998.
16. Morley, J.E., Decreased food intake with aging, *J. Gerontol. A Biol. Sci. Med. Sci.*, 56, 81, 2001.
17. Wakimoto, P. and Block, G., Dietary intake, dietary patterns, and changes with age: an epidemiological perspective, *J. Gerontol. A Biol. Sci. Med. Sci.*, 56, 65, 2001.
18. Morley, J.E. and Silver, A.J., Anorexia in the elderly, *Neurobiol. Aging*, 9, 9, 1988.
19. DeCastro, J.M., Age-related changes in the social, psychological, and temporal influences on food intake in free-living, healthy, adult humans, *J. Gerontol. Med. Sci.*, 57A, M368, 2002.
20. Roberts, S.B., Fuss, P., Heyman, M.B., et al., Control of food intake in older men, *JAMA*, 272, 1601, 1994.
21. Schiffman, S.S., Chemosensory impairment and appetite commentary on "impaired sensory functioning in elders: the relation with its potential determinants and nutritional intake," *J. Gerontol. A Biol. Sci. Med. Sci.*, 54, B332, 1999.
22. Suzuki, Y., Critchley, H.D., Suckling, J., et al., Functional magnetic reasonance imaging of odor identification: the effect of aging, *J. Gerontol. A Biol. Sci. Med. Sci.*, 56, M756, 2001.
23. Wynne, K., Stanley, S., McGowan, B., et al., Appetite control, *J. Endocrinol.*, 184, 291, 2005.
24. Farr, S.A., Banks, W.A., Kumar, V.B., et al., Orexin A-induced feeding is dependent on nitric oxide, *Peptides*, 26, 759, 2005.
25. Morley, J.E. and Baumgartner, R.N., Cytokine-related aging process, *J. Gerontol. A Biol. Sci. Med. Sci.*, 59, M924, 2004.
26. Chapman, I.M., MacIntosh, C.G., Morley, J.E., et al., The anorexia of aging, *Biogerontology*, 3, 67, 2002.
27. Clarkston, W.K., Pantano, M.M., Morley, J.E., et al., Evidence for the anorexia of aging: gastrointestinal transit and hunger in healthy elderly vs. young adults, *Am. J. Physiol.*, 272, R243, 1997.
28. MacIntosh, C.G., Morley, J.E., Wishart, J., et al., Effect of exogenous cholecystokin (CCK)-8 on food intake and plasma CCK, leptin, and insulin concentrations in older and young adults: evidence for increased CCK activity as a cause of the anorexia of aging, *J. Clin. Endocrinol. Metab.*, 86, 5830, 2001.
29. Banks, W.A., Coon, A.B., Robinson, S.M., et al., Triglycerides induce leptin resistance at the blood-brain barrier, *Diabetes*, 53, 1253, 2004.
30. Morley, J.E., Thomas, D.R., and Wilson, M.M., Cachexia: pathophysiology and clinical relevance, *Am. J. Clin. Nutr.*, 83, 735, 2006.

31. Chapman, I.M., Gobie, E.A., Wittert, G.A., et al., Effect of intravenous glucose and euglycemic insulin infusions on short-term appetite and food intake, *Am. J. Physiol.*, 274, R596, 1998.

9 Water Metabolism

David R. Thomas, M.D.
John E. Morley, M.B., B.Ch.

CONTENTS

Water accounts for about 60% of body weight in an average human, varying mainly with degree of adiposity. As the percentage of body fat increases, the amount of body water decreases. Water is distributed in virtual compartments in the body, moving between compartments by osmosis or pumps. Total body water (TBW) is about 42 l in a 70-kg person, or 600 ml/kg. TBW is divided into intracellular fluids (two thirds TBW, 400 ml/kg) and extracellular fluids (one third TBW, 200 ml/kg). About 75% of the extracellular fluid is distributed interstitially between cells (150 ml/kg), and about 25% of extracellular fluid is found in the intravascular space (50 ml/kg).[1]

The spaces define the clinical syndromes of fluid loss. The principal regulator of extracellular water is sodium, because of active transport of sodium into this space. The principal regulator of the larger intracellular compartment is the effective osmolarity of the extracellular fluid. By osmosis, essentially equal tonicity is maintained across both compartments. Intravascular volume depletion leads to hypotension, compensatory tachycardia, decreased tissue perfusion, and shock. The intravascular volume is highly protected to prevent these complications, primarily regulated by a sodium pump. Water is transferred to the intravascular volume from the extracellular compartment and the intracellular compartment.

Loss from the extracellular compartment is termed intravascular volume depletion, while loss from the intracellular compartment is termed dehydration. Loss from both compartments is termed hypovolemia.

9.1 WATER LOSS

Water can be lost from the body via renal, cutaneous, respiratory, and gastrointestinal routes. The kidney is the main controller of body water. The kidneys filter about 150 l of fluid a day, but only about 1% (1.5 l) is excreted as urine. Cutaneous water loss, through sweating, is a major thermoregulatory mechanism. Large amounts of heat are dissipated by sweat. The volume of water loss is usually around 500 ml per day, but can increase substantially in the presence of fever, high environmental temperatures, increased physical activity, increased metabolism, or burns. A relatively small amount of water (around 200 ml per day) can be lost through respiration. This loss is affected by ventilatory volume and the environmental relative humidity. A large amount of water passes through the intestines each day and is recovered by the colon. Because of this, a relatively small amount of water (about 100 ml per day) is lost through feces. However, gastrointestinal loss can increase significantly in the presence of diarrhea, vomiting, or other gastrointestinal pathology and cause severe dehydration.

9.2 REGULATION OF WATER BALANCE

The balance between water loss and water repletion is regulated by arginine vasopressin. Arginine vasopressin (AVP) works as an antidiuretic hormone, thereby regulating water excretion and also stimulating thirst, which regulates water ingestion. This balance is so carefully maintained that the osmolarity varies only between 282 and 298 milliosmil per kilogram. Disorders of this careful balance can lead to severe illness and death.

AVP, the main water-regulating hormone, is controlled by osmotic sensors in the hypothalamus and, to a lesser extent, by baroreceptor (pressure) signals. AVP levels increase rapidly with small increases in osmolality and produce sensations of thirst. The osmotic level for stimulation of AVP appears to be 284 milliosmol/kg, with sensations of thirst appearing at a threshold of 294 milliosmol/kg.[2] However, the data suggest that other nonosmotic triggers for thirst occur when the osmolarity is in the normal range. Moreover, there appears to be an individual set point that varies from person to person.[3]

Increased water loss due to exposure to heat, fever, insufficient fluid consumption, and physical activity results in an increase in osmolality and a decrease in plasma volume (hyperosmotic hypovolemia), the main cause of dehydration. In such situations, dehydration stimulates both thirst and increases in AVP levels. This results in thirst, which increases fluid ingestion (when access is available), and a decrease in urinary output due to increased tubular water reabsorption in the nephron. Because of urine concentration, the urine becomes a darker yellowish color. Changes in urine color, urine osmolality, and urine specific gravity have been used to estimate levels of hydration.

The act of drinking rapidly suppresses the release of AVP, through a reflex mechanism in the oropharynx. Water balance is also affected by changes in intravascular volume. A loss of about 10% of circulating intravascular volume also stimulates the osmoreceptors. Loss of intravascular volume directly stimulates thirst and water intake through baroreceptors located in the vascular system. The renin–angiotensin–aldosterone system is also activated by stimulation of the baroreceptors, with an effect to increase salt intake.

Negative feedback loops operate in conjunction with these systems. Osmotic dilution shuts off the thirst stimulus and AVP secretion. Continued osmotic dilution also stimulates the renin–angiotensin–aldosterone system to retain sodium and restore osmolarity. The renin–angiotensin system controls salt intake and thereby controls intravascular volume. Other hormones, such as atrial natriuretic peptide, have a negative feedback to decrease AVP secretion and the renin–angiotensin–aldosterone system. Urodilatin and the oropharyngeal swallowing reflex also appear to play a role. A simplified diagram of volume regulation is shown in Figure 9.1.

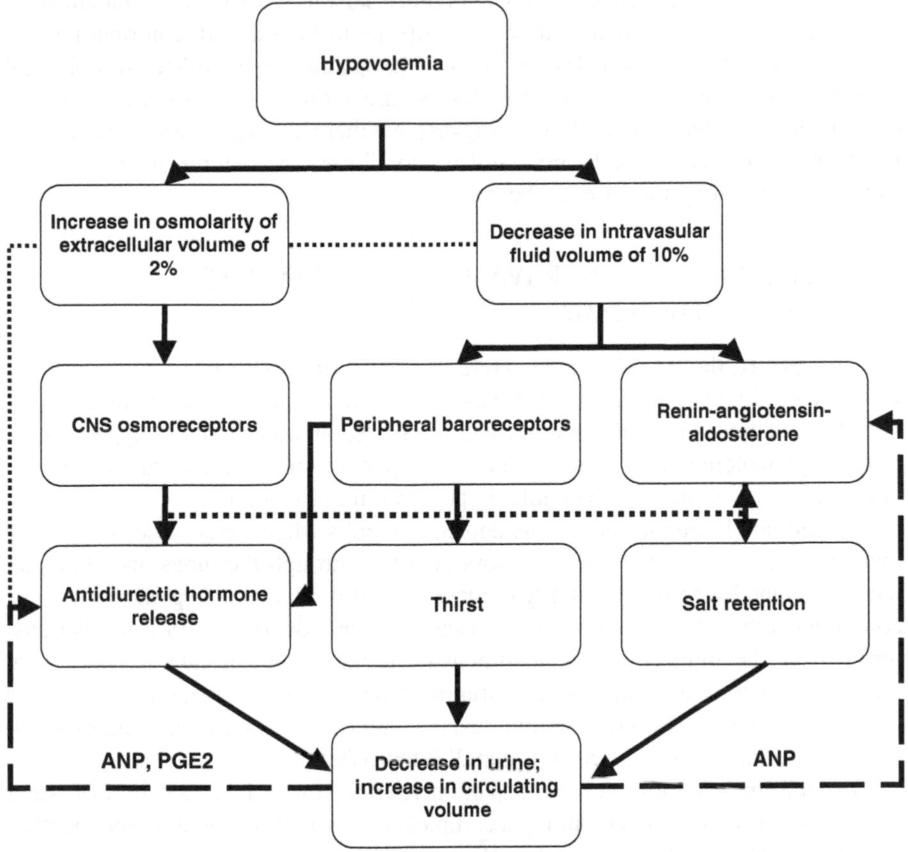

CNS=central nervous system; ANP=atrial naturectic peptide; PGE2=prostaglandin E2

FIGURE 9.1 Simplified regulation of water balance.

9.3 WATER REGULATION IN OLDER ADULTS

In older persons, the regulation of water balance appears to be impaired. There is a diminished thirst response in older persons to water deprivation,[4] or infusion of hypertonic saline.[5] When older and younger men were restricted in water intake over a 24-h period that produced equal weight loss, healthy men age 67 to 75 years were less thirsty and drank less water over 2 h compared to younger men.[6] In studies using heat stress and exercise to induce hyperosmolarity and a volume deficit, older individuals tend to operate at a higher plasma osmolality, indicating a shift in the set point of the regulatory system.[7] Again, the perception of thirst was not different in older men. Other studies have found that older men perceived a greater thirst, but drank the same amount of water as younger men in response to passive heat stress.[8]

In the face of water loss producing either a osmoreceptor or a baroreceptor stimulus, older persons exhibit a decreased thirst sensation and reduced fluid intake. Fluid replacement is effective but slower in older persons. Chronic fluid maintenance in response to repetitive dehydration also appears to be reduced, contributing to a decrease in ability to expand plasma volume. The age differences in the physiological control systems associated with dehydration are more closely associated with a decrease in thirst perception. The data suggest that there is a higher osmotic operating point for thirst sensation under normal daily conditions and a diminished sensitivity to thirst triggered by the vascular baroreceptors.[9]

9.4 DEHYDRATION, INTRAVASCULAR FLUID LOSS, AND HYPOVOLEMIA

Physiologically, the term *dehydration* refers specifically to a decrease in intracellular water. A loss in the intravascular compartment results in intravascular volume depletion. Loss of both intracellular water and intravascular water is more appropriately termed hypovolemia. Dehydration is always hypernatremic, while intravascular volume depletion can be hypernatremic, hyponatremic, or isotonic.

Hypertonic intravascular volume depletion results when water losses are greater than sodium losses. Fever results in loss of water through the lungs and skin and, when combined with limited ability to increase oral fluid intake, is perhaps the most common cause of hypernatremic intravascular volume depletion. As water is transferred from the intracellular compartment to maintain intravascular volume, total body water decreases, causing dehydration. Characteristic laboratory parameters include hypernatremia (serum sodium levels greater than 145 mmol/l) and hyperosmolality (serum osmolality greater than 300 mmol/kg).

Isotonic intravascular volume depletion results from a balanced loss of water and sodium, which can occur during a complete fast. Vomiting and diarrhea, because of large amounts of both water and electrolytes in gastric contents, will result in isotonic dehydration.

Hypotonic intravascular volume depletion occurs when sodium loss exceeds water loss. This type of dehydration occurs primarily with overuse of diuretics, causing excess loss of sodium. The serum sodium is decreased (less than 135 mmol/l) and the serum osmolality is low (less than 280 mmol/kg).

9.5 DIAGNOSIS OF DEHYDRATION

There is no accepted definition of dehydration. A number of parameters have been used to suspect or define dehydration, but all have limitations.[10]

9.5.1 Body Composition

The components of body water can be accurately measured by research techniques such as radiological dilution. Bioelectrical impedance[11–13] can determine total body water and extracellular water, estimating the intracellular water by subtraction. Bioelectrical impedence is based on the fact that fat-free mass has a much greater electrical than fat mass. However, the standard error of the fluid compartment estimates may be as high as ±2 l. Moreover, these modalities may not be readily available in clinical settings.

9.5.2 Body Weight

A useful definition of dehydration is loss of 3% or more of body weight. However, this presumes knowing the stable body weight prior to dehydration. This is useful in atheletes and younger persons, but is not practical in older individuals. Weight fluctuations due to disease or drugs may be misleading, and the lower body weights in older persons may be a total of 3 to 4 pounds, which is in the standard error of measurement of most scales.

9.5.3 Physical Examination

The physical signs of dehydration are often confusing, particularly in older adults. Clinical signs of extravascular volume deficit are often misleading. The most helpful physical findings are either severe postural dizziness such that the patient cannot assume an upright position or a postural pulse increment of 30 beats/min or more. The presence of either finding has a poor sensitivity for moderate intravascular volume depletion due to blood loss (22%) but a much greater sensitivity for large blood loss (97%). Supine hypotension and tachycardia are frequently absent in extravascular fluid loss, and the finding of mild postural dizziness has no proven value. The presence of a dry axilla supports the diagnosis of dehydration (positive likelihood ratio, 2.8; 95% confidence interval (CI), 1.4 to 5.4), and a moist mucous membrane and a tongue without furrows argue against the presence of dehydration (negative likelihood ratio, 0.3; 95% CI, 0.1 to 0.6 for both findings). In adults, the capillary refill time and poor skin turgor have no proven diagnostic value.[14]

9.5.4 Laboratory Parameters

Given the paucity of sensitive clinical signs, laboratory evaluation provides the clinical gold standard. The diagnosis of extracellular volume depletion can be suspected from history and careful physical examination, but requires the support of adjunctive data from laboratory studies. The diagnosis of intracellular volume depletion cannot be established without laboratory analysis of serum sodium or calculation of serum tonicity.[15]

Serum osmolarity is very sensitive, rising in dehydration with as little as a 1% change in body weight.[16] During dehydration due to insufficient fluid intake, both plasma sodium and osmolarity are significantly elevated. Serum osmolarity can be measured directly or estimated by the formula.

REFERENCES

1. Koeppen BM, Stanton BA. *Renal Physiology*, 3rd ed. Mosby Year Book, St. Louis, 2000.
2. Roberton GL. Disorders of thirst in man. In *Thirst, Physiological and Pathological Aspects*, Ramsey DJ, Booth DA, Eds. Springer Verlag, London, 1991, pp. 453–477.
3. McKenna K, Thompson C. Osmoregulation in clinical disorders of thirst appreciation. *Clin. Endocrinol.*, 1998;49:139–152.
4. Phillips PA, Rolls BJ, Ledingham JGG, Forsling ML, Crowe JJ, Walner L. Reduced thirst after water deprivation in healthy elderly men. *N. Engl. J. Med.*, 1984;12:753–759.
5. Davis I, O'Neil PA, McLean KA, Catania J, Bennett D. Age-associated alterations in thirst and arginine vasopressin in response to a water or sodium load. *Age Aging*, 1995;24:151–159.
6. Phillips PA, Rolls BJ, Ledingham ML, et al. Reduced thirst after water deprivation in healthy elderly men. *N. Engl. J. Med.*, 1984;311:753–759.
7. Mack GW, Weseman CA, Langhans GW, Scherzer H, Gillen CM, Nadel ER. Body fluid balance in dehydrated healthy older men: thirst and renal osmoregulation. *J. Appl. Physiol.*, 1994;76:1615–1623.
8. Miescher E, Fortney SM. Responses to dehydration and rehydration during heat exposure in young and older men. *Am. J. Physiol.*, 1989;257:R1050–R1056.
9. Kenney WL, Chiu P. Influence of age on thirst and fluid intake. *Med. Sci. Sports Exerc.*, 2001;33:1524–1532.
10. Kavouras SA. Assessing hydration status. *Curr. Opin. Clin. Nutr. Metab. Care*, 2002;5:519–524.
11. Ritz P. Bioelectrical impedance analysis estimation of water compartments in elderly diseased patients: the source study. *J. Gerontol. A Biol. Sci. Med. Sci.*, 2001;56:M344–M348.
12. O'Brien C, Baker-Fulco CJ, Young AJ, Sawka MN. Bioimpedance assessment of hypohydration. *Med. Sci. Sports Exerc.*, 1999;31:1466–1471.
13. Olde Rikkert MG, Deurenberg P, Jansen RW, van't Hof MA, Hoefnagels WH. Validation of multi-frequency bioelectrical impedance analysis in detecting changes in fluid balance of geriatric patients. *J. Am. Geriatr. Soc.*, 1997;45:1345–1351.
14. McGee S, Abernethy WB III, Simel DL. Is this patient hypovolemic? *JAMA* 1999;281:1022–1029.
15. Mange K, Matsuura D, Cizman B, Soto H, Ziyadeh FN, Goldfarb S, Neilson EG. Language guiding therapy: the case of dehydration versus volume depletion. *Ann. Intern. Med.*, 1997;127:848–853.
16. Popowski LA, Oppliger RA, Patrick Lambert G, et al. Blood and urinary measures of hydration status during progressive acute dehydration. *Med. Sci. Sports Exerc.*, 2001;33:747–753.

10 Vitamin Disorders

Ramzi R. Hajjar, M.D.
Zeina Nahhas, Pharm.D.

CONTENTS

10.1 INTRODUCTION

Nutrition plays an increasingly important role in health and disease as we age. The prevalence of protein-energy malnutrition (PEM) increases with age and frailty and is associated with poor outcome. Nutrition-related disorders in Western societies more often conjure images of nutritional excess and obesity rather than malnutrition. Nonetheless, with advancing age, multiple well-documented age-related conditions converge to put the geriatric population at risk for nutritional deficits (Morley and Silver 1995, Thomas and Morley 2001). Weight loss in the elderly may not receive the attention and sense of urgency it commands, in part due to the compulsion during earlier adult life to achieve just such a weight loss. While undernutrition may be the cause or the end result of a specific disease process, it more often represents a single facet of multiple complex interacting physiological changes, resulting in progressive functional decline, as seen in anorexia of aging and adult failure to thrive (Morley and Silver 1985). It is estimated that up to 16% of Americans over the age of 65 consume less than 1000 kcal/day, and 30 to 40% of individuals over the age of 75 are at least 10% below their ideal body weight (Third National Health and Nutritional Examination Survey 1994, Wakimoto and Block 2001, Joshi and Morley 2006). Overt malnutrition is encountered in 5 to 12% of ambulatory community-dwelling elderly, 20 to 37% of home-bound elderly, and 32 to 50% of hospitalized older adults. In the long-term-care setting, the prevalence of undernutrition may be as high as 85% (Drinka and Goodwin 1991, Zulkowski 2000, Johnson et al. 2002, Abbasi 1995, Abbasi and Rudman 1993, Ritchie et al. 1997, Garry et al. 1984).

As caloric intake decreases, so does the quantity and quality of micronutrients. A daily dietary intake of 1000 kcal is unlikely to provide sufficient vitamins, particularly in diets deficient in fresh fruits and vegetables. Approximately 50% of all older adults ingest less than the recommended dietary allowance of vitamins and minerals, and 10 to 53% have levels below normal (Foote et al. 2000, Souba 1997). The Second National Health and Nutrition Examination Survey (NHANES II) found that only 10% of the elderly consume the recommended five-a-day servings of fruits and vegetables (Block 1991, Third National Health and Nutritional Examination Survey 1994). Of the 12,000 adults surveyed, 41% consumed no fruits and 17% no vegetables on the day of the survey. Individual deficiencies vary widely by setting and vitamin type. As might be expected, the highest deficiency prevalence occurred in hospitalized and institutionalized persons. Fat-soluble vitamin A deficiency was rare, occurring in less than 1% of older adults, despite decreased intake in 4 to 17% of the population. Vitamin D deficiency, in contrast, was found in 2.6 to 6.8% of independent elderly and 35% of nursing home residents. Body stores of vitamins may also vary with age. Decreasing lean body mass (LBM) and the accompanying increase in body fat are normal age-associated changes in body composition. LBM begins to decline as early as age 30, and the rate of decline accelerates in late life. Consequently, as a general rule, fat-soluble vitamins can be stored in the body in large amounts and do not necessarily need to be taken daily. Water-soluble vitamins, on the other hand, lack large body stores and may be depleted in a few weeks, with the exception of vitamin B_{12}, which is stored in the liver. Vitamins B_1 and B_6, for example, were found to be deficient in 13 to 43% and 5 to 56% of independent elderly, respectively.

Classical deficiency states such as scurvy, beriberi, and pellagra rarely occur in the geriatric population. Public health measures have led to a near elimination of these extreme deficiency states in industrialized countries. In today's nutritionally enriched environment, vitamin deficiencies are suffered mainly by the decrepit who cannot eat or digest a normal diet, or the faddist who will not (Gordon 1993). Consequently, vitamin deficiencies in the elderly typically do not develop in isolation, but rather in combination with other micronutrient and macronutrient disorders. They may present with vague or atypical symptoms, masked by coexisting disease, or be mistaken for the aging process itself. Symptoms remain enigmatic and treatment delayed, if the diagnosis is based solely on clinical manifestations. In most cases, hematological tests are required to establish the diagnosis unequivocally.

Currently available assays, however, have their own limitations. Serum levels may not accurately reflect total body stores (e.g., vitamin A) or tissue levels (e.g., vitamin B_{12}). Assigning cutoff limits below which a diagnosis is made imposes an artificial break in the measurement continuum. Statistically derived limits are generated from population-based observational studies and are best suited for epidemiological work. Stringent diagnostic limits do not account for changes in vitamin requirements that occur with age, comorbidities, LBM, and lifestyle.

Not all vitamin disorders in the elderly are attributed to poor intake. Changes in vitamin requirements, altered metabolism, and hypervitaminosis complete the spectrum of vitamin disorders. Vitamin requirements are not static throughout life and have only recently been studied in the geriatric population despite avid interest in this area by academicians and laypersons alike. The requirements of some fat-soluble vitamins, such as vitamin A, decrease with age. Other vitamins, such a vitamins D, B_6, and B_{12}, are required in larger quantities. New reference intake guidelines developed by the Food and Nutrition Board of the Institute of Medicine were released in three publications between 1998 and 2001 and for the first time included recommendations for individuals 70 years and older (Institute of Medicine 1998, 2000, 2001). However, heterogeneity among individuals above the age of 70 increases rapidly, and the recommendations were meant to be applied as guidelines for the group, and not as a gold standard for individuals. Perhaps future recommendations will account for comorbidities, risk factors, and lifestyle patterns, rather than age alone.

Over the past two decades, evidence has emerged suggesting that vitamin supplementation may provide benefits beyond simply preventing the deficiency state. Vitamins are being studied for their potential protective effect against many conditions that afflict the elderly, including cancer, atherosclerotic disease, neurodegenerative disorders, infections, cataracts, blood disorders, and possibly the aging process itself. As life expectancy in industrialized countries forges into the ninth decade, opportunities to impact health status easily and inexpensively become very appealing. Vitamin supplementation is one such measure—at least in theory. With the identification and synthesis of vitamins during the first half of the 20th century, several affordable vitamin preparations have become readily available. Subsequently, the vitamin pharmaceutical industry has grown into a multi-billion-dollar annual enterprise, fueled by the debatable assumption that "more is better." Widespread use of vitamin supplements for health maintenance in older individuals is driven by consumers who have become disenchanted with the medical establishment, and by a growing tendency toward homeopathic therapy. Daily vitamin supplements, often multiple and in combinations, are consumed by approximately 20 to 60% of the elderly (Vitolins et al. 2000, Massey 2002, Radimer et al. 2004, Third National Health and Nutritional Examination Survey 1994). Such practice is not always beneficial or even benign. Vitamin toxicities are rare but do occur—most seriously with A and B_6. Drug–vitamin interactions are also a concern, particularly with the high prevalence of polypharmacy in the elderly. Many vitamin consumers do not view their supplements as medications. Surreptitious and inadvertent vitamin overuse may go unnoticed without a judicious vitamin history.

10.2 BRIEF HISTORICAL PERSPECTIVE

The year was 1911. Casimir Funk (1884–1967), a Polish-born chemist working at the Lister Institute in London, had isolated a pyrimidine compound that when fed to experimental pigeons cured them of beriberi. Earlier, Christiaan Eijkman (1858–1930), a Dutch physician, observed that feeding chicken polished rice resulted in a peculiar polyneuropathy that was promptly cured by introducing unpolished rice or adding extracts of rice husk to the diet. In 1905, English physician William Fletcher (1844–1925) demonstrated similar findings in a nutritional experiment conducted on asylum inmates in Malaysia, then a British colony. Nearly one quarter of the inmates who were fed polished rice developed symptoms of beriberi, whereas only 2% of those fed unpolished rice were similarly affected, all dietary components otherwise being similar. The following year, Sir Frederick Hopkins (1861–1947) concluded that foods contain "accessory factors" or "growth factors" needed in small amounts to sustain growth and life itself. Funk initially theorized the vital dietary components to be ammonia derivatives and proposed the name *vitamines*, derived from the Latin for life (*vita*) and amines. The trailing *e* was later dropped to deemphasize the amine nature of these compounds, when it became clear that not all vitamins contained amine moieties. In 1929, Eijkman and Hopkins shared the Nobel Prize for their work on vitamin B_1 (thiamin). It was the first of three Nobel Prizes issued for work on vitamins.

It had long been known that certain dietary components were capable of preventing or curing certain disease conditions. As early as 1500 B.C., the ancient Egyptians recognized that night blindness could be treated with specific foods, notably liver, now known to be rich in vitamin A. Scribes of the ancient city states of Mesopotamia noted that food could affect health in more subtle ways than simply sustaining life. Despite early insight, little further progress was made in the field of nutrition until the middle of the 18th century. The turning point came when Scottish naval surgeon James Lind (1716–1794) discovered that an unknown component of citrus fruits helped prevent scurvy, a particularly gruesome and deadly disease at that time, most common among seafaring people. Vasco da Gama (1469–1524), first to round the Cape of Good Hope in 1497, lost 100 of 160 deck hands to scurvy. In 1536, Jacques Cartier (1491–1557), in search of a northern passage to the Orient, describes in his journal: "An unknown sickness began to spread itself among us in the strangest sort that ever was heard of or seen." He continues to recount that "out of 110 that we were, not ten were well enough to help the others, a thing pitiful to see." By the mid-1700s, more British sailors were being lost to scurvy than to war.

No one knew what caused scurvy. Reports exist of sailors being left for dead ashore tropical islands only to be found thriving upon the return voyage. Sailors noted that tropical fruits eaten ashore cured scurvy, as did scurvy grass, a coastal plant of the cruciferae family related to turnips, radishes, cabbage, and watercress. Cartier cured his men with a brew from the bark and needles of the white cedar tree bordering the St. Lawrence after he learned of a dying Indian who was cured within a week by this remedy. It was not until 1747, however, that James Lind discovered that scurvy could not only be cured, but prevented, by oranges and lemons. He published his *Treaties on the Scurvy* in 1753 and recommended that rations of lemons and limes be consumed by all sailors after 6 weeks at sea. He had found a remedy, with no notion of how it worked, to a disease for which nobody remotely knew the reason (Gordon 1993). Incredibly, his breakthrough was ignored for another 40 years, at the cost of untold thousands of lives.

By the dawn of the 20th century, nutritional science was entering a new era. It was previously believed that an adequate diet consisted of proteins, carbohydrates, fats, and inorganic salts, and that humans could survive on these components alone. In 1881, Nikolai Lunin (1853–1937) found that mice did not survive when fed adequate amounts of the separate milk constituents known at that time, whereas those fed whole milk developed normally. He concluded that natural foods contained small amounts of unknown substances essential for life. Meanwhile, the germ theory of disease became in vogue after Louis Pasteur (1822–1895) discovered that many diseases were caused by microbes. Despite the pioneer work of Lind and Lunin, many vitamin deficiency states were still thought to be of infectious origin, even in the early 1900s. With increasing numbers of vitamins being identified, however, the critical role of vitamins in disease prevention could no longer be ignored. A growth-promoting factor in butter was discovered in 1913 and later designated vitamin A. Vitamin C was isolated in 1932 and was the first vitamin to be synthesized in the laboratory. In the early 1920s, vitamin D was discovered as a cure for rickets. And so it went. A flurry of activity resulted in the 13 vitamins known to us today. Vitamins were found to be a heterogeneous group of compounds, and to simplify nomenclature, they were assigned letters roughly in order of their discoveries. The skipped letters represent vitamins that were later found not to meet the criteria for vitamins, or were reclassified, such as vitamin G, which was renamed vitamin B_2 (riboflavin). The parallel effort of biochemists to artificially produce vitamins in the laboratory led to the availability of affordable nutritional supplements. Widespread use of vitamins ensued as a result of intensive public health campaigns and the supplementation of common foods, such as vitamin D in milk. Together with advances in infectious diseases, nutritional sciences accounted for the unprecedented amelioration in health and longevity seen during the 20th century. For the first time, it was believed that consuming vitamins in abundance could prevent other diseases.

The latter half of the 20th century ushered in two further developments that once again changed the way vitamins were viewed. First, the free radical theory of aging was developed. When first conceived by Dr. Denham Harman in 1954, the theory of oxidative damage was met with skepticism, but soon thereafter it was embraced as a leading theory of aging. Antioxidant vitamins were suddenly thrust to the forefront of antiaging research. Second, Americans grew old. For the first time in the history of mankind, life expectancy extended decades beyond the reproductive years—but with it came chronic disease. Together, these forces set the pace and direction of much of the vitamin research to follow. The expectation was that chronic diseases afflicting the elderly could be delayed or even prevented by the use of pharmacological doses of antioxidant vitamins. Answers were not to emerge that easily, as will be discussed later. The widespread use of vitamin supplements beyond what is necessary to prevent deficiency disease was abetted by evidence that vitamins consumed in their natural form decreased the incidence of cardiovascular disease and cancer, and by the endorsement of high-profile scientists, such as the double

Nobel Prize winner Linus Pauling, who touted the antiaging effects of megadoses of vitamin C. Observational studies supporting an inverse relation between consumption of fresh fruits and vegetables and the incidence of cancer was so compelling that in 1996 the American Cancer Society launched the five-a-day campaign urging the consumption of no less than five servings of fruits and vegetables each day (American Cancer Society Advisory Committee 1996). Some experts now recommend increasing the daily servings to eight, particularly in high-risk persons (Smith-Warner et al. 2000, McEligol 2002), a rather inane point since 90% of the elderly do not achieve the five-a-day goal (Block 1991).

10.3 DIETARY REFERENCE INTAKES

Since 1941, the Recommended Dietary Allowances (RDAs) have been the most authoritative reference on nutrient levels necessary to maintain health. The 11th revision of the RDAs was completed in 2001. The Food and Nutrition Board of the Institute of Medicine, National Academy of Science, established the new guidelines based on the most recent understanding of nutrient requirements necessary to optimize health and prevent chronic disease, not just prevent nutrient deficiency (Institute of Medicine 1998, 2000, 2001). Four categories of reference values were described, collectively referred to as the Dietary Reference Intakes (DRIs). The new recommendations took into consideration vitamin source and bioavailability—the body being able to better utilize natural rather than synthetic vitamins. While megadose vitamins cannot be achieved by diet alone, natural foods may contain necessary cofactors or vitamin complexes (e.g., vitamins A and E), making natural foods the preferred method of attaining vitamins. DRIs also addressed levels above which vitamins produce harmful side effects. Perhaps the most substantial way in which the DRIs parted from previous recommendations, however, is that age and gender were taken into consideration, with separate and distinct recommendations for each group when applicable. The recommendation categories include:

- Estimated Average Requirement (EAR): The amount of a nutrient intake necessary to meet the requirements of 50% of healthy individuals in a group.
- Recommended Dietary Allowance (RDA): Set at two standard deviations above the EAR and represents the average daily amount of nutrient intake necessary to meet the requirements of 98% of healthy individuals in a group. The RDA serves as a guide for individual assessment and diet planning.
- Adequate Intake (AI): When the RDA cannot be established due to lack of sufficient clinical evidence, the Adequate Intake level is used. AI levels are derived from experimental or observed effects of nutrient intake on specific health outcomes, based on the judgment of a panel of experts.
- Tolerable Upper Intake Level (TUL): The upper limit of daily nutrient intake that is not likely to produce adverse effects in 98% of individuals in a group. The TUL is not intended to be used for recommended levels of intake, but as a safety limit above which there is a likelihood of toxicity. Total intake from all sources should not exceed the TUL.

DRI recommendations (Table 10.1) are considered to be average values that apply to healthy people. Although a margin of safety is built in to the DRIs, specific requirements may change with disease and lifestyle.

10.4 FAT-SOLUBLE VITAMINS

Vitamins A, D, E, and K are fat soluble. As a general rule, they can be stored in the body in relatively large amounts, and are therefore less likely to be depleted than water-soluble vitamins. In fact, with advancing age, vitamin stores may accumulate, increasing the risk of toxicity. Vitamins A and E are potent antioxidants, as is the water-soluble vitamin C. The potential risks and benefits of using vitamins as antioxidants to impede the aging process will be discussed in the final section of this chapter.

10.4.1 Vitamin A and Carotenoids

Vitamin A (retinol) is a general term that refers to preformed retinol and carotenoids that are converted to retinol. Vitamin A can be ingested as retinol or synthesized in the body from a diverse group of natural pigment precursors collectively referred to as carotenoids. Preformed retinol is found exclusively in animal products. Food sources of preformed retinol include fish, meat, liver, egg yolks, butter, fortified milk, and other animal sources. Preformed vitamin A is absorbed by the intestinal epithelial cell by a carrier-mediated mechanism and transported via the lymphatics to the liver, where it is stored. In order to reach its target organ, vitamin A binds to retinol-binding protein (RBP) and is released into the circulation as a RBP–retinol complex. The liver holds 50 to 95% of the body's store of vitamin A. Retinol blood levels are tightly controlled, and greater intake in well-nourished persons has little effect on circulating levels. Thus, serum levels of vitamin A do not necessarily reflect dietary intake or vitamin A balance. Circulating levels are largely maintained by release of vitamin A from the large liver stores, and a drop in serum levels only occurs in severe deficiency states, when liver stores become depleted.

Carotenoids, on the other hand, cannot be synthesized by the human body. We are dependent exclusively on dietary intake for these micronutrients. Of the more than 600 naturally occurring pigments, all can function as antioxidants, but only approximately 10% have vitamin A-like activity, beta-carotene being the most prominent. Carotenoids are found in yellow, orange, and red plant compounds and green leafy vegetables. Unlike retinol, carotinoids are passively absorbed by the intestinal epithelium. In the intestine, the carotenoid precursors break down into retinaldehyde molecules, which in turn can be reduced to retinol by hepatic aldehyde reductase and stored in the liver. Less than one third of ingested carotenoid is absorbed by the body, and a small amount of that is eventually converted to retinol. Unlike retinol, carotenoids are stored in various tissues. Beta-carotene is the major carotenid in the liver, adrenal glands, kidney, ovary, and adipose tissue, whereas lycopene is predominantly found in the testes. Oxycarotenoids, like zeaxanthin and lutein, are present in the macula in the virtual absence of beta-carotene.

Retinol is the precursor of two bioactive metabolites: retinal (retinaldehyde), which is critical for proper vision, and retinoic acid, an intracellular messenger

TABLE 10.1
Dietary Reference Intake for Micronutrients

	Vitamin	Common Chemical Name	Recommended Daily Allowance or Adequate Intakes*				Tolerable Upper Level			
			51–70 Years		>70 Years		51–70 Years		>70 Years	
			Male	Female	Male	Female	Male	Female	Male	Female
Fat soluble	Vitamin A	Carotenoids	900 μg	700 μg	900 μg	700 μg	3000 μg	3000 μg	3000 μg	3000 μg
	Vitamin D*	Calciferols	10 μg	10 μg	15 μg	15 μg	50 mg	50 mg	50 mg	50 mg
	Vitamin E	—	15 mg	15 mg	15 mg	15 mg	1000 mg	1000 mg	1000 mg	1000 mg
	Vitamin K*	—	120 μg	90 μg	120 μg	90 μg	ND	ND	ND	ND
Watersoluble	Vitamin B_1	Thiamin	1.2 mg	1.1 mg	1.2 mg	1.1 mg	ND	ND	ND	ND
	Vitamin B_2	Riboflavin	1.3 mg	1.1 mg	1.3 mg	1.1 mg	ND	ND	ND	ND
	Vitamin B_3	Niacin	16 mg	14 mg	16 mg	14 mg	35 mg	35 mg	35 mg	35 mg
	Vitamin B_6	Pyridoxin	1.7 mg	1.5 mg	1.7 mg	1.5 mg	100 mg	100 mg	100 mg	100 mg
	Vitamin B_9	Folic acid	400 μg	400 μg	400 μg	400 μg	1000 μg	1000 μg	1000 μg	1000 μg
	Vitamin B_{12}	Cyanocobalamine	2.4 μg	2.4 μg	2.4 μg	2.4 μg	ND	ND	ND	ND
	Vitamin C	Ascorbic acid	90 mg	75 mg	90 mg	75 mg	2000 mg	2000 mg	2000 mg	2000 mg

Source: Institute of Medicine, *Dietary Reference Intakes for Thiamin, Riboflavin, Niacin, Vitamin B6, Folate, Vitamin B12, Pantothenic Acid, Biotin, and Choline* (1998), *Dietary Reference Intakes for Vitamin C, Vitamin E, Selenium and Carotenoids* (2000), *Dietary Reference Intakes for Vitamin A, Vitamin K, Arsenic, Boron, Chromium, Copper, Iodine, Manganese, Molybdenum, Nickel, Silicon, Vanadium, and Zinc* (2001), National Academy Press, Washington, DC.

* Indicates adequate intake values; all others are Recommended Daily Allowances.

ND: not determined.

affecting gene transcription. The main biological functions of vitamin A are to promote good vision by maintaining photoreceptor pigment, ensure normal cellular differentiation and integrity, maintain an efficient immune function, and prevent squamous metaplasia of the epithelium. Vitamin A is also important for gene expression, and wound healing. By virtue of their antioxidant activity, carotenoids have been shown to limit oxidative damage from free radical reactions and contribute to the protection of membranes from lipid peroxidation.

The current RDA for vitamin A is 700 μg for women and 900 μg for men over the age of 50, depicting a decrease from previous recommendations. Worldwide, it is the third most common nutritional deficiency, causing blindness, ill health, and mortality in over 100,000 children annually. In developed countries, deficiency occurs very rarely, particularly in the elderly. Prolonged periods of diminished intake is necessary for a deficiency state to develop. Conditions responsible for deficiency include fat malabsorption of any etiology, liver disease (reduced storage of retinol esters and impaired synthesis of retinol and RBP), decreased dietary intake, and nephrotic syndrome due to urinary loss of RBP. Deficiency results in:

- Night blindness due to loss of rhodopsin in rods, complete blindness due to loss of iodopsin in cones, and xerophthalmia.
- Bitot's spots (abnormal squamous cell proliferation and keratinization of the conjunctiva), corneal perforation, and keratomalacia—all more common in children.
- Xerodermia, follicular hyperkeratosis (phrynoderma), squamous metaplasia of hair follicles, and possibly impaired wound healing.
- Increased susceptibility to and severity of infections due to impaired immunity secondary to decreased natural killer cell number and function. Increased susceptibility to pneumonia and bronchitis is further exacerbated by squamous metaplasia of the respiratory epithelium.

Although only two thirds of those 65 to 75 years old in the U.S. consume the RDA for vitamin A, mean and median liver levels of vitamin A do not drop with advancing age (Hoppner 1968). Some studies have indicated increased absorption (Hollander and Morgan 1979) and decreased clearance (Krasinski et al. 1990) in the elderly, making the likelihood of toxicity greater if supplements or fortified foods are included in the daily diet. Elderly persons taking vitamin A supplements have been found to have higher levels of circulating retinyl esters, the toxic indicator, than elderly not taking supplements (Krasinski et al. 1989). Toxicity can result from chronic intake of retinol at levels as low as three to four times the RDA (3000 μg), and acutely with higher doses. Impaired renal and hepatic function increased risk of toxicity (Chernoff 2005), whereas excess vitamin E imparts some protection. Symptoms of toxicity include nausea, vomiting, anorexia, headaches, dizziness, drowsiness, and irritability. Chronic toxicity presents with anorexia, alopecia, fatigue, hypothyroidism, bone and muscle pain, hepatosplenomegaly, and increased intracranial pressure. Hypervitaminosis A in the elderly also presents with bone pain, bone inflammation, and hypercalcemia. Vitamin A enhances the activity of vitamin D and parathyroid hormone and a negative calcium balance may occur. Increased osteoclastic activity and decreased bone mineral density at the femoral neck and lumbar spine have been documented (Kneissel et al. 2005, Rohde and DeLuca 2003, Promislow et al. 2002, Melhus et al. 1998). Dietary intake of 1500 μg or more per day is associated with osteoporosis and an increased risk of hip fractures (Melhus et al. 1998, Michaelsson et al. 2003, Feskanich et al. 2002, Lips 2003), in some instances as much as doubling the risk. These findings were only noted with excess intake of preformed vitamin A (retinol) and not beta-carotene.

There is no known deficiency state for carotenoids and no RDAs. Beta-carotein is also widely considered to be nontoxic, and humans tolerated high doses without apparent harm. There is no evidence that conversion of beta-carotene to vitamin A contributes to toxicity of the latter, even when beta-carotene is ingested in large amounts. The only undesirable effect of high beta-carotene intake is a yellowish discoloration of the skin, or carotehnemia, which occurs only at extremely high intake (Mathews-Roth 1986).

10.4.2 Vitamin D

Vitamin D is not a true vitamin. It can be synthesized in the human body, and therefore functions more as a pro-hormone. Vitamin D is a general term referring to the final biologically active product as well as its numerous precursors. It is a lipid-soluble compound related in structure to the cholesterol molecule. The two forms of vitamin D are ergocalciferol (D_2) and cholecalciferol (D_3). Vitamin D_2 is formed by the ultraviolet irradiation of ergosterol and is found in plants, while vitamin D_3 is primarily found in animal products. It was previously believed that both forms have similar metabolism and biological function, but Armas et al. (2004) recently showed that vitamin D_3 is over three times more potent than D_2. Dietary sources of vitamin D_3 include egg yolks, fish liver oils, and fortified foods. The major source, however, is synthesized in the skin by converting 7-dehydrocholesterol to vitamin D_3 with adequate sunlight exposure. Vitamin D from either source is bound to vitamin D-binding protein and transported to the liver, where it is hydroxylated by 25-vitamin D-hydroxylase to 25-hydroxy-vitamin D, or calcidiol. In the kidneys, 25(OH)D is further hydroxylated by 1-alpha-hydroxylase to 1,25-dihydroxy-vitamin D (1,25$(OH)_2$D), or calcitriol. A smaller amount of relatively inactive 24,25$(OH)_2$D is also synthesized in the liver. Calcitriol is the most active form of vitamin D. The affinity of the nuclear receptor for 1,25$(OH)_2$D is approximately 1000 times that for 25(OH)D. Serum levels of calcitriol, however, do not necessarily reflect total body stores of the vitamin due to the relatively short half-life of 4 to 6 hours. Calcidiol, on the other hand, has a half-life of approximately 3 weeks (Thomas and Demay 2000) and is a better measure of vitamin D status (Johnson et al. 2002).

Vitamin D deficiency is common in the elderly and can have serious consequences. Despite the ability to store vitamin D, studies have shown that both 1,25$(OH)_2$D and 25(OH)D serum levels decline with age. Up to 25% of community-dwelling elderly may have vitamin D deficiency, and the prevalence can be as high as 80% in residents of long-term-care facilities. Several changes associated with aging result in age being a risk factor for vitamin D deficiency. Decreased exposure to sunlight and decreased amounts of 7-dehydrocholesterol levels in the aging skin deprive the elderly of the major source of vitamin D that younger adults enjoy. In the absence of adequate photoconversion, dietary intake becomes a much more crucial source of vitamin D. This, however, occurs at a time when dairy products and other vitamin D-rich foods constitute a declining part of the typical geriatric diet. Decreased renal conversion of 25(OH)D to 1,25$(OH)_2$D and, to a lesser degree, decreased hepatic hydroxylation of D to 25(OH)D further limit availability of the active form of vitamin D. Finally, several medications disrupt vitamin D absorption, activation, or function. Most notable are anticonvulsants, rifampin, ketoconazole, primidone, and many other drugs that can impair hydroxylation or accelerate elimination by activating the cytochrome P-450 system. The new DRIs account for these age-related changes. The Adequate Intake (AI) is set at 400 IU (10 μg) for individuals age 51 to 70 years and 600 IU (15 μg) for those over the age of 70. High-risk elderly may benefit from 800 IU/day, which has been shown to increase bone mineral density and decrease the risk of bone fracture. These levels of intake can easily be achieved with a multivitamin (most containing 200 IU) twice a day or a plain vitamin D supplement. Concurrent calcium supplementation is advised since the typical adult diet does not meet calcium requirements (Kamel and Hajjar 2003). Most vitamin D preparations are supplemented with 250 to 600 mg calcium.

Biochemical manifestations of vitamin D deficiency include hypocalcemia, hypophosphatemia, and elevated alkaline phosphatase. With prolonged hypocalcemia, secondary hyperparathyroidism may develop, which further decreases phosphorus levels and promotes bone resorption by stimulating osteoclasts. Clinical features of these changes include accelerated osteoporosis and an increased risk of vertebral and long bone fracture. Vitamin D deficiency may also present with any of the symptoms of hypocalcemia, such as neuromuscular irritability, neuropathy, hyperesthesia, and proximal myopathy or pain.

The benefits of supplementing vitamin D in the elderly have been documented in many studies. In a study of 3270 elderly women (mean age, 84 years; SD, 6 years), Chapuy et al. (1992) demonstrated a 43% decrease in hip fractures (p = 0.043) and a 32% decrease in total nonvertebral fractures ($p = 0.015$) in the treatment group compared to the placebo group. Treatment consisted of 800 IU vitamin D with 1200 mg calcium daily for 18 months. In a subgroup analysis (n = 56), bone mineral density (BMD) at the proximal femur increase by 2.7% in the treatment group, compared to a decrease of 4.6% in the placebo group ($p < 0.001$). The preventive effect of calcium and cholecalciferol supplementation on fracture risk continued after an additional 18 months of follow-up (Chapuy et al. 2002). At 3 years total follow-up, hip fractures and all nonvertebral fractures were reduced in the treatment group by 29 and 24%, respectively ($p < 0.01$ in both cases). The intention to treat analysis showed 17.2% fewer subjects with at least one vertebral fracture ($p < 0.02$) and 23.0% fewer subjects with hip fractures ($p < 0.02$).

Similar results have been reported by other investigators, though not consistently. Dawson-Hughes et al. (1991) showed that in wintertime, when vitamin D levels dip, spinal bone loss was significantly less in postmenopausal women consuming at least 500 IU vitamin D plus calcium compared to the control group. During the summer months, supplementation was associated with a net gain in BMD. The same group of investigators later showed that daily supplementation with a low dose of vitamin

D (100 IU) plus calcium was sufficient to limit spinal bone loss at 2 years follow-up, but higher doses (700 IU) were necessary to minimize bone loss from the femoral neck (Dawson-Hughes et al. 1995). Since then, the RDA for vitamin D was increased, as discussed earlier. These trials, however, should not lull the public into a false sense of complacency, as the benefit of vitamin D and calcium on BMD does not continue unabashed. The natural history of osteoporosis is one of a gradual continuous bone loss, starting in early adulthood, and preventive interventions only retard the rate of bone loss, not prevent it. In a follow-up study, the effect of 700 IU vitamin D and 500 mg calcium on BMD of the femoral neck and spine was statistically significant compared to placebo after 1 year, but not in the second or third year of follow-up (Dawson-Hughes et al. 1997).

Since most interventional studies combined various amounts of vitamin D and calcium supplements, it is not clear how much benefit is derived from each component. It has been suggested that a significant component of the benefit is due to calcium supplementation in calcium-deficient elderly. In a 4-year study of 438 elderly subjects with a baseline median calcium intake of 546 mg/day and median serum 25(OH)D of 59 nmol/l (normal > 75 to 80 nmol/l), Peacock et al. (2000) supplemented subjects daily with 750 mg calcium or 15 μg (600 IU) 25(OH)D. At 4 years follow-up, calcium reduced bone loss, secondary hyperparathyroidism, and bone turnover, whereas 25(OH)D was intermediate between placebo and calcium. Fracture rates were similar among the groups. The authors concluded that the beneficial effect of vitamin D is due to the reversal of calcium insufficiency. Findings are in line with those of Lips et al. (1996), who showed no decrease in the incidence of hip fractures and other peripheral fractures with vitamin D supplementation (400 IU/day) after a median follow-up of 3.5 years. The mean baseline dietary intake of calcium from dairy products was 868 mg/day, and the mean serum 25(OH)D concentration in the third year of the study was 60 nmol/l in the vitamin D group. It is quite possible, though, that these results reflect dose-related outcomes. In a recent meta-analysis of randomized controlled trials (RCTs) a vitamin D dose of 700 to 800 IU/day reduced the relative risk (RR) of hip fractures by 26% (RR, 0.74; 95% confidence interval (CI), 0.61 to 0.88) and nonvertebral fractures by 23% (RR, 0.77; 95% CI, 0.68 to 0.87) vs. calcium and placebo (Bischoff-Ferrari et al. 2005). No significant benefit was observed in the RTCs with 400 IU/day vitamin D supplement. Based on currently available evidence, most experts advise supplementing high-risk individuals, which includes most of the geriatric population, with no less than 400 to 600 IU vitamin D and 800 to 1000 mg calcium daily, with the remaining balance obtained by diet. While daily oral supplementation is the preferred means of administering vitamin D, high-dose biannual oral replacement (10,000 to 100,000 IU) or annual intramuscular injections (150,000 IU) have been used and appear to be well tolerated (Heikenheimo et al. 1991, Holick 1994).

Other effects of vitamin D replacement have been studied. Vitamin D nuclear receptors are found in most human cells and tissues, including skeletal muscles. It is not unexpected, therefore, to anticipate various systemic effects of vitamin D, due to either direct receptor activation or indirect effect of calcium metabolism. Vitamin D serum levels have been found to correlate with muscle strength (Bischoff et al. 1999), and supplementation improved functional outcome as measured by the Frail

Elderly Functional Assessment (FEFA) questionnaire (Gloth et al. 1995). In frail elderly women with a mean age of 85.3 years, daily vitamin D (800 IU) plus calcium (1200 mg) over a 3-month period reduced the risk of falls by 49% compared to calcium alone (Bischoff et al. 2003). The investigators hypothesized that the impact of vitamin D on falls could be related to the observed improvement in musculoskeletal function. The reduced fall risk in women appears to continue beyond the short term. A 3-year trial of cholecalciferol (700 IU) and calcium (500 mg) dietary supplementation reduced the odds of falling in ambulatory older women by 46% (odds ratio (OR), 0.54; CI, 0.30 to 0.97), but not in men (OR, 0.93; CI, 0.50 to 1.72) (Bischoff-Ferrari et al. 2006). In less active women, fall reduction was even greater. The gender discrepancy is not fully explained, though mean baseline 25(OH)D in men was significantly higher than in women, falling in the low-normal range. In a meta-analysis of RCTs, vitamin D supplementation appeared to reduce the risk of falls among all older individuals by more than 20% (Bischoff-Ferrari et al. 2004). From the pooled risk difference, the number needed to treat was 15 (95% CI, 8 to 53) to prevent one fall. While these early studies show promising results, they are limited by the relatively small number of participants and short follow-up period. Clearly more clinical trials are needed prior to establishing evidence-based clinical recommendations with any degree of confidence.

Vitamin D toxicity is rare but does occur. Most commonly, toxicity is due to prolonged ingestion of high doses of vitamin D, usually 50 to 100 times the daily requirement in the elderly (Johnson et al. 2002). Chronic renal insufficiency, parathyroid disease, hypercalcemia, and granulomatous diseases increase the risk of toxicity. Symptoms generally are those of hypercalcemia. Serum and urine calcium levels should be monitored as an indicator of vitamin D toxicity. Excessive sunlight exposure will not lead to vitamin D toxicity with normal oral intake.

10.4.3 Vitamin E

Vitamin E exists in nature as eight related fat-soluble compounds, the tocopherols and tocotrienols, each in alpha, beta, gamma, and delta form. All are potent antioxidants. Alpha-tocopherol is the most biologically active of the tocopherols, though gamma-tocopherol is more prevalent in the human diet. Human trials have almost exclusively been conducted with alpha-tocopherol due to its potency. Dosing and RDA for vitamin E are reported either in milligrams as alpha-tocopherol equivalents (ATE), to account for different activities of the various forms of vitamin E, or in international units (IU). For conversion, 1 mg ATE equals 1.5 IU. Vitamin E is marketed with a *d* or *dl* designation, indicating the natural or synthetic form, respectively. The natural form, also known as RRR-alpha-tocopherol, is more active and better absorbed. Sources of vitamin E include egg yolk, leafy vegetables, wheat germ, various nuts, vegetable oils, margarine, and legumes. As with other fat-soluble compounds, intestinal absorption of vitamin E requires micelle and chylomicron formation and adequate production of bile acid. In the bloodstream, vitamin E is dispersed by a variety of lipoprotein transportation pathways after chylomicrons are broken down by lipoprotein lipase. Chylomicron remnant reuptake occurs in the liver in a process that is not fully explained, and vitamin E is excreted back into the bloodstream primarily bound to very low density lipoproteins (VLDLs). Approximately 90% of vitamin E is ultimately stored in adipose tissue. Adrenal glands, cell membranes, and circulating lipoproteins also accumulate vitamin E.

Three quarters of a century after its discovery, the diverse functions of vitamin E are still being studied and are incompletely understood. The hydroxyl group on the aromatic ring is responsible for the remarkable antioxidant property of the vitamin E molecule. Vitamin E is important in preventing peroxidation of polyunsaturated fatty acids, a major structural components of cell membranes. Blood cells and lung membranes particularly benefit from the antioxidant effect. Decreased incidence of some types of malignancies is thought to be due to decreased free radical cellular damage and stimulation of the humoral immune system. Apart from the antioxidant function, vitamin E has been shown to suppress production of leukotrienes, and thus inflammation, by inhibiting lypoxygenase. At a higher dose, vitamin E modifies the production of prostaglandins, such as thromboxane, and consequently inhibits platelet aggregation. Following activity as a free radical scavenger, nascent vitamin E can be regenerated by interacting with vitamin C or other antioxidants. Alternatively, vitamin E can be sequentially oxidized to a hydroquinone, conjugated to glucuronic acid, and excreted in bile.

Although the highest concentration of natural vitamin E is in foods that are not generally consumed in large amounts (e.g., oils, nuts), it is present ubiquitously, and deficiency does not commonly occur in the elderly. Prolonged fat malabsorption of any etiology, such as chronic pancreatic insufficiency, cholestasis, celiac disease, and inflammatory bowel disease, may lead to vitamin E deficiency. Due to the diverse activity of this vitamin, deficiency symptoms are widespread throughout the body and may include:

- Mild anemia related to increased erythrocyte hemolysis.
- Easy bruisability and prolonged clotting time.
- Degenerative myopathy presenting as muscle weakness.
- Neuronal degeneration and spinocerebellar dysfunction, more commonly encountered in children but may develop in the elderly. May present as spinocerebellar ataxia, decreased proprioception and vibratory perception, diminished deep tendor reflexes, and peripheral neuropathy. Ataxia is a basic manifestation of vitamin E deficiency, though many other causes may result in ataxia in the elderly.
- Extraocular muscle paresis and retinopathy.
- Ceroidosis and brown bowel syndrome due to accumulation of lipofuscin in the muscularis propria of the GI tract.

The RDA for vitamin E in adults is 15 mg/day. The elderly have taken much large doses of vitamin E (400 to 800 mg/day) without apparent ill effect. In persons taking >1000 mg/day, muscle weakness, fatigue, nausea, and diarrhea have been reported. In animal models, impaired absorption of vitamins A and K has been observed with large doses of vitamin E. The most significant clinical effect of supplementing vitamin E at doses over 1000 mg/day is the increased risk of hemorrhage in subjects on oral coumarin and other anticoagulant or antiplatelet agents.

10.4.4 Vitamin K

Vitamin K is a generic term for two groups of molecules that have in common a methylated naphthoquinone ring structure but vary in the aliphatic side chain. Vitamin K_1, or phylloquinone, is the natural form found in green leafy vegetables, cabbage, cauliflower, soy beans, cereals, vegetable oils, and liver. Vitamin K_2, or menaquinones, are synthesized by intestinal bacteria. Both forms are necessary to maintain adequate vitamin levels. Body stores of vitamin K are relatively small and concentrate mostly in the liver. Trabecular and cortical bone also contain significant concentrations. Vitamin K is necessary for the hepatic formation of coagulation factors II (prothrombin), VII (proconvertin), IX (Christmas factor), and X. It functions primarily as a cofactor for the enzyme gamma-glutamylcarboxylase, which converts glutamate (Glu) to gamma-carboxyglutamate (Gla), necessary for binding calcium and for activation of the coagulation factors. Other coagulation factors dependent on vitamin K for activation are protein C, protein S, and the thrombin-targeting protein Z. Two bone matrix proteins, osteocalcin and matrix-Gla protein, necessary for normal bone metabolism, are also vitamin K dependent. Common to these proteins is the posttranslational requirement for carboxylation of glutamic acid residues in order to become biologically active.

The daily requirement of vitamin K is 90 µg for women over the age of 50 and 120 µg for men over 50. Despite low body stores, deficiency occurs rarely in adults because vitamin K is widely distributed in plants and animal tissues. Furthermore, the vitamin K cycle conserves the vitamin and allows for its reutilization, and the gastrointestinal flora produces significant amounts of menoquinones. Deficiency can occur in:

- Persons with marginal dietary intake, particularly if they undergo significant trauma, extensive surgery, or prolonged parenteral nutrition
- Prolonged treatment with broad-spectrum antibiotics
- Persons with fat malabsorption of any cause
- Persons on medications that may interfere with vitamin K absorption or metabolism, such as anticonvulsants, anticoagulants, antibiotics, salicylates, and megadose vitamin A or E
- Malnutrition and starvation

In all cases, vitamin K deficiency is manifested by a prolonged prothrombin time (PT) and activated partial thromboplastin time (aPTT). Measuring serum levels has not proven helpful, especially without knowledge of vitamin K intake. The main clinical symptoms relate to bleeding propensity and are easy bruisability, mucosal bleeding including epistaxis and gastrointestinal hemorrhage, menorrhagia, hematuria, and spontaneous hemarthrosis in advanced cases. Hypoprothrombinemia is the feature differentiating vitamin K-related bleeding from other diseases, such as scurvy, allergic purpura, leukemia, and thrombocytopenia. Vitamin K is not contraindicated in the elderly undergoing warfarin therapy, but daily vitamin K intake from all sources should be kept relatively constant to avoid wide fluctuations in the prothrombin time. Even at 500 times the RDA, vitamin K is nontoxic in the elderly.

In recent years, the role of vitamin K in maintaining bone health has received considerable attention. The Gla-protein osteocalcin is synthesized by osteoblasts and regulated by $1,25(OH)_2D_3$. The mineral-binding capacity of osteocalcin, however, requires vitamin K-dependent gamma-carboxylation of three glutamic acid residues. Undercarboxylated osteocalcin rises markedly with age and correlates strongly with hip fractures (Szulc et al. 1993). Low-dose vitamin K supplementation can decrease serum levels of undercarboxylated osteocalcin and decrease urinary loss of calcium (Vermeer et al. 1992). Clinical evidence supporting the putative benefit of vitamin K on bone health is starting to emerge. In a study of over 72,000 women, low vitamin K intake increased the risk of hip fractures (Feskanich et al. 1999). This study, however, was conducted on younger women (age 38 to 63 years) and utilized a food frequency questionnaire. In a smaller study of men and women with an average age of 75.2 years, low vitamin K intake was associated with an increased incidence of hip fractures in both genders (Booth et al. 2000). No association was found between vitamin K intake and BMD in this study, but in a follow-up trial by the same investigators, low dietary vitamin K intake was associated with low BMD in women but not men (Booth et al. 2003). Finally, vitamin K_1 serum levels were shown to correlate with BMD in the hemiplegic limb (and to a lesser extent contralateral limb) of stroke patients, independent of vitamin D status (Sato et al. 1999).

10.5 WATER-SOLUBLE VITAMINS

10.5.1 Vitamin B_1 (Thiamin)

Thiamin pyrophosphate (TPP), the biologically active form of thiamin, functions as a coenzyme for a small number of crucial reactions necessary for cellular energy production via the Kreb's cycle. Oxydative decarboxylation of pyruvate and alpha-ketoglutarate, to form acetyl-coenzyme A and succinyl-coenzyme A, respectively, requires enzymes that are TPP dependent. Transketolase, the pentose phosphate pathway enzyme, is also dependent on TPP for proper function. One of the most important intermediates of this pathway is ribose-5-phophate, a precursor for the energy-rich ribonucleotide adenosine triphosphate (ATP) and nucleic acids (DNA and RNA). Since transketolase activity decreases early in thiamin deficiency, the erythrocyte transketolase activation coefficient (ETK-AC) has been used to assess thiamin status. ETK-AC is a functional assay affected by various factors, including other nutritional deficiencies, diabetes, liver disease, and age (Telwar et al. 2000). The newer direct measurement of thiamine pyrophosphate in erythrocytes is a more precise measurement, particularly in the deficiency state.

Sources of thiamin include whole grains, nuts, legumes, pork, liver, and yeast. White (milled) rice and flour are fortified with thiamin since most of the vitamin is lost during the processing of these foods. A varied diet should provide most of the elderly with sufficient thiamin intake. In the NHANES I study, however, up to 46% of the elderly had intake of vitamin B_1 less than two thirds of the RDA, and intake correlated with caloric consumption (Abraham et al. 1979). The incidence of thiamin deficiency has been estimated at 13 to 43% in community-dwelling elderly and 5% of nursing home residents (Joshi and Morley 2006). Race, income, and institutionalization were significant risk factors for thiamin deficiency. The decreased incidence in some nursing home populations may be due to the common practice of administering multivitamin supplements to all at-risk residents of long-term-care facilities. Another cause—the primary cause one in industrialized countries—of thiamin deficiency is alcoholism. With alcohol abuse, increased urinary loss (due to high fluid intake and urine production) exacerbates poor nutritional intake. Prolonged diuretic use in renal insufficiency may prevent renal tubular reabsorption of thiamin (Suter et al. 2000), and renal failure with hemodialysis or peritoneal dialysis may accelerate thiamin loss (Hung et al. 2001). Increased utilization of thiamin may be seen with vigorous activity, prolonged fever, and physiologic stress, such as major operation, and may precipitate a deficiency state in those with marginal levels. Refeeding after starvation and administering glucose to thiamin-depleted persons require thiamin supplementation due to the metabolic demand of glucose utilization.

Early symptoms of thiamin deficiency may be vague or insidious and include constipation, anorexia, nausea, fatigue, and peripheral neuropathy. The severe deficiency state, known as beriberi, is not commonly seen in developed countries. In Southeast Asia, it is the result of a diet rich in carbohydrates that has been stripped of nutrients, such as polished rice. The purported etymology of beriberi is from the Sinhalese word for "weakness," depicting the peripheral neuropathy that accompanies the disease. Symptoms can generally be classified into four categories:

- Peripheral neuropathy, or dry beriberi: May affect motor or sensory pathways and generally presents with paresthesia, hyperreflexia, weakness, and diminished sensation in the arms or legs.
- Cardiac failure, or wet beriberi: Symptoms may include tachycardia, cardiomegaly, dyspnea due to pulmonary congestion or edema, and generalized edema. This is a high-output cardiac failure and may progress rapidly.
- Wernicke's encephalopathy: Represents central nervous system involvement and may present with abnormal eye movements (extraocular muscular palsy, nystagmus), gait and balance abnormalities, and declining mental function. If untreated, the clinical course may rapidly deteriorate to vomiting, hypothermia, hypotension, stupor, coma, and death.
- Korsakoff's psychosis (or Korsakoff amnestic syndrome): A profound memory disorder presenting with impairment of the ability to acquire new knowledge or information, to form new memories, and to retrieve previous memories.

Wernicke's encephalopathy and Korsakoff's psychosis are generally viewed as different stages of the same disorder. The latter typically tends to develop as Wernicke's symptoms diminish and, as such, represents the chronic phase of the disorder. At this late stage, the symptoms are not likely to fully reverse with thiamin replacement. Some experts use the term *Wernecke's disease* when central nervous involvement is present without amnestic symptoms and *Wernicke–Korsakoff syndrome* (WKS) when amnestic symptoms exist alongside the nystagmus and ataxia. Central or cerebral beriberi has also been used to refer to both conditions.

Because thiamin deficiency can lead to WKS and long-lasting cognitive impairment, its relation to Alzheimer's dementia has been questioned. No randomized controlled trials have satisfactorily addressed this question to date, but early studies provide some insight. In a cross-sectional observational study, plasma thiamine deficiency was associated with Alzheimer's dementia but not with Parkinson's disease (Gold et al. 1998). Thiamin supplementation at several times the RDA dose resulted in moderate cognitive improvement (Meador et al. 1993, Benton et al. 1995, Mimori et al. 1996) or no cognitive improvement (Nolan et al. 1991, Rodriguez-Martin et al. 2001) in patients with early stages of Alzheimer's dementia. Finally, a controlled trial in 80 older females with marginal baseline thiamin levels suggested that thiamin supplementation improved overall quality of life as measured by improved appetite, sleep pattern, activity level, and decreased fatigue (Smidt et al. 1991). Thiamin is well tolerated at many times the RDA and toxicity is rare; excess thiamin is rapidly excreted in the urine.

10.5.2 Vitamin B_2 (Riboflavin)

Riboflavin is an integral component of coenzymes flavin mononucleotide (FMN) and flavin adenine dinucleotide (FAD), both of which are essential for oxidation–reduction reactions in multiple metabolic pathways. FAD is involved in ATP production via the mitochondrial oxidative phoshporylation cascade. As a component of glutathione reductase in the pentose–phosphate pathway, riboflavin is important in the production of reduced glutathione, a potent intracellular antioxidant. Flavins also participate in the hepatic metabolism of drugs and toxins, in conjunction with cytochrome P-450. Sources of riboflavin include dairy products, fortified cereals, meat, liver, eggs, cheese, fish, and green leafy vegetables. Riboflavin is heat stable, but is destroyed by exposure to light.

Vitamin B_2 deficiency, or ariboflavinosis, is relatively common in the U.S. and may result from insufficient dietary intake or disease conditions such as persistent diarrhea, liver disease, or alcohol abuse. It rarely occurs in isolation and is more likely to be seen in conjunction with other water-soluble vitamin deficiencies. Riboflavin deficiency may present with inflammation of the oral mucosa, cheilosis, angular stomatitis, magenta tongue (inflammation and redness of the tongue), seborrheic dermatitis, revascularization of the cornea, and normochromic normocytic anemia. These symptoms are not pathognomonic of ariboflavinosis, as some may occur with other other vitamin B-complex deficiencies.

The role of riboflavin in the pathogenesis of age-related cataracts has recently been studied. Opacification due to oxidative damage of lens proteins can theoretically be reduced with nutritional antioxidants. In controlled studies, cataract formation was inversely related to riboflavin intake (Cumming et al. 2000) and riboflavin levels (Leske et al. 1995) as measured by red blood cell glutathione reductase activity. In both studies, however, cataract prevention also correlated with other antioxidant vitamins and protein nutritional status. A third prospective study of over 50,000 women failed to show any correlation between riboflavin and cataracts (Hankinson et al. 1992). This last study, however, had a narrow range between the highest and lowest intake quintiles, and median intake for the lowest quintile was above the RDA.

10.5.3 Vitamin B_3 (Niacin)

Like riboflavin, niacin and its derivatives play a central role in cellular oxidation–reduction reactions. Niacin refers to nicotinic acid and nicotinamide, which are precursors of coenzymes nicotinamide adenine dinucleotide (NAD) and nicotinamide adenine dinucleotide phospate (NADP). Many enzymes require NAD and NADP as coenzymes for the transfer of electrons in the catabolic production of energy from carbohydrates, fats, and proteins, or the anabolic synthesis of fatty acids and cholesterol. Dietary sources of niacin include meat, fish, legumes, yeast, nuts, and seeds. Niacin can also be synthesized in the liver from dietary tryptophan, or by the intestinal flora. In natural cereal grains such as corn, millet, and wheat, niacin may be bound to sugars in the form of glycosides, which severely limits bioavailability (Gregory 1998). Thus, many commercially available cereals are fortified with niacin.

Niacin deficiency can result from diets deficient in niacin or tryptophan, or rich in maize and millet. Comorbid conditions contributing to a negative vitamin B_3 balance include alcoholism, chronic diarrhea, and cirrhosis. In carcinoid syndrome, increased synthesis of serotonin from tryptophan may lead to a relative deficiency of the latter. Consequently, less tryptophan is available for niacin synthesis. Hartnup's disease is a rare autosomal recessive disease often diagnosed early in life and caused by defective intestinal absorption and renal reuptake of tryptophan and other amino acids. Symptom severity varies and is generally attributed to the resultant niacin deficiency. The past two decades has seen a resurgence of tuberculosis. Prolonged treatment with the antituberculosis drug isoniazid, and other drugs, may result in niacin deficiency. The incidence of vitamin B_3 deficiency is difficult to establish and varies greatly by various estimates. This is in part due to diagnostic challenges. Symptoms are predictable but nonspecific, and a diagnosis based on clinical features is not sensitive or specific. Measurements of serum levels have not proven helpful, and nutritional intake questionnaires only provide inexact quantitation of intake and body stores due to bioavailability, absorption, and utilization variables. The most effective diagnostic test currently available is measurement of urinary metabolite N-methyl-2-pyridone-5-carboxamide by liquid chromatography (Moore et al. 2000).

Full-blown niacin deficiency presenting as pellagra is uncommon in Western societies, but might occasionally be seen in immigrant groups and extreme cases of PEM. Pellagra is characterized by the three D's: diarrhea, dermatitis, and dementia. Diarrhea is the most prominent gastrointestinal symptom, resulting from mucosal inflammation and ulceration. A red-tinged tongue and vomiting may also occur, and vaginal mucosa may be involved. Dermatitis takes various forms but most often presents as hyperpigmented symmetrical lesions in sun-exposed areas. Dementia of pellagra may develop alongside a host of neurological disorders. In early stages, these include delirium, headaches, loss of appetite, irritability, confusion, and amnesia. Psychiatric disorders such as depression, paranoia, anxiety, or apathy may also be present. If left untreated, symptoms may progress to frank encephalopathy. Involvement of the central nervous system is also characterized by cogwheel rigidity and uncontrollable sucking and grasping reflexes. Differentiating these symptoms from those of thiamin deficiency can be difficult, and the two may coexist. Extreme cases of niacin deficiency can ultimately be fatal, sometimes referred to as the fourth D of pellagra (i.e., death).

The RDA for vitamin B_3 is 14 mg/day for females over the age of 50 years and 16 mg/day for males. At higher doses (500 to 3000 mg/day), niacin has been effective in the management of dyslipidemia and cardiovascular disease (Knopp 1999, Miller 2003). The cholesterol-lowering effect of niacin was first reported as early as 1955 (Altschul et al. 1955). Since then, niacotinic acid has been shown to increase serum levels of high-density lipoprotein (HDL) cholesterol, and to lower triglycerides, lipoprotein(a), and, to a lesser extent, low-density lipoprotein (LDL) cholesterol and total cholesterol (Canner et al. 1986, Carlson and Rosenhamer 1988, Cheung et al. 2001, Brown et al. 2001, Coronary Drug Project Research Group 1975, Knopp et al. 1985, 1998). Clinically, nicotinic acid has been proven effective in reducing cardiovascular morbidity when used alone (Coronary Drug Project Research Group 1975, Canner et al. 1986) or in combination with statin drugs (Brown et al. 2001, Cheung et al. 2001), fibrates (Carlson and Rosenhamer 1988), or bile-acid-binding resins (Blankenhorn et al. 1987, Brown et al. 1990, Kane et al. 1990). The benefits of combining niacin with other lipid-lowering agents are better control of LDL cholesterol and better tolerability due to lower dosing. Adverse effects of nicotinic acid are more likely with higher doses and are sufficiently disturbing to result in discontinuation of the medication in over 25% of users (Miller 2003). Flushing of the skin due to nonspecific histamine release is the most prominent side effect. Pruritis, nasal congestion, gastrointestinal disturbance, diarrhea, and conjunctivitis may also occur. Administration of aspirin before each dose of niacin may alleviate the prostaglandin-mediated flush. Patients should be urged to continue the use of niacin during the initial symptomatic period since tachyphylaxis and tolerance develop, and aspirin can be discontinued in a few days (Knopp 1999). Sustained-release formulations are designed to minimize cutaneous flushing, but are associated with increased hepatic toxicity and may be less effective (Knopp et al. 1985, Knopp 2000, McKenney et al. 1994).

10.5.4 Vitamin B_6

Vitamin B_6 refers to three compounds structurally related to pyridine (pyridoxine, pyridoxal, and pyridoxamine) and their phosphorylated derivatives. Of these compounds, pyridoxal 5'-phosphate (PLP) is the most important coenzyme and is involved in a large number of diverse metabolic reactions. PLP is intimately involved in amino acid metabolism, including transamination, decarboxylation, and desulfuration reactions necessary for the synthesis of certain amino acids and neurotransmitters, such as serotonin, norepinephrin, and -aminobutyric acid (GABA). PLP is required for the synthesis of niacin from tryptophan. PLP also functions as a coenzyme for glycogen phosphorelase, an enzyme necessary for the release of glucose from stored glycogen in muscles and, for gluconeogenesis reactions, the process of generating glucose from amino acids. Production of the heme precursor aminolevulinic acid is dependent on PLP, as is the formation of sphyngolipids necessary for the development of the myelin sheath surrounding nerve cells.

Dietary sources of vitamin B_6 include meat, fish, nuts, whole grain, fortified cereal, and leafy vegetables. Bioavailability varies by food types, with pyridoxine glucoside being the least bioavailable. Glycosylated pyridoxine constitutes 5 to 75% of vitamin B_6 obtained from plant sources, but is virtually absent in vitamin B_6 from animal products. Vitamin B_6 is absorbed by passive diffusion from the lumen of the upper small intestine. Absorption is enhanced by an acidic milieu. The body does not store large amounts of the vitamin, and frequent intake is necessary to maintain metabolic requirements. Vitamin B_6 deficiency may result from decreased intake, malabsorption, alcoholism, liver cirrhosis, or dialysis. Medications such as isoniazide, hydralazine, penicillamine, cycloserine, and theophylline may bind or antagonize vitamin B_6. For this reason, supplementation with vitamin B_6 is recommended when isonizide is prescribed for prolonged periods. Clinical manifestations of vitamin B_6 deficiency include angular stomatitis, cheilosis, glossitis, peripheral neuropathy, irritability, confusion, and anemia. In the elderly, vitamin B_6 deficiency often occurs with other nutritional disorders. Symptoms are not specific to vitamin B_6. The diagnosis can be made by measuring plasma PLP or erythrocyte transaminase activity. Pyridoxine-dependent transaminase activity is decreased in vitamin B_6 deficiency, but the wide range of values in healthy persons make interpreting results difficult (Johnson et al. 2002).

The effect of vitamin B_6 on cardiovascular disease, cognitive function, and the immune system has recently been studied. Elevated serum homocysteine levels have been linked to increased risk of cardiovascular disease (Boushey et al. 1995, Eikelboom et al. 1999), and vitamin B_6 deficiency is associated with increased homocysteine levels. Whether homocysteine is an independent risk factor for cardiovascular disease or simply a marker of some other pathophysiological process continues to be debated. A large body of evidence alludes to the fact that homocysteine may promote intimal damage, atherosclerosis, and thrombosis (Gerhard and Duell 1999), but a direct causal relationship has not been demonstrated. In other words, it is not known if hyperhomocysteinemia per se, in the absence of vitamin B_6, B_{12}, and folate deficiency, is pathogenic. Several observational as well as prospective studies provide ample clinical support for the benefit of supplementing vitamin B_6 above the current RDA for primary prevention of cardiovascular disease. In a study of 80,000 women with no previous history of cardiovascular disease, hypercholesterolemia, or diabetes, Rimm et al. (1998) demonstrated the importance of vitamin B_6 and folate, individually and in combination, in the prevention of coronary heart disease. After controlling for cardiovascular risk factors, the relative risk of coronary heart disease between extreme quintiles of vitamin B_6 intake was 0.67 (95% CI, 0.53 to 0.85) after 14 years of follow-up. Another large prospective trial found higher levels of PLP to be associated with decreased risk of cardiovascular disease (Folsom et al. 1998). Furthermore, these findings were independent of homocysteine levels, shedding uncertainty on conclusions derived mostly from cross-sectional observational studies that homocysteine is a major causative risk factor for heart disease (Folsom et al. 1998, Eikelboom et al. 1999). Similar findings were noted in a controlled trial of over 1500 subjects (Robinson et al. 1998). Both folate and vitamin B_6 plasma levels were inversely related to the risk of cardiovascular disease. Low levels of vitamin B_6, but not folate, were associated with increased risk of disease independent of homocysteine. On the other hand, in a smaller controlled study of subjects hospitalized for myocardial infarction, homocysteine was found to be an independent risk factor (Verhoef et al. 1996). Interpreting these results is complicated by observations that in contrast to folate and vitamin B_{12}, supplementing vitamin B_6 alone does not necessarily lower fasting homocysteine levels significantly. After oral methionine loading, however, vitamin B_6 effectively decreased serum homocysteine levels (Ubbink et al. 1994, 1996). Furthermore, few geriatric subjects were included in these studies.

The effect of vitamin B_6 deficiency on the immune system resembles that of PEM in many ways. Low vitamin B_6 levels are associated with decreased number and function of circulating lymphocytes, as well as decreased production of interleukin 2 (Meydani et al. 1991, Talbott et al. 1987). In a small 3-week controlled trial of hospitalized elderly patients with acute infections, vitamin B_6 levels were lower in the study group than in the control group at days 7 and 14 of the study (Pfitzenmeyer et al. 1997). The authors, however, make no causative conclusions, but speculate that an acute catabolic state, like infection, may influence vitamin B_6 metabolism. Nevertheless, Meydani et al. (1991) demonstrated that impairment of the cellular immune system associated with vitamin B_6 deficiency can be reversed with vitamin repletion, but at doses above the RDA.

Observational studies have demonstrated a correlation between loss of cognitive function in the elderly and declining vitamin B_6 levels, and thus elevated homocysteine levels (Selhub et al. 2000). In one cross-sectional observational study, higher plasma concentrations of vitamin B_6 were associated with better performance on two measures of memory, but not 18 other measures of cognitive function (Riggs et al. 1996). Interventional trials in older subjects have been somewhat disappointing. In a trial of 76 men, age 70 to 79 years, the control group (n = 38) received 20 mg vitamin B_6 daily (RDA = 1.7 mg) for 3 months (Deijen et al. 1992). A modest but significant improvement in memory was noted. In a more recent 5-week trial, 12 women, age 65 to 92, were allocated to the vitamin B_6 segment of a four-arm trial, and no statistically significant benefits from vitamin B_6 on mood or cognition were observed (Bryan et al. 2002). Both trials were limited by the small number of study subjects and short follow-up period, and at present it is unclear whether declining vitamin B_6 levels in the elderly contribute to age-associated cognitive impairment, or whether both arise from a third confounding variable.

10.5.5 Folate

The terms *folate* and *folic acid* are often used interchangeably and are also known as vitamin B_9. Natural folate occurs in over 35 forms and is ubiquitous in nature. Natural folate is highly susceptible to oxidative and heat destruction, and 50 to 95% of the food content of folate is lost by excessive cooking and canning (Johnson et al. 2002). While most foods contain folate, the highest concentrations are found in green leafy vegetables, citrus fruits, legumes, yeast, liver, and other organ meats. Folic acid, the pharmacologic form of the vitamin, is more stable and bioavailable than folate, but rarely occurs in natural foods. It is the form most often used in vitamin supplements and fortified foods.

The various functions of folate in humans appear to be centered around the transfer of single-carbon units. The folate coenzyme acts as an acceptor and donor of one-carbon groups required mainly for the metabolism of amino acids and nucleic acids. Folate is required for the synthesis of methionine, and hence the regeneration of the universal methyl donor S-adenosylmethionine (SAM). SAM is a methyl donor involved in many biological reactions, including methylation of RNA and DNA, which may play a role in cancer prevention. The remethylation of homocysteine into methionine is dependent on folate as well as vitamin B_{12}. Folate deficiency results in accumulation of homocysteine, increasing the risk of cardiovascular disease. Of the three vitamins involved in homocysteine metabolism (folate, vitamin B_6, and B_{12}), folate is the most effective in lowering serum levels.

Folate is absorbed from the small intestine by both passive and active mechanisms. In the circulation, folate is loosely bound to albumin as 5-methyltetrahydrofolate and taken up by various cells via a high-affinity folate receptor. Folates undergo enterohepatic recirculation, and excess folates are excreted in the urine. The body does not hold extensive stores of folate. Folate deficiency may occur after just a few days of diminished intake, though symptoms may take longer to develop. It is estimated that 2.5 to 34% of the elderly experience folate deficiency (Joshi and Morley 2006). Beyond decreased intake and malnutrition, folate deficiency may occur with excessive alcohol intake, smoking, atrophic gastritis, inflammatory bowel disease, and certain medication use, such as methotrexate, triamterene, and antiepileptic drugs (Kishi et al. 1997). Individual folate status can be assessed by direct serum folate measurement. With recent changes in dietary intake, red cell folate levels may be a better indicator of body stores. Rapidly dividing cells are the most susceptible to the effects of low folate levels. Folate deficiency can present with macrocytic anemia, leukopenia, and thrombocytopenia. Hypersegmented neutrophils may be seen on microscopic examination of a peripheral blood smear. Because of the 3-month life span of red blood cells, full-blown megaloblastic anemia may take many weeks to become apparent. Other clinical sequelae of folate deficiency include loss of appetite, fatigue, diarrhea, glossitis, and delirium.

Due to the high prevalence of folate deficiency in the elderly, and the potential benefit of folate in the mitigation of cancer, atherosclerotic vascular disease, and dementia, the 1998 RDA for folate was increased to 400 μg for men and women, double that of previous recommendations. Folate supplementation at 5 mg/day has been associated with decreased markers of colorectal cancer, as measured by DNA methylation and DNA strand breaks (Cravo et al. 1998, Kim et al. 2001). Epidemiological studies as well as prospective controlled trials have found a similar inverse relationship between folate intake and the incidence of colon cancer (Freudenheim et al. 1991, Ferraroni et al. 1994, Su and Arab 2001, Terry et al. 2002, White et al. 1997, Giovannucci et al. 1993, 1998), though the relationship was weaker (Giovannucci et al. 1998) or absent (Su and Arab 2001) in women. Alcohol consumption interferes with the absorption and metabolism of folate (Herbet 1999). In a large prospective study, greater than two alcoholic drinks per day doubled the risk of colorectal cancer, and the risk increased further with low folate intake (Giovannucci et al. 1995). The consumption of 650 μg/day or more of folate, however, appeared to cancel the increased alcohol-related risk of colon cancer. A similar finding was noted with breast cancer. Three studies have shown that increased folate intake reduces the risk of breast cancer in women who consume alcohol regularly (Rohan et al. 2000, Sellers et al. 2001, Zhang et al. 1999).

As previously mentioned, serum homocysteine is associated with cardiovascular disease. In fact, over 80 studies have found that even moderately elevated levels of homocysteine increase the risk of cardiovascular disease (Gerhard and Duell 1999). A meta-analysis of 38 observational studies estimated that lowering homocysteine blood levels by 1 μmol/l reduced the risk of coronary artery disease (CAD) by 10% (Boushey et al. 1995). The odds ratio for CAD of a 5 μmol/l increment in serum homocysteine was 1.6 (95% CI, 1.4 to 1.7) for men and 1.8 (95% CI, 1.3 to 1.9) for women (Boushey et al. 1995). What is not yet known is whether lowering homocysteine levels with folate will decrease the risk of cardiovascular disease (Stampfer and Malinow 1995). Several randomized placebo-controlled trials are currently being conducted to specifically answer this question. In a 10-year prospective cohort study of 1980 Finnish men age 42 to 60 years, the relative risk reduction for acute coronary events in men in the highest quintile of folate intake was 55% compared to the lowest quintile (RR, 0.45; 95% CI, 0.25 to 0.81; p = 0.008) (Voutilainen et al. 2001). Until results of controlled clinical trials become available, the emphasis should be placed on meeting current RDAs for folate, as well as vitamins B_6 and B_{12}, by intake of fresh fruits and vegetables (Malinow et al. 1999). For high-risk patients, the Nutrition Committee of the American Heart Association recommends daily supplementation with 0.4 mg folic acid, 2 mg vitamin B_6, and 6 µg vitamin B_{12}, with the goal of lowering homocysteine levels below 10 μmol/l (Malinow et al. 1999).

In recent years, several investigators have focused attention on the association between decreased folate intake and cognitive impairment in the elderly (Weir and Molloy 2000). In a cross-sectional Canadian study of subjects 65 years or older, low folate levels were associated with depression, short-term memory impairment, and dementia of all kinds (Ebly et al. 1998). Low folate was also associated with increased risk of institutionalization, low body mass index (BMI), and low serum albumin levels, but it is not clear to what extent these findings reflect poor nutritional intake in elderly frail patients with dementia. Other studies have shown an association between decreased serum folate levels (Snowdon et al. 2000, Wang et al. 2001) or increased homocysteine levels (Seshadri et al. 2002) and Alzheimer's disease. With baseline homocysteine levels greater than 14 μmol/l in elderly subjects without dementia, the risk of developing Alzheimer's disease nearly doubled over an 8-year follow-up period (Seshadri et al. 2002). In another study, low serum folate levels were similarly associated with doubling the risk of developing Alzheimer's dementia in 370 elderly subjects followed for 3 years (Wang et al. 2001). Furthermore, low serum folate was strongly associated with atrophy of the cerebral cortex related to Alzheimer's disease (Snowdon et al. 2000). Other types of dementia might also be affected by low folate levels. In the Health Professional Follow-up Study, increased folate intake was associated with a decreased risk of ischemic stroke in men (He et al. 2004). It is quite possible that vascular and other forms of dementia are more prevalent with folate deficiency (Ebly et al. 1998), but more extensive trials are needed to delineate the magnitude of the effect.

There are no known adverse or toxic effects associated with excessive folate intake. Large doses of folic acid, however, may mask vitamin B_{12} deficiency. Megaloblastic anemia occurs with vitamin B_{12} deficiency and is indistinguishable from that of folate deficiency. Consumption of large amounts of folic acid in individuals with undiagnosed B_{12} deficiency could correct the anemia without addressing the underlying deficiency (Higdon 2002). Progressive and irreversible neurological damage may result. For this reason and others, the Food and Nutrition Board of the Institute of Medicine advises that all adults limit their intake of folic acid from all sources to 1000 μg daily.

10.5.6 Vitamin B_{12} (Cobalamin)

Vitamin B_{12} is a complex molecule consisting of a tetrapyrrol ring structure (corrin ring) connected through an aminopropanol bridge to a ribonucleotide. The ring center contains a molecule of the metal ion cobalt. The principal forms of vitamin B_{12} in the human body are methylcobalamin and 5-deoxyadenosylcobalamin. Cyanocobalamin is the form used for food fortification and vitamin supplements and is readily converted to 5-deoxyadenosylcobalamin and methylcobalamin (Higdon 2003). Vitamin B_{12} is an important cofactor required for the proper function of the enzymes methionine synthase and L-methylmalonyl-CoA mutase. Methionine synthase is needed for the conversion of homocysteine to methionine. This process involves a methyl group transfer from 5-methylene tetrahydrofolate to cobalamin, resulting in the formation of methylcobalamin and tetrahydrofolate. Methylcobalamin in turn donates its methyl group to homocysteine to form methionin, and in the process cobalamin is regenerated. As previously discussed, methionin is required for the synthesis of S-adenosylmethionine (SAM), the methyl group donor necessary for many cellular methylation reactions, including the methylation of RNA and DNA. The other main function of vitamin B_{12} is the synthesis of succinyl-CoA from L-methylmalonyl-CoA by the enzyme L-methylmalonyl-CoA mutase, which requires 5-deoxyadenosylcobalamin as a coenzyme. Succinyl-CoA is essential for energy production in the Kreb's cycle, and for the synthesis of hemoglobin.

Dietary sources of vitamin B_{12} include fish, meat, chicken, milk, and cheese. The vitamin is generally not found in plants or yeast. The RDA for vitamin B_{12} in the elderly is 2.4 μg. An 8-ounce cup of milk contains approximately 0.9 μg of vitamin B_{12} and may be an important source of the vitamin for vegetarians (Institute of Medicine 1998). Gastric acid and enzymes are required to free protein-bound vitamin B_{12} from ingested food, allowing it to bind proteins called haptocorrin or R-proteins. In the small intestine, R-proteins are degraded by pancreatic proteases and B_{12} binds to intrinsic factor (IF), a transport glycoprotein produced by gastric parietal cells. The IF–B_{12} complex is absorbed from the terminal ileum via receptors on the enterocytes. The vitamin enters the portal circulation bound to transcobalamine II and is transported to the liver for storage. About 1% of vitamin B_{12} is absorbed by passive diffusion, independent of IF.

Unlike folate, where deficiency is typically due to decreased intake, vitamin B_{12} deficiency in the elderly is generally the result of decreased absorption, with the exception of strict vegans. Owing to large hepatic stores and efficient enterohepatic recirculation, the effective half-life of vitamin B_{12} is long, and a deficiency state may take several years to develop. Deficiency in the elderly ranges between 4 and 43% (Baik and Russell 1999, Joshi and Morley 2006), depending on the population studied and the serum marker and cutoff points used to define deficiency. Because the release of protein-bound dietary vitamin B_{12} is dependent on gastric acid, conditions resulting in hypochlorhydria may lead to deficiency. Atrophic gastritis effects up to 30% of older adults (Baik and Russell 1999, linus) and may result in decreased absorption of vitamin B_{12} due to decreased acid secretion. Prolonged use of histamine (H_2) receptor antagonists or proton pump inhibitors can potentially have a similar effect. In both cases, supplemental vitamin B_{12}, which is not bound to proteins, continues to be well absorbed, provided IF secretion is not affected. Bacterial overgrowth in the small intestine, due to hypochlorhydria or other causes, may result in B_{12} deficiency because of bacterial competition for uptake of the vitamin. Other conditions affecting intestinal digestion of vitamin B_{12} include pancreatic insufficiency (due to decreased degradation of R-protein), ileal resection or bypass, Crohn's disease, tropical sprue, celiac sprue, and malignancy. Total gastrectomy results in B_{12} deficiency secondary to loss of intrinsic factor and acidity. Approximately 10 to 30% of patients who undergo partial gastrectomy have inadequate B_{12} absorption (Sumner et al. 1996). Pernicious anemia may affect 2 to 5% of individuals over the age of 60 years and may be more prevalent in certain populations (Carmel 1996, Institute of Medicine 2001, Joshi and Morley 2006). Among family members of patients with pernicious anemia, approximately 20% will also develop the disease. Pernicious anemia is caused by autoimmune damage to gastric parietal cells, resulting in diminished acid secretion and IF production. Autoantibodies are directed against hydrogen–potassium adenosine triphosphatase (proton pump), IF, or both (Pruthi and Tefferi 1994). Since enteric vitamin supplementation is poorly absorbed, intramuscular vitamin B_{12}, usually hydroxycobalamine, is necessary to treat the deficiency state associated with pernicious anemia.

Regardless of the cause, vitamin B_{12} deficiency is diagnosed by hematological tests. Direct serum measurement of vitamin B_{12} can be used to assess for deficiency, but serum levels are not a sensitive indicator of tissue levels or total body stores (Lindenbaum et al. 1990). Elevated blood levels of homocysteine and methylmalonic acid (MMA) are an earlier and more reliable indicator of cobalamin deficiency. These metabolites accumulate due to impaired methionine synthase and L-methylmalonyl-CoA mutase function. Homocysteine levels can also be elevated because of renal failure or folate or vitamin B_6 deficiency. Elevated MMA levels, on the other hand, do not occur with these conditions and are more indicative of B_{12} deficiency. Clinical symptoms of vitamin B_{12} deficiency, and megaloblastic anemia, are not reliable diagnostic tools. They typically are late manifestations of vitamin B_{12} deficiency and could result from an array of other conditions. Neurologic deficits include paresthesia and abnormal position or vibratory sense. Progression to weakness and ataxia may occur if untreated. Subacute combined degeneration refers to involvement of both posterior and lateral columns of the spinal cord. Central nervous system manifestations also include mental confusion, memory loss, and depression. Clinical symptoms may develop without the presence of macrocytic anemia. The Shilling's test is rarely used in the workup of vitamin B_{12} deficiency in the elderly. Although it was devised to shed light on the specific cause of the deficiency, it is cumbersome to administer and interpret and is fraught with multiple potential sources of error in the frail elderly (Fairbanks et al. 1983). Perhaps the best means of detecting tissue depletion of vitamin B_{12} is the transcobalamin assay (Stabler 1995, Metz et al. 1996); however, this test is costly and generally not reimbursed by third-party payers (Johnson et al. 2002). Since supplementation is safe and cost-effective, it would seem clinically prudent to supplement all older individuals who have elevated MMA or homocystein levels, even if serum B_{12} levels are normal.

Traditionally, the treatment for vitamin B_{12} deficiency consisted of intramuscular injections of cyanocobalamin. Once body stores are repleted, a maintenance dose of 1000 μg is equally effective in preventing recurrence when administered every 1, 2, or 4 months (Hajjar et al. 2000). More recently, however, enteral supplementation is favored, despite the age-associated decreased absorption of vitamin B_{12}. Even in pernicious anemia, passive absorption of oral supplementation will prevent recurrence of deficiency if administered in sufficient amounts (Kuzminski et al. 1998). In such cases, it is recommended that overt deficiency be corrected with parenteral supplementation, and that the daily oral maintenance dose be 1000 μg rather than the usual 100 to 500 μg. An alternate to high-dose oral therapy in persons lacking IF is B_{12} nasal gel.

As with folate and vitamin B_6 deficiency, hyperhomocysteinemia due to vitamin B_{12} deficiency is associated with increased risk of cardiovascular disease. In a meta-analysis of 12 trials, folate supplementation at 0.5 to 5 mg/day was found to have the greatest effect on lowering homocysteine blood levels, followed by vitamin B_{12} supplementation at 500 μg/day (Homocysteine Lowering Trialists' Collaboration 1998), though some evidence suggests that vitamin B_{12} is an increasingly important determinant of elevated homocysteine in the elderly (Stabler et al. 1997). Although studies have shown a decreased risk of cardiovascular disease with high levels of folate and vitamin B_6, no such findings have yet been shown with vitamin B_{12} (Joshi and Morley 2006, Eikelboom et al. 1999).

Vitamin B_{12} deficiency has also been implicated as a risk factor for malignancy and neuropsychiatric disorders. In findings similar to those of folate deficiency, impaired DNA methylation and DNA damage may result from vitamin B_{12} deficiency. Increased serum levels of homocysteine and decreased levels of vitamin B_{12} were associated with biomarkers of chromosome damage, and supplementing folate and vitamin B_{12} at 3.5 times the RDA diminished these markers (Fenech 1999). These findings, however, were observed mostly in younger individuals, and it is not entirely clear as to which vitamin predominantly influences risk. In a case-control observational study, postmenopausal women with vitamin B_{12} levels in the lowest quintile had more than twice the risk of breast cancer compared to those in higher quintiles (Wu et al. 1999). The investigators found no such correlation between breast cancer and serum levels of folate, vitamin B_6, or homocysteine. A causal relationship between breast cancer and vitamin B_{12} deficiency cannot be made from this observational study.

Vitamin B_{12} deficiency and elevated homocysteine blood levels have also been linked to Alzheimer's disease (Clarke et al. 1998, Wang et al. 2001, Seshadri et al. 2002) and depression (Hutto 1997, Penninx et al. 2000, Tiemeier et al. 2002).

Approximately 30% of patients hospitalized for depression were found to be deficient in the vitamin (Hutto 1997), and community-dwelling women over the age of 65 years with vitamin B_{12} deficiency were twice as likely to experience severe depression (Penninx et al. 2000). The reason for the association between vitamin B_{12} and neuropsychiatric disorders is unclear. Several explanations have been proposed. Vitamin B_{12} is necessary for the methylation and synthesis of myelin sheath and certain neurotransmitters. Decreased synthesis of methionine and S-adenosylmethionine will affect this function. Although decreased nutritional intake resulting from depression or dementia undoubtedly plays a central role in nutritional deficiencies, the association appears to be more complex than that. After controlling for nutritional status, one study indicated that the association between homocysteine or B_{12} levels and Alzheimer's dementia was not solely due to dementia-associated malnutrition (Clarke et al. 1998). Nutritional factors as a *cause* of dementia and depression are less well studied, but some experts believe that vitamin B_{12} and general nutrition play a protective role, not yet fully understood, in the development of these conditions (Nourhashemi et al. 2000). Finally, it is worth noting that neuropsychiatric disorders due to cobalamin deficiency may develop in the absence of anemia or elevated mean corpuscular volume of red cells (Lindenbaum et al. 1988).

10.5.7 Vitamin C (Ascorbic Acid)

Vitamin C is synthesized as L-ascorbic acid in most plants and animals, but not in humans. The D-enantiomer has no known biological activity. It is found in many fruits and vegetables in varying concentrations, most notably kiwi, citrus fruits, strawberries, currant berries, red pepper, broccoli, tomatoes, potatoes, and raw leafy vegetables such as parsley. The concentration of vitamin C in a single food source varies depending on season, shelf time prior to consumption, method of storage, and cooking practices. For example, supermarket broccoli can lose a third of its vitamin C content compared to wholesaler or fresh broccoli, and boiling vegetables can cause a 50 to 80% loss of the vitamin (Johnson et al. 2002). Prolonged boiling may destroy vitamin C, but the majority of vitamin loss from cooking is due to leaching of the vitamin into the cooking water. Vegetable soups, therefore, may not be as deficient in vitamin C as once thought. Steaming vegetables, using microwave ovens, or cooking with minimal amounts of water will decrease vitamin C loss.

Vitamin C is absorbed in the small intestine through an energy-dependent transport process. Absorption, and hence bioavailability, is inversely related to dose. A total daily dose of 200 mg of pure vitamin C ingested in divided doses would have nearly complete bioavailability (Levine et al. 1999). With increasing doses, the percent absorption decreases, even as the absolute amount absorbed increases. Food components such as glucose might decrease bioavailability by decreasing absorption. The biological half-life of vitamin C in the blood is rather short—generally 30 to 60 minutes. A number of medications are known to lower vitamin C blood levels, by either decreasing absorption or increasing excretion. For example, two aspirin taken four times a day has been shown to lower white blood cell vitamin C levels by 50% within 1 week, primarily due to increased renal excretion (Basu 1982). Vitamin C undergoes glomerular filtration and concentration-dependent active tubular reabsorption (Levine et al. 1999). Though no organ system functions as a storage site for vitamin C per se, the adrenal glands, pituitary, thymus, and retina can concentrate the vitamin at over 50 times serum levels (Jacob 1999). The brain, spleen, testicles, liver, thyroid, leukocytes, pancreas, and kidneys normally contain 5 to 25 times the blood levels of vitamin C (Groff et al. 1995, Jacob 1999). Cellular accumulation of ascorbic acid is mediated by active transport, and cells may saturate at lower doses (100 mg/day) despite low plasma levels. As a general rule, vitamin C levels are approximately 20% higher in women than in men, and nonsmokers have higher levels than smokers (Institute of Medicine 2000, Johnson et al. 2002). Consequently, the RDA for men is 90 mg/day (75 mg/day for women), and smokers need an additional 35 mg/day of vitamin C above the requirement of nonsmokers (Institute of Medicine 2000). Deficiency may occur in up to 5% of frail elderly and is caused by insufficient dietary intake (Joshi and Morley 2006). Vitamin C status is best evaluated by measuring plasma or leukocyte levels.

The multiple effects of vitamin C can be classified according to three main functional categories:

- Ascorbate as a synthetic compound. Vitamin C is essential for the synthesis and integrity of collagen, which is a crucial structural component of blood vessels, tendons, ligaments, and bone, and is important in wound healing. Vitamin C also plays an important role in the synthesis of norepinephrine and carnithine, the latter being necessary for transfer of fat into mitochondria for energy production.
- Ascorbate as an antioxidant. Vitamin C is an effective antioxidant that limits the harmful effects of free radicals generated during normal metabolism or exposure to pollutants and toxins such as smoking. Vitamin C protects DNA, proteins, lipids, and carbohydrates against oxidative damage.
- Ascorbate as a chemical reductant. Vitamin C facilitates absorption of iron in the duodenum and the conversion of methemoglobin to hemoglobin by reducing ferric iron (Fe^{3+}) to the ferrous form (Fe^{2+}). Vitamin C is also involved in the reduction of nitrates. Decreased formation of mutagenic nitrosamines possibly confers protection against gastric cancer.

Vitamin C deficiency results in decreased collagen cross-linking, which leads to diminished collagen tensile strength. Decreased wound healing and weakened blood vessels cause hemostasis abnormalities. Clinical manifestations include painful subperiosteal hemorrhages, hemarthrosis, hemorrhagic perifolliculitis, gingival bleeding, and petechia or ecchymoses. Some of these findings are common in the elderly and may be attributed to age-related physiologic changes, medications, or comorbidities, rather than vitamin deficiency (Joshi and Morley 2006). Another consequence of structurally abnormal collagen is structurally abnormal bone. Scurvy, the full-blown deficiency syndrome, develops with vitamin C intake of less than 10 mg/day for as little as 3 months. In addition to the previously mentioned physical findings, scurvy involves the development of corkscrew hairs, glossitis, gingival hyperplasia and bleeding, and poor dentition or loss of teeth due to periodontal disease. Iron deficiency anemia can also occur. Terminal features include icterus, edema, hypotension, convulsions, and death. Scurvy is rarely encountered in modern-day societies, but the existence of a milder form of the disease known as chronic subclinical scurvy and presenting as senile purpura has been debated (Stone 1972).

Being water soluble, vitamin C has few toxic effects, and adverse effects are related to intake dose (Levine et al. 1995). Ingestion of more than 2000 mg daily, the Tolerable Upper Limit, can cause gastrointestinal symptoms such as nausea, abdominal cramps, and diarrhea (Miller and Hays 1982). Abnormal vitamin B_{12} absorption and increased blood levels of estrogen replacement hormone can also occur. Excess vitamin C may interfere with a number of laboratory tests and may cause false-negative results on stool guaiac tests and on urine dipstick evaluation for blood, glucose, bilirubin, nitrites, and leukocyte esterase. Because vitamin C enhances iron absorption, patients suffering from hemochromatosis, thalassemia major, sideroblastic anemia, or other conditions requiring multiple red blood cell transfusion should monitor their vitamin C intake (Levine et al. 1999).

High-dose vitamin C supplementation has been proposed as a remedy for the common cold (Pauling 1970), and numerous placebo-controlled trials have been conducted to address this question. A meta-analysis of 30 trials conducted over the past 35 years found that supplementing vitamin C in doses up to 2000 mg/day had no perceptible effect on reducing the incidence of colds except in select cases of subjects exposed to extreme exercise or cold (Douglas et al. 2004). The duration of cold symptoms in adults was shortened by 8% (95% CI, 3 to 13%) with preventive use of vitamin C, but when therapy was started with the onset of symptoms at doses up to 4000 mg/day, no change was noted in the duration of symptoms in seven trials.

Megadose vitamin C supplementation continues to be recommended by some experts for the prevention of cardiovascular disease and cancer in the elderly despite limited evidence to support such claims. The protective role of vitamin C in delaying age-related lens opacities is supported in most studies (Hankinson et al. 1992, Simon and Hudes 1999, Jacques et al. 2001, Mares-Perlman et al. 2000) but not all (AREDS Research Group 2001). Since megadose vitamin C given chronically appears to have little additional benefit in delaying the aging process and might have adverse effects, it seems prudent to ingest enough vitamin C to keep tissue stores saturated. This can be achieved with around 100 to 140 mg/day. Diets rich in vitamin C (200 mg or more) from natural sources are associated with lower cancer risk and can easily be attained with five daily servings of fruits and vegetables. The potential benefits of vitamin C and other antioxidants in prevention of cardiovascular disease and cancer are briefly discussed next.

10.6 VITAMINS AS ANTIOXIDANTS

The oxidative stress hypothesis of aging has triggered a large number of investigations examining the effect of antioxidant vitamins on various aspects of health and aging. These investigations include epidemiological studies and clinical trials of vitamins in their natural as well as supplemental forms. The resulting body of literature is too extensive to comprehensively review in this chapter; key trials have been reviewed elsewhere (Thomas 2004, Asplund 2002, Pearce et al. 2000, McCall and Frei 1999, Morris and Carson 2003, Jha et al. 1995, Steinmetz and Potter 1996). Despite intensive investigations, confusion and controversy abound.

A large body of evidence suggests that diets rich in antioxidant vitamins protect against the development of various age-associated diseases. The origin of the National Cancer Institute's "five-a-day for better health" campaign arose from such observations. Based on epidemiological studies, the inverse relationship between fruit/vegetable consumption and the risk of developing atherosclerotic vascular disease has been strong and consistent, and appears evident, albeit somewhat less vigorous, for cancer prevention (Gillman et al. 1995, Hung et al. 2004, Joshipura et al. 1999, 2001, Liu et al. 2000, 2001, Sauvaget et al. 2003, Hajjar 2004). In a study of over 40,000 subjects followed for 18 years, daily intake of green-yellow vegetables was associated with a statistically significant 26% reduction in the risk of mortality from all strokes, compared with intake of once or less per week (Sauvaget et al. 2003). Furthermore, the incidence of stroke in daily consumers of fruits was reduced by 35% in men and 25% in women. In another 14-year prospective cohort study that combined over 100,000 participants, fruit and vegetable consumption was associated with a modest, although not statistically significant, reduction in cardiovascular disease, but not cancer (Hung et al. 2004). In a smaller trial, dependence in self-care had a strong negative association with lycopene, but was not clearly related to other carotenoids in elderly nuns living in a controlled setting (Snowdon et al. 1996).

Epidemiological associations, however, cannot prove causality and are replete with potential methodological problems. Food frequency recall questionnaires may be unreliable (Ferro-Luzzi 2002) and do not necessarily reflect nutritional intake during the duration of a trial. Data on dietary intake recorded once at the onset of a trial (Sauvaget et al. 2003) or updated every few years (Hung et al. 2004) are used to predict risk of disease many years later. By the nature of these trials, confounding factors are ill controlled for and individual components of a healthy diet are difficult to identify. Despite these limitations, the clear inverse association between fruit and vegetable intake and the risk of cardiovascular disease and some types of cancer is firmly established. As strong as this association may be, one cannot make the intuitive leap linking any specific nutrient type or dose with a particular disease process. For this type of determination, randomized controlled clinical trials are needed.

The strong association between dietary vitamin intake and disease prevention seen in epidemiologic studies has not been borne out in clinical trials (Thomas 2004). In fact, two trials, the Alpha-Tocopherol Beta-Carotene (ATBC) Cancer Prevention Study (ATBC Cancer Prevention Study Group 1994) and the Carotenoid and Retinol Efficacy Trial (CARET) (Omenn et al. 1996), found an increase in the incidence of lung cancer in smokers who were administered beta-carotene. No such effect was noted in nonsmokers. The efficacy of beta-carotene in prevention of atherosclerosis has been similarly disappointing (ATBC Cancer Prevention Study Group 1994). Vitamin E supplementation in human controlled trials showed a reduction in mortality and morbidity from atherosclerotic disease in the Cambridge Heart Antioxidant Study (Ness and Smith 1999) but not in the Primary Prevention Project (Collaborative Group of the Primary Prevention Project 2001), the Heart Outcomes Prevention Evaluation Study (Yusuf et al. 2000), or the Italian GISSI-Prevenzione Study (Valagussa et al.

1999). Furthermore, in the HDL–atherosclerosis trial, an antioxidant cocktail including vitamin E inhibited the ability of niacin and simvastatin to increase HDL (Brown et al. 2001), and progression of atherosclerosis was not prevented by vitamin E in the SECURE trial (Lonn et al. 2001). Similarly, the Heart Protection Study failed to show a significant reduction in heart disease with a daily combination of vitamins E and C and beta-carotene (Heart Protection Study Collaborative Group 2002). Despite the tremendous zeal for the therapeutic properties of vitamin C in pharmacological doses, no interventional study has demonstrated any major beneficial effect against cancer or atherosclerotic disease (Hercberg et al. 1998). In fact, high doses of vitamin C may exhibit pro-oxidant effects, as levels of 8-oxoadenine are increased (Podmore et al. 1998), but the clinical significance of this finding is yet to be determined. Finally, Virtamo et al. (2003) found a nonsignificant decline in prostate cancer with the use of alpha-tocopherol in 25,390 elderly men followed for 6 years, and no effect of beta-carotene on the incidence of prostate cancer.

Overall, these studies are not supportive of the ability of antioxidant vitamins in supplemental form to deter the development of atherosclerotic disease or cancer in the elderly. The discrepancy between epidemiological observations and controlled clinical trials is likely rooted in the nature and limitations of the trial designs themselves, and in the fact that dietary vitamins and supplemental vitamins are not physiologically equivalent. For example, synthetic vitamins A and E do not encompass the spectrum of compounds that comprise the natural form of these vitamins. Fresh fruits and vegetables may include yet unidentified components responsible for the improved health outcome in those who consume them. Finally, risk reduction may not solely be due to the vitamins themselves, but in part to decreased intake of harmful compounds, resulting from the substitution of dietary meat and fat with fruits and vegetables (Jha et al. 1995).

10.7 CONCLUSION

Despite the near elimination of vitamin deficiency syndromes from Western societies over the past century, older individuals continue to experience vitamin deficiencies at relatively high rates. Failure to diligently screen and treat at-risk populations is a failure to provide optimal care and maintain function in an already frail population. As vitamin supplementation moved from the realm of preventing deficiency conditions to management of chronic disease, a wide array of age-associated conditions, and indeed the aging process itself, have been thought to be influenced by vitamin use. The promise of warding off disease with vitamins has led to their widespread use, often in megadoses. While these health benefits continue to be studied, current consensus is for obtaining vitamins in their natural rather than synthetic form, as the latter have proven less promising in preventing disease thus far. Many disease-specific exceptions exist, such as the clear benefit of vitamin supplements in slowing the progression of osteoporosis and macular degeneration, and the management of pernicious anemia with large doses orally of vitamin B_{12}. The best recommendation today is to heed mother's age-old advice to "eat your vegetables," no less than five servings each day.

REFERENCES

Abbasi A. Nutrition in the nursing home. In *Annual Review of Gerontology and Geriatrics*, Vol. 15, Morely JE, Miller DK, Eds. Springer Publishing Company, New York, 1995, pp. 54–66.

Abbasi AA, Rudman D. Observations on the prevalence of protein calorie undernutrition in VA nursing homes. *J Am Geriatric Soc* 1993;41:117–121.

Abraham S, Carroll MD, Dressler CM, Johnson CL. *Dietary Intake Source Data, United States, 1971–1974*, PHS 79-1221. Hayattsville, MD: U.S. Department of Health, Education, and Welfare, Public Health Service, 1979.

Age-Related Eye Disease Study Research Group. A randomized, placebo-controlled, clinical trial of high-dose supplementation with vitamins C and E and beta carotene for age-related cataract and vision loss: AREDS report no. 9. *Arch Ophthalmol* 2001;119:1439–1452.

Alpha-Tocopherol Beta Carotene Cancer Prevention Study Group. The effect of vitamin E and beta carotene on the incidence of lung cancer and other cancers in male smokers. *N Engl J Med* 1994;330:1029–1035.

Altschul R, Hoffer A, Stephen JD. Influence of nicotinic acid on serum cholesterol in man. *Arch Biochem Biophys* 1955;54:558–559.

American Cancer Society Advisory Committee on Diet, Nutrition and Cancer Prevention. Guidelines on diet, nutrition and cancer prevention: reducing the risk of cancer with healthy food choices and physical activity. *Cancer* 1996;46:325.

Armas LAG, Hollis BW, Heaney RP. Vitamin D2 is much less effective than vitamin D3 in humans. *J Clin Endocrinol Metab* 2004;89:5387–5391.

Asplund K. Antioxidant vitamins in the prevention of cardiovascular disease: a systematic review. *J Intern Med* 2002;251:372–392.

Baik HW, Russell RM. Vitamin B_{12} deficiency in the elderly. *Annu Rev Nutr* 1999;19:357–377.

Basu TK. Vitamin C-aspirin interactions. *Int J Vitam Nutr Res Suppl* 1982;23:83–90.

Benton D, Fordy J, Haller J. The impact of long-term vitamin supplementation on cognitive functioning. *Psychopharmacology* 1995;117:298–305.

Bischoff HA, Stahelin HB, Dick W, Akros R, Knecht M, et al. Effect of vitamin D and calcium supplementation on falls: a randomized controlled trial. *J Bone Miner Res* 2003;18:343–351.

Bischoff HA, Stahelin HB, Urscheler N, Ehrsam R, Vonthein R, et al. Muscle strength in the elderly: its relation to vitamin D metabolites. *Arch Phys Med Rehabil* 1999;80:54–58.

Bischoff-Ferrari HA, Dawson-Hughes B, Willett WC, Staehelin HB, Bazemore MG, Zee RY, Wong JB. Effect of vitamin D on falls: a meta-analysis. *JAMA* 2004;291:1999–2006.

Bischoff-Ferrari HA, Orav EJ, Dawson-Hughes B. Effect of cholecalciferol plus calcium on falling on ambulatory older men and women: a 3-year randomized controlled trial. *Arch Intern Med* 2006;166:424–430.

Bischoff-Ferrari HA, Willett WC, Wong JB, Giovannucci E, Dietrich T, Dawson-Hughes B. Fracture prevention with vitamin D supplementation: a meta-analysis of randomized controlled trials. *JAMA* 2005;293:2257–2264.

Blankenhorn DH, Nessim SA, Johnson RL, Sanmarco ME, Azen SP, Cashin-Hemphill L. Beneficial effects of combined colestipol-niacin therapy on coronary atherosclerosis and coronary venous bypass grafts. *JAMA* 1987;257:3233–3240.

Block G. Dietary guidelines and results of food consumption surveys. *Am J Clin Nutr* 1991;53:356S–357S.

Booth SL, Broe KE, Gagnon DR, Tucker KL, Hannan MT, et al. Vitamin K intake and bone mineral density in women and men. *Am J Clin Nutr* 2003;77:512–516.

Booth SL, Tucker KL, Chen H, Hannan MT, et al. Dietary vitamin K intakes are associated with hip fracture but not with bone mineral density in elderly men and women. *Am J Clin Nutr* 2000;71:1201–1208.

Boushey CJ, Beresford SA, Omenn GS, Motulsky AG. A quantitative assessment of plasma homocysteine as a risk factor for vascular disease. Probable benefits of increasing folic acid intakes. *JAMA* 1995;274:1049–1057.

Brown BG, Zhao XQ, Chait A, et al. Simvastatin and niacin, antioxidant vitamins, or the combination for the prevention of coronary disease. *N Engl J Med* 2001;345:1583–1592.

Brown G, Albers JJ, Fisher LD, et al. Regression of coronary artery disease as a result of intensive lipid-lowering therapy in men with high levels of apolipoprotein B. *N Engl J Med* 1990;323:1289–1298.

Bryan J, Calvaresi E, Hughes D. Short-term folate, vitamin B-12 or vitamin B-6 supplementation slightly affects memory performance but not mood in women of various ages. *J Nutr* 2002;132:1345–1356.

Carlson LA, Rosenhamer G. Reduction of mortality in the Stockholm Ischaemic Heart Disease Secondary Prevention Study by combined treatment with clofibrate and nicotinic acid. *Acta Med Scand* 1988;223:405–418.

Carmel R. Prevalence of undiagnosed pernicious anemia in the elderly. *Arch Intern Med* 1996;156:1097–1100.

Canner PL, Berge KG, Wenger NK, Stamler J, Friedman L, Prineas RJ, et al. Fifteen year mortality in coronary drug project patients: long-term benefit with niacin. *J Am Coll Cardiol* 1986;8:1245–1255.

Chapuy MC, Arlot ME, Delmans PD, Meunier PJ. Effect of calcium and cholecalciferol treatment for three years on hip fractures in elderly women. *BMJ* 1994;308:1081–1082.

Chapuy MC, Arlot ME, Duboeuf F, Brun J, Crouzt B, Arnaud S et al. Vitamin D3 and calcium to prevent hip fractures in elderly women. *N Engl J Med* 1992;327:1637–1642.

Chapuy MC, Pamphile R, Paris E, Kempf C, Schlichting M, Arnaud S, Garnero P, Meunier PJ. Combined calcium and vitamin D3 supplementation in elderly women: confirmation of reversal of secondary hyperparathyroidisim and hip fracture risk: the Decalyos II study. *Osteoporos Int* 2002;3:257–264.

Chernoff R. Micronutrient requirements in older women. *Am J Clin Nutr* 2005;81:1240s–1245s.

Cheung MC, Zhao XQ, Chait A, Albers JJ, Brown BG. Antioxidant supplements block the response of HDL to simvastatin-niacin therapy in patients with coronary artery disease and low HDL. *Arterioscler Thromb Vasc Biol* 2001;21:1320–1326.

Clarke R, Smith AD, Jobst KA, Refsum H, Sutton L, Ueland PM. Folate, vitamin B_{12}, and serum total homocysteine levels in confirmed Alzheimer disease. *Arch Neurol* 1998;55:1449–1455.

Collaborative Group of the Primary Prevention Project (PPP). Low-dose aspirin and vitamin E in people at cardiovascular risk: a randomised trial in general practice. *Lancet* 2001;357:89–95.

Coronary Drug Project Research Group. Clofibrate and niacin in coronary heart disease. *JAMA* 1975;231:360–381.

Cravo ML, Pinto AG, Chaves P, et al. Effect of folate supplementation on DNA methylation of rectal mucosa in patients with colonic adenomas: correlation with nutrient intake. *Clin Nutr* 1998;17:45–49.

Cumming RG, Mitchell P, Smith W. Diet and cataract: the Blue Mountains Eye Study. *Ophthalmology* 2000;107:450–456.

Dawson-Hughes B, Dallal GE, Krall EA, et al. Effect of vitamin D supplementation on wintertime and overall bone loss in healthy post menopausal women. *Ann Intern Med* 1991;115:505–512.

Dawson-Hughes B, Harris SS, Krall EA, Dallal GE, Falconer G, Green CL. Rates of bone loss in postmenopausal women randomly assigned to one of two dosages of vitamin D. *Am J Clin Nutr* 1995;61:1140–1145.

Dawson-Hughes B, Harris SS, Krall EA, Dallal GE. Effects of calcium and vitamin D supplementation on bone density in men and women 65 years or age or older. *N Engl J Med* 1997;337:670–676.

Deijen JB, van der Beek EJ, Orlebeke JF, et al. Vitamin B-6 supplementation in elderly men: effects on mood, memory, performance and mental effort. *Psychopharmacology* 1992;109:489–496.

Douglas RM, Hemila H, D'Souza R, Chalker EB, Treacy B. Vitamin C for preventing and treating the common cold. *Cochrane Database Syst Rev* 2004;4:CD000980.

Drinka P, Goodwin JS. Prevalence and consequence of vitamin deficiencies in the nursing home: a critical review. *J Am Geriatr Soc* 1991;39:1008–1017.

Ebly EM, Schaefer JP, Campbell NR, Hogan DB. Folate status, vascular disease and cognition in elderly Canadians. *Age Ageing* 1998;27:485–491.

Eikelboom JW, Lonn E, Genest J, Hankey G, Yusuf S. Homocyst(e)ine and cardiovascular disease: a critical review of the epidemiologic evidence. *Ann Intern Med* 1999;131:363–375.

Fairbanks VF, Wahner HW, Phyliky RL. Tests for pernicious anemia: the "Shilling test." *Mayo Clin Proc* 1983;58:541–544.

Fenech M. Micronucleus frequency in human lymphocytes is related to plasma vitamin B_{12} and homocysteine. *Mutat Res* 1999;428:299–304.

Ferraroni M, La Vecchia CL, D'Avanzo B, Negri E, Franceschi S, Decarli A. Selected micronutrient intake and the risk of colorectal cancer. *Br J Cancer* 1994;70:1150–1155.

Ferro-Luzzi A. Individual Food Intake Survey Methods. Paper presented at the International Scientific Symposium; Food and Agriculture Organization of the United Nations, Rome, June 26–28, 2002. Accessed at http://www.fivims.net/EN/ISS.htm.

Feskanich D, Singh V, Willett WC, Colditz GA. Vitamin A intake and hip fractures among postmenopausal women. *JAMA* 2002;287:47–54.

Feskanich D, Weber P, Willett WC, Rockett H, Booth SL, Colditz GA. Vitamin K intake and hip fractures in women: a prospective study. *Am J Clin Nutr* 1999;69:74–79.

Folsom AR, Nieto FJ, McGovern PG, Tsai MY, Malinow MR, Eckfeldt JH, Hess DL, Davis CE. Prospective study of coronary heart disease incidence in relation to fasting total homocysteine, related genetic polymorphisms, and B vitamins: the Atherosclerosis Risk in Communities (ARIC) study. *Circulation* 1998;98:204–210.

Foote JA, Giuliano AR, Harris RB. Older adults need guidance to meet nutritional recommendations. *J Am Coll Nutr* 2000;19:628–640.

Freudenheim JL, Graham S, Marshall JR, Haughey BP, Cholewinski S, Wilkinson G. Folate intake and carcinogenesis of the colon and rectum. *Int J Epidemiol* 1991;20:368–374.

Garry PJ, Goodwin JS, Hunt WC. Folate and B12 status in the healthy elderly population. *J Am Geriatr Soc* 1984;32:719–726.

Gerhard GT, Duell PB. Homocysteine and atherosclerosis. *Curr Opin Lipidol* 1999;10:417–428.

Gillman MW, Cupples A, Gagnon D, Posner BM, Ellison RC, Castelli WP, Wolf PA. Protective effect of fruits and vegetables on development of stroke in men. *JAMA* 1995;273:1113–1117.

Giovannucci E, Rimm EB, Ascherio A, Stampfer MJ, Colditz GA, Willett WC. Alcohol, low-methionine–low-folate diets, and risk of colon cancer in men. *J Natl Cancer Inst* 1995;87:265–273.

Giovannucci E, Stampfer MJ, Colditz GA, Hunter DJ, Fuchs C, Rosner BA, Speizer FE, Willett WC. Multivitamin use, folate, and colon cancer in women in the Nurses' Health Study. *Ann Intern Med* 1998;129:517–524.

Giovannucci E, Stampfer MJ, Colditz GA, Rimm EB, Trichopoulos D, Rosner BA, Speizer FE, Willett WC. Folate, methionine, and alcohol intake and risk of colorectal adenoma. *J Natl Cancer Inst* 1993;85:875–884.

Gloth FM, Smith CE, Hollis BW, Tobin JD. Functional improvement with vitamin D replenishment in a cohort of frail, vitamin D-deficient older people. *JAGS* 1995;43:1269–1271.

Gold M, Hauser RA, Chen MF. Plasma thiamine deficiency associated with Alzheimer's disease but not Parkinson's disease. *Metab Brain Dis* 1998;13:43–53.

Gordon R. *The Alarming History of Medicine*. St. Martin's Griffin, New York, 1993.

Gregory JF, 3rd. Nutritional properties and significance of vitamin glycosides. *Annu Rev Nutr* 1998;18:277–296.

Groff JL, Gropper SS, Hunt SM. The water soluble vitamins. In *Advanced Nutrition and Human Metabolism*. West Publishing Company, Minneapolis, 1995, pp. 222–237.

Hankinson SE, Stampfer MJ, Seddon JM, et al. Nutrient intake and cataract extraction in women: a prospective study. *BMJ* 1992;305:335–339.

Hajjar RR. Cancer in the elderly: is it preventable? *Clin Geriatr Med* 2004;20:293–316.

Hajjar RR, Stewart R, Meitzler D. The effect of dosing intervals of intramuscular vitamin B12 on serum levels in B12-deficient elderly after loading (abstract). *J Am Geriatr Soc* 2000;48:S23.

He K, Merchant A, Rimm EB, Rosner BA, Stampfer MJ, Willett WC, Ascherio A. Folate, vitamin B6, and B12 intakes in relation to risk of stroke among men. *Stroke* 2004;35:169–174.

Heart Protection Study Collaborative Group. MRC/BHF Heart Protection Study of antioxidant vitamin supplementation in 20563 high-risk individuals: a randomised-controlled trial. *Lancet* 2002;360:23–33.

Heikenheimo RJ, Haavisto MV, Harju EJ, et al. Serum vitamin D levels after annual intramuscular injection of ergocalciferol. *Calcif Tissue Int* 1991;49(Suppl.):S87.

Herbert V. Folic acid. In *Nutrition in Health and Disease*, 9th ed., Shils M, Olson JA, Shike M, Ross AC, Eds. Williams & Wilkins, Baltimore, 1999, pp. 433–446.

Hercberg S, Galan P, Preziosi P, Alfarez MJ, Vazquez C. The potential role of antioxidant vitamins in preventing cardiovascular diseases and cancer. *Nutrition* 1998;14:513–520.

Higdon J. Folic acid. Linus Pauling Institute—Micronutrient Information Center, 2002. http://lpi.oregonstate.edu/infocenter/vitamins/fa/. Accessed August 8, 2006.

Higdon J. Vitamin B12. Linus Pauling Institute—Micronutrient Information Center, 2003. http://lpi.oregonstate.edu/infocenter/vitamins/vitaminB12/. Accessed August 20, 2006.

Holick MF. McCollum Award Lecture 1994: Vitamin D: new horizons for the 21st century. *Am J Clin Nutr* 1994;60:619–630.

Hollander D, Morgan D. Aging: its influence on vitamin A intestinal absorption *in vivo* by rat. *Exp Gerontol* 1979;14:301–305.

Homocysteine Lowering Trialists' Collaboration. Lowering blood homocysteine with folic acid based supplements: meta-analysis of randomised trials. Homocysteine Lowering Trialists' Collaboration. *BMJ* 1998;316:894–898.

Hoppner K, Phillips WE, Murray TK, Campbell JS. Survey of liver vitamin A stores of Canadians. *Can Med Assoc J* 1968;99:983–6.

Hung HC, Joshipura KJ, Jiang R, et al. Fruit and vegetable intake and risk of major chronic disease. *J Natl Cancer Inst* 2004;96:1577–1584.

Hung SC, Hung SH, Tarng DC, Yang WC, Chen TW, Huang TP. Thiamine deficiency and unexplained encephalopathy in hemodialysis and peritoneal dialysis patients. *Am J Kidney Dis* 2001;38:941–947.

Hutto BR. Folate and cobalamin in psychiatric illness. *Comp Psychiatry* 1997;38:305–314.

Institute of Medicine. *Dietary Reference Intakes for Thiamin, Riboflavin, Niacin, Vitamin B6, Folate, Vitamin B12, Pantothenic Acid, Biotin, and Choline*. National Academy Press, Washington, DC, 1998.

Institute of Medicine. *Dietary Reference Intakes for Vitamin C, Vitamin E, Selenium and Carotenoids*. National Academy Press, Washington, DC, 2000.

Institute of Medicine. *Dietary Reference Intakes for Vitamin A, Vitamin K, Arsenic, Boron, Chromium, Copper, Iodine, Manganese, Molybdenum, Nickel, Silicon, Vanadium, and Zinc*. National Academy Press, Washington, DC, 2001.

Jacob RA. Vitamin C. In *Modern Nutrition in Health and Disease*, 9th ed., Shils M, Olson J, Shike M, Ross AC, Eds. Williams & Wilkins, Baltimore, 1999, pp. 467–482.

Jacques PF, Chylack LT, Jr., Hankinson SE, et al. Long-term nutrient intake and early age-related nuclear lens opacities. *Arch Ophthalmol* 2001;119:1009–1019.

Jha P, Flather M, Lonn E, Farkouh M, Yusuf S. The antioxidant vitamins and cardiovascular disease: a critical review of epidemiologic and clinical trial data. *Ann Intern Med* 1995;123:860–872.

Johnson KA, Bernard MA, Fundeburg K. Vitamin nutrition in older adults. *Clin Geriatr Med* 2002;18:773–799.

Johnson LE. Vitamin nutrition in the elderly. In *Geriatric Nutrition: A Comprehensive Review*, 2nd ed., Morley JE, Glick Z, Rubenstein LZ, Eds. Raven Press, New York, 1995, pp. 79–105.

Joshi S, Morley JM. Vitamins and minerals in the elderly. In *Principles and Practice of Geriatric Medicine*, 4th ed., Pathy MSJ, Sinclair AJ, Morley JE, Eds. John Wiley & Sons, Chishester, England, 2006, 329–46.

Joshipura JH, Hu FB, Manson JE, Stampfer MJ, Rimm EB, Speizer, FE, Colditz G, Ascherio A, Rosner B, Spiegelman D, Walter WC. The effect of fruit and vegetable intake on risk for coronary heart disease. *Ann Intern Med* 2001;134:1106–1114.

Joshipura KJ, Ascherio A, Manson JE, Stampfer MJ, Rimm EB, Speizer FE, Hennekens CH, Spiegelman D, Willett WC. Fruit and vegetable intake in relation to risk of ischemic stroke. *JAMA* 1999;282:1233–1239.

Kamel H, Hajjar RR. Osteoporosis for the home care physician. II. Management. *J Am Med Dir Assoc* 2003;5:259–262.

Kane JP, Malloy MJ, Ports TA, Phillips NR, Diehl JC, Havel RJ. Regression of coronary atherosclerosis during treatment of familial hypercholesterolemia with combined drug regimens. *JAMA* 1990;264:3007–3012.

Kim YI, Baik HW, Fawaz K, et al. Effects of folate supplementation on two provisional molecular markers of colon cancer: a prospective, randomized trial. *Am J Gastroenterol* 2001;96:184–195.

Kishi T, Fujita N, Eguchi T, et al. Mechanism for reduction of serum folate by antiepileptic drugs during prolonged therapy. *J Neurosci* 1997;145:109–112.

Kneissel M, Studer A, Cortesi R, Susa M. Retinoid induced bone thinning is caused by subperiosteal osteoclast activity in adult rodents. *Bone* 2005;36:202–214.

Knopp RH. Drug treatment of lipid disorders. *N Engl J Med* 1999;341:498–511.

Knopp RH. Evaluating niacin in its various forms. *Am J Cardiol* 2000;86:51L–56L.

Knopp RH, Alagona P, Davidson M, et al. Equivalent efficacy of a time-release form of niacin (Niaspan) given once-a-night vs. plain niacin in the management of hyperlipidemia. *Metabolism* 1998;47:1097–1104.

Knopp RH, Ginsberg J, Albers JJ, et al. Contrasting effects of unmodified and time-release forms of niacin on lipoproteins in hyperlipidemic subjects: clues to mechanism of action of niacin. *Metabolism* 1985;34:642–650.

Krasinski S, Cohn J, Schaefer E, Russell R. Postprandial plasma retinyl ester response is greater in older subjects compared with younger subjects. *J Clin Invest* 1990;85:883–892.

Krasinski SD, Russell RM, Otradovec CL, et al. Vitamin A and E intake: relationship to fasting plasma retinol, retinol-binding protein, retinyl ester, carotene and alpha tocopherol levels in the elderly and young adults. *Am J Clin Nutr* 1989;49:112–120.

Kuzminski AM, Del Giacco EJ, Allen RH, Stabler SP, Lindenbaum J. Effective treatment of cobalamin with oral cobalamin. *Blood* 1998;92:1191–1198.

Leske MC, Wu SY, Hyman L, et al. Biochemical factors in the lens opacities. Case-control study. The Lens Opacities Case-Control Study Group. *Arch Ophthalmol* 1995;113:1113–1119.

Levine M, Dhariwal KR, Welch RW, et al. Determination of optimal vitamin C requirements in humans. *Am J Clin Nutr* 1995;62(Suppl.):1347S–1356S.

Levine M, Rumsey SC, Daruwala R, et al. Criteria and recommendations for vitamin C intake. *JAMA* 1999;281:1415–1423.

Lindenbaum J, Healton EB, Savage DG, et al. Neuropsychiatric disorders caused by cobalamin deficiency in the absence of anemia or macrocytosis. *N Engl J Med* 1988;318:1720–1728.

Lindenbaum J, Savage DG, Stabler SP, et al. Diagnosis of cobalamin deficiency. II. Relative sensitivity of serum cobalamin, methylmalonic acid, and total homocysteine concentrations. *Am J Hematol* 1990;34:99–107.

Lips P. Hypervitaminosis A and fractures. *N Engl J Med* 2003;348:347–349.

Lips P, Graafmans WC, Ooms ME, Bezemer PD, Bouter LM. Vitamin D supplementation and fracture incidence in elderly persons: a randomized, placebo-controlled clinical trial. *Ann Intern Med* 1996;124:400–406.

Liu S, Lee IM, Ajani U, Cole SR, Buring JE, Manson JE. Intake of vegetables rich in carotenoids and risk of coronary heart disease in men: the Physicians' Health Study. *Int J Epidemiol* 2001;30:130–135.

Liu S, Manson JE, Lee IM, Cole SR, Hennekens CH, Willett WC, Buring JE. Fruit and vegetable intake and risk of cardiovascular disease: the Women's Health Study. *Am J Clin Nutr* 2000;72:922–928.

Lonn E, Yusuf S, Dzavik V, Doris I, Yi Q, et al. for the SECURE Investigators. Effects of ramipril and of vitamin E on atheroslerosis: results of the prospective randomized Study to Evaluate Carotid Ultrasound Changes in Patients Treated with Ramipril and Vitamin E (SECURE). *Circulation* 2001;103:919–925.

Malinow MR, Bostom AG, Krauss RM. Homocyst(e)ine, diet, and cardiovascular diseases: a statement for healthcare professionals from the Nutrition Committee, American Heart Association. *Circulation* 1999;99:178–182.

Mares-Perlman JA, Lyle BJ, Klein R, et al. Vitamin supplement use and incident cataracts in a population-based study. *Arch Ophthalmol* 2000;118:1556–1563.

Massey PB. Dietary supplements. *Med Clin North Am* 2002;86:127–147.

Mathews-Roth MM. Beta-carotene therapy for erythropoietic protoporphyria and other photosensitivity diseases. *Biochimie* 1986;68:875–884.

McCall MR, Frei B. Can antioxidant vitamins maternally reduce oxidative damage in humans? *Free Radic Biol Med* 1999:26:1034–1053.

McEligol AJ. Nutrition research: high fiber diet should not cause gut problems. *J Am Diet Assoc* 2002;102:549–551.

McKenney JM, Proctor JD, Harris S, Chinchili VM. A comparison of the efficacy and toxic effects of sustained- vs. immediate-release niacin in hypercholesterolemic patients. *JAMA* 1994;271:672–677.

Meador K, Loring D, Nichols M, et al. Preliminary findings of high-dose thiamine in dementia of Alzheimer's type. *J Geriatr Psychiatry Neurol* 1993;6:222–229.

Melhus H, Michaelsson K, Kindmark A, et al. Excessive dietary intake of vitamin A is associated with reduced bone mineral density and increased risk for hip fracture. *Ann Intern Med* 1998;129:770–778.

Metz J, Bell AH, App B, et al. The significance of subnormal serum vitamin B12 concentrations in older people: a case control study. *J Am Geriatr Soc* 1996;44:1355–1357.

Meydani SN, Ribaya-Mercado JD, Russell RM, Sahyoun N, Morrow FD, Gershoff SN. Vitamin B-6 deficiency impairs interleukin 2 production and lymphocyte proliferation in elderly adults. *Am J Clin Nutr* 1991;53:1275–1280.

Michaelsson K, Lithell H, Vessby B, Melhus H. Serum retinol levels and the risk of fracture. *N Engl J Med* 2003;348:287–294.

Miller DR, Hays KC. Vitamin excess and toxicity. In *Nutritional Toxicology*, Vol. 1, Hathcock JN, Ed. Academic Press, New York, 1982, 81–133.

Miller M. Niacin as a component of combination therapy for dyslipidemia. *Mayo Clin Proc* 2003;78:735–742.

Mimori Y, Katsuoka H, Nakamura S. Thiamine therapy in Alzheimer's disease. *Metab Brain Dis* 1996;11:89–94.

Moore WP, Bolton CH, Downs L, Gilmor HA, Gale EA. Measurement of N-methyl-2-pyridone-5-carboxamide in urine by high performance liquid chromatography. *Biomed Chromatogr* 2000;14:69–71.

Morley JE, Silver AJ. Anorexia in the elderly. *Neurobiol Aging* 1985;9:9–16.

Morley JE, Silver AJ. Nutritional issues in nursing home care. *Ann Intern Med* 1995;123:850.

Morris C, Carson S. Routine vitamin supplementation to prevent cardiovascular disease: a summary of the evidence for the U.S. Preventive Services Task Force. *Ann Intern Med* 2003;139:56–70.

Ness A, Smith GD. Mortality in the CHAOS trial. Cambridge Heart Antioxidant Study. *Lancet* 1999;353:1017–1018.

Nolan KA, Black RS, Sheu KF, Langberg J, Blass JP. A trial of thiamin in Alzheimer's disease. *Arch Neurol* 1991;48:81–83.

Nourhashemi F, Gillette-Guyonnet S, Andrieu S, et al. Alzheimer disease: protective factors. *Am J Clin Nutr* 2000;71:643S–649S.

Omenn GS, Goodman GE, Thornquist, MD, Balmes J, Cullen MR, Glass A, et al. Effects of a combination of beta-carotene and vitamin A on lung cancer and cardiovascular disease. *N Engl J Med* 1996;334:1150–1155.

Pauling LC. *Vitamin C and the Common Cold.* W.H. Freeman, San Francisco, 1970.

Peacock M, Liu G, Carey M, McClintock R, et al. Effect of calcium or 25OH vitamin D_3 dietary supplementation on bone loss at the hip in men and women over the age of 60. *J Clin Endocrinol Metab* 2000;85:3011–3019.

Pearce KA, Boosalis MG, Yeager B. Update on vitamin supplements for the prevention of coronary disease and stroke. *Am Fam Physician* 2000;62:1359–1366.

Penninx BW, Guralnik JM, Ferrucci L, Fried LP, Allen RH, Stabler SP. Vitamin B(12) deficiency and depression in physically disabled older women: epidemiologic evidence from the Women's Health and Aging Study. *Am J Psychiatry* 2000;157:715–721.

Pfitzenmeyer P, Guilland JC, d'Athis P. Vitamin B6 and vitamin C status in elderly patients with infections during hospitalization. *Ann Nutr Metab* 1997;41:344–352.

Podmore ID, Griffiths HR, Herbert KE, Mistry N, Mistry P, Lunec J. Vitamin C exhibits pro-oxidant properties. *Nature* 1998;392:559.

Promislow JH, Goodman-Gruen D, Slymen DJ, Barrett-Connor E. Retinol intake and bone mineral density in the elderly: the Rancho Bernardo Study. *J Bone Miner Res* 2002;17:1349–1358.

Pruthi, RK, Tefferi, A. Pernicious anemia revisited. *Mayo Clin Proc* 1994;69:144–150.

Radimer K, Bindewald B, Hughes J, et al. Dietary supplement use by US adults: data from the National Health and Nutrition Examination Survey, 1999–2000. *Am J Epidemiol* 2004;160:339–349.

Riggs KM, Spiro A, 3rd, Tucker K, Rush D. Relations of vitamin B-12, vitamin B-6, folate, and homocysteine to cognitive performance in the Normative Aging Study. *Am J Clin Nutr* 1996;63:306–314.

Rimm EB, Willett WC, Hu FB, Sampson L, Colditz GA, Manson JE, Hennekens C, Stampfer MJ. Folate and vitamin B6 from diet and supplements in relation to risk of coronary heart disease among women. *JAMA* 1998;279:359–364.

Ritchie CS, Burgio KL, Locher JL, et al. Nutritional status of urban homebound older adults. *Am J Clin Nutr* 1997;66:815.

Robinson K, Arheart K, Refsum H, et al. Low circulating folate and vitamin B_6 concentrations: risk factors for stroke, peripheral vascular disease, and coronary artery disease. *Circulation* 1998;97:437–443.

Rodriguez-Martin JL, Qizilbash N, Lopez-Arrieta JM. Thiamine for Alzheimer's disease (Cochrane review). *Cochrane Database Syst Rev* 2001;2:CD001498.

Rohan TE, Jain MG, Howe GR, Miller AB. Dietary folate consumption and breast cancer risk. *J Natl Cancer Inst* 2000;92:266–269.

Rohde CM, DeLuca H. Bone resorption activity of all-trans retinoic acid is independent of vitamin D in rats. *J Nutr* 2003;133:777–783.

Sato Y, Tsuru T, Oizumi K, Kaki M. Vitamin K deficiency and osteopenia in disuse-affected limbs of vitamin D-deficient elderly stroke patients. *Am J Phys Med Rehabil* 1999;78:317–322.

Sauvaget C, Nagano J, Allen N, Kodama K. Vegetable and fruit intake and stroke mortality in the Hiroshima/Nagasaki Life Span Study. *Stroke* 2003;34:2355–2360.

Selhub J, Bagley LC, Miller J, Rosenberg IH. B vitamins, homocysteine, and neurocognitive function in the elderly. *Am J Clin Nutr* 2000;71:614S–620S.

Sellers TA, Kushi LH, Cerhan JR, et al. Dietary folate intake, alcohol, and risk of breast cancer in a prospective study of postmenopausal women. *Epidemiology* 2001;12:420–428.

Seshadri S, Beiser A, Selhub J, et al. Plasma homocysteine as a risk factor for dementia and Alzheimer's disease. *N Engl J Med* 2002;346:476–483.

Simon JA, Hudes ES. Serum ascorbic acid and other correlates of self-reported cataract among older Americans. *J Clin Epidemiol* 1999;52:1207–1211.

Smidt LJ, Cremin FM, Clifford AJ. Influence of thiamin supplementation on the health and general well-being of an elderly Irish population with marginal thiamin deficiency. *J Gerontol* 1991;46:M180.

Smith-Warner SA, Elmer PJ, Tharp TM, et al. Increasing vegetable and fruit intake: randomized intervention and monitoring in an at-risk population. *Cancer Epidemiol Biomarkers Prev* 2000;9:307–317.

Snowdon DA, Gross MD, Buttler SM. Antioxidants and reduced functional capacity in the elderly: findings from the nun study. *J Gerontol A Biol Sci Med Sci* 1996;51:M10–M16.

Snowdon DA, Tully CL, Smith CD, Riley KP, Markesbery WR. Serum folate and the severity of atrophy of the neocortex in Alzheimer disease: findings from the nun study. *Am J Clin Nutr* 2000;71:993–998.

Souba WW. Nutritional support. *N Engl J Med* 1997;336:41–48.

Stabler SP. Progress in geriatrics: screening the older population for cobalamin (vitamin B12) deficiency. *J Am Geriatr Soc* 1995;43:1290–1297.

Stabler SP, Lindenbaum J, Allen RH. Vitamin B-12 deficiency in the elderly: current dilemmas. *Am J Clin Nutr* 1997;66:741–749.

Stampfer MJ, Malinow MR. Can lowering homocysteine levels reduce cardiovascular risk? *N Engl J Med* 1995;332:328–329.

Steinmetz KA, Potter JD. Vegetables, fruit, and cancer prevention: a review. *J Am Diet Assoc* 1996;96:1027–1039.

Stone, I. *The Healing Factor: Vitamin C against Disease.* Grosset Dunlap, New York, 1972.

Su LJ, Arab L. Nutritional status of folate and colon cancer risk: evidence from NHANES I epidemiologic follow-up study. *Ann Epidemiol* 2001;11:6–72.

Sumner AE, Chin MM, Abrahm JL, Berry GT, Gracely EJ, Allen RH, et al. Elevated methylmalonic acid and total homocysteine levels show high prevalence of vitamin B_{12} deficiency after gastric surgery. *Ann Intern Med* 1996;124:46–76.

Suter PM, Haller J, Hany J, Vetter W. Diuretic use: a risk for subclinical thiamine deficiency in elderly patients. *J Nutr Health Aging* 2000;4:6–71.

Szulc P, Chapuy MC, Meunier PJ, et al. FERUM undercarboxylated osteocalcin is a marker of the risk of hip fractures in elderly women. *J Clin Invest* 1993;91:176–174.

Talbott MC, Miller LT, Kerkvliet NI. Pyridoxine supplementation: effect on lymphocyte responses in elderly persons. *Am J Clin Nutr* 1987;46:559–64.

Talwar D, Davidson H, Cooney J, St. JO'Reilly. Vitamin B_1 status assessed by direct measurement of thiamin pyrophosphate in erythrocytes or whole blood by HPLC: comparison with erythrocyte transketolase activation assay. *Clin Chem* 2000;46:70–10.

Terry P, Jain M, Miller AB, Howe GR, Rohan TE. Dietary intake of folic acid and colorectal cancer risk in a cohort of women. *Int J Cancer* 2002;97:864–867.

Third National Health and Nutritional Examination Survey, Phase III. Daily dietary fat and total food energy intake. *MMWR* 1994;43:116–125.

Thomas DR, Morley JE. Assessing and treating undernutrition in older medical outpatients. *Clin Geriatr* 2001;9(Suppl.):1–4.

Thomas DR. Vitamins in health and aging. *Clincs in Geriatric Med* 2004;20:259–74.

Thomas MK, Demay MB. Vitamin D deficiency and disorders of vitamin D metabolism. *Endocrinol Metabol Clin North Am* 2000;29:611–627.

Tiemeier H, van Tuijl HR, Hofman A, Meijer J, Kiliaan AJ, Breteler MM. Vitamin B12, folate, and homocysteine in depression: the Rotterdam study. *Am J Psychiatry* 2002;159:2099–2101.

Ubbink JB, Van der Merwe A, Delport R, Allen RH, Stabler SP, Riezler R, et al. The effect of a subnormal vitamin B-6 status on homocysteine metabolism. *J Clin Invest* 1996;98:177–184.

Ubbink JB, Vermaak WJ, van der Merwe A, Becker PJ, Delport R, Potgieter HC. Vitamin requirements for the treatment of hyperhomocysteinemia in humans. *J Nutr* 1994;124:1927–1933.

Valagussa F, Franzosi MG, Geraci E, et al. Dietary supplementation with n-3 polyunsaturated fatty acids and vitamin E after myocardial infarction: results of the GISSI-Prevenzione trial. *Lancet* 1999;354:447–455.

Verhoef P, Stampfer MJ, Buring JE, Gaziano JM, Allen RH, et al. Homocysteine metabolism and risk of myocardial infarction: relation with vitamins B6, B12, and folate. *Am J Epidemiol* 1996;143:845–859.

Vermeer C, Knapen MHJ, Jie KSG. Physiologic importance of extra-hepatic vitamin K-dependent carboxylation reactions. *Ann NY Acad Sci* 1992;669:21–33.

Virtamo J, Pietinen P, Huttunen JK, Korhonen P, Malila N, Virtanen MJ, et al. Incidence of cancer and mortality following alpha-tocopherol and beta-carotene supplementation: a postintervention follow-up. *JAMA* 2003:290;476–485.

Vitolins MZ, Quandt SA, Case LD, Bell RA, Arcury TA, McDonald J. Vitamin and mineral supplement use by older rural adults. *J Gerontol Med Sci* 2000;55A:M613–M617.

Voutilainen S, Rissanen TH, Virtanen J, Lakka TA, Salonen JT. Low dietary folate intake is associated with an excess incidence of acute coronary events: the Kuopio Ischemic Heart Disease Risk Factor Study. *Circulation* 2001;103:2674–2680.

Wakimoto P, Block G. Dietary intake, dietary patterns, and changes with age: an epidemiological perspective. *J Gerontol A Med Sci* 2001;56A:65–80.

Wang HX, Wahlin A, Basun H, Fastbom J, Winblad B, Fratiglioni L. Vitamin B(12) and folate in relation to the development of Alzheimer's disease. *Neurology* 2001;56:1188–1194.

Weir DG, Molloy AM. Microvascular disease and dementia in the elderly: are they related to hyperhomocysteinemia? *Am J Clin Nutr* 2000;71:859–860.

White E, Shannon JS, Patterson RE. Relationship between vitamin and calcium supplement use and colon cancer. *Cancer Epidemiol Biomark Prev* 1997;6:769–774.

Wu K, Helzlsouer KJ, Comstock GW, Hoffman SC, Nadeau MR, Selhub J. A prospective study on folate, B_{12}, and pyridoxal 5'-phosphate (B6) and breast cancer. *Cancer Epidemiol Biomarkers Prev* 1999;8:209–217.

Yusuf S, Dagenais G, Pogue J, Bosch J, Sleight P. Vitamin E supplementation and cardiovascular events in high-risk patients. The Heart Outcomes Prevention Evaluation Study Investigators. *N Engl J Med* 2000;345:154–160.

Zhang S, Hunter DJ, Hankinson SE, et al. A prospective study of folate intake and the risk of breast cancer. *JAMA* 1999;281:1632–1637.

Zulkowski K. Examining the nutritional status of independently living elderly. *Ostomy/Wound Manage* 2000;46:415–460.

11 Trace Elements

John E. Morley, M.B., B.Ch.

CONTENTS

Trace elements play an important role in the maintenance of multiple enzyme reactions and are essential for the maintenance of tissue structure. Table 11.1 summarizes the major functions of the trace elements and the effects of aging on them.

11.1 ARSENIC

Arsenic has a biologic function in the metabolism of arginine and zinc.[1] Arsenic deprivation retards growth in the presence of marginal zinc status. Arsenic also plays a role in the modulation of kidney arginase activity, alkaline phosphatase activity, and plasma levels of triglycerides, uric acid, and urea. Based on animal studies, the human arsenic requirement appears to be between 12 and 25 μg daily. The role of arsenic in human malnutrition has been extrapolated from animal studies. The effect of aging on arsenic has not been studied.

TABLE 11.1
Functions of Trace Elements and the Effects of Aging on These Trace Elements

Trace Element	Function	Effect of Aging
Arsenic	Urea cycle, myocardial muscle function, triglyceride synthesis	Unknown
Boron	Bone structure, mineral metabolism	Unknown
Chromium	Glucose homeostasis, lipid metabolism	Decrease
Cobalt	Vitamin B_{12}, erythropoiesis, triglyceride synthesis	No change
Copper	Cholesterol metabolism erythropoiesis, collagen, cross-linking, conversion of dopamine to norepinephrine, electron transport chain, coagulation factor V	Increase in serum; decrease in saliva, hair, and heart
Fluoride	Bone structure, tooth enamel	Increase to 60, then decline in skeleton
Iodine	Thyroid hormones	Unknown
Lead	Toxicity leads to dementia, hypertension, and anemia	Increase in serum after 45
Lithium	Endocrine secretory function	Unknown
Manganese	Protein and energy metabolism, mucopolysaccharides; Parkinsonism with excess intake	No change in serum; reduced in kidney and heart
Molybdenum	Uric acid production, oxidation of sulfite to sulfate	Unknown
Nickel	RNA and DNA structure, membrane stabilization, iron absorption and metabolism, pituitary function	Increase in lung
Selenium	Constituent of glutathione peroxidase, T and B cell function, muscle metabolism	Decrease
Silicon	Bone structure, connective tissue structure	Decrease in aorta and skin
Tin	Induces hemoxygenase and carbon monoxide production	Increase in Alzheimer's disease
Vanadium	Cholesterol synthesis, catalysis of oxidation–reduction reactions	Unknown
Zinc	Immune function, taste, oxidative metabolism, sexuality, skin integrity	None

11.2 BORON

In *Drosophilia*, moderate levels of boron increase life span while higher levels decrease it.[2] Boron appears to interact with cholecalciferol in the maintenance of bone structure.[1] It also interacts with magnesium. In postmenopausal women on a low-magnesium diet, boron supplementation (3 mg/day) reduced the urinary excretion of calcium, magnesium, and phosphorus.[3] Boron supplementation also resulted in an increase in serum testosterone and 17-estradiol in these women. A second study found that a low-boron diet was associated with hypercalcemia.[4] Increasing boron intake failed to alter sex steroid hormone levels or urinary excretion of pyrrolidinium cross-link markers of bone turnover. These studies have led to the perhaps premature claim that boron supplementation may play a role in the prevention of calcium loss and bone demineralization in postmenopausal women.

11.3 CHROMIUM

Chromium is an essential trace element that may play a role in glucose homeostasis.[5] Deficiency of chromium or its biologically active form, glucose tolerance factor (a dinicotinic acid–glutathionine complex), has been shown to result in glucose intolerance.[6] The glucose tolerance factor is poorly characterized. The richest sources of it are brewer's yeast, liver, and kidney.

Hyperglycemia, which responds to chromium replacement, has been reported to occur in patients on total parenteral nutrition.[7–9] However, the role of chromium in the hyperglycemia of aging remains controversial. Skeptics totally reject its role, whereas others embrace it wholeheartedly. One well-controlled study of 16 patients 65 years of age and older found that chromium in combination with nicotinic acid caused a 15% decrease in the integrated glucose area in response to a glucose load.[10] Numerous studies continue to produce contradictory studies on the effect of chromium on diabetic control.[11–15] A low-chromium diet was shown to produce deterioration in glucose tolerance in some subjects, and this was improved by chromium supplementation.[16]

Chromium deficiency has been associated with hypercholesterolemia in some but not all studies.[5] Two of three studies have found an increase in high-density lipoprotein (HDL) cholesterol with chromium supplementation.[17–19]

Chromium deficiency in humans has been associated with weight loss, atoxia, and peripheral neuropathy, as well as with hyperglycemia in patients on total parenteral nutrition.

Tissue and serum chromium levels decline with age[20–22] and may do so more dramatically in Western societies that eat refined foods and are somewhat deficient in chromium.[23] There is increased urinary excretion of chromium with aging and in diabetics.[24] The Recommended Daily Allowance (RDA) for chromium is between 50 and 200 μg.[25] However, Bunker et al.[26] reported that healthy volunteers ingesting 13.6 to 47.7 μg/day were able to maintain a positive chromium balance. In a study of institutionalized older individuals, the average chromium content of food offered (not eaten) was 52 μg/day.[27] Urinary excretion of chromium increases with age.[28]

11.4 COBALT

Cobalt tissue concentrations are unchanged with age.[29] Cobalt is an essential portion of the vitamin B_{12} molecule. Cobalt therapy increases hemoglobin in anemic patients on dialysis.[30] However, this response may be associated with an increase in tumorigenesis. Cobalt therapy also increases triglyceride levels.[31] High cobalt levels in beer have been associated with the development of a cardiomyopathy.[32] Cobalt may reduce thyroid function when given in pharmacologic doses.[33] Elevated cobalt levels can be found in both the blood and urine of patients with metallic hip replacements.[34]

11.5 COPPER

Copper is involved in iron absorption and mobilization. It acts as a catalyst in multiple enzymatic reactions, including the superoxidase dismutase reaction, the cross-linking of collagen, the lipyloxidase enzyme, the electron transport chain through cytochromic oxidase, coagulation factor V, and the conversion of dopamine to norepinephrine. Copper deficiency is associated with hypercholesterolemia, perhaps through an increased rate of cholesterol release from the liver.[35] Copper deficiency also leads to an impairment of glucose tolerance,[36] and copper has been shown to act synergistically with insulin to drive the incorporation of glucose into fat cells.[37] In humans, a weak association between serum copper levels and fasting blood glucose has been demonstrated.[38,39] Klevay[40] suggested that atherosclerosis is related to the rate of zinc to copper levels. However, the evidence that copper deficiency is associated with atherosclerosis is extremely weak. A recent study did demonstrate higher serum copper levels in persons who had a myocardial infarction than in age-matched controls.[41] Systolic blood pressure is positively correlated with urinary copper excretion.[42] Copper deficiency has been associated with anemia, neutropenia, and osteoporosis.[36] Lower levels of serum copper were found in elderly patients with femoral neck fractures.[43] In addition, it may cause muscle weakness and a bleeding tendency. Symptoms of congenital copper deficiency (Menkes syndrome) include arterial disease, abnormal hair, osteoporosis, cerebellar atoxia, and other brain damage. Copper deficiency in older individuals has usually been associated with total

TABLE 11.2
Possible Clinical Syndromes Associated with Copper Deficiency in Humans

Anemia and neutropenia
Osteoporosis
Arterial disease
Pigmentation loss
Muscle weakness
Bleeding tendency
Cardiomyopathy vs. atherosclerotic heart disease
Brain degeneration
Impaired glucose tolerance
Myelopathy

parenteral nutrition. Symptoms in two patients on total parenteral nutrition with severe copper deficiency responded to copper supplementation.[44]

Serum copper levels tend to increase with aging,[45] although there is no change in leukocyte copper levels.[46] A recent study found an increase in serum copper levels in men but a decrease in women.[47] In the locus coeruleus of the brain copper levels decrease.[48]

The increase in serum copper with advancing age is accompanied by an increase in ceruloplasmin.[49] Ceruloplasmin in older persons is oxidatively modified, resulting in conformational changes around the copper-binding sites.[50] In contrast, copper levels decrease in salivary sediment and hair with aging.[51] Copper levels are also significantly reduced in the heart tissue of older subjects.[52] Absorption of copper is similar in young and old men[53] and women.[49] Biologic half-life increases in men but not in women with advancing age.

Although older subjects ingest significantly lower amounts of copper than younger subjects, they appear to have no problem in maintaining metabolic balance.[53] In the presence of type II diabetes mellitus, both copper and ceruloplasmin levels are elevated, and this elevation is more pronounced with advancing age.[36]

Overall, copper metabolism seems to be conserved with aging. The potential pathophysiologic role of copper deficiency in atherosclerosis and the hyperglycemia of aging warrants further study. The potential effects of mild copper deficiency are summarized in Table 11.2. Recently copper deficiency has been recognized to produce a myelopathy similar to subacute combined degeneration.[54]

11.6 FLUORIDE

Fluoride plays a role in the hydroxyapatite of bone and tooth enamel. Circulating fluoride levels tend to rise after middle age because of the decrease in renal function and an increased release of fluoride from bone.[55]

Fluoride has been used in the therapy of osteoporosis to reduce the fracture rate.[56] However, during the early course of fluoride therapy, microfractures may occur in the lower limbs, resulting in pain in the lower extremities. An increase in hip fractures has been reported in some patients receiving fluoride therapy. Fluoride therapy can cause exacerbations of rheumatoid arthritis as well as gastrointestinal bleeding and painful joints.

11.7 IODINE

Iodine is an integral part of the thyroid hormones. Iodine deficiency can lead to the development of goiter. There are no studies on iodine metabolism with advancing age.

11.8 LEAD

Animal studies have suggested that aging produces enhanced vulnerability to the behavioral effects of lead.[57] Lead levels increase throughout life, with levels being higher in males than in females.[58]

Adult exposure to lead is associated with a decline in cognitive function; smaller brain volume and increased white matter lesions are seen with magnetic resonance imaging (MRI).[59] Lead exposure, as a fetus can be associated with developmental reprogramming of the amyloid precursor protein to overproduce amyloid beta protein.[60] Lead exposure is also associated with development of hypertension, age-related cataract, and decreased hemoglobin levels.[61–63]

11.9 LITHIUM

Animal studies have suggested a role for lithium as an essential trace element.[1] Lithium appears to be involved in the regulation of pituitary, adrenal, and thyroid hormone secretion and water metabolism. Pharmacologic amounts of lithium used for the treatment of depression can result in hypothyroidism. Chronic lithium therapy has been associated with hypoproteinemia.[64] Increased sodium–lithium countertransport in erythrocytes predicted increased susceptibility to the development of hypertension.[65] Studies on lithium metabolism with aging have not been carried out.

11.10 MANGANESE

Manganese is essential for protein and energy metabolism and the formation of mucopolysaccharides. A deficiency of manganese can result in impaired glucose tolerance and bone abnormalities. Two studies have failed to show any effects of age on manganese concentrations.[66,67] Tissue manganese levels are reduced in the heart and kidney of older persons (mean age, 80 years) compared with younger persons (mean age, 29 years).[52] Manganese levels have been reported to be elevated in diabetic patients age 61 to 70 years old.[56,68] These elevated manganese levels may cause increased hepatic arginase activity in diabetics, resulting in increased amino acid metabolism and urea synthesis.[69]

Excessive manganese in the existing water is associated with neurologic deterioration.[64] Manganese intoxication can result in Morvan's fibrillary chorea, hyperhidrosis, insomnia, and hallucinations, which appear to be due to inhibition of acetylcholinesterase activity resulting in cholenergic hyperactivity.[70] Manganese excess is associated with a Parkinson's-like syndrome and increased body sway.[71]

11.11 MOLYBDENUM

Molybdenum deficiency has been reported in a 24-year-old patient with Crohn's disease on total parenteral nutrition (TPN).[72] He had symptoms of intolerance to the TPN solution as a source of nutrients. He had high urinary levels of sulfite, thiosulfate, hypoxanthine, and xanthine, and low levels of sulfate and uric acid. Biochemical and symptomatic normalization occurred with molybdenum supplementation.

Molybdenum intakes of 0.15 mg/day appear adequate to maintain molybdenum balance. Molybdenum toxicity (10 to 15 mg/day) is associated with elevated xanthine oxidase activity and uric acid levels.[73] Molybdenum excess increases the urinary excretion of copper. Clinically, molybdenum toxicity presents with anorexia, weight loss, skin changes, anemia, and diarrhea. No studies on molybdenum with aging have been conducted. It has been suggested that tissue damage that occurs during postischemic injury is related to dehydrogenase-to-oxidase conversion of the molybdenum-dependent enzyme, xanthine dehydrogenase.[73]

11.12 NICKEL

Stabilization of RNA and DNA and membrane structure requires nickel. Nickel may also be involved in hormonal release from the pituitary. Most ingested nickel is excreted in the feces, with only small amounts excreted. Grains and vegetables are the major source of nickel. Phytates in the grains appear to interfere with the absorption of nickel.

Nickel concentrations in lung tissue increase with age and are higher in men than in women.[74] Diabetes does not alter serum levels of nickel.[75] Nickel is increased in lungs of patients with bronchial cancer, and smoking is associated with increased nickel accumulation.[76] Environmental nickel exposure is associated with an increased lung cancer incidence.

11.13 SELENIUM

Selenium was first recognized to be an essential trace element in 1957. The most fully characterized biochemical effect of selenium is its inclusion in the glutathione peroxidase molecule. The major physiologic role of flutathione peroxidase is to maintain appropriately low levels of hydrogen peroxides within cells, thus decreasing potential free radical damage. Selenium deficiency is accompanied by a decrease in glutathione peroxidase activity and results in an increase in hepatic glutathione-S-transferase activity. Glutathione-S-transferase catalyzes the conjugation of electrophilic compounds and metabolites with glutathione, which is an important hepatic detoxification mechanism. Glutathione-S-transferase is also involved in the storage of heme and bilirubin. Selenium deficiency also increases liver glutathione synthesis, which can lead to a depletion of cysteine and impairment of protein synthesis.

Selenium has also been demonstrated to alter other drug (xenobiotic)-metabolizing enzymes in addition to gluthathione-S-transferase.[77] In particular, selenium deficiency is associated with a decrease in some of the isoenzymes of cytochrome P-450. In contrast, it is also associated with an increase in uridine diphosphate (UDP) glucuronyl transferase activity. Thus, selenium deficiency clearly affects the ability of an individual to metabolize drugs. Because of its different effects on different enzymes' systems, selenium deficiency may be associated with increased toxicity of some drugs and decreased efficiency of others.

The selenium content of food is directly dependent on the soil concentration of selenium. Selenium intakes vary widely throughout the world, with intakes between 7 and 38,000 μg/day having been reported. An adequate selenium intake has been estimated at 50 μg/day, with toxic levels estimated to occur with intakes of the order of 350 to 700 μg/day. It appears that selenium in the form of selenomethionine (the form found in wheat) results in better selenium retention than does selenate or selenite.[78]

TABLE 11.3
Disease States Possibly Associated with Selenium Deficiency

Keshan disease
Cardiomyopathy in patients on total parenteral nutrition
Muscle weakness and pain
Nail changes
T and B cell dysfunction
Cancer?
Coronary artery disease?

Note: ? = uncertain association.

Some controversy exists concerning the effects of age on selenium levels. Circulating selenium concentrations either fall slightly[79] or remain stable with aging.[80,81] Elderly residents in long-term-care settings who are tube fed have both low selenium levels and a reduction in red blood cell glutathione peroxidase levels.[82] Selenium in hair has been found to decline from a mean of 0.76 μg/g of hair in 11- to 15-year-olds to a mean of 0.55 μg/g in 61- to 70-year-olds.[83] Dietary intake of selenium is high in adolescents and declines to 65 μg/day in individuals over 70 years of age.

Selenium deficiency may be associated with a number of pathologic conditions (Table 11.3). The disease state best shown to be produced by selenium deficiency is a cardiomyopathy of children and young women (Keshan disease). Although selenium deficiency provides the necessary setting for the development of cardiomyopathy, other factors, such as viral infections, seem to play a role in the pathogenesis of this disease.[84] Cardiomyopathy has also been found in some patients receiving total parenteral nutrition who are selenium deficient.[85–87] Whether selenium deficiency plays a role in the pathogenesis of heart failure in some older individuals is unknown.

One of the highest concentrations of selenium in the body is in the thyroid gland. Selenium plays a role through glutathione peroxidase in iodination of thyroglobulin. The enzyme responsible for conversion of thyroxine to triodothyronine is selenium dependent. Selenium is inversely correlated with thyroid peroxidase antibody. The effects of borderline selenium deficiency on thyroid function are minimal.[88]

Patients receiving hyperalimentation have been reported to develop a syndrome of muscle weakness or pain and nail changes.[89–91] This syndrome responded to selenium administration.

Selenium deficiency has been implicated in carcinogenesis. There is a lower prevalence of cancer in countries with a high selenium concentration in the soil, such as Venezuela. Many case-controlled prospective studies have suggested a relationship of selenium deficiency to cancer risk.[92] However, not all studies have demonstrated such a correlation.[93] A study from Finland suggested that a major cancer risk existed for persons with low selenium and vitamin E levels.[94] This finding is in keeping with an *in vitro* study of irradiated cells that suggested both selenium and vitamin E act at different sites to attenuate radiation-induced damage.[95] Numerous animals studies have shown that high-selenium diets can prevent the development of cancer.[96]

In a meta-analysis of nine studies, low levels of serum selenium were predictive of those who developed cancer of the lung, bladder, stomach, and pancreas.[97] The Nutritional Prevention Cancer Trial was a double-blind placebo-controlled trial of the ability of 200 μg of selenized yeast to prevent recurrence of nonmelanoma skin cancer.[98] There was a 25% decrease in total cancer and a 42% decrease in prostate cancer. Reductions in cancer were most prominent in smokers and those who had the lowest selenium levels. Two controlled trials in China also suggested that selenium supplementation reduced cancer occurrence.[99] The Nurses' Health Study showed no effect of selenium on breast cancer.[100] There is some suggestive data that selenium may prevent colorectal cancer.[101] Selenium may also be useful in preventing chemotherapy toxicity.

In the Women's Health and Aging Studies high-serum selenium was associated with a mortality HR of 0.71 in women age 70 to 79.[102] In the EVA study the relative risk of death in older men and women with low selenium was 1.56.[103] Serum selenium is inversely associated with homocysteine with lower levels of interleukin 6.[104]

Selenium deficiency increases thromboxane B_2, which causes platelet aggregation, while decreasing prostacyclin, which prevents aggregation.[78] This gives a biochemical mechanism by which selenium deficiency could enhance the development of atherosclerotic cardiovascular disease.[78] A weak correlation of low selenium levels and coronary vascular disease was reported in one study,[105] but not in another.[106] In the study where the association with low selenium levels was found, the major dietary source of selenium was fish, suggesting that the correlation may have been spurious and related to fish intake. This observation was supported by the finding that serum selenium levels correlated with the eicospentanoic acid concentrations.[107]

Suppressed cellular and humoral immune function has been associated with selenium deficiency.[108] In animals, selenium deficiency has been associated with impaired defense against candidiasis.[108] The putative role of selenium deficiency in the immune dysfunction often found in elderly nursing home residents has not been evaluated.

Studies in children have suggested that selenium-deficient kwashiorkor patients may fail to thrive until they receive selenium supplementation.[78] Again, the role of selenium supplementation in older subjects with protein-energy malnutrition has not been evaluated.

Selenium toxicity was reported in subjects in the U.S. who ingested an over-the-counter "health food" supplement that mistakenly contained 180 times more selenium than stated on the label.[78] These subjects experienced nail changes, hair loss, and peripheral neuropathy. An early sign of selenium overexposure is the development of a garlic odor on the breath. Other toxic effects include gastrointestinal disturbances, dizziness, and sweating.

The future role of selenium in human nutrition of the elderly is uncertain. Controlled trials of selenium's effects in nutritionally depleted older individuals need to be carried out. Selenium supplementation or choosing a selenium-supplemented formula should be considered in elderly subjects who are tube fed.

11.14 SILICON

Silicon is important for maintaining the structural integrity of bone and connective tissue. Silicon deficiency may play a role in the development of such degenerative diseases as osteoarthritis or atherosclerosis. The silicon content of certain animal tissues, such as the aorta, skin, and thymus, decreases with aging, whereas the content is unchanged in most tissues.[33] Silicon content in the human aorta decreases with age, and this decrease is more marked in association with atherosclerosis.[109] Animal studies suggest a decreased absorption of silicon with advancing age.[110] Silicon levels are reduced in patients with diabetes mellitus.[36] Further studies on the role of silicon with aging are indicated. Inhalation of silica particles can lead to the lung disease silicosis.

11.15 TIN

The adult daily tin intake has decreased from 17 mg/day in 1940 to 3.5 mg/day today due to improvement in tinning techniques. Tin excess is associated with hepato- and neurotoxicity. Tin stimulates the production of hemoxygenase, which results in the elaboration of endogenous carbon monoxide. Recently, carbon monoxide has been suggested to play a role as a neurotransmitter and may play a role in appetite regulation. Tin compounds have been found to be elevated in patients with Alzheimer's disease.[111]

11.16 VANADIUM

Vanadium deficiency in animals leads to elevated cholesterol levels.[33] Data on humans are controversial, with two studies failing to show an effect of vanadium on cholesterol[112,113] and one study suggesting that vanadium could lower cholesterol levels.[114] Vanadium is an important element in the regulation of tumor necrosis factor-alpha.[115] It also has insulinomimetic actions.[116]

Vanadate is a potent inhibitor of sodium- and potassium-activated adenosine triphosphatase (Na^+ K^+ ATPase) *in vitro* and may play a role in the physiologic regulation of the sodium pump and energy metabolism.[1] *In vivo* evidence for this hypothesis is presently lacking. The average daily human intake of vanadium is 2 mg. Studies on alterations in the intake or excretion of vanadium in older individuals have not been undertaken.

11.17 ZINC

Zinc is essential for many biochemical reactions. It plays a key role in four areas: cell proliferation and growth, apoptosis, immune function, and oxidative metabolism. Zinc has been shown to play a role in modulating some of the polymorphisms associated with longevity, e.g., IL-6-174 G/C locus and those associated with worsening atherosclerosis, e.g., 1267 Hsp 70-2A/B and severe infections, e.g., TNF-alpha-308 G/A.[117] The main clinical manifestations of zinc deficiency are growth retardation, hypogonadism and erectile dysfunction, hypogeusia, diarrhea, anorexia, immune deficiencies, hair loss, acrodematiles, poor wound healing, and poor dark adaptation (Table 11.4).

TABLE 11.4
Possible Clinical Syndromes Associated with Zinc Deficiency in Humans

Growth retardation
Hypogonadism
Erectile dysfunction
Hypogeusia
Diarrhea
Anorexia and weight loss
Immune deficiency
Poor wound healing
Acrodermatitis
Poor dark adaptation
Macular degeneration?
Osteoporosis?

Note: ? = uncertain association.

Measurement of zinc status is difficult with multiple factors from infection to exercise altering serum zinc levels. For this reason, making a diagnosis of zinc deficiency requires a cellular, e.g., hair or leukocyte level, and some evidence of excessive loss or poor zinc absorption or alteration in a zinc-dependent enzyme, e.g., 5′-nucleotidase. Dietary studies in older persons suggest that on the average they ingest less than the estimated average requirement of 9.4 mg/day for women and 11 mg/day for men.[118,119] Overall, zinc absorption appears to be similar in young and older persons.[119,120] However, older persons on chelating agents, laxatives, antacids, and iron calcium supplements will have decreased zinc absorption. Diuretics, diabetes mellitus, lung cancer, and cirrhosis of the liver are associated with hyperzincuria. Given that these conditions are relatively common in older persons, it is not surprising that the National Health and Nutrition Examination Survey (NHANES) II estimated that zinc deficiency was present in about 12% of older persons.[121]

Despite a strong basic science literature supporting the importance of zinc in maintaining health, there is a paucity of adequate studies to provide a strong evidence base for zinc replacement in older persons. Three double-blind studies support the concept that zinc replacement improves cellular immunity in zinc-deficient older persons.[122–124] There is inadequate data to recommend zinc for the treatment of pressure ulcers,[125] although many believe it should be used in zinc-deficient persons. A single trial (AREDS in the U.S.) has supported the beneficial effect of zinc in treating macular degeneration,[126] but this was associated with increased urinary problems. Excess zinc (40 mg/day) leads to impaired immune responses, abnormal copper metabolism, and adverse cholesterol patterns. High levels of zinc have been associated with precipitation of amyloid-beta peptide in Alzheimer's disease.[127] In animal models of Alzheimer's disease, the metal-complexing agent, dioquinol, decreased brain amyloid plaque burden. There is a clear need for adequately powered trials of zinc replacement in older persons with zinc deficiency to demonstrate its utility in improving the quality of life of older persons.

11.18 TRACE ELEMENT INTERACTION

The effects of each trace element are heavily dependent on one another. Thus, high intakes of zinc, cadmium, or copper interfere with the utilization and tissue storage of iron.[128] Similarly, zinc supplements have been shown to cause anemia secondary to hypocupremia.[129] Tetrathiomolybdate inhibits copper absorption.[128] Low concentrations of dietary iron enhance the absorption not only of dietary iron but also of lead, zinc, cadmium, cobalt, and manganese.[128] The potentiating effect of selenium deficiency on lipid peroxidation and thus free radical damage is enhanced in some tissues by concurrent deficiency of copper or manganese.[128]

An antioxidant index was demonstrated to correlate significantly with a reduction in age-related macular degeneration risk, while selenium levels alone showed no such significant relationships.[130] The role of these trace element interactions requires intensive study in older individuals who may be on one trace element supplement, such as zinc, have a poor dietary intake, and be receiving drugs (e.g., diuretics) that cause trace element loss in the urine.

11.19 CONCLUSION

Many of these trace elements appear to be important for the maintenance of normal glucose homeostatis and lipid metabolism. Others play an important role in the maintenance of bone structure. Enzymes involved in collagen cross-linking, one of the benchmarks of aging, are often catalyzed by trace elements. Selenium deficiency may play a role in carcinogenesis, is associated with immune dysfunction, and occurs commonly in tube-fed patients. Selenium is essential for the activity of glutathionine peroxidase, which protects against free radical damage by decreasing the formation of hydroxy radicals. Zinc appears to play an important role in immunity, macular degeneration, anorexia, taste abnormalities, and wound healing. Little is known about the role of drugs, especially diuretics, and intercurrent illness on the development of trace mineral deficiency with advancing age. Also, the interactions of trace elements with one another—particularly in the situation where the decision is made to replace a single trace element—need further investigation. Overall, there is a need for increased study of the role of trace elements in the aging process.

REFERENCES

1. Nielsen, F.H., Ultratrace elements in nutrition, *Ann. Rev. Nutr.*, 4, 21, 1984.
2. Massie, H.R., Whitney, S.J., Aiello, V.R., et al., Changes in boron concentrations during development and ageing of *Drosophilia* and effect of dietary boron on life span, *Mech. Ageing Dev.*, 53, 1, 1990.
3. Nielsen, F.H., Effect of dietary boron on mineral, estrogen, and testosterone metabolism in postmenopausal women, *FASEB J.*, 1, 394, 1987.

4. Beattie, J.H. and Peace, H.S., The influence of a low-boron diet and boron supplementation on bone, major mineral and sex steroid metabolism in postmenopausal women, *Br. J. Nutr.*, 69, 871, 1993.
5. Offenbacher, E.G. and Pi-Sunyer, F.X., Chromium in human nutrition, *Ann. Rev. Nutr.*, 8, 543, 1988.
6. Schwarz, K. and Mertz, W., A glucose tolerance factor and its differentiation from factor 3, *Arch. Biochem. Biophys.*, 72, 515, 1957.
7. Jeejeebhoy, K.N., Chu, R.C., Marliss, E.B., et al., Chromium deficiency, glucose intolerance, and neuropathy reversed by chromium supplementation, in a patient receiving long-term total parenteral nutrition, *Am. J. Clin. Nutr.*, 30, 531, 1977.
8. Freund, H., Atamian, S., and Fischer, J.E., Chromium deficiency during total parenteral nutrition, *JAMA*, 241, 496, 1979.
9. Brown, R.O., Forloines-Lynn, S., Cross, R.E., et al., Chromium deficiency after long-term total parenteral nutrition, *Dig. Dis. Sci.*, 31, 661, 1986.
10. Urberg, M. and Zemel, M.B., Evidence for synergism between chromium and nicotinic acid in the control of glucose tolerance in elderly humans, *Metab. Clin. Exp.*, 36, 896, 1987.
11. Pei, D., Hsieh, C.H., Hung, Y.J., et al., The influence of chromium chloride-containing milk to glycemic control of patients with type 2 diabetes mellitus: a randomized, double-blind, placebo-controlled trial, *Metab. Clin. Exp.*, 55, 923, 2006.
12. Rabinovitz, H., Friedensoh, A., Leibovitz, A., et al., Effect of chromium supplementation on blood glucose and lipid levels in type 2 diabetes mellitus in elderly patients, *Int. J. Vitamin Nutr. Res.*, 74, 178, 2004.
13. Vladeva, S.V., Terzieva, D.D., and Arabadjiiska, D.T., Effect of chromium on the insulin resistance in patients with type II diabetes mellitus, *Folia Med.*, 47, 59, 2005.
14. Racek, J., Trefil, L., Rajdl, D., et al., Influence of chromium-enriched yeast on blood glucose and insulin variables, blood lipids, and markers of oxidative stress in subjects with type 2 diabetes mellitus, *Biol. Trace Elem. Res.*, 109, 215, 2006.
15. Kleefstra, N., Houweling, S.T., Jansman, F.G., et al., Chromium treatment has no effect in patients with poorly controlled, insulin-treated type 2 diabetes in an obese Western population: a randomized, double-blind, placebo-controlled trial, *Diabetes Care*, 29, 521, 2006.
16. Anderson, R.A., Polansky, M.M., Bryden, N.A., et al., Supplemental-chromium effects on glucose, insulin, glucagons, and urinary chromium losses in subjects consuming controlled low-chromium diets, *Am. J. Clin. Nutr.*, 54, 909, 1991.
17. Roeback, J.R., Jr., Hla, K.M., Chambles, L.E., et al., Effects of chromium supplementation on serum high-density lipoprotein cholesterol levels in men taking beta-blockers. A randomized, controlled trial, *Ann. Intern. Med.*, 115, 917, 1991.
18. Gordon, J.B., An easy and inexpensive way to lower cholesterol? *West. J. Med.*, 154, 352, 1991.
19. Offenbacher, E.G., Chromium in the elderly, *Biol. Trace Elem. Res.*, 32, 123, 1992.
20. Schroeder, H., Balassa, J.J., and Tipton, I.H., Abnormal trace metals in man: chromium, *J. Chronic Dis.*, 15, 941, 1962.
21. Schroeder, H.A., Nason, A.P., and Tipton, I.H., Chromium deficiency as a factor in atherosclerosis, *J. Chronic Dis.*, 23, 123, 1970.
22. Davies, S., McLaren, H.J., Hunnisett, A., et al., Age-related decreases in chromium levels in 51,665 hair, sweat, and serum samples from 40,872 patients: implications for the prevention of cardiovascular disease and type II diabetes mellitus, *Metab. Clin. Exp.*, 46, 469, 1997.

23. Pi-Sunyer, F.X. and Offenbacher, E.G., in *Nutrition Reviews: Present Knowledge in Nutrition*, 4th ed., Hegsted, D.M., Chichester, C.O., Darby, W.J., et al., Eds., Nutrition Foundation, New York, 1976, p. 571.
24. Ding, W., Chai, Z., Duan, P., et al., Serum and urine chromium concentrations in elderly diabetes, *Biol. Trace Elem. Res.*, 63, 231, 1998.
25. World Health Organization, *Evaluation of Certain Food Additives and the Contaminants Mercury, Lead and Cadmium*, Technical Report Series 505, Geneva, 1972.
26. Bunker, V.W., Lawson, M.S., Delvers, H.T., et al., The intake and excretion of lead and cadmium by the elderly, *Am. J. Clin. Nutr.*, 39, 803, 1984.
27. Shaper, A.G., Pocock, S.J., Walker, M., et al., Effects of alcohol and smoking on blood lead in middle-aged British men, *Br. Med. J.*, 284, 299, 1982.
28. Offenbacher, E.G., Riinko, C.J., and Pi-Sunyer, F.X., The effects of inorganic chromium and brewer's yeast on glucose tolerance, plasma lipids, and plasma chromium in elderly subjects, *Am. J. Clin. Nutr.*, 42, 454, 1985.
29. Schroeder, H.A., Nason, A.P., and Tipton, I.H., Essential trace metals in man: cobalt, *J. Chronic Dis.*, 20, 869, 1967.
30. Duckham, J.M. and Lee, H.A., The treatment of refractory anaemia of chronic renal failure with cobalt chloride, *Q. J. Med.*, 45, 277, 1976.
31. Taylor, A., Marks, V., Shabaan, A.A., et al., Cobalt induced lipaemia and erythropoiesis, in *Clinical Chemistry and Chemical Toxicology of Metal*, Amsterdam, Elsevier, 1977, p. 105.
32. Alexander, C.S., Cobalt-beer cardiomyopathy: a clinical and pathologic study of twenty-eight cases, *Am. J. Med.*, 53, 395, 1972.
33. Udipi, S.A. and Watson, R.R., Trace element requirements of the elderly, in *Handbook of Nutrition in the Aged*, CRC Press, Boca Raton, FL, 1985, p. 145.
34. Coleman, R.F., Herrington, J., and Scales, J.T., Concentration of wear products in hair, blood and urine after total hip replacement, *Br. Med. J.*, 1, 527, 1973.
35. Klevay, L.M., Inman, L., Johnson, L.K., et al., Increased cholesterol in plasma in a young man during experimental copper depletion, *Metab. Clin. Exp.*, 33, 1112, 1984.
36. Mooradian, A.D. and Morley, J.E., Micronutrient status in diabetes mellitus, *Am. J. Clin. Nutr.*, 45, 877, 1987.
37. Fields, M., Reiser, S., and Smith, J.C., Jr., Effect of copper or insulin on diabetic copper-deficient rats, *Proc. Soc. Exp. Biol. Med.*, 173, 137, 1983.
38. Kanabrocki, E.L., Case, L.F., Graham, L., et al., Non-dialyzable manganese and copper levels in serum of patients with various diseases, *J. Nucl. Med.*, 8, 166, 1967.
39. Batista, M.N., Cuppari, L., and deFatima Campos Pedrosa, L., Effect of end-stage renal disease and diabetes in zinc and copper status, *Biol. Trace Elem. Res.*, 112, 1, 2006.
40. Klevay, L.M., Coronary heart disease: the zinc/copper hypothesis, *Am. J. Clin. Nutr.*, 28, 764, 1975.
41. Tan, I.K., Chua, K.S., and Toh, A.K., Serum magnesium, copper, and zinc concentrations in acute myocardial infarction, *J. Clin. Lab. Anal.*, 6, 324, 1992.
42. Staessen, J., Sartor, F., Roels, H., et al., The association between blood pressure, calcium and other divalent cations: a population study, *J. Hum. Hypertens.*, 5, 485, 1991.
43. Conlan, D., Korula, R., and Tallentire, D., Serum copper levels in elderly patients with femoral-neck fractures, *Age Ageing*, 19, 212, 1990.
44. Oliver, A., Allen, K.R., and Taylor, J., Trace element concentrations in patients on home enteral feeding: two cases of severe copper deficiency, *Ann. Clin. Biochem.*, 42, 136, 2005.
45. Yunice, A.A., Lindeman, R.D., Czerwinski, A.W., et al., Influence of age and sex on serum copper and ceruloplasmin levels, *J. Gerontol.*, 29, 277, 1974.

46. Bunker, V.W., Hinks, L.J., Lawson, M.S., et al., Assessment of zinc and copper status of healthy elderly people using metabolic balance studies and measurement of leucocyte concentrations, *Am. J. Clin. Nutr.*, 40, 1096, 1984.
47. Benes, B., Spevackova, V., Smid, J., et al., Effects of age, BMI, smoking and contraception on levels of Cu, Se and Zn in the blood of the population in the Czech Republic, *Cent. Eur. J. Public Health*, 13, 202, 2005.
48. Zecca, L., Stroppolo, A., Gatti, A., et al., The role of iron and copper molecules in the neuronal vulnerability of locus coeruleus and substantia nigra during aging, *Proc. Natl. Acad. Sci. U.S.A.*, 101, 9843, 2004.
49. Milne, D.B. and Johnson, P.E., Assessment of copper status: effect of age and gender on reference ranges in healthy adults, *Clin. Chem.*, 39, 883, 1993.
50. Musci, G., Bonaccorsi di Patti, M.C., Fagiolo, U., et al., Age-related changes in human ceruloplasmin. Evidence for oxidative modifications, *J. Biol. Chem.*, 268, 13388, 1993.
51. Bales, C.W., Freeland-Graves, J.H., Askey, S., et al., Zinc, magnesium, copper, and protein concentrations in human saliva: age- and sex-related differences, *Am. J. Clin. Nutr.*, 51, 462, 1990.
52. Martin, B.J., Lyon, T.D., and Fell, G.S., Comparison of inorganic elements from autopsy tissue of young and elderly subjects, *Trace Elem. Electrol.*, 5, 203, 1991.
53. Turnlund, J.R., Michel, M.C., Keyes, W.R., et al., Copper absorption in elderly men determined by using stable 65 Cu, *Am. J. Clin. Nutr.*, 36, 587, 1982.
54. Kumar, N., Gross, J.B., Jr., and Ahlskog, J.E., Copper deficiency myelopathy produces a clinical picture like subacute combined degeneration, *Neurology*, 63, 33, 2004.
55. Husdan, H., Vogl, R., Oreopoulos, D., et al., Serum ionic fluoride: normal range and relationship to age and sex, *Clin. Chem.*, 22, 1884, 1976.
56. Morley, J.E., Gorbien, M.J., Mooradian, A.D., et al., UCLA geriatric grand rounds: osteoporosis, *J. Am. Geriatr. Soc.*, 36, 845, 1988.
57. Cory-Slechta, D.A., Pokora, M.J., and Widzowski, D.V., Behavioral manifestations of prolonged lead exposure initiated at different stages of the life cycle. II. Delayed spatial alternation, *Neurotoxicology*, 12, 761, 1991.
58. Staessen, J.A., Lauwerys, R.R., Buchet, J.P., et al., Impairment of renal function with increasing blood lead concentrations in the general population. The Cadmibel Study Group, *N. Engl. J. Med.*, 327, 151, 1992.
59. Stewart, W.F., Schwartz, B.S., Davatzikos, C., et al., Past adult lead exposure is linked to neurodegeneration measured by brain MRI, *Neurology*, 66, 1464, 2006.
60. Basha, M.R., Murali, M., Siddiqi, H.K., et al., Lead (Pb) exposure and its effect on APP protealysis and abetea aggregation, *FASEB J.*, 19, 2083, 2005.
61. Schaumberg, D.A., Mendes, F., Balaram, M., et al., Accumulated lead exposure and risk of age-related cataract in men, *JAMA*, 292, 2750, 2004.
62. Hu, H., Watanabe, H., Payton, M., et al., The relationship between bone lead and hemoglobin, *JAMA*, 272, 1512, 1994.
63. Hu, H., Aro, A., Payton, M., et al., The relationship of bone and blood lead to hypertension. The Normative Aging Study, *JAMA*, 275, 1171, 1996.
64. Fukue, M., Nakahara, T., and Sarai, K., Hypoproteinemia related with chronic lithium therapy in two patients, *Jpn. J. Psychiatry Neurol.*, 44, 55, 1990.
65. Turner, S.T., Weidman, W.H., Michels, V.V., et al., Distribution of sodium-lithium countertransport and blood pressure in Caucasians five to eighty-nine years of age, *Hypertension*, 13, 378, 1989.
66. Pleban, P.A. and Pearson, K.H., Determination of manganese in whole blood and serum, *Clin. Chem.*, 25, 1915, 1979.

67. Schroeder, H.A. and Nason, A.P., Interactions of trace metals in rat tissues. Cadmium and nickel with zinc, chromium, copper, manganese, *J. Nutr.*, 104, 167, 1974.
68. Lisun-Lobanova, V.P., Trace elements (manganese, copper, and zinc), *Zdavookhr Beloruss*, 9, 49, 1963.
69. Hirsch-Kolb, H., Kolb, H.J., and Greenberg, D.M., Nuclear magnetic resonance studies of manganese binding of rat liver arginase, *J. Biol. Chem.*, 246, 395, 1971.
70. Haug, B.A., Schoenle, P.W., Karch, B.J., et al., Morvan's fibrillary chorea. A case with possible manganese poisoning, *Clin. Neurol. Neurosurg.*, 91, 53, 1989.
71. Hudnell, H.K., Effects from environmental Mn exposures: a review of the evidence from non-occupational exposure studies, *Neurotoxicology*, 20, 379, 1999.
72. Abumrad, N.N., Schneider, A.J., Steel, D., et al., Amino acid intolerance during prolonged total parenteral nutrition reversed by molybdate therapy, *Am. J. Clin. Nutr.*, 34, 2551, 1981.
73. Rajagopalan, K.V., Molybdenum: an essential trace element in human nutrition, *Ann. Rev. Nutr.*, 8, 401, 1988.
74. Kollmeier, H., Seemann, J.W., Rothe, G., et al., Age, sex, and region adjusted concentrations of chromium and nickel in lung tissue, *Br. J. Ind. Med.*, 47, 682, 1990.
75. Yarat, A., Nokay, S., Ipbuker, A., et al., Serum nickel levels of diabetic patients and healthy controls by ASS with a graphite furnace, *Biol. Trace Elem. Res.*, 35, 273, 1992.
76. Akslen, L.A., Myking, A.O., Morkve, O., et al., Increased content of chromium and nickel in lung tissues from patients with bronchial carcinoma, *Pathol. Res. Pract.*, 186, 717, 1990.
77. Burk, R.F., Biological activity of selenium, *Annu. Rev. Nutr.*, 3, 53, 1983.
78. Levander, O.A., A global view of human selenium nutrition, *Annu. Rev. Nutr.*, 7, 227, 1987.
79. Erden-Inal, M., Sunal, E., and Kanbak, G., Age-related changes in the glutathione redox system, *Cell Biochem. Funct.*, 20, 61, 2002.
80. Lane, H.W., Warren, D.C., Taylor, B.J., et al., Blood selenium and glutathione peroxidase levels and dietary selenium of free-living and institutionalized elderly subjects, *Proc. Soc. Exp. Biol. Med.*, 173, 87, 1983.
81. Miller, L., Mills, B.J., Blotcky, A.J., et al., Red blood cell and selenium concentrations as influenced by age and selected diseases, *J. Am. Coll. Nutr.*, 2, 331, 1983.
82. Feller, A.G., Rudman, D., Erve, P.R., et al., Subnormal concentrations of serum selenium and plasma carnitine in chronically tube-fed patients, *Am. J. Clin. Nutr.*, 45, 476, 1987.
83. Ganapathy, S.N. and Thimaya, S., in *Trace Elements in Human Health and Disease*, Vol. 3, Watson, R.R., Ed., CRC Press, Boca Raton, FL, 1985, p. 111.
84. Diplock, A.T., Trace elements in human health with special reference to selenium, *Am. J. Clin. Nutr.*, 45, 1313, 1987.
85. Levander, O.A. and Burk, R.F., Report on the 1986 A.S.P.E.N. Research Workshop on selenium in clinical nutrition, *J. Parenter. Enteral Nutr.*, 10, 545, 1986.
86. Fleming, C.R., Lie, J.T., McCall, J.T., et al., Selenium deficiency and fatal cardiomyopathy in a patient on home parenteral nutrition, *Gastroenterology*, 83, 689, 1982.
87. Johnson, R.A., Baker, S.S., Fallon, J.T., et al., An occidental case of cardiomyopathy and selenium deficiency, *N. Engl. J. Med.*, 304, 1210, 1981.
88. Thomson, C.D., McLachlan, S.K., Grant, A.M., et al., The effect of selenium on thyroid status in a population with marginal selenium and iodine status, *Br. J. Nutr.*, 94, 962, 2005.
89. Brown, M.R., Cohen, H.J., Lyons, J.M., et al., Proximal muscle weakness and selenium deficiency associated with long term parenteral nutrition, *Am. J. Clin. Nutr.*, 43, 549, 1986.

90. Kien, C.L. and Ganther, H.E., Manifestations of chronic selenium deficiency in a child receiving total parenteral nutrition, *Am. J. Clin. Nutr.*, 37, 319, 1983.
91. vanRij, A.M., Thomson, C.D., and McKenzie, J.M., et al. Selenium deficiency in total parenteral nutrition, *Am. J. Clin. Nutr.*, 32, 2076, 1979.
92. Morley, J.E., Mooradian, A.D., Silver, A.J., et al., Nutrition in the elderly, *Ann. Intern. Med.*, 109, 890, 1988.
93. Menkes, M.S., Comstock, G.W., Vuilleumier, J.P., et al., Serum beta-carotene, vitamins A and E, selenium, and the risk of lung cancer, *N. Engl. J. Med.*, 315, 1250, 1986.
94. Brown, M.R., Cohen, H.J., Lyons, J.M., et al., Proximal muscle weakness and selenium deficiency associated with long term parenteral nutrition, *Am. J. Clin. Nutr.*, 43, 549, 1986.
95. Borek, C., Ong, A., Mason, H., et al., Selenium and vitamin E inhibit radiogenic and chemically induced transformation *in vitro* via different mechanisms, *Proc. Natl. Acad. Sci. U.S.A.*, 83, 1490, 1986.
96. Dworkin, B.M., Rosenthal, W.S., Wormser, G.P., et al., Selenium deficiency in the acquired immunodeficiency syndrome, *J. Parenter. Enteral Nutr.*, 10, 405, 1986.
97. Burney, P.G., Comstock, G.W., and Morris, J.S., Serologic precursors of cancer: serum micronutrients and the subsequent risk of pancreatic cancer, *Am. J. Clin. Nutr.,* 49, 895–900, 1989.
98. Duffield-Lillico, A.J., Reid, M.E., Turnbull, B.W., et al., Baseline characteristics and the effect of selenium supplementation on cancer incidence in a randomized clinical trial: a summary report of the Nutritional Prevention of Cancer Trial, *Cancer Epidemiol. Biomarkers Prev.*, 11, 630, 2002.
99. Yu, S.Y., Zhu, Y.J., and Li, W.G., Protective role of selenium against hepatitis B virus and primary liver cancer in Qidong, *Biol. Trace Elem. Res.*, 56, 117, 1997.
100. Li, B., Taylor, P.R., Li, J.Y., et al., Linxian nutrition intervention trials. Design, methods, participant characteristics, and compliance, *Ann. Epidemiol.*, 3, 577, 1993.
101. Clark, L.C., The epidemiology of selenium and cancer, *Fed. Proc.*, 44, 2584, 1985.
102. Ray, A.L., Semba, R.D., Walston, J., et al., Low serum selenium and total carotenoids predict mortality among older women living in the community: the women's health and aging studies, *J. Nutr.*, 136, 172, 2006.
103. Akbaraly, N.T., Arnaud, J., Hininger-Favier, I., et al., Selenium and mortality in the elderly: results from the EVA study, *Clin. Chem.*, 51, 2117, 2005.
104. Walston, J., Xue, Q., Semba, R.D., et al., Serum antioxidants, inflammation, and total mortality in older women, *Am. J. Epidemiol.*, 163, 18, 2006.
105. Virtamo, J., Valkeila, E., Alfthan, G., et al., Serum selenium and the risk of coronary heart disease and stroke, *Am. J. Epidemiol.*, 122, 276, 1985.
106. Kok, F.J., deBruijn, A.M., Vermeeren, R., et al., Serum selenium, vitamin antioxidants, and cardiovascular mortality: a 9-year follow-up study in the Netherlands, *Am. J. Clin. Nutr.*, 45, 462, 1987.
107. Smith, D.K., Teague, R.J., McAdam, P.A., et al., Selenium status of malnourished hospitalized patients, *J. Am. Coll. Nutr.*, 5, 243, 1986.
108. Watson, R.R., Moriguchi, S., McRae, B., et al., Effects of selenium *in vitro* on human T-lymphocyte functions and K-562 tumor cell growth, *J. Leukoc. Biol.*, 39, 447, 1986.
109. Loeper, J. and Lemaire, A., Study of silicium in animal biology and during atheroma (English, original version French), *Presse Med.*, 74, 865, 1966.
110. Schwarz, K., New essential trace elements (Sn, V, F, Si): progress report and outlook, in *Trace Element Metabolism in Animals*, Vol. 2, Butterworths, London, 1975, p. 355.
111. Corrigan, F.M., Van Rhijn, A.G., Ijomah, G., et al., Tin and fatty acids in dementia, *Prostaglandins Leukot. Essent. Fatty Acids*, 43, 229, 1991.

112. Diamond, E.G., Caravaca, J., and Benchimol, A., Vanadium: excretion, toxicity, lipid effect in man, *Am. J. Clin. Nutr.*, 12, 49, 1963.
113. Hopkins, L.L., Jr., and Mohr, H.E., Proceedings: vanadium as an essential nutrient, *Fed. Proc.*, 33, 1773, 1974.
114. Curran, G.L., Azarnoff, D.L., and Bolinger, R.E., Effect of cholesterol synthesis inhibition in normocholesteremic young men, *J. Clin. Invest.*, 38, 1251, 1959.
115. Mukherjee, B., Patra, B., Mahapatra, S., et al., Vanadium: an element of atypical biological significance, *Toxicol. Lett.*, 150, 135, 2004.
116. Srivastava, A.K. and Mehdi, M.Z., Insulino-mimetic and anti-diabetic effects of vanadium compounds, *Diabet. Med.*, 22, 2, 2005.
117. Mocchegiani, E., Costarelli, L., Giacconi, R., et al., Nutrient-gene interaction in ageing and successful ageing. A single nutrient (zinc) and some target genes related to inflammatory/immune response, *Mech. Ageing. Dev.*, 127, 517, 2006.
118. Bunker, V.W., Hinks, L.J., Stansfield, M.F., et al., Metabolic balance studies for zinc and copper in housebound elderly people and the relationship between zinc balance and leukocyte zinc concentrations, *Am. J. Clin. Nutr.*, 46, 353, 1987.
119. Gibson, R.S., Martinez, O.B., and MacDonald, A.C., The zinc, copper, and selenium status of a selected sample of Canadian elderly women, *J. Gerontol.*, 40, 296, 1985.
120. Couzy, F., Kastenmayer, P., Mansourian, R., et al., Zinc absorption in healthy elderly humans and the effect of diet, *Am. J. Clin. Nutr.*, 58, 690, 1993.
121. Fosmire, G., Trace metal requirements, in *Geriatric Nutrition*, 3rd ed., Chernoff, R., Ed., Jones and Bartlett, Sudbury, 2006, p. 95.
122. Bogden, J.D., Influence of zinc on immunity in the elderly, *J. Nutr. Health Aging*, 8, 48, 2004.
123. Boukaiba, N., Flament, C., Acher, S., et al., A physiological amount of zinc supplementation: effects on nutritional, lipid, and thymic status in an elderly population, *Am. J. Clin. Nutr.*, 57, 566, 1993.
124. Prasad, A.S., Fitzgerald, J.T., Hess, J.W., et al., Zinc deficiency in elderly patients, *Nutrition*, 9, 218, 1993.
125. Langer, G., Schloemer, G., Knerr, A., et al., Nutritional interventions for preventing and treating pressure ulcers, *Cochrane Database Syst. Rev.*, 4, CD003216, 2003.
126. Evans, J.R., Antioxidant vitamin and mineral supplements for slowing the progression of age-related macular degeneration, *Cochrane Database Syst. Rev.*, 2, CD000254, 2006.
127. Religa, D., Strozyk, R.A., Cherny, I., et al., Elevated cortical zinc in Alzheimer disease, *Neurology*, 67, 69, 2006.
128. Mills, C.F., Dietary interactions involving the trace elements, *Annu. Rev. Nutr.*, 5, 173, 1985.
129. Prasad, A.S., Brewer, G.J., Schoomaker, E.B., et al., Hypocupremia induced by zinc therapy in adults, *JAMA*, 240, 2166, 1978.
130. Anonymous, Antioxidant status and neovascular age-related macular degeneration. Eye Disease Case-Control Study Group, *Arch Ophthalmol.*, 111, 104, 1993.

12 Nutritional Assessment in Older Persons

David R. Thomas, M.D.

CONTENTS

> Thousands of patients are annually starved in the midst of plenty.
>
> **—Florence Nightingale, 1859**

> Doctors and nurses frequently fail to recognize undernourishment because they are not trained to look for it.
>
> **—J.E. Lennard-Jones, 1992**

The nutritional status of older adults living at home is poor. On average, persons over the age of 70 years consume one third less calories than younger persons. Energy intakes of older men (40 to 74 years old) range from 2100 to 2300 calories/day compared to younger men (24 to 34 years old), who consume 2700 calories/day.[1] Ten percent of older men and twenty percent of older women have intakes of protein below the U.S. Recommended Daily Allowance (RDA), and one third consume fewer calories than the RDA. Fifty percent of older adults have intakes of minerals and vitamins less than the RDA, and ten to thirty percent have subnormal levels of minerals and vitamins.[2] Sixteen to eighteen percent of community-dwelling elderly persons consume less than 1000 kcal daily.[3]

Undernutrition reportedly occurs in 5 to 12% of community-dwelling older persons.[4–6] Up to 11% of adults attending a medical outpatient clinic are malnourished.[7] In higher-risk populations, such as sheltered housing, the proportion increases to 20%.[8] Thirty to forty percent of men and women over 75 are at least ten percent underweight. Acute illness is characterized by a spontaneous decrease in food intake,[9] a paradoxical response in the face of a need for increased nutrients during healing. A reduction in food intake accompanying acute illness occurs both before and during hospitalization. In the month before hospitalization, 65% of the males and 69% of the females had an insufficient energy intake, and undernutrition was present in 53% of males and 61% of females by the time of admission to the hospital.[10]

Inadequate intake of nutrients often continues during hospitalization. In 286 general medical subjects, 27% became malnourished during hospital admission. These subjects were more likely to consume less than 40% of prescribed food and were more likely to have lower Mini-Mental Status Examination scores, functional impairment, lower total lymphocyte counts, and lower serum albumin levels.[11] In hospitalized subjects, ranges of undernutrition prevalence of 32 to 50% have been reported.[12,13] Reasons for this high prevalence include poor recognition and monitoring of nutritional status[14–17] and forced inadequate intake of nutrients for days at a time.[18,19] In this setting, severity of illness and other factors limit the patient's ability to consume an adequate diet. When patients who had no current nutritional deficits and no predicted risk of developing deficits at hospital admission were followed, significant decreases in albumin, total lymphocyte count, triceps skinfold thickness, and mid-arm circumference occurred in all patients by 3 weeks. The only nutritional parameter remaining unchanged at 3 weeks was percent of ideal body weight.[20]

Over 90% of older persons admitted to a skilled care facility after hospitalization either have or are at high risk for undernutrition.[21] Among those patients newly admitted to a long-term-care setting, a point prevalence of 54% malnutrition was observed.[22] Prevalence rates for protein-energy malnutrition in nursing home residents range from 23 to 85%.[23,24] Variables widely associated with undernutrition, including body weight, mid-arm muscle circumference, and visceral protein levels are low in at least 50% of nursing home patients, suggesting widespread protein-energy malnutrition. Blood levels are frequently low for both water-soluble and fat-soluble vitamins.[25]

These data suggest that a large number of older adults are undernourished, with prevalence increasing to over half of older adults in selected populations.

12.1 CONSEQUENCES OF UNDERNUTRITION

Undernutrition clearly is associated with adverse health outcomes. Persons who are identified as undernourished have higher mortality, a higher rate of life-threatening complications, longer hospital stays, higher comorbidities, more infections, and oxidative stress leading potentially to degenerative disease than persons who are considered well nourished[26–28] (see Table 12.1).

Weight loss of more than 5% in women 60 to 74 years old has been associated with a two-fold increase in risk of disability over time, compared to women who did not lose weight.[29] This effect persists when adjusted for age, smoking, education,

TABLE 12.1
Association of Nutritional Parameters with Outcomes

Population	Measures	Results
Community-dwelling older persons[100,101]	BMI < 22	15% higher 1-year mortality and poorer functional status
Community-dwelling women 60 to 74 years old[102]	>5% loss of body weight	Two-fold increased risk of disability, adjusted for age, smoking, education, study duration, and health conditions
Homebound older adults[103]	Weight loss	76% increase in mortality, adjusted for initial BMI, smoking, health status, and functional status
Hospitalized patients[104]	BMI < 20 and decreased functional status	Higher in-hospital mortality
Hospitalized patients[105]	BMI < 15 percentile	Higher 180-day mortality, adjusted for recent weight loss, serum albumin, severity of illness score, and patient demographics
Hospitalized veterans[106]	>5% loss of body weight in the preceding 6 months	Higher life-threatening in-hospital complications
Hospitalized veterans[107]	BMI < 20 and weight as a percentage of usual weight ≤85%	Higher 1-year mortality, adjusted for illness severity and functional status
Hospitalized patients[108]	Serum albumin, % ideal body weight, dressing, cardiac arrhythmia	Higher 1-year posthospital mortality
Hospitalized patients[109]	Serum albumin < 35 g/l	14% mortality vs. 4% among patients with albumin > 35 g/l
Rehabilitation patients[110]	Serum albumin, BMI, blood urea nitrogen > 30 mg/l, Katz Index of Activities of Daily Living score, amount of weight loss in the year prior to admission	Higher life-threatening complications
Rehabilitation patients[111]	Albumin < 30 g/l or BMI < 19	Higher mortality at 4.5 years
Nursing home residents[112]	>10% loss of body weight in preceding 6 months	Higher mortality in next 6 months
Nursing home residents[113]	5% loss of body weight	4.6 times higher mortality in 1 year
Nursing home residents[114]	5% loss of body weight in 1 month	10 times higher mortality

Note: BMI = body mass index (weight divided by height squared).

study duration, and health conditions. Age and gender-adjusted body mass index (BMI) below 19 in men and below 19.4 in women is associated with higher mortality.[20] The increase in mortality is linear—the lower the BMI, the greater the risk. Increased risk of death has been shown to begin at a body mass index of <23.5 in men and <22.0 in women.[30]

12.2 CAUSES OF INVOLUNTARY WEIGHT LOSS IN OLDER ADULTS

Body composition is mediated by three interactive control mechanisms. Minute-to-minute changes reflect the metabolic state. Hormonal regulators, such as insulin and glucagon, control day-to-day changes. Other hormones, such as estrogens and androgens, growth hormone, prolactin, thyroid hormones, catecholamines, and corticosteroids, control life cycle-related body composition. Finally, immunological mediators, such as interleukin-1, tumor necrosis factor, and interleukin-6, control a number of other metabolic factors, such as muscle regeneration, body fat, and nitrogen regulation.

Involuntary weight loss in older adults usually occurs for one of three reasons: starvation, sarcopenia, or cachexia. Starvation results from failure to consume adequate protein and energy. The reasons for starvation include lack of access to food, inability to consume adequate calories because of mechanical limitations, such as inability to swallow, or inability to absorb ingested nutrients.

The drive to find food, designated by the term *hunger*, is essential in all species. Hunger is controlled by chemical mediators, signaling when to stop eating (*satiation*) and when to resume searching for food (*satiety*), which defines the interval between meals. *Appetite*, the enjoyment of food for itself, rather than for physiological need, is conditioned by a number of social, cultural, and psychological factors, as well as by disease states. Even in the presence of adequate food, older adults often fail to consume adequate protein and energy. Accumulating evidence points toward *anorexia*, the decline in appetite, as a major contributor to weight loss and undernutrition of older persons.[31]

Sarcopenia is defined as the loss of muscle protein mass, muscle function, and muscle quality that accompanies advancing age.[32] The term *sarcopenia* is most commonly used to refer to body composition changes in elderly persons, but can also occur in patients who have repeatedly tried to lose weight by dieting, patients with growth hormone deficiency, or patients with very limited physical activity.

Observations over considerable time have demonstrated that dynamic, static, and isokinetic muscle strength decreases with age.[33] This decline in muscle mass occurs in both sedentary and active aging adults.[34] Sarcopenia, a term first coined in 1988, is operationally defined as a lean body mass more than two standard deviations below the young normal mean.[35] This reduction in muscle mass and strength that occurs with aging may be independent of total body mass.[36] Although the loss of skeletal muscle mass generally results in weight loss, this loss of muscle mass may occur even in obese subjects, making the diagnosis inapparent. Whether or not body mass measured by body weight declines, sarcopenia is associated with about a four-fold increase in the risk of disability in at least three of the Instrumental Activities of Daily Living, a two- to three-fold increase in the risk of having a balance disorder, and about a two-fold greater likelihood for men of having to use a cane or walker.[37]

Cachexia is a syndrome of muscle wasting and weight loss, resembling marasmus. A number of chronic disease conditions have been associated with muscle wasting and weight loss, including cancer,[38] end-stage renal disease,[39] chronic pulmonary disease,[40] congestive heart failure,[41] rheumatoid arthritis,[42] and AIDS.[43] A common feature of cachexia is the presence of proinflammatory cytokines.

Disease-associated cytokines directly result in feeding suppression and lower intake of nutrients. Interleukin-1 beta and tumor necrosis factor act on the glucose-sensitive neurons in the ventromedial hypothalamic nucleus (a satiety site) and the lateral hypothalamic area (a hunger site).[44] Thus, increased cytokine levels commonly associated with disease conditions characterized by cachexia may play a role in appetite suppression, mortality, and weight loss. Cytokine-induced anorexia is the most common cause of poor caloric intake observed in the acute care setting,[45] and affects community-dwelling older persons as well.

12.3 ASSESSING NUTRITIONAL STATUS

Historically, undernutrition has been divided into clinical syndromes of kwashiokor, marasmus, or a mixture of both. Kwashiorkor, first defined in children, occurs when carbohydrate is the major dietary energy source and protein is relatively absent from the diet for a prolonged period. A key component of the diagnosis of kwashiorkor includes hypoalbuminemia. Other clinical features include edema, ascites, dermatitis, thin brittle hair, hepatomegaly, and muscle wasting.[46] Adipose tissue remains preserved. Marasmus, on the other hand, is a chronic deprivation of adequate dietary energy characterized by extreme weight loss and muscle wasting. Marasmius results in stunted growth in children, loss of adipose tissue, and generalized wasting of lean body mass without edema.[47] Both of these conditions directly result from inadequate food intake and are reversible by refeeding.

Since serum albumin, along with other hepatic proteins such as transthyretin and transferrin, and body weight are easily measured, the paradigm was applied to adults in hospital, institutional, and community settings. Hypoalbuminemia, or other abnormalities, such as total lymphocyte count, were judged to result from a kwashiokor-like nutritional deficiency in protein intake. Weight loss, muscle wasting, and low anthropometric measures compared to population normals were attributed to a deficient energy intake. Using this diagnostic paradigm, the vast majority of patients in the American healthcare system are undernourished, with estimates ranging up to 70% of hospitalized adults and up to 85% of long-term-care residents.[48,49]

12.3.1 Risk Assessment Tools

Generally, nutritional problems are identified using various biochemical or anthropometric parameters, including body weight,[50] serum concentrations of proteins produced by the liver,[51] mid-arm circumference or triceps skinfold thickness,[52–54] body mass index,[55] grip strength,[56] anergy,[57] and immunologic functions.[58] No single measurement is highly sensitive and specific in identifying malnutrition.[59]

Several indices, including both biochemical and anthropometric parameters, have been suggested to define undernutrition.[60–63] The characteristics of a successful nutritional tool include (1) a reliable scale, (2) a clear definition of thresholds, (3) compatibility with skills of a generalist assessor, (4) minimal bias due to data collector, (5) acceptability to patients, and (6) relatively inexpensive in time and energy costs.

Currently available instruments include two types. The first aims at identifying persons at risk for malnutrition but is not used to diagnose clinical undernutrition. The Nutritional Screening Initiative serves as an example of these instruments.[64,65] Other screening tools for nutrition risk include the Meals on Wheels (Table 12.2) and SCALES (Table 12.3) acrostics.

The second type of instrument has been developed to evaluate nutritional risks in hospitalized subjects with an eye toward predicting future complications. The Subjective Global Assessment (SGA)[66,67] and the Prognostic Nutritional Index (PNI)[68] are examples of these instruments. The Mini-Nutritional Assessment (MNA) was developed to assess undernutrition in elderly populations.[69]

TABLE 12.2
Meals on Wheels Mnemonic for Undernutrition

Medications
Emotional problem (depression)
Anorexia, elder abuse, alcoholism
Late-life paranoia
Swallowing disorders
Oral factors
No money or nosocomical infections, e.g., tuberculosis, *C. difficile*, *H. pylori*
Wandering (dementia)
Hyperthyroidism, hyperparathyroidism, hypoadrenalism, hypertension (pheochromocytoma)
Enteric problems (malabsorption)
Eating problems (inability to self-feed)
Low-salt, low-cholesterol diet
Social problems and stones

TABLE 12.3
SCALES: An Instrument for the Detection of Malnutrition Risk

Sadness (Geriatric Depression Scale)
Cholesterol < 160 mg/dl
Albumin < 3.5 mg/dl
Loss of 5% of body weight
Eating problems (physical or cognitive)
Shopping/food preparation

12.3.2 Subjective Global Assessment

The Subjective Global Assessment was developed to assess risk of hospital complications in patients undergoing gastrointestinal surgery.[70,71] The instrument contains four elements of history and three elements of examination (Figure 12.1). No laboratory

		S GA Score		
Part 1: Medical History		A	B	C
1. Weight Change				
A. Overall change in past 6 months	_____kilograms			
B. Percent change	gain or less than 5% loss			
	5-10% loss			
	greater than 10% loss			
2. Dietary intake				
A. Overall change	no change			
	change			
C. Type of change	suboptimal solid diet			
	full liquid diet			
	hypocaloric liquid			
	starvation			
3. Gastrointestinal Symptoms (persisting for >2 weeks)	none			
	nausea			
	vomiting			
	diarrhea			
	anorexia			
4. Functional Impairment (nutritionally related)				
Overall impairment	none			
	moderate			
	severe			

Part 2: Physical Examination	SGA Score			
5. Evidence of	Normal	Mild	Moderate	Severe
Loss of subcutaneous fat				
Muscle wasting				
Edema				
Ascites (hemo only)				

Part 3. SGA Rating (Check one)		
A__ Well Nourished	B__ Mildly-Moderately Malnourished	C__Severely Malnourished

FIGURE 12.1 Parameters used in subjective global assessment.

data are required. Subjects are grouped into three classes: class A, well nourished; class B, moderately (or suspected of being) malnourished; and class C, severely malnourished. No numerical score exists for combining these data. The elements are combined subjectively into an overall global assessment.

The Subjective Global Assessment is useful in predicting surgical complications. In 102 hospitalized subjects, 42% were classified as well nourished, 17% as mildly to moderately malnourished, and 41% as severely malnourished. The likelihood ratios for major complications, septic complications, and pneumonia in the three groups were 0.53 in the well nourished, 0.69 in the mildly to moderately malnourished, and 1.8 in the severely malnourished.[72] Using the Subjective Global Assessment, subjects with severe malnutrition (class C) had a higher rate of major infectious complications and noninfectious complications in the Veterans Affairs Perioperative Total Parenteral Nutrition trial.[73]

12.3.3 Mini-Nutritional Assessment

The Mini-Nutritional Assessment (MNA) consists of several anthropomorphic measurements, six global assessment questions, eight dietary questions, and subjective perception of health questions (Figure 12.2). The total score sums to 30 points. The MNA was developed and validated in elderly, long-term-care populations. In the development phase, determination of malnutrition by the two clinical experts was compared to determination of malnutrition by a battery of anthropomorphical and biochemical indices. A total of 125 hospitalized subjects were evaluated. Independent variables included energy intake, protein intake, lipid intake, carbohydrate intake, transferrin, albumin, alpha1 acid glycoprotein, transthyretin, ceruloplasmin, retinol binding protein, C-reactive protein, gamma-glutamyl transferase, total protein, cholesterol, triglycerides, folate, vitamins B12, A, and E, zinc, copper, weight, body mass index, calf circumference, mid-arm circumference, and triceps and subscapular skinfolds. Discriminate analysis was used to test the MNA compared to the independently obtained clinical diagnosis. The analysis demonstrated that clinical status misclassified only 3 subjects of 125. Thus, determination of nutritional status clinically compares favorably with determination of nutritional status by a battery of anthropomorphical and biochemical indices.

Two additional cross-validation studies were used to confirm the instrument. In the first, 90 of 115 (78%) subjects were correctly classified. In the second, 100 of 139 (72%) subjects were correctly classified.[74] These studies indicate that approximately 75% of elderly subjects can be correctly classified using the MNA without using any biochemical parameters. However, 25 to 30% of subjects fall into an intermediate zone between well nourished and undernourished. These subjects are classified as borderline or at risk of undernutrition and require further assessment by biochemical markers or additional clinical evaluation. Using the validated cutoffs of adequate nutritional status (MNA score ≥ 24), at risk for undernutrition (MNA score = 17 to 23.5), and undernutrition (MNA score < 17), the sensitivity is 96%; specificity, 98%; and positive predictive value, 97% for undernutrition.[75]

NESTLÉ NUTRITION SERVICES

Nestlé

Mini Nutritional Assessment
MNA®

Last name: First name: Sex: Date:

Age: Weight, kg: Height, cm: I.D. Number:

Complete the screen by filling in the boxes with the appropriate numbers.
Add the numbers for the screen. If score is 11 or less, continue with the assessment to gain a Malnutrition Indicator Score.

Screening

A Has food intake declined over the past 3 months due to loss of appetite, digestive problems, chewing or swallowing difficulties?
0 = severe loss of appetite
1 = moderate loss of appetite
2 = no loss of appetite ☐

B Weight loss during last months
0 = weight loss greater than 3 kg (6.6 lbs)
1 = does not know
2 = weight loss between 1 and 3 kg (2.2 and 6.6 lbs)
3 = no weight loss ☐

C Mobility
0 = bed or chair bound
1 = able to get out of bed/chair but does not go out
2 = goes out ☐

D Has suffered psychological stress or acute disease in the past 3 months
0 = yes 2 = no ☐

E Neuropsychological problems
0 = severe dementia or depression
1 = mild dementia
2 = no psychological problems ☐

F Body Mass Index (BMI) (weight in kg) / (height in m)²
0 = BMI less than 19
1 = BMI 19 to less than 21
2 = BMI 21 to less than 23
3 = BMI 23 or greater ☐

Screening score (subtotal max. 14 points) ☐☐
12 points or greater Normal – not at risk – no need to complete assessment
11 points or below Possible malnutrition – continue assessment

Assessment

G Lives independently (not in a nursing home or hospital)
0 = no 1 = yes ☐

H Takes more than 3 prescription drugs per day
0 = yes 1 = no ☐

I Pressure sores or skin ulcers
0 = yes 1 = no ☐

J How many full meals does the patient eat daily?
0 = 1 meal
1 = 2 meals
2 = 3 meals ☐

K Selected consumption markers for protein intake
- At least one serving of dairy products (milk, cheese, yogurt) per day? yes ☐ no ☐
- Two or more servings of legumes or eggs per week? yes ☐ no ☐
- Meat, fish or poultry every day yes ☐ no ☐

0.0 = if 0 or 1 yes
0.5 = if 2 yes
1.0 = if 3 yes ☐.☐

L Consumes two or more servings of fruits or vegetables per day?
0 = no 1 = yes ☐

M How much fluid (water, juice, coffee, tea, milk...) is consumed per day?
0.0 = less than 3 cups
0.5 = 3 to 5 cups
1.0 = more than 5 cups ☐.☐

N Mode of feeding
0 = unable to eat without assistance
1 = self-fed with some difficulty
2 = self-fed without any problem ☐

O Self view of nutritional status
0 = view self as being malnourished
1 = is uncertain of nutritional state
2 = views self as having no nutritional problem ☐

P In comparison with other people of the same age, how does the patient consider his/her health status?
0.0 = not as good
0.5 = does not know
1.0 = as good
2.0 = better ☐.☐

Q Mid-arm circumference (MAC) in cm
0.0 = MAC less than 21
0.5 = MAC 21 to 22
1.0 = MAC 22 or greater ☐.☐

R Calf circumference (CC) in cm
0 = CC less than 31 1 = CC 31 or greater ☐

Assessment (max. 16 points) ☐☐.☐

Screening score ☐☐

Total Assessment (max. 30 points) ☐☐.☐

Malnutrition Indicator Score
17 to 23.5 points at risk of malnutrition ☐
Less than 17 points malnourished ☐

Ref.: Guigoz Y, Vellas B and Garry PJ. 1994. Mini Nutritional Assessment: A practical assessment tool for grading the nutritional state of elderly patients. *Facts and Research in Gerontology*. Supplement #2:15-59.
Rubenstein LZ, Harker J, Guigoz Y and Vellas B. Comprehensive Geriatric Assessment (CGA) and the MNA: An Overview of CGA, Nutritional Assessment, and Development of a Shortened Version of the MNA. In: "Mini Nutritional Assessment (MNA): Research and Practice in the Elderly". Vellas B, Garry PJ and Guigoz Y., editors. Nestlé Nutrition Workshop Series. Clinical & Performance Programme, vol. 1. Karger, Bâle, in press.

FIGURE 12.2 Mini-Nutritional Assessment.

12.3.4 Simplified Nutritional Appetite Questionnaire (SNAQ)

Appetite is a key component of involuntary weight loss. Defects in appetite often precede the onset of weight loss and complicate treatment with hypercaloric supplements or feeding. A tool for the assessment of appetite has been developed and validated (Table 12.4).[76] The SNAQ identifies older subjects with a decrease in

TABLE 12.4
Simplified Nutritional Appetite Questionnaire (SNAQ)

Question	1	2	3	4	5	Score
1. My appetite is	Very poor	Poor	Average	Good	Very good	
2. When I eat	I feel full after eating only a few mouthfuls	I feel full after eating about a third of my meal	I feel full after eating over half of a meal	I feel full after eating most of the meal	I hardly ever feel full	
3. Food tastes	Very bad	Bad	Average	Good	Very good	
4. Normally I eat	Less than one meal a day	One meal a day	Two meals a day	Three meals a day	More than three meals a day	
Total						

Source: Wilson, M.M. et al., *Am. J. Clin. Nutr.*, 82, 1074–1081, 2005. With permission.

appetite and prospectively predicts weight loss over the next 6 months. The sensitivity and specificity were 81 and 76% for predicting a 5% weight loss and 88 and 84% for a 10% weight loss. Early identification of older persons with abnormalities in appetite who are at high risk for ensuing weight loss with a four-question instrument may allow prompt intervention to ameliorate nutritional problems.

12.3.5 Comparison of Risk Assessment Instruments

Serum albumin and the Subjective Global Assessment are both strongly predictive of prognosis, but it is not clear whether they measure similar or different clinical information. Discordance between albumin and the SGA is common. In a study of hospitalized subjects older than 70 years, 38% of patients with albumin levels of 4.0 g/dl or higher were classified as moderately malnourished on the Subjective Global Assessment, whereas 28% of patients with albumin levels lower than 3.0 g/dl were classified as well nourished. No single albumin level was associated with acceptable sensitivity and specificity as a predictor of Subjective Global Assessment classification. The ability of either measure to predict the other measure was only marginally better than chance (0.58). Thus, both measures are limited as markers of nutritional status and may reflect fundamentally different clinical processes.[77]

The Determine checklist, proposed by the Nutrition Screening Initiative (NSI), has been compared to the Mini-Nutritional Assessment using retrospective data from the Survey in Europe of Nutrition in the Elderly, a Concerted Action (SENECA). Based on variables collected in 1988, 19.3% of subjects were classified at high nutritional risk, 51% were considered at moderate risk, and 29.7% were within the normal range using the NSI. Using the MNA, 78.4% of subjects were classified as well nourished compared to 21.6% who were at nutritional risk. Using mortality rates completed in 1993, subjects with a normal baseline score had a lower mortality risk (0.35; 95% confidence interval (CI), 0.18 and 0.66) than subjects with an abnormal MNA score. In contrast, the NSI was not a predictor of subsequent mortality. The subjects judged to be at risk by the MNA had more frequent acute illness ($p < 0.05$), need for more assistance, and more weight loss during the period 1988 to 1995.[78]

Using the 1993 SENECA data, the MNA was compared to the NSI in 1161 subjects in another study. The MNA classified 55% of subjects as normal, 44% as at risk of malnutrition, and 1% as malnourished. The NSI differed considerably, finding only 11% classified as normal, 41% as moderate risk, and 48% as high nutritional risk. The MNA was found to be 96% sensitive and 60% specific for body weight loss. The NSI was 75% sensitive and 54% specific for body weight loss. Neither instrument correlated well with the Quick Nutritional Index or with biochemical changes.[79] Thus, comparison between instruments developed to date suggests that the MNA is a superior instrument.

It is critical to understand that these nutritional risk assessment instruments are predictive of only hospital complications or future mortality. When used in this way, the instruments are highly predictive of persons at risk for these outcomes. However, it is not clear that these instruments are measuring true nutritional status or simply sicker individuals. While these instruments indicate that they measure undernutrition or nutritional risk, it is not clear that they do so. These instruments do not indicate which persons will respond to nutritional interventions. The results of most clinical trials of refeeding or energy-dense nutritional supplements have not shown that the measured adverse outcomes can be corrected.

12.3.6 Diagnosing Undernutrition

Undernutrition is a state induced by nutrient deficiency that may be improved solely by administration of nutrients.[80] By this definition, provision of adequate protein and energy sources should reverse the clinical presentation and correct the problem. However, a large number of patients who appear to be undernourished (that is, who exhibit the phenotype of kwashiokor or marasmus) fail to respond to refeeding in published nutritional intervention trials.

A meta-analysis of 55 randomized controlled trials with 9187 older participants evaluated the effect of nutritional supplements across a variety of healthcare settings.[81] Nutritional supplementation produced a small but significant percentage weight gain of 1.8% (95% CI, 1.1 to 2.3) in hospitalized subjects. Percentage weight change for subjects in long-term-care settings was 2.5% (95% CI, 1.7 to 3.2), and 2.3% (95% CI, 1.7 to 2.7) for older people living at home. Mortality in the supplemented group was reduced, although the reduction was only borderline statistically significant (odds ratio, 0.9; 95% CI, 0.7 to 1.0).

For short-term hospital stays, mortality was not reduced (odds ratio, 0.9; 95% CI, 0.7 to 1.0). However, a reduction in mortality was seen in trials that only included undernourished subjects (odds ratio, 0.7; 95% CI, 0.5 to 0.9). A reduction in mortality was not seen in supplemented residents in long-term-care settings (odds ratio, 0.7; 95% CI, 0.4 to 1.0) or for people living at home (odds ratio, 1.1; 95% CI, 0.6 to

2.0). Hospitalized patients who were given supplements had a statistically significant decrease in complications (odds ratio, 0.7; 95% CI, 0.5 to 0.9), but supplementation did not have an effect on morbidity or complications in residents in long-term care (odds ratio, 0.9; 95% CI, 0.6 to 1.5) or at home (odds ratio, 1.0; 95% CI, 0.6 to 1.6).

Oral nutritional supplements have been evaluated in subjects with Alzheimer's type dementia. In a prospective controlled study, 91 subjects older than 65 years with dementia of the Alzheimer's type who were at risk of undernutrition by the Mini-Nutritional Assessment instrument and who had lost more than 5% of their body weight were randomized to receive either an oral supplement or usual care. Despite a significant improvement in dietary intakes and body weight in the intervention group, no significant changes were found for biological markers of nutrition, functional status, or cognitive function.[82] Assistance with eating by trained personnel over a mean of 16 weeks did not improve markers of nutritional status, Barthel score, grip strength, length of stay, or mortality in acutely ill older adults.[83]

Enteral nutritional support in persons diagnosed with undernutrition has shown only modest benefits.[84] In patients who cannot eat for more than 10 to 14 days, nutritional support is indicated to prevent morbidity and mortality from starvation. In patients with major trauma and in severely malnourished patients undergoing major elective surgery, the reduction in major complications has been demonstrated. However, the use of nutritional support is not associated with a reduction in the length of the hospital stay.[85] Furthermore, there has been little improvement in specific disease states, such as cancer, AIDS, or hemodialysis patients.[86]

Nutritional parameters were compared among 44 hospitalized, bed-confined subjects over age 65 years, with and without tube feeding, and 41 age-matched free-eating elders in a nursing home. Tube-fed subjects received 26 kcal/kg/day and 1.0 g of protein/day, an amount calculated to equal the predicted total energy expenditure. However, the incidence of protein energy undernutrition, as evidenced by decreased arm muscle circumference (<80% of normal) and hypoalbuminemia (<35 g/l), was significantly higher in the patients with tube feeding than in the orally fed older persons. Thus, undernutrition was still demonstrable in patients fed energy and protein that approximated calculated predicted values.[87] Survival for a period of 24 months was not different in nursing home residents with progressive dementia compared to residents who were and were not enterally fed.[88]

Using the definition of undernutrition as state reversible by providing adequate energy and protein, these subjects are not undernourished. This suggests that a proportion of persons who are labeled as undernourished may in fact have another clinical syndrome.

12.4 TOWARD A NEW PARADIGM

A developing understanding of the acute phase response to illness and the role of cytokines in the pathophysiology of chronic illness has challenged the current diagnostic paradigm of undernutrition. The effect of acute and chronic cytokine-mediated conditions on hepatic proteins, muscle wasting, and weight loss has led to considerable confusion about the diagnosis of undernutrition.

The major hepatic proteins, albumin, transthyretin (prealbumin), and transferrin, as well as a large number of other less well known proteins, act as acute phase reactants. These acute phase biochemical markers are not specific for nutritional status. Serum levels of these proteins fall quickly in response to infection, injury, or trauma and slowly increase with recovery from the same conditions.[89] For example, hypoalbuminemia occurs in disease states such as hepatic disease, renal disease, congestive heart failure,[90] and stress,[91] and after 8 hours of bed rest.[92] This acute phase decrease in serum hepatic protein levels occurs despite adequate intake of nutrients prior to the illness or injury.[93] Moreover, the acute phase serum hepatic protein levels do not increase in response to the provision of protein and energy.[94] Other nutritional markers, such as the total lymphocyte count, correlate poorly with both the body cell mass and the nutritional state measured by the Nae-to-Ke ratio, producing a false-positive rate of 34% and a false-negative rate of 50% for diagnosing undernutrition.[95]

In contrast to cytokine-mediated disease states, few changes occur in biochemical markers in simple starvation. Serum albumin remains normal in both short-term and long-term fasting.[96] In fact, after 9 weeks on a diet of about half of the normal dietary intake of protein, serum albumin remained normal despite changes in lean body mass and immune status.[97] Serum albumin levels in anorexia nervosa, a condition of chronic energy deficiency, remain normal and serum cholesterol levels increase in one third of anorexia patients. However, chronic inadequate intake of protein (kwashiorkor) does lead to a decline in serum albumin levels, although much later in the course of starvation.

It is likely that the acute phase response and chronic cachexia are responsible for the association of adverse mortality and morbidity outcomes reported in clinical studies, rather than undernutrition per se. Inclusion of patients with cachexia may explain the inconsistent effect of hypercaloric feeding on nutritional outcome measures in clinical trials. Indeed, in several clinical trials, hypercaloric feeding in acute illness has been associated with an increase in morbidity and mortality.[98]

Nutritional assessment, particularly if it encompasses or focuses on physiological function, may be an overall marker of illness that is not caused solely by inadequate intake or reversed by nutritional supplementation. This may explain why the clinical trials of total parenteral nutrition in a variety of clinical circumstances have in some cases produced disappointing results in improving outcomes.[99]

A summary of the differentiation of weight loss is shown in Figure 12.3. Table 12.5 shows the differential diagnosis of starvation and cachexia.

12.5 SUMMARY AND CONCLUSIONS

It is imperative that we revise our paradigm thinking about undernutrition to distinguish starvation, which is responsive to refeeding, from cachexia, which is resistent to refeeding. Nutrition should be provided to every person, with the expectation that

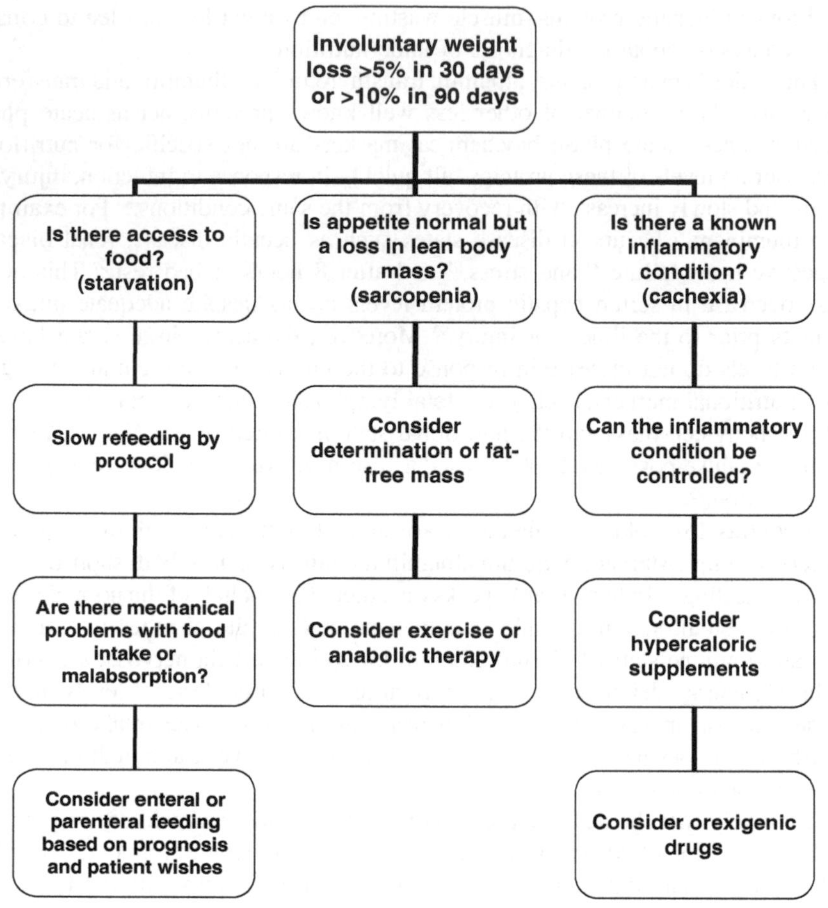

FIGURE 12.3 Approach to nutritional assessment.

TABLE 12.5
Distinguishing Starvation from Cachexia

	Starvation	Cachexia
Appetite	Suppressed in late phase	Suppressed in early phase
Body mass index	Not predictive of mortality	Predictive of mortality
Serum albumin	Low in late phase	Low in early phase
Transthyretin	Low in late phase	Low in early phase
Transferrin	Low	Low
Retinol binding protein	Low	Low
Cholesterol	May remain normal	Low
Total lymphocyte count	Low, responds to refeeding	Low, unresponsive to refeeding
C-reactive protein	Little data	Elevated
Inflammatory disease	Usually not present	Present
Response to refeeding	Reversible	Resistant

starvation will respond to nutrition but conditions associated with cachexia may not. Labeling the acute phase response and chronic cachexia under the umbrella of an outdated undernutrition paradigm can lead to inappropriate medical therapy. Failure to distinguish starvation from cachexia can result in a failure to address the underlying pathophysiology, expose patients to unnecessary risks, or result in failure to improve the condition. In patients with medical conditions known to be associated with cachexia or cytokine induction, a diagnosis of marasmus should be made only after thoughtful deliberation. Further research into whether anti-inflammatory or anticytokine interventions may impact appetite, increase food intake, or reverse effects of cachexia is essential.

REFERENCES

1. McGandy RB, Barrows CH Jr, Spanias A, Meredity A, Stone JL, Norris AH. Nutrient intake and energy expenditure in men of different ages. *J Gerontol* 1966;21:581–587.
2. Ritchie CR, Thomas DR. Aging. In *Handbook of Clinical Nutrition*, 3rd ed Heimburger DC, Weinsier RL, Eds. Mosby, St. Louis, 1997.
3. Abraham S, Carroll MD, Dresser CM, et al. *Dietary Intake of Persons 1–74 Years of Age in the United States.* Advance Data from Vital and Health Statistics of the National Center for Health Statistics No. G, Rockville, MD, Public Health Service, March 30, 1977.
4. Silver AJ. Malnutrition. In *Geriatrics Review Syllabus. A Core Curriculum in Geriatric Medicine*, Book 1, *Syllabus and Questions*, Beck JC, Ed. American Geriatrics Society, New York, 1991.
5. McCormack P. Undernutrition in the elderly population living at home in the community: a review of the literature. *J Adv Nurs* 1997;26:856–863.
6. Guigoz Y, Vellas BJ. Malnutrition in the elderly: the Mini Nutritional Assessment (MNA). *Ther Umschcriffen* 1997;54:345–350.
7. Wilson MM, Vaswani S, Liu D, Morley JE, Miller DK. Prevalence and causes of undernutrition in medical outpatients. *Am J Med* 1998;104;56–63.
8. Irving GF, Olsson BA, Cederholm T. Nutritional and cognitive status in elderly subjects living in service flats, and the effect of nutrition education on personnel. *Gerontology* 1999;45:187–194.
9. Plata-Salaman CR. Anorexia during acute and chronic disease. *Nutrition* 1996;12:69–76.
10. Mowe M, Bohmer T, Kindt E. Reduced nutritional status in an elderly population (> 70 y) is probable before disease and possibly contributes to the development of disease. *Am J Clin Nutr* 1994;59:317–324.
11. Incalzi RA, Gemma A, Capparella O, Cipriani L, Landi F, Carbonin P. Energy intake and in-hospital starvation. A clinically relevant relationship. *Arch Intern Med* 1996;156:425–429.
12. Willard MD, Gilsdorf RB, Price RA. Protein-calorie malnutrition in a community hospital. *JAMA* 1980;243:1720–1722.
13. Bistrian BR, Blackburn GL, Vitale J, Cochran D, Naylor J. Prevalence of malnutrition in general medical patients. *JAMA* 1976;235:1567–1570.
14. Prevost EA, Butterworth CE. Nutritional care of hospitalized patients. *Am J Clin Nutr* 1974;27:432.

15. Sullivan DH, Moriarty MS, Chernoff R, et al. Patterns of care: an analysis of the quality of nutritional care routinely provided to elderly hospitalized veterans. *J Parent Enteral Nutr* 1989;13:249–254.
16. McNab H, Restivo R, Ber L, et al. Dietetic quality assurance practices in Chicago area hospitals. *J Am Diet Assoc* 1987;85:635–637.
17. Kamath SK, Lawler M, Smith AE, et al. Hospital malnutrtion: a 33-hospital screening study. *J Am Diet Assoc* 1986;86:203–206.
18. Tobias AL, Van Itallie TB. Nutritional problems of hospitalized patients. *J Am Diet Assoc* 1977;71:253–257.
19. Riffer J. Malnourished patients feeding rising costs. *Hospitals* 1986;60:86.
20. Pinchcofsky GD, Kaminski MV Jr. Increasing malnutrition during hospitalization: documentation by a nutritional screening program. *J Am Coll Nutr* 1985;4:471–479.
21. Thomas DR, Zdrowski CD, Wilson MM, Conright KC, Lewis C, Tariq S, Morley JE. Malnutrition in subacute care. *Am J Clin Nutr* 2002;75:308–313.
22. Thomas DR, Verdery RB, Gardner L, Kant AK, Lindsay J. A prospective study of outcome from protein-energy malnutrition in nursing home residents. *J Parent Enteral Nutr* 1991;15:400–404.
23. Sliver AJ, Morley JE, Strome LS, Jones D, Vickers L. Nutritional status in an academic nursing home. *J Am Geriatr Soc* 1988;36:487–491.
24. Shaver HJ, Loper JA, Lutes RA. Nutritional status of nursing home patients. *J Parent Enteral Nutrition* 1980;4:367–370.
25. Drinka PJ, Goodwin JS. Prevalence and consequences of vitamin deficiency in the nursing home: a critical review. *J Am Geriatr Soc* 1991;39:1008–1017.
26. Young ME. Malnutrition and wound healing. *Heart Lung* 1988;17:60–67.
27. Dempsey DT, Mullen JL, Buzby GP. The link between nutritional status and clinical outcome: can nutritional intervention modify it? *Am J Clin Nutr* 1988;47(Suppl):352–356.
28. Detsky AS, Baker JP, O'Rourke K, et al. Predicting nutrition-associated complications for patients undergoing gastrointestinal surgery. *J Parent Enteral Nutrition* 1987;11:440–446.
29. Launer LJ, Harris LT, Rumpel C, Madans J. Body mass index, weight change and risk of mobility disability in middle-aged and older women. *JAMA* 1994;271:1083–1098.
30. Calle EE, Thun MJ, Petrilli JM, Rodriguez C, Heath CW Jr. Body-mass index and mortality in a prospective cohort of U.S. adults. *N Engl J Med* 1999;341:1097–1105.
31. Morley JE. Decreased food intake with aging. *J Gerontol A Biol Sci Med Sci* 2001;56:81–88.
32. Zinna EM, et al. Exercise treatment to counteract protein wasting of chronic diseases. *Curr Opin Clin Nutr Metab Care* 2003;61:87.
33. Aniansson A, Sperling L, Rundgren A, Lehnberg E. Muscle function in 75-year old men and women: A longitudinal study. *Scand J Rehab Med* 1983;9:92–102.
34. Davies C, Thomas D, White M. Mechanical properties of young and elderly human muscle. *Acta Med Scand Suppl* 1985;711:216–219.
35. Baumgartner RN, Waters DL, Gallagher D, Morley JE, Garry PJ. Predictors of skeletal muscle mass in elderly men and women. *Mech Ageing Dev* 1999;107(2):123–126.
36. Lauretani F, Russo CR, Bandinelli S, Bartali B, Cavazzini C, Di Iorio A, Corsi AM, Rantanen T, Guralnik JM, Ferrucci L. Age-associated changes in skeletal muscles and their effect on mobility: an operational diagnosis of sarcopenia. *J Appl Physiol* 2003;95:1851.
37. Baumgartner RN, Waters DL, Gallagher D, Morley JE, Garry PJ. Predictors of skeletal muscle mass in elderly men and women. *Mech Ageing Dev* 1999;107(2):123–126.

38. Shike M, Russell DM, Detsky AS, Harrison JE, McNeill KG, Shepherd FA, et al. Changes in body composition in patients with small-cell cancer. The effect of total parenteral nutrition as an adjunct to chemotherapy. *Ann Intern Med* 1984;101:303–309.
39. Mitch WE. Mechanisms causing loss of lean body mass in kidney disease. *Am J Clin Nutr* 1998;67:359–366.
40. Hedlund J, Hansson LO, Ortqvist A. Short- and long-term prognosis for middle-aged and elderly patients hospitalized with community-acquired pneumonia: impact of nutritional and inflammatory factors. *Scand J Infect Dis* 1995;27:32–37.
41. Toth MJ, Gottlieb SS, Goran MI, Fisher ML, Poehlman ET. Daily energy expenditure in free-living heart failure patients. *Am J Physiol* 1997;272:469–475.
42. Roubenoff R, Roubenoff RA, Cannon JG, Kehayias JJ, Zhuang H, Dawson-Hughes B, et al. Rheumatoid cachexia: cytokine-driven hypermetabolism accompanying reduced body cell mass in chronic inflammation. *J Clin Invest* 1994;93:2379–2386.
43. Kotler DP, Wang J, Pierson RN. Body composition studies in patients with the acquired immunodeficiency syndrome. *Am J Clin Nutr* 1985;42:1255–1265.
44. Espat NJ, Moldawer LL, Copeland EM 3rd. Cytokine-mediated alterations in host metabolism prevent nutritional repletion in cachectic cancer patients. *J Surg Oncol* 1995;58:77–82.
45. Rote NS. Inflammation. In *Pathophysiology: The Biological Basis for Disease in Adults and Children*, McCance KL, Huether SE, Eds. Mosby, St. Louis, 1998, pp. 205–236.
46. Golden MH, Golden BE. Severe malnutrition. In *Human Nutrition and Dietetics*, 10th ed., Garrow JS, James WPT, Ralph A, Eds. Churchill Livingston, Edinburgh, 2000, pp. 515–526.
47. McNurlan MA, Garlick PJ. Protein synthesis and degradation. In *Biochemical and Physiological Aspects of Human Nutrition*, Stipanuk MA, Ed. W.B. Saunders Company, Philadelphia, 2000, pp. 211–232.
48. Thomas DR. Starving in the hospital. *Nutrition* 2003;19:907–908.
49. Shaver HJ, Loper JA, Lutes RA. Nutritional status of nursing home patients. *J Parent Enteral Nutrition* 1980;4:367–370.
50. Windsor JA, Hill GL. Risk factors of postoperative pneumonia: the importance of protein depletion. *Ann Surg* 1988;208:209–214.
51. Herrmann FR, Safran C, Levkoff SE, Minaker KL. Serum albumin level on admission as a predictor of death, length of stay, and readmission. *Arch Intern Med* 1992;152:125–130.
52. Bistrian BR, Blackburn GL, Vitale J, Cochran D, Naylor J. Prevalence of malnutrition in general medical patients. *JAMA* 1976;235:1567–1570.
53. Bistrian BR, Blackburn GL, Hallowell E, Heddle R. Protein status of general surgical patients. *JAMA* 1974;230:858–860.
54. Weinsier RL, Hunker EM, Krumdieck CL, Butterworth CE Jr. Hospital malnutrition: a prospective evaluation of general medical patients during the course of hospitalization. *Am J Clin Nutr* 1979;32:418–426.
55. Heymsfield SB, Tighe A, Wang ZM. Nutritional assessment by anthropometric and biochemical methods. In *Modern Nutrition in Health and Disease*, 8th ed., Shils ME, Olson JA, Shike M, Eds. Lea & Fibiger, Philadelphia, 1994, pp. 812–841.
56. Klidjian AM, Foster KJ, Kammerling RM, Cooper A, Karran SJ. Relation of anthropometric and dynamometric variables to serious postoperative complications. *BMJ* 1980;281:899–901.
57. Christou NV, Meakins JL, Gordon J, et al. The delayed hypersensitivity response and host resistance in surgical patients: 20 years later. *Ann Surg* 1995;222:534–548.

58. Chandra RK. Nutrition, immunity, and infection: present knowledge and future directions. *Lancet* 1983;1:688–691.
59. Souba WW. Drug therapy: nutritional support. *N Engl J Med* 1997;336:41–48.
60. Thomas DR, Verdery RB, Gardner L, Kant AK, Lindsay J. A prospective study of outcome from protein-energy malnutrition in nursing home residents. *J Parent Enteral Nutr* 1991;15:400–404.
61. Blackburn GL, Bistrian BR, Maini BS, Schlamm HT, Smith MF. Nutritional and metabolic assessment of the hospitalized patient. *J Parent Enteral Nutr* 1977;1:11–22.
62. Roubenoff R, Roubenoff RA, Preto J, Balke CW. Malnutrition among hospitalized patients. *Arch Intern Med* 1987;147:1462–1465.
63. Dimant J, Solow BA. Nutritional assessment in nursing home patients. *J Long-Term Care Admin* 1988:3:7–9.
64. White JV, Dwyer JT, Posner BM, Ham RJ, Lipschitz DA, Wellman NS. Nutrition Screening Initiative: development and implementation of the public awareness checklist and screening tools. *J Am Diet Assoc* 1992;92:163–167.
65. Dwyer JA. Vital sign: progress and prospects in nutrition screening of older Americans. *Aging Clin Exp Res* 1993;5S:13–21.
66. Detsky AS, McLaughlin JR, Baker JP, Johnston N, Whittaker S, Mendelson RA, JeeJeebhoy KN. What is Subjective Global Assessment of the nutritional status. *J Parent Enteral Nutr* 1987;11:8–13.
67. Detsky AS, Smalley PS, Chang J. Is this patient malnourished? *JAMA* 1994;27:54–58.
68. Buzby GP, Mullern JL, Matthews DC, Hobbs CL, Rosato EF. Prognostic nutritional index in gastrointestinal surgery. *Am J Surg* 1980;39:160–167.
69. Guigoz Y, Vellas B, Garry PJ. Mini-Nutritional Assessment: a practical assessment tool for grading the nutritional state of elderly patients. *Facts Res Gerontol* 1994;2S:15–59.
70. Detsky AS, Baker JP, O'Rourke K, et al. Predicting nutrition-associated complications for patients undergoing gastrointestinal surgery. *J Parentl Enteral Nutr* 1987;11:440–446.
71. Detsky AS, McLaughlin JR, Baker JP, et al. What is Subjective Global Assessment of nutritional status? *J Parent Enteral Nutr* 1987;11:8–13.
72. Windsor JA, Hill GL. Weight loss with physiologic impairment: a basic indicator of surgical risk. *Ann Surg* 1988;207:290–296.
73. Veterans Affairs Total Parenteral Nutrition Cooperative Study Group. Perioperative nutrition in surgical patients. *N Engl J Med* 1991;325:525–532.
74. Guigoz Y, Vellas B, Garry PJ. Mini-Nutritional Assessment: a practical assessment tool for grading the nutritional state of elderly patients. *Facts Res Gerontol* 1994;2S:15–59.
75. Guigoz Y, Vellas B. The Mini-Nutritional Assessment for Grading the Nutritional State of Elderly Patients: Presentation of the MNA, History and Validation. Nestle Nutrition Workshop Series, Clinical and Performance Program 1, Denges, Switzerland, 1998, pp. 1–2.
76. Wilson MM, Thomas DR, Rubenstein LZ, Chibnall JT, Anderson S, Baxi A, Diebold MR, Morley JE. Appetite assessment: simple appetite questionnaire predicts weight loss in community-dwelling adults and nursing home residents. *Am J Clin Nutr* 2005;82:1074–1081.
77. Covinsky KE, Covinsky MH, Palmer RM, Sehgal AR. Serum albumin concentration and clinical assessments of nutritional status in hospitalized older people: different sides of different coins? *J Am Geriatr Soc* 2002;50:631–637.
78. Beck AM, Ovesen L, Osler M. The Mini-Nutritional Assessment and the Determine Your Nutritional Health Checklist (NSI Checklist) as predictors of morbidity and mortality in an elderly Danish population. *Br J Nutr* 1999;81:31–36.

79. de Groot LC, Beck AM, Schroll M, van Staveren WA. Evaluating the DETERMINE Your Nutritional Health Checklist and the Mini Nutritional Assessment as tools to identify nutritional problems in elderly Europeans. *Eur J Clin Nutr* 1998;52:877–883.
80. A.S.P.E.N. Board of Directors and the Clinical Guidelines Task Force. Guidelines for the use of parenteral and enteral nutrition in adult and pediatric patients. *J Parent Enteral Nutr* 2002;26(Suppl):S1–S138.
81. Milne AC, Avenell A, Potter J. Meta-analysis: protein and energy supplementation in older people. *Ann Intern Med* 2006;144:37–48.
82. Lauque S, Arnaud-Battandier F, Gillette S, Plaze JM, Andrieu S, Cantet C, Vellas B. Improvement of weight and fat-free mass with oral nutritional supplementation in patients with Alzheimer's disease at risk of malnutrition: a prospective randomized study. *J Am Geriatr Soc* 2004;52:1702–1707.
83. Hickson M, Bulpitt C, Nunes M, Peters R, Cooke J, Nicholl C, Frost G. Does additional feeding support provided by health care assistants improve nutritional status and outcome in acutely ill older in-patients? A randomised control trial. *Clin Nutr* 2004;23:69–77.
84. Haddad RY, Thomas DR. Enteral nutrition and tube feeding: a review of the evidence. *Geriatr Clin North Am* 2002;18:867–882.
85. Montejo JC, Zarazaga A, Lopez-Martinez J, Urrutia G, Roque M, Blesa AL, Celaya S, Conejero R, Galban C, Garcia de Lorenzo A, Grau T, Mesejo A, Ortiz-Leyba C, Planas M, Ordonez J, Jimenez FJ, Spanish society of intensive care medicine and coronary units. Immunization in the intensive care unit: A systematic review and consensus statement. *Clin Nutr* 2003;22(3):221–33.
86. Souba WW. Drug therapy: nutritional support. *N Engl J Med* 1997;336:41–48.
87. Okada K, Yamagami H, Sawada S, Nakanishi M, Tamaki M, Ohnaka M, Sakamoto S, Niwa Y, Nakaya Y. The nutritional status of elderly bed-ridden patients receiving tube feeding. *J Nutr Sci Vitaminol* 2001;47:236–241.
88. Mitchell, SL, Kiely, DK, Lipsitz LA. The risk factors and impact on survival of feeding tube placement in nursing home residents with severe cognitive impairment. *Arch Intern Med* 1997;157:327–332.
89. Schweigert FJ. Inflammation-induced changes in the nutritional biomarkers serum retinol and carotenoids. *Curr Opin Clin Nutr Metab Care* 2001;4(6):477–81.
90. Friedman PJ, Campbell AJ, Caradoc-Davies TH. Hypoalbuminemia in the elderly is due to disease not malnutrition. *J Clin Exp Gerontol* 1985;7:191–293.
91. Ingenblick Y, Carpentier YA. A prognostic inflammatory and nutritional index scoring critically ill patients. *Int J Vitamin Nutr Res* 1985;55:91–101.
92. Hyltoft PP, Felding P, Horder M, Tryding N. Effects of posture on concentration of serum proteins in healthy adults. *Scand J Clin Lab Invest* 1980;40:623–628.
93. Johnson AM. *Clin Chem Lab Med* 1999;37:91.
94. O'Keefe SJ, et al. *Eur J Clin Nutr* 1988;42:41.
95. Forse RA, Rompre C, Crosilla P, O-Tuitt D, Rhode B, Shizgal HM. Reliability of the total lymphocyte count as a parameter of nutrition. *Can J Surg* 1985;28:216–219.
96. Hoffer LJ, Bistrian BR, Young VR, Blackburn GL, Wannemacher RW. Metabolic effects of carbohydrate in low-calorie diets. *Metab Clin Exp* 1984;33:820–825.
97. Castaneda C, Charnley JM, Evans WJ, Crim MC. Elderly women accommodate to a low-protein diet with losses of body cell mass, muscle function, and immune response. *Am J Clin Nutr* 1995;62:30–39.
98. Montejo JC, Zarazaga A, Lopez-Martinez J, Urrutia G, Roque M, Blesa AL, Celaya S, Conejero R, Galban C, Garcia de Lorenzo A, Grau T, Mesejo A, Ortiz-Leyba C, Planas M, Ordonez J, Jimenez FJ, Spanish society of intensive care medicine and coronary units. Immunization in the intensive care unit: A systematic review and consensus statement. *Clin Nutr* 2003;22(3):221–33.

99. Detsky AS, Smalley PS, Chang J. Is this patient malnourished? *JAMA* 1994;271:54–58.
100. Landi F, Zuccala G, Gambassi G, Incalzi RA, Manigrasso L, Pagano F, Carbonin P, Bernabei R. Body mass index and mortality among older people living in the community. *J Am Geriatr Soc* 1999;47:1072–1076.
101. Calle EE, Thum MJ, Petrelli JM, Rodriguez C, Heath CW. Body-mass index and mortality in a prospective cohort of U.S. adults. *New Engl J Med* 1999;341:1097–1105.
102. Launer LJ, Harris LT, Rumpel C, Madans J. Body mass index, weight change and risk of mobility disability in middle-aged and older women. *JAMA* 1994;271:1083–1098.
103. Payette H, Coulombe C, Boutier V, Gray-Donald K. Weight loss and mortality among free-living frail elders: a prospective study. *J Gerontol A Biol Sci Med Sci* 1999;54:M440–M445.
104. Thomas DR, Kamel H, Azharrudin M, Ali AS, Khan A, Javaid U, Morley JE. The relationship of functional status, severity of illness, and nutritional markers to in-hospital mortality and length of stay. *J Nutr Health Aging* 2005;9:169–175.
105. Galanos AN, Pieper CF, Kussin PS, Winchell MT, Fulkerson WJ, Harrell FE Jr, Teno JM, Layde P, Connors AF Jr, Phillips RS, Wenger NS. Relationship of body mass index to subsequent mortality among seriously ill hospitalized patients. SUPPORT Investigators. The Study to Understand Prognoses and Preferences for Outcome and Risks of Treatments. *Crit Care Med* 1997;25:1962–1968.
106. Sullivan DH, Bopp MM, Roberson PK. Protein-energy undernutrition and life-threatening complications among the hospitalized elderly. *J Gen Intern Med* 2002;17:923–932.
107. Liu L, Bopp MM, Roberson PK, Sullivan DH. Undernutrition and risk of mortality in elderly patients within 1 year of hospital discharge. *J Gerontol A Biol Sci Med Sci* 2002;57:M741–M746.
108. Sullivan DH, Walls RC, Bopp MM. Protein-energy undernutrition and the risk of mortality within one year of hospital discharge: a follow-up study. *J Am Geriatr Soc* 1995;43:507–512.
109. Herrmann FR, Safran C, Levkoff SE, Minaker KL. Serum albumin level on admission as a predictor of death, length of stay, and readmission. *Arch Intern Med* 1992;152:125–130.
110. Sullivan DH, Walls RC. The risk of life-threatening complications in a select population of geriatric patients: the impact of nutritional status. *J Am Coll Nutr* 1995;14:29–36.
111. Sullivan DH, Walls RC. Protein-energy undernutrition and the risk of mortality within six years of hospital discharge. *J Am Coll Nutr* 1998;17:571–578.
112. Murden RA, Ainslie NK. Recent weight loss is related to short-term mortality in nursing homes. *J Gen Intern Med* 1994;9:648–650.
113. Ryan C, Bryant E, Eleazer P, Rhodes A, Guest K. Unintentional weight loss in long-term care: predictor of mortality in the elderly. *South Med J* 1995;88:721–724.
114. Sullivan DH, Johnson LE, Bopp MM, Roberson PK. Prognostic significance of monthly weight fluctuations among older nursing home residents. *J Gerontol A Biol Sci Med Sci* 2004;59:M633–M639.

13 Geriatric Assessment and Its Interaction with Nutrition

Julie Gammack, M.D.

CONTENTS

ABSTRACT

Nutritional disorders are common in the older population. Chronic medical conditions and geriatric syndromes frequently coexist with these nutritional disorders. It is important to assess older adults for the presence of nutritional deficiencies, especially in the setting of weight loss or anorexia. The use of a comprehensive approach is especially beneficial in this population given the extent and complexity of medical illnesses. Comprehensive Geriatric Assessment (CGA) is a specialized assessment of older adults who already have or are at risk for developing functional disabilities, cognitive impairment, geriatric syndromes, or psychosocial deficits. CGA can uncover important medical and nutritional conditions that may otherwise be undetected.

KEY POINTS

- Nutritional disorders frequently coexist with geriatric syndromes.
- Comprehensive Geriatric Assessment is a specialized evaluation of older adults who are at risk for developing functional decline.
- The key domains in Comprehensive Geriatric Assessment are medical, cognitive, functional, and psychosocial.
- Geriatric syndromes are defined as diseases, disabilities, or functional impairments, often of multifactorial etiology, that are commonly observed in the aging population.
- Geriatric syndromes include polypharmacy, falls, weight loss, incontinence, delirium, dementia, and depression.

13.1 INTRODUCTION

As the U.S. population ages, a greater percentage of individuals will be living into their eighth and ninth decades of life. Many of these individuals will develop functional and cognitive impairments; however, many are expected to "age successfully" with few disabilities until late in life. At this time, less than one third of community-residing people age 85 years or older need assistance with activities of daily living.

As with younger individuals, older adults are at ongoing risk of developing acute and chronic illnesses. As a result of physiologic changes of aging, older adults have less functional reserve and are more likely to develop complications from medical illnesses and medications. Many of these illnesses have a direct impact on nutritional health. Prevention and early detection of illness and disease are critical in the care of older adults.

Nutritional health is complex and requires a multidimensional approach in the older population. Many medical conditions affect diet and nutrition. Conversely, nutrition directly and substantially affects chronic disease management in the elderly. Older adults are more susceptible to the adverse effects of nutritional deficiencies. Weight loss and undernutrition are especially troublesome and predict poor health outcomes. Older adults must be monitored carefully for evidence of nutritional disorders. A comprehensive approach can be useful in screening this population for common medical and nutritional illnesses.

13.2 COMPREHENSIVE GERIATRIC ASSESSMENT

Comprehensive Geriatric Assessment (CGA) is a specialized assessment of older adults who already have or are at risk for developing functional disabilities, cognitive impairment, geriatric syndromes, or psychosocial disorders. This interdisciplinary method is used to identify and treat the multiple and complex problems found in the frail elderly population. The assessment includes functional evaluation, screening for geriatric syndromes, cognitive evaluation, and thorough review of social support systems (Table 13.1). CGA uses a variety of assessment and screening tools that are fast and easy to administer.

Comprehensive Geriatric Assessment was first introduced in the 1980s as a multidisciplinary patient-centered model of care for high-risk elderly in the hospital setting. The model has since evolved to include the outpatient clinic and home care settings. The core members of the assessment team include the physician, social worker, and gerontological nurse. Other key members include the dietician, physical, occupational, and speech therapists, and pharmacist.

What makes CGA different from a standard office visit is the specific focus on functional abilities, geriatric syndromes, and aging-related conditions. CGA emphasizes

TABLE 13.1
Components of a Comprehensive Geriatric Assessment

Medical Evaluation	Psychosocial Evaluation
Geriatric syndrome screening	Social service review
Polypharmacy	Advance care planning
Medication review	Family support
Medication counseling	Safety
Falls/dizziness	Caregivers/caregiving
Weight loss	Financial resources
Nutritional evaluation	Cognitive services
Incontinence assessment	Neuropsychiatric testing
Cognitive evaluation	Family and patient counseling
Delirium	Dementia education
Dementia	Stress management
Depression	Community resource management
Functional assessment	Identifying available resources
ADLs and IADLs	Enrollment in programs
Gait assessment	Transportation services
Sensory evaluation	Case management
Health maintenance/screening	
Chronic disease management	

the domains of **medical**, **cognitive**, **functional**, and **psychosocial health**. These domains have a significant impact on the ability of an elderly individual to maintain satisfactory quality of life, independence, and health status. The CGA approach adds critical dimensions to the traditional disease-based approach to medical care.

CGA has important implications for dietary management and nutritional assessment. Screening for nutritional disorders is a standard component of the CGA and is useful in identifying problems such as weight loss and impaired appetite. Conversely, nutritional impairments may prompt the clinician to conduct a CGA and identify risk factors or comorbidities that contribute to nutritional compromise. Undernutrition and weight loss are the focus in CGA. Weight loss is especially worrisome in the frail and institutionalized population and is a predictor of functional decline and mortality. Obesity, although a serious health concern, does not carry the same health implications as underweight in the older population. Obesity is specifically addressed elsewhere in this textbook.

13.3 ASSESSMENT OF NUTRITIONAL STATUS: MEDICAL EVALUATION

13.3.1 Geriatric Syndromes

The key medical component of a CGA is the screening for geriatric syndromes. Commonly accepted geriatric syndromes include polypharmacy, falls, weight loss, incontinence, delirium, dementia, and depression. Geriatric syndromes are defined as diseases, disabilities, or functional impairments, often of multifactorial etiology, that are commonly observed in the aging population. The development of nutritional deficiencies can precede the development of geriatric syndromes, and the presence of geriatric syndromes can increase the likelihood of nutritional insufficiency. Many tools are available to screen for geriatric syndromes. When identified, these syndromes may prompt additional screening for related nutritional concerns (Table 13.2). It is important to screen for these syndromes in older adults to identify previously undiagnosed conditions and risks for imminent health decline. Once identified, interventions to treat or reduce the morbidity of these syndromes should be employed.

13.3.1.1 Polypharmacy

Inappropriate medication use (often broadly termed polypharmacy) is defined as the overuse, underuse, and inappropriate use of medication in elderly adults. Due to physiologic changes of aging, the older population is more sensitive to medication effects and more likely to experience side effects. These effects can have a significant impact on nutritional status.

Overuse of medications includes the use medications without clear ongoing medical need. In nursing home care, the Centers for Medicare and Medicaid Services (CMS) has established a threshold of nine medications as a potential state of medication overuse. The more medications administered, the more likely that drug–drug or drug–food interactions will impact nutritional status.

TABLE 13.2
Screening for Geriatric Syndromes and Related Nutritional Concerns

Syndrome	Screening Tool	Related Nutritional Concerns
Polypharmacy	Beers' criteria Number of medications	Anorexia Medication side effects
Falls	Up-and-go test Tinnetti Gait/Balance Test	Vitamin D and calcium Micronutrient deficiencies
Weight loss	Mini-Nutritional Assessment Simplified Nutritional Appetite Questionnaire (SNAQ) Body mass index	Weight monitoring Nutritional evaluation Management of contributing conditions
Incontinence	Incontinence questionnaire Voiding dairy	Bladder irritants
Delirium	Confusion Assessment Method *Diagnostic and Statistical Manual IV* criteria	Swallowing safety Adequate caloric intake
Dementia	Mini-Mental State Examination St. Louis University Mental State Examination Clock drawing task	Progressive weight loss Dysphagia and aspiration Micronutrient deficiencies
Depression	Geriatric Depression Scale Cornell Scale for Depression in Dementia Hamilton Dementia Rating Scale	Adequate caloric intake Weight monitoring

Many drugs and drug classes are associated with anorexia, including antidepressants, opioids, benzodiazepines, neuroleptics, antihistamines, proton pump inhibitors, anticonvulsants, and digoxin. It is important to note that virtually any medication can cause anorexia, and in persons losing weight, all medications need to be carefully reviewed. In extreme cases, a large number of medications taken simultaneously can reduce appetite due to the volume of tablets "filling up" the stomach.

Underuse of medication can impact nutritional status when chronic medical conditions are inadequately managed. The undertreatment of pain and depression are common examples of conditions that can impair eating if not properly managed. Inappropriate prescribing can also impact nutrition, usually due to medication side effects, when an alternative safer medication could be utilized. In some cases, a medication may improve appetite or nutritional status, such as a patient using a proton pump inhibitor for severe gastric upset due to gastric reflux. In other patients, the adverse effects of this same medication (alteration in taste) may cause anorexia. It is therefore important to correlate the use of medications with the onset of nutritional or dietary effects.

Drugs can impair nutrient absorption, particularly those that alter gastric pH (histamine and proton pump inhibitors), bind directly to micronutrients (antacids, bile acid sequestants), or promote excessive gastrointestinal transit (laxatives, promotility agents). Excessive metabolic stimulation (central stimulants, thyroid hormone) can reduce appetite or invoke weight loss due to a hypercatabolic state.

TABLE 13.3
Nutritional Causes of Sensory Loss

B1 (thiamine) deficiency
B6 (pyridoxine) deficiency or toxicity
B12 (cyanocobalamin) deficiency
Folate deficiency
Hypophosphatemia
Vitamin E deficiency
Vitamin A toxicity
Copper deficiency
Hyperglycemia (diabetes)
Hypercalcemia
Heavy metal toxicity
Alcohol toxicity

Medications that cause oversedation can worsen weight loss by reducing the time awake needed for food consumption.

13.3.1.2 Falls

Severe nutritional deficiencies have been associated with falling or increased risk of falls. Micronutrient deficiencies or intoxications that cause sensory neuropathy lead to impaired balance and increased fall risk (Table 13.3). When falls or sensory loss is noted, screening for nutritional causes of neuropathy is warranted.

Vitamin D deficiency is associated with falls, functional decline, and nursing home placement.[1,2] In one study, vitamin D deficiency was found in 10% of community-dwelling seniors and an additional 37% had low vitamin D levels.[1] Many elders have insufficient dietary intake of vitamin D and have limited exposure to the sunlight necessary for production of vitamin D. Older adults are encouraged to take 800 IU of vitamin D in order to reduce weakness, falls, and fractures. Repletion of vitamin D has been associated with decreased risk of future falls.[3–5]

Many older adults have insufficient dietary intake of calcium due to lactose intolerance or aversion to dairy products. Adequate intake of calcium via supplementation, along with vitamin D, is therefore needed for most older adults. Intake of 1500 mg of elemental calcium each day is recommended for both older men and women. Inadequate calcium intake can result in osteoporosis and fractures, which cause pain, weakness, and risk of falling. All older adults should be asked about falls annually and those with a single fall evaluated using an up-and-go gait assessment. Those with an abnormal gait or with multiple falls should undergo a comprehensive falls evaluation.[6]

13.3.1.3 Weight Loss

Nutritional and dietary factors associated with weight loss are discussed throughout this chapter. Weight loss is usually multifactorial in etiology and associated with

TABLE 13.4
Meals on Wheels Mnemonic as an Easy Method to Screen for Causes of Weight Loss in Older Persons

Medications (e.g., digoxin, theophylline, cimetidine)
Emotional (e.g., depression)
Alcoholism, elder abuse, anorexia tardive
Late-life paranoia
Swallowing problems
Oral factors
Nosocomial infections (e.g., tuberculosis)
Wandering and other dementia-related factors
Hyperthyroidism, hypercalcemia, hypoadrenalism
Enteral problems (e.g., gluten enteropathy)
Eating problems
Low-salt, low-cholesterol, and other therapeutic diets
Stones (cholecystitis)

Source: Reproduced from Morley, J.E. and Silver, A.J., *Ann. Intern. Med.*, 123, 850–859, 1995. With permission. American College of Physicians is not responsible for the accuracy of the translation.

chronic medical conditions, medication side effects, malignancies, and psychosocial conditions. The Meals on Wheels mnemonic (Table 13.4), developed by St. Louis University physicians, is a useful tool to recall potentially reversible causes of weight loss in older adults.[7]

Significant weight loss is usually defined as unintentional 5% one-month or 10% six-month loss in body weight. Most unintentional weight loss is not due to the presence of malignancy.[8,9] Unlike younger adults, older adults lose more muscle relative to fat with unintentional weight loss. Loss of muscle mass increases the risk of falls, functional disability, and mortality.[10–12]

Weight loss is an independent predictor of mortality among older adults.[13,14] Anorexia is also an independent predictor of mortality (hazard ratio, 2.9; 95% confidence interval (CI), 1.1 to 7.4).[15]

The Mini-Nutritional Assessment (MNA) is a commonly used tool to assess nutritional status. This tool has been used to predict mortality and weight loss; however, it is fairly time consuming and requires self-assessment, calculation of physical parameters, and cognitive evaluation. The Simplified Nutritional Appetite Questionnaire (SNAQ) is a brief, four-item survey that can be self-administered or given by nonmedical personnel (Table 13.5). This tool predicts weight loss in both community-dwelling and institutionalized individuals.[16]

Diseases such as end-stage cardiac and lung disease, depression, dementia, endocrine dysfunction, and gastrointestinal disorders are common contributors to weight loss. The specialized diets prescribed to manage these diseases can also result in decreased dietary intake. In long-term care, therapeutic diets often lead to weight loss and their efficacy has been questioned.[17,18] It is no longer acceptable to routinely prescribe therapeutic diets for the majority of older persons in nursing homes.

TABLE 13.5
Simplified Nutritional Appetite Questionnaire (SNAQ)

Name: ______________________________ Sex (circle): Male Female
Age: ____________ Weight: ________________ Height: ____________
Date: ____________________

Administration Instructions: Ask the subject to complete the questionnaire by circling the correct answers and then tally the results based upon the following numerical scale: a = 1, b = 2, c = 3, d = 4, e = 5. The sum of the scores for the individual items constitutes the SNAQ score. *SNAQ score ≤14 indicates significant risk of at least 5% weight loss within six months.*

1. **My appetite is**
   a. very poor
   b. poor
   c. average
   d. good
   e. very good
2. **When I eat**
   a. I feel full after eating only a few mouthfuls
   b. I feel full after eating about a third of a meal
   c. I feel full after eating over half a meal
   d. I feel full after eating most of the meal
   e. I hardly ever feel full
3. **Food tastes**
   a. very bad
   b. bad
   c. average
   d. good
   e. very good
4. **Normally I eat**
   a. less than one meal a day
   b. one meal a day
   c. two meals a day
   d. three meals a day
   e. more than three meals a day

Source: Reproduced from Wilson, M.M. et al., *Am. J. Clin. Nutr.*, 82, 1074–1081, 2005. With permission.

13.3.1.4 Incontinence

Identifying urinary incontinence can bring important nutritional factors to light. Certain foods are considered urinary irritants and can worsen urge incontinence. Spicy or acidic foods such as citrus fruits and peppers can irritate the bladder mucosa. Caffeine causes increased urinary production and can worsen detrusor instability by irritating the bladder lining. Inappropriate water intake can exacerbate urinary symptoms. Reduced water intake causes concentrated urine, which is a bladder irritant. Conversely, excessive liquid intake results in polyuria and can worsen incontinence in some individuals. Polyuria may also occur with poorly controlled diabetes mellitus due to hyperglycemia. In older adults with new or long-standing urinary incontinence, nutritional screening should be a part of the Comprehensive Geriatric Assessment to determine if these dietary factors are contributing to urinary symptoms.

13.3.2 Sensory Assessment

13.3.2.1 Vision

Visual assessment is a component of the initial CGA visit. Identifying visual disorders can lead to a diagnosis of nutritional deficits. Treatment of vision loss may require a focus on specific nutritional repletion. Diseases that affect nutritional status such as diabetes mellitus and alcoholism may increase the risk for developing cataracts and glaucoma. Vitamin deficiencies such as vitamin A and beta-carotene can result in a decline in visual functioning. There is a weak association between macular degeneration (MD) and dietary fat intake, diabetes, hyperlipidemia, intake of carotenoids, and intake of omega-3 fatty acids.

Correcting nutritional deficiencies or overreplacing micronutrient stores has been postulated to improve visual deficits. The use of antioxidant vitamins has been especially promising in the management of macular degeneration. Research on antioxidants and micronutrients has focused on the prevention and treatment of MD. In one study, subjects randomized to lutein ± antioxidant vitamins showed improvement in visual acuity and contrast sensitivity compared with placebo.[19] In another study, incident MD was reduced (hazard ratio, 0.65; 95% CI, 0.46 to 0.92) for individuals taking a combination of the antioxidants (vitamins C and E, beta-carotene) and zinc.[20]

13.3.2.2 Hearing

Over time, the subtle loss of high-frequency sounds may result in clinically significant hearing loss. Screening questionnaires, such as the Hearing Handicap Inventory for the Elderly, can identify those in need of further evaluation. Portable audiometers can be used by trained medical staff in screening for hearing loss during the CGA. Examination of the ear canal and removal of wax can improve hearing and balance and should be performed prior to an audiology evaluation or referral.

Although most hearing loss in older adults is associated with noise exposure or presbycusis, some data indicate that micronutrients may have a role in hearing acuity. In a study of healthy older women, those with hearing impairment had 38 and 31% lower serum vitamin B12 and red cell folate levels, respectively ($p = 0.01$; $p = 0.008$).[21,22]

As in MD, antioxidants are also thought to have protective effects on hearing. The use of antioxidant vitamins to reduce the ototoxicity of certain medications has been fairly well studied in animal models. In one human study, cancer patients exposed to cisplatin treatment with the highest plasma concentrations of antioxidant micronutrients had significantly less high-tone hearing loss.[23] In another study, two antioxidants were provided to individuals with prebycusis. Hearing was improved after 8 weeks of treatment.[22]

13.3.2.3 Taste/Smell

It is not uncommon for the older adult to complain of loss of taste (sweet and salty) and smell.[24] These symptoms are important to note in individuals who are losing weight or are malnourished. Studies have revealed an association between impaired olfaction and cognitive impairment.[25] Impaired smell/taste is also associated with deficiency in vitamins B12 and A. Inquiry about smell/taste changes should be made during CGA in individuals at risk for weight loss or having cognitive deficits. Chemosensory disorders have been associated with decreases in food acceptability, weight loss, and distorted or phantom smell or taste sensations. Certain medications, such as antihistamines, calcium channel blockers, antibiotics, and anticonvulsants, alter taste perception and may reduce oral intake due to poor appetite.

13.3.3 Prevention/Screening

Too often, elderly individuals miss appropriate opportunities for screening under a misperception that they are "too old" for benefits. Conversely, some individuals with serious and life-limiting illnesses continue to receive screening interventions that offer little overall benefit. For this reason, a series of functionally dependent screening and prevention guidelines were created to assist clinicians in approaching this decision making in older adults. Rather than age, these clinical "Glidepaths" divide older adults into categories of (1) healthy, (2) frail, (3) demented, and (4) end of life. Recommendations are provided for health maintenance interventions, such as screening lipid profiles, mammography, and fecal occult blood testing. The Glidepaths suggest screening approaches based on function and physiologic age rather than chronologic age.[26]

13.3.4 Cognitive Assessment

13.3.4.1 Delirium

Delirium is a state of altered cognition with impaired level of consciousness. The presence of delirium is associated with incident development of comobidities, including weight loss.[27] Delirious individuals are often acutely ill and may be hospitalized with a medical condition (such as pneumonia or myocardial infarction) that can further reduce nutritional intake. Delirium itself may make it impossible for an individual to consume adequate nutrition. When altered, the delirious patient is often too confused, somnolent, or agitated to swallow liquid or solid food safely. Patient inattention may lead to incomplete consumption of meals or supplements. The clinician must be aware of the potential for delirium as a cause of acute nutritional decline. When inadequate meal intake is noted, additional calories may be necessary through oral supplements, enteral feeding, or parenteral feeding if nutritional/delirium recovery will be prolonged.

13.3.4.2 Dementia

Most irreversible and progressive causes of dementia, such as Alzheimer's disease, Lewy body disease, and frontal-temporal dementia, will eventually result in nutritional impairment. This is an eventual progression of the dementia process in which the brain eventually fails to trigger normal food consumption. Loss of weight is one of the features used to qualify those with end-stage dementia for the benefit of hospice care. Dementia also causes neurologic degeneration with impairment in the swallowing mechanism, recurrent aspiration, pneumonia, and hypoxic events. Despite the natural instinct to feed these individuals via artificial enteral methods, mortality, morbidity, and functional status are not improved with tube feeding.[28,29] Despite similar caloric intake, individuals with dementia are more likely to lose weight than nondemented individuals. This suggests that mechanisms beyond food consumption are impacting weight maintenance in this population.[30]

There is growing evidence that weight loss may predate the development of dementia and that this sign should thus prompt close monitoring for cognitive impairment.[31] In mild to moderate dementia, nutritional deficiency may develop as a result of psychosocial circumstances. Individuals may withdraw from friends and family who provide assistance with meal planning and grocery shopping. Demented adults tend to be more isolated, which contributes to lower food consumption. As memory declines further, cooking becomes impaired and disorganized, leading to nutritionally inadequate meals.

Of the reversible causes of dementia, several are associated with nutritional disorders. Folate, vitamin B12, niacin, and thiamine deficiency are associated with cognitive impairment that may (but not always) be improved by correcting the micronutrient deficit. Derangements of calcium, phosphorus, and glucose can resemble dementia when serum levels are transiently or persistently abnormal due to nutritional or endocrine disorders. The hypercatabolic state of hyperthyroidism due to autoimmune process or overreplacement of thyroid hormone is associated with cognitive impairment and may result in weight loss. In a study of 60 hospitalized elders (average age, 80 years) with hyperthyroidism, 83% had weight loss and 52% had a diagnosis of cognitive impairment.[32]

13.3.4.3 Depression

Depression is associated with physical decline in community-dwelling, hospitalized, and institutionalized older adults. It is also associated with weight loss and decreased survival.[33] Screening for depression during a CGA is very important given the atypical presentations of this disorder in the elderly population.

Depression appears to be the most common cause of weight loss in older persons.[34] Depression increases the corticotrophin-releasing factor within the hypothalamus, which is a potent anorectic agent. Individuals not only have a decrease in appetite, but depression potentially impairs the motivation needed to obtain, prepare, and consume adequate nutrition. Every older adult who is losing weight requires screening for depression to exclude this condition as a cause of weight loss.

Certain medical conditions are associated with depression and thus should prompt the clinician to monitor for weight loss. Chronic pain is associated with a host of psychiatric conditions, including depression. Elders who have experienced a stroke have nearly a 65% 3-month incidence of depression.[35] Individuals with a history of chronic congestive heart failure have up to a 50% incidence of depression. In this population, weight loss may not be the most accurate marker of nutritional deficiency given the potential for weight fluctuation with heart failure.[36]

13.3.5 Functional Assessment

Functional status generally refers to the ability of an individual to participate in everyday tasks with or without the assistance of another person, use of an assistive device, or benefit of adaptive equipment. Functional assessment is a core component of the geriatric assessment. The primary scales for measuring functional status are the Activities of Daily Living (ADLs) and the Instrumental Activities of Daily Living (IADLs) (Table 13.6).

Several components of these tools specifically address nutritional status, including eating (ADL), cooking (IADL), and shopping (IADL). When evaluated, a person is identified as fully independent, needing assistance, or fully dependent in these specific activities. If not fully independent, a person requires assistance, oversight, or a support structure to maintain the current level of functioning.

Individuals who have experienced or are at risk of functional decline may be considered frail. Frailty has been specifically defined as a clinical syndrome in which three or more of the following criteria were present: unintentional weight loss (10 lb in past year), self-reported exhaustion, weakness (grip strength), slow walking speed, and low physical activity.[37] Body mass index (BMI) is not a criterion, and thus frailty may be present in elders who are overweight, underweight, or at an ideal body weight. In the Women's Health Initiative cohort of elderly women (n = 40,657), 16% were found to be frail at baseline, with a 5% yearly incident development of frailty. In this study, frailty was associated with an increased risk of death, hip fracture, ADL disability, and hospitalization.[38]

Nutritional decline, especially weight loss, is a key component in the development of frailty; however, other dietary deficiencies have been associated with this syndrome. Women with frailty were more likely to have two or more micronutrient deficiencies, including carotenoids, vitamin E, vitamin D, and vitamin B6.[39] Of 749 women independent in ADLs at baseline, 25% were found to be frail. By 3 years, 56% of frail women were then dependent in ADLs compared with 20% of nonfrail women.[40]

TABLE 13.6
ADL and IADL Components

ADL	Toileting
	Bathing
	Eating
	Dressing
	Continence
	Transferring
IADL	Cooking
	Laundry
	Housework
	Shopping
	Medication management
	Telephoning
	Transportation
	Money management

Functional status may decline due to muscular or skeletal weakness alone, with or without meeting the full criteria of frailty. Declines in muscle mass (sarcopenia) and bone mass (osteopenia) are normal physiologic changes of aging. When muscle loss results in fatigue, weakness, or inability to perform ADLs or IADLs, this is not a normal aging process. Likewise, when bone mass declines to a level –2.5 standard deviations below peak bone mass or a fracture occurs, this is not a normal aging process.

Many medical conditions, medications, and nutritional deficiencies in older adults contribute to loss of muscle and bone mass. Malnutrition and weight loss result in hypoalbuminemia. Without proper protein stores, muscle mass cannot be maintained and weakness develops. When functional deficits or weakness are reported, nutritional assessment should take place. Micro- and macronutrient serum markers may reveal deficits, including calcium, phosphorus, magnesium, albumin, prealbumin, total cholesterol, and lymphocyte count. Glucose should be drawn to exclude hypo- or hyperglycemia.

13.4 ASSESSMENT OF NUTRITIONAL STATUS: PSYCHOSOCIAL EVALUATION

13.4.1 Social Factors

Many psychosocial factors affect nutritional health (Table 13.7). These factors must be carefully evaluated in older adults with nutritional disorders. Frail older adults may rely heavily, if not exclusively, on others for nutritional support. Social networks provide a support structure for those requiring nutritional assistance. Community organizations, friends, family, neighbors, and health professionals may be of assistance in supporting nutritional health (Table 13.8). A spouse or direct caregiver often provides these necessary services. Major illness or death of a caregiver can drastically alter the nutritional health of at-risk elders.

Eating is a social activity. Simply sharing mealtime can increase food intake and pleasure of eating in both community and institutionalized seniors.[41,42] The mealtime environment also contributes to the quantity of food consumption. A pleasantly set

TABLE 13.7
Psychosocial Factors Affecting Nutritional Health

Financial resources
Medical insurance
In-home services
Spiritual needs
Caregiver role/health
Transportation
Family structure/support
Community connections
Cultural practices

TABLE 13.8
Potential Nutritional Support Needs

Transportation to store
Grocery shopping
Meal preparation
Cooking
Feeding
Hot/frozen meal delivery
Providing snacks or supplements
Mealtime visits
Weight monitoring
Nutritional/dietary counseling

table with garnishes, food choices, noninstitutional utensils, music, comfortable temperature, and pleasant aromas makes meal consumption more pleasing and effective.

13.4.2 Financial Factors

During the CGA, it is important to assess financial resources, as these impact diet and nutritional status. Many seniors live on limited monthly incomes that can restrict food choices. High-quality and fresh foods may be too costly for regular purchase. Less expensive prepared or processed foods are generally high in fat and sodium. Lack of available or low-cost transportation can limit access to grocery shopping. As the number and cost of medications increase, seniors may be forced to choose between purchasing medications or purchasing food. Nutritional supplements may help replace caloric deficiencies; however, these cost around $1 each and are infrequently covered by insurance plans. Those at highest risk socially for nutritional deficiencies are at the greatest risk of lacking high-quality food or dietary supplements.

Many communities offer free or low-cost meal delivery programs for elderly or disabled individuals who are homebound or impoverished. These meals are well balanced, fresh or frozen, and may be modified for dietary preferences or restrictions. The social worker is most helpful in referring patients for food support programs. He or she can assist in enrolling qualified patients for financial services and low-cost support programs.

13.4.3 Cultural Factors

A CGA attempts to uncover cultural preferences that can impact health and nutrition. When assessing nutritionally at-risk or deficient older adults, it is important to understand the cultural aspects of eating. Older individuals may be more accustomed to certain types of food or eating patterns based on their ethnicity, geographic location (costal, agricultural), and personal beliefs (vegan, vegetarian). Elderly immigrants tend to maintain dietary habits of the country of origin. Moving to a new state or country may limit the availability and affordability of ethnic foods and cooking styles. Institutionalization usually provides a diet consistent with the surrounding geographic/ethnic demography and may not be desirable to some individuals. A culturally sensitive caregiver or cook may be needed to prepare meals or meet the dietary preferences of the patient.

13.4.4 Spiritual Factors

The spiritual history should be a part of a CGA and may reveal factors that affect nutritional health. The spiritual practices of older adults may be more nutritionally challenging than for younger adults. Long periods of fasting can limit caloric consumption and result in weight loss. Healthy older adults may tolerate fasting without difficulty; however, frail or elderly individuals may not have the nutritional reserve needed to avoid weight loss during this period of dietary restraint.

Avoidance of certain foods or changes in diet for religious observances may result in less caloric intake or poorer-quality dietary substitutions. This is especially problematic when institutionalized seniors have minimal available food alternatives to the regularly provided meal.

13.5 CONCLUSION

Nutritional disorders are common in the older population. Chronic medical conditions and geriatric syndromes frequently coexist with these nutritional disorders. It is important to assess older adults for the presence of nutritional deficiencies, especially in the setting of weight loss or anorexia. The use of a comprehensive approach is especially beneficial in this population given the extent and complexity of medical illnesses.

CGA is a specialized assessment of older adults who already have or are at risk for developing functional disabilities, cognitive impairment, geriatric syndromes or psychosocial deficits. The focus of CGA is functional status with the goal to promote wellness and maintain independence. Using screening tools and an interdisciplinary approach can assist in the evaluation of older adults who are experiencing or at risk for nutritional decline. CGA can uncover important medical and nutritional conditions that may otherwise be undetected.

REFERENCES

1. Visser M, Deeg DJ, Puts MT, et al. Low serum concentrations of 25-hydroxyvitamin D in older persons and the risk of nursing home admission. *Am J Clin Nutr* 2006;84:616–622; quiz, 671–672.
2. Sato Y, Iwamoto J, Kanoko T, et al. Low-dose vitamin D prevents muscular atrophy and reduces falls and hip fractures in women after stroke: a randomized controlled trial. *Cerebrovasc Dis* 2005;20:187–192.
3. Flicker L, MacInnis RJ, Stein MS, Scherer SC, Mead KE, Nowson CA, Thomas J, Lowndes C, Hopper JL, Ward JD. Should older people in residential care receive vitamin D to prevent falls? Results of a randomized trial. *J Am Geriatr Soc* 2005;53:1881–1888.

4. Bischoff-Ferrari HA, Willett WC, Wong JB, Giovannucci E, Dietrich T, Dawson-Hughes B. Fracture prevention with vitamin D supplementation: a meta-analysis of randomized controlled trials. *JAMA* 2005;293:2257–2264.
5. Bischoff-Ferrari HA, Dawson-Hughes B, Willett WC, Staehelin HB, Bazemore MG, Zee RY, Wong JB. Effect of Vitamin D on falls: a meta-analysis. *JAMA* 2004;291:1999–2006.
6. American Geriatrics Society, British Geriatrics Society, and American Academy of Orthopaedic Surgeons Panel on Falls Prevention. Guideline for the prevention of falls in older persons. *J Am Geriatr Soc* 2001;49:664–672.
7. Morley JE, Silver AJ. Nutritional issues in nursing home care. *Ann Intern Med* 1995;123:850–859.
8. Lankisch P, Gerzmann M, Gerzmann JF, Lehnick D. Unintentional weight loss: diagnosis and prognosis. The first prospective follow-up study from a secondary referral centre. *J Intern Med* 2001;249:41–46.
9. Thompson MP, Morris LK. Unexplained weight loss in the ambulatory elderly. *J Am Geriatr Soc* 1991;39:497–500.
10. Moreland JD, Richardson JA, Goldsmith CH, Clase CM. Muscle weakness and falls in older adults: a systematic review and meta-analysis. *J Am Geriatr Soc* 2004;52:1121–1129.
11. Metter EJ, Talbot LA, Schrager M, Conwit R. Skeletal muscle strength as a predictor of all-cause mortality in healthy men. *J Gerontol A Biol Sci Med Sci* 2002;57:B359–B365.
12. Janssen I, Heymsfield SB, Ross R. Low relative skeletal muscle mass (sarcopenia) in older persons is associated with functional impairment and physical disability. *J Am Geriatr Soc* 2002;50:889–896.
13. Payette H, Coulombe C, Boutier V, Gray-Donald K. Weight loss and mortality among free-living frail elders: a prospective study. *J Gerontol A Biol Sci Med Sci* 1999;54:M440–M445.
14. White H, Pieper C, Schmader K. The association of weight change in Alzheimer's disease with severity of disease and mortality: a longitudinal analysis. *J Am Geriatr Soc* 1998;46:1223–1227.
15. Cornali C, Franzoni S, Frisoni GB, Trabucchi M. Anorexia as an independent predictor of mortality. *J Am Geriatr Soc* 2005;53:354–355.
16. Wilson MM, Thomas DR, Rubenstein LZ, Chibnall JT, Anderson S, Baxi A, Diebold MR, Morley JE. Appetite assessment: simple appetite questionnaire predicts weight loss in community-dwelling adults and nursing home residents. *Am J Clin Nutr* 2005;82:1074–1081.
17. Tariq SH, Karcic E, Thomas DR, Thomson K, Philpot C, Chapel DL, Morley JE. The use of a no-concentrated-sweets diet in the management of type 2 diabetes in nursing homes. *J Am Diet Assoc* 2001;101:1463–1466.
18. Niedert KC, American Dietetic Association. Position of the American Dietetic Association: liberalization of the diet prescription improves quality of life for older adults in long-term care. *J Am Diet Assoc* 2005;105:1955–1965.
19. Richer S, Stiles W, Statkute L, Pulido J, Frankowski J, Rudy D, Pei K, Tsipursky M, Nyland J. Double-masked, placebo-controlled, randomized trial of lutein and antioxidant supplementation in the intervention of atrophic age-related macular degeneration: the Veterans LAST study (Lutein Antioxidant Supplementation Trial). *Optometry* 2004;75:216–230.
20. van Leeuwen R, Boekhoorn S, Vingerling JR, Witteman JC, Klaver CC, Hofman A, de Jong PT. Dietary intake of antioxidants and risk of age-related macular degeneration. *JAMA* 2005;294:3101–3107.

21. Houston DK, Johnson MA, Nozza RJ, Gunter EW, Shea KJ, Cutler GM, Edmonds JT. Age-related hearing loss, vitamin B-12, and folate in elderly women. *Am J Clin Nutr* 1999;69:564–571.
22. Takumida M, Anniko M. Radical scavengers: a remedy for presbyacusis. A pilot study. *Acta Otolaryngol* 2005;125:1290–1295.
23. Weijl NI, Elsendoorn TJ, Lentjes EG, Hopman GD, Wipkink-Bakker A, Zwinderman AH, Cleton FJ, Osanto S. Supplementation with antioxidant micronutrients and chemotherapy-induced toxicity in cancer patients treated with cisplatin-based chemotherapy: a randomised, double-blind, placebo-controlled study. *Eur J Cancer* 2004;40:1713–1723.
24. Murphy C, Schubert CR, Cruickshanks KJ, Klein BE, Klein R, Nondahl DM. Prevalence of olfactory impairment in older adults. *JAMA* 2002;288:2307–2312.
25. Eibenstein A, Fioretti AB, Simaskou MN, et al. Olfactory screening test in mild cognitive impairment. *Neurol Sci* 2005;26:156–160.
26. Flaherty JH, Morley JE, Murphy DJ, Wasserman MR. The development of outpatient clinical glidepaths. *J Am Geriatr Soc* 2002;50:1886–1901.
27. Fick D, Foreman M. Consequences of not recognizing delirium superimposed on dementia in hospitalized elderly individuals. *J Gerontol Nurs* 2000;26:30–40.
28. Finucane TE, Christmas C, Travis K. Tube feeding in patients with advanced dementia: a review of the evidence. *JAMA* 1999;282:1365–1370.
29. Meier DE, Ahronheim JC, Morris J, Baskin-Lyons S, Morrison RS. High short-term mortality in hospitalized patients with advanced dementia: lack of benefit of tube feeding. *Arch Intern Med* 2001;161:2385–2386.
30. Wang PN, Yang CL, Lin KN, Chen WT, Chwang LC, Liu HC. Weight loss, nutritional status and physical activity in patients with Alzheimer's disease. A controlled study. *J Neurol* 2004;251:314–320.
31. Johnson DK, Wilkins CH, Morris JC. Accelerated weight loss may precede diagnosis in Alzheimer disease. *Arch Neurol* 2006;63:1312–1327.
32. Martin FI, Deam DR. Hyperthyroidism in elderly hospitalised patients. Clinical features and treatment outcomes. *Med J Aust* 1996;164:200–203.
33. Gallo JJ, Bogner HR, Morales KH, Post EP, Ten Have T, Bruce ML. Depression, cardiovascular disease, diabetes, and two-year mortality among older, primary-care patients. *Am J Geriatr Psychiatry* 2005;13:748–755.
34. Morley JE, Kraenzle D. Causes of weight loss in a community nursing home. *J Am Geriatr Soc* 1994;42:583–585.
35. Johnson JL, Minarik PA, Nystrom KV, Bautista C, Gorman MJ. Poststroke depression incidence and risk factors: an integrative literature review. *J Neurosci Nurs* 2006;38(Suppl):316–327.
36. Haworth JE, Moniz-Cook E, Clark AL, Wang M, Waddington R, Cleland JG. Prevalence and predictors of anxiety and depression in a sample of chronic heart failure patients with left ventricular systolic dysfunction. *Eur J Heart Fail* 2005;7:803–808.
37. Fried LP, Tangen CM, Walston J, Newman AB, Hirsch C, Gottdiener J, Seeman T, Tracy R, Kop WJ, Burke G, McBurnie MA, Cardiovascular Health Study Collaborative Research Group. Frailty in older adults: evidence for a phenotype. *J Gerontol A Biol Sci Med Sci* 2001;56:M146–M156.
38. Woods NF, LaCroix AZ, Gray SL, Aragaki A, Cochrane BB, Brunner RL, Masaki K, Murray A, Newman AB, Women's Health Initiative. Frailty: emergence and consequences in women aged 65 and older in the Women's Health Initiative Observational Study. *J Am Geriatr Soc* 2005;53:1321–1330.

39. Michelon E, Blaum C, Semba RD, Xue QL, Ricks MO, Fried LP. Vitamin and carotenoid status in older women: associations with the frailty syndrome. *J Gerontol A Biol Sci Med Sci* 2006;61:600–607.
40. Boyd CM, Xue QL, Simpson CF, Guralnik JM, Fried LP. Frailty, hospitalization, and progression of disability in a cohort of disabled older women. *Am J Med* 2005;118:1225–1231.
41. Locher JL, Robinson CO, Roth DL, Ritchie CS, Burgio KL. The effect of the presence of others on caloric intake in homebound older adults. *J Gerontol A Biol Sci Med Sci* 2005;60:1475–1478.
42. Wright L, Hickson M, Frost G. Eating together is important: using a dining room in an acute elderly medical ward increases energy intake. *J Hum Nutr Diet* 2006;19:23–26.

14 Nutritional Assessment in the European Community

Juergen Martin Bauer
Dorothee Volkert

CONTENTS

14.1 INTRODUCTION

The World Health Organization (WHO) European Region includes 52 member states with 879 million people.[1] It covers a wide spectrum of cultures and societies with different ethnic and religious backgrounds, different economic and health situations. During the last decades, in many of these countries changes in health status and disease patterns occurred with increasing economic wealth, followed by demographic changes. Life expectancy, for example, increased in the 25 countries of today's European Union (EU-25) by nearly 3 years during the last 10 decades. In 2002, it amounted to 75 years for men and 81 years for women, and thus was higher than that in the U.S. but lower than that in Japan or Canada.[2] The proportion of people age 65 years or older also increased and is expected to double between 1995 and 2050. It presently ranges from 11% in Ireland and Slowakia to 19% in Italy and

Greece and is anticipated to be more than 20% in 2015 in Italy, Greece, Germany, Finland, and Sweden. In the EU-25 more than 86 million people and in the WHO European Region more than 135 million people will then be older than 65 years.[1]

14.2 NUTRITIONAL INTAKE AND NUTRITIONAL STATUS IN THE ELDERLY

14.2.1 Independently Living Elderly

According to great cultural, economic, and health differences, the nutritional habits and status and the food pattern of elderly Europeans show broad variations.

The most comprehensive information about the nutritional situation of independently living elderly people in Europe originates from the Survey in Europe of Nutrition in the Elderly, a Concerted Action (SENECA) study.[3,4] This study was designed to assess regional or cross-cultural differences in nutrition, lifestyle, health, and performance in elderly Europeans. It started in 1988 in 19 traditional towns in 12 European countries with 2586 participants born between 1913 and 1918. In a first follow-up in 1993, about 1125 subjects from 13 towns took part, and in the SENECA finale in 1999, around a quarter of the original study population (n = 627) could be reassessed. Participating countries were Belgiuim, Denmark, France, Greece, Hungary, Italy, the Netherlands, Norway, Poland, Portugal, Spain, and Switzerland. Data were assessed in a uniform standardized manner.

14.2.1.1 Dietary Intake

For all dietary components, great variation between the 18 SENECA towns is reported. Using a modified dietary history method, including a 3-day estimated record and a food frequency list for dietary assessment, energy intakes between 7.6 MJ/day in central France and 11.8 MJ/day in Poland were observed in men, and between 6.0 MJ/day in Portugal and 10.1 MJ/day in Poland in women.[5] Five years later, the same picture was evident in the surviving participants: for men, mean intakes between 7.9 and 12.1 MJ/day are reported, and for women between 6.3 and 10.2 MJ/day. For both sexes, intakes were lowest in Yverdon, Switzerland, and highest in Marki, Poland.[6]

In several other nationwide studies, for example, in Finland,[7] the Netherlands,[8] Germany,[9] and Great Britain,[10] energy intakes were generally in the same magnitude.

Regarding nutrients, there also was an enormous variability between different centers and even within most research sites. Variability in intake was particularly evident for vitamins A and C. In general, the lowest median intakes were above the lowest European Recommended Dietary Intake (ERDI); exceptions were vitamin B_2 (lowest ERDI, 1.0 mg/day), vitamin A (lowest ERDI, 700 μg retinol equivalents/day), and iron (lowest ERDI, 8 mg/day).[11] In some towns, considerable proportions of elderly men and women failed to meet the lowest ERDI for vitamins C, B_1, and B_2, calcium, and iron. This suggests that in some towns a considerable percentage might be at risk of vitamin or mineral deficiency.

In a recent German nationwide nutrition survey for the elderly, median intake was well above the recommended amount for all nutrients except dietary fiber, calcium, vitamin D, and folate, where 38, 35, 75, and 37%, respectively, did not reach two thirds of the recommended amount.[9] In several other studies, low intakes of these nutrients are also reported.[12–18] In addition, dietary intake of vitamins B_6[19,20] and B_2[13,18,20] is repeatedly reported to be inadequate.

14.2.1.2 Food and Meal Pattern

Not only energy and nutrient intake but also food and meal patterns are clearly different beween European countries. As for younger adults, the food pattern in southern countries is characterized by high intakes of grain, vegetables, fruit, lean meat, and olive oil. In northern countries a high consumption of milk products is typical, and Polish elderly, for example, consume great amounts of meat products.[21] Concerning fruit and vegetable consumption, a clear north–south difference was apparent in the SENECA study. In northern towns only about 10% of men and women recorded five or more servings per day, whereas in southern towns about one third did so. Differences between men and women were generally small; however, a constant trend could be noted that men recorded fewer servings of fruits and vegetables than women.[22]

The number of meals eaten per day ranges from six in Denmark to three in the south of France. In the south of Europe the cooked meal seems to mediate the beneficial effects of the Mediterranean diet.[23] Also, meal size is much different between northern and southern European countries, with a higher calorie intake around noon in the second group.

14.2.1.3 Nutritional Status

Regarding nutritional status, again great variation across Europe is reported. In the SENECA baseline study mean BMI values varied from 24.4 ± 3.8 to 30.3 ± 5.2 kg/m^2 among men and from 23.9 ± 3.6 to 30.5 ± 5.1 kg/m^2 among women age 70 to 75 years—with the lowest mean values reported from Norway (men) and central France (women) and the highest from central Italy (men and women) and Poland (women).[24]

Underweight—defined as BMI of <20 kg/m^2—was only occasionally reported in the SENECA study. At baseline, 5% of men and 6% of women were affected, with the highest prevalence for men in Hungary (15%) and Norway (13%) and for women in central France (17%) and on Crete (14%).[24] Ten years later, 4% of male and 7% of female surviving participants (now between 80 and 85 years of age) were underweight.[25]

Overweight, in contrast, was widespread. Over all study centers, in 1989 18% of men and 28% of women showed BMI values of ≥30 kg/m^2. In some towns more than 40% of the participants were overweight. The highest prevalence was observed in central Italy (43% of men, 56% of women) and Poland (41% of men, 54% of women).[24]

In a German random sample of 1550 elderly men and women stratified in three age groups (65 to 74, 75 to 84, 85+ years) 2% of male and 6% of female participants were underweight and 13 and 18%, respectively, were obese. With increasing age, the prevalence of underweight significantly increased in both sexes, while the prevalence of overweight decreased.[26]

In a recent project gathering information about nutrition and lifestyle of elderly people in the Baltic, central, and eastern regions of the European Community, in these countries less than 10% of men and women were affected from undernutrition, whereas overnutrition was reported in several countries and age groups in more than 30%. Women seem to be generally more often afflicted with obesity than men.[27]

14.2.2 Institutionalized Elderly

In contrast to healthy free-living persons, elderly subjects suffering from multiple acute and chronic illnesses are often undernourished. Among the elderly admitted to the hospital, malnutrition is widespread and one of the most frequent and serious attendant symptoms. Prevalence figures up to 65% have been reported, depending on the patient characteristics and method used.[28–33]

In a recent multicenter study in Germany, the German Hospital Malnutrition Study, with around 2000 patients older than 18 years, the prevalence of malnutrition assessed by Subjective Global Assessment (SGA) was 27% in the total study population and clearly increased with age. By far the highest prevalence of malnutrition was observed in geriatric patients: 56% of 306 patients age 75 years or older from 3 geriatric departments were judged to be malnourished.[34]

This proportion is in accordance with other studies in Europe using the SGA, where 45,[35] 48,[36] and 56%[37] of geriatric patients were found to be malnourished.

In European long-term-care facilities several studies have shown a wide variation of malnutrition using the Mini-Nutritional Assessment (MNA) for nutritional assessment (Table 14.1).

The most comprehensive of these surveys was performed by Suominen et al.,[45] who studied malnutrition and associated factors among all aged residents living in

TABLE 14.1
Prevalence of Malnutrition (MNA < 17) and Risk of Malnutrition (MNA = 17 to 23.5) in Nursing Homes

First Author (year)	Country	n	Age (year)	MNA < 17	MNA = 17 to 23.5
Baldelli (2004)[38]	Italy	352	81 ± 8	38%	55%
Compan (1999)[39]	France	423	83 ± 10	25%	50%
Gerber (2003)[40]	Switzerland	78	86 ± 6	15%	58%
Griep (2000)[41]	Belgium	81	83 ± 7	2%	37%
Lamy (1998)[42]	Switzerland	120	81 ± 8	6%	57%
Ruiz-Lopez (2003)[43]	Spain	89	72–98	8%	62%
Salva (1999)[44]	Sweden	87	80 ± 9	6%	47%
Suominen (2005)[45]	Finland	2114	82 ± 9	29%	60%

Note: * indicates mean.

nursing homes in Helsinki, Finland. According to the MNA, one third of the 2114 residents (mean age, 82 years) suffered from malnutrition and 60% were at risk. In a logistic regression analysis malnutrition was associated with impaired functioning, swallowing difficulties, dementia, constipation, and eating less than half of the offered portion.

In a Swedish study, the nutritional status in institutionalized elderly in different settings was studied: service flat, old people's homes, group living for the demented, and nursing home. With increasing dependence and need for assistance, nutritional status worsened. The prevalence of malnutrition (MNA <17) increased from 21% in service flats up to 71% in nursing homes.[46]

14.3 DIAGNOSING UNDERNUTRITION IN EUROPE

The practice of diagnosing undernutrition in the elderly varies considerably across the European countries. It also differs greatly between institutions caring for geriatric patients. In many European countries, resources have not been available for the diagnosis and treatment of nutrition-related diseases to an extent necessary to develop successful strategies. Therefore, screening and assessment tools have to be quick and practical. Otherwise, they will not be used in daily routine. This holds true for all settings.

In 2003, the Council of Europe passed a resolution on food and nutritional care in hospitals. It pointed to an "unacceptable number of undernourished hospital patients in Europe," which is especially true for the population of geriatric patients. The council mentioned that "undernutrition of hospital patients leads to extended hospital stays, prolonged rehabilitation, diminished quality of life and unnecessary costs to health care." Furthermore, it declared the "access to a safe and healthy variety of food a fundamental human right." The effects of proper food service and nutritional care in hospitals on the recovery of patients and their quality of life were regarded as beneficial.

Based on these assumptions, the governments of the member states were recommended, among other aspects:

a. To draw up and implement national recommendations on food and nutritional care in hospitals, including nutritional assessment and treatment
b. To promote the implementation and take steps toward the application of principles and measures concerning nutritional assesment and treatment in hospitals
c. To ensure the widest possible dissemination of this resolution among all parties concerned

Three years later some important steps were taken toward the realization of some of these aspects, but in most European countries the recommendations of the Council of Europe have not been put in practice yet.

Bearing in mind that the highest prevalence rate of undernutrition is constantly observed among geriatric hospital patients, the resolution is of special importance for all those involved in the nutritional care for the elderly in this setting.

The knowledge about individual parameters reflecting a person's nutritional status, like oral intake, weight loss, absolute weight, anthropometric data, and hepatic plasma proteins, is widely spread over all European countries. National and international societies as well as international publications have helped to bring forward the most important facts on this topic. The general European opinion on most of these items should not be different from the way things are seen in the U.S. or elsewhere.

When evaluating the nutritional status in an elderly person it is necessary not to concentrate on a single parameter but to get a broader view combining the available information on energy stores (fat mass), muscle mass, micronutrient deficiencies, and disease-related weight loss.[47] For simple diagnosis of undernutrition in the elderly, a BMI below 22 kg/m^2, weight loss (>5% in 3 months, >10% in 6 months), oral energy intake, and disease-related energy requirements are essential.

Among the anthropometric measurements, calf circumference may be regarded as very valuable because it is significantly associated with an individual's muscle mass and functionality.[48,49]

With regard to anthropometric parameters for exact interpretation, the ethnic diversity within Europe should be considered. At present, study data reflecting this heterogenity, especially for the elderly population, are lacking.

Furthermore, no single parameter will allow the diagnosis of undernutrition in the elderly with sufficient sensitivity and specificity. In a recent study from Sweden that used a BMI of <22 kg/m^2 or weight loss of >5% of body weight as a criterion for malnutrition in patients at risk, no association between malnutrition and length of stay, discharge destination, or aid from the social welfare system could be demonstrated.[50] More specific assessments may be necessary. Therefore, it has been a logical aim to establish a screening and assessment tool that combines the answers to several key questions with a number of measurements.

In Europe the most established tools for application in the elderly are the Mini-Nutritonal Assessment (MNA), the Nutritional Risk Screening 2002 (NRS 2002), and the Subjective Global Assessment (SGA).

On a scientific level, no universally accepted tool has been implemented up to now with regard to the screening and assessment of undernutrition in the elderly.

In 2003, the European Society for Clinical Nutrition and Metabolism (ESPEN) published guidelines for nutrition screening.[51] They include a set of standards that are applicable for general use within the present healthcare resources. The key concepts of these guidelines will be outlined below.

According to ESPEN, the purpose of nutrition screening is to predict not only the probability of a better or worse outcome due to nutritional factors, but also, if not even more important, whether nutritional treatment is likely to influence this. Outcome has to be assessed with regard to the improvement or prevention of deterioration in mental and physical function, reduced number or severity of complications, accelerated recovery, and reduced consumption of resources.

In this context, the authors stress the importance of predicitve validity for the screening tools. The screened individual who has been tested as malnourished or at risk must have a high probability to benefit from measures taken on the basis of the test result. According to ESPEN, the tests also should be practical and offer a high reliability. Each institution where nutrition screening is routinely undertaken should produce a standard care plan for the malnourished and those at risk, which reflects local resources and which offers individual adaptability. Monitoring the outcome should be part of the whole process.[51]

The typical ESPEN screening tool should include three to four essential components:

- Description of the present condition (e.g., BMI)
- Description of the stability of the condition (weight loss)
- Probability of deterioration of the condition (oral intake)
- Influence of disease processes on the condition (especially in hospitals)

The Malnutrition Universal Screening Tool (MUST) (Figure 14.1) and NRS 2002 (Figure 14.2) are highly based on these assumptions.

The measurement of weight and height in sick elderly persons may be difficult. Therefore, a screening tool not relying on these measurements may be advantageous. The MUST was originally developed by the British Association for Parenteral and Enteral Nutrition (BAPEN) for use in the community.[52] It includes three clinical parameters and rates each parameter as 0, 1, or 2 as follows: BMI of >20 kg/m^2 = 0, 18.5 to 20.0 kg/m^2 = 1, <18.5 kg/m^2 = 2; weight loss of <5% = 0, 5 to 10% = 1,

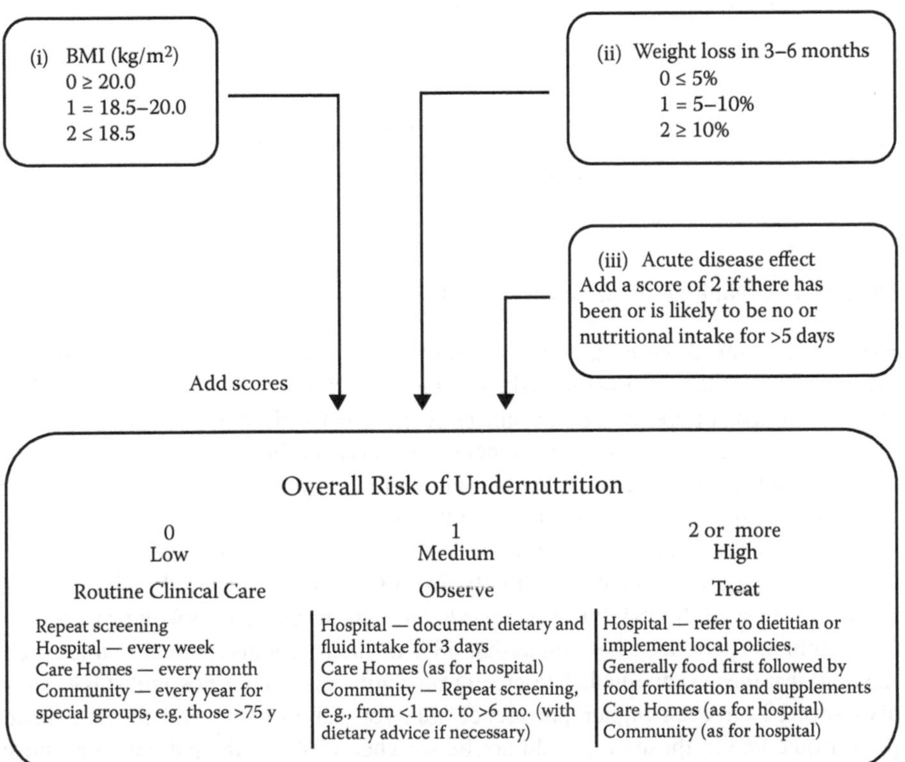

FIGURE 14.1 Malnutrition Universal Screening Tool (MUST) for adults.

Table 1 Initial screening			
		Yes	No
1	Is BMI <20.5?		
2	Has the patient lost weight within the last 3 months?		
3	Has the patient had a reduced dietary intake in the last week?		
4	Is the patient severely ill ? (e.g. in intensive therapy)		

Yes: If the answer is 'Yes' to any question, the screening in Table 2 is performed.
No: If the answer is 'No' to all questions, the patient is re-screened at weekly intervals. If the patient e.g. is scheduled for a major operation, a preventive nutritional care plan is considered to avoid the associated risk status.

Table 2 Final screening			
	Impaired nutritional status		**Severity of disease (≈ increase in requirements)**
Absent **Score 0**	Normal nutritional status	Absent **Score 0**	Normal nutritional requirements
Mild **Score 1**	Wt loss >5% in 3 mths or Food intake below 50–75% of normal requirement in preceding week	Mild **Score 1**	Hip fracture* Chronic patients, in particular with acute complications: cirrhosis*, COPD*. *Chronic hemodialysis, diabetes, oncology*
Moderate **Score 2**	Wt loss >5% in 2 mths or BMI 18.5 – 20.5 + impaired general condition or Food intake 25–60% of normal requirement in preceding week	Moderate **Score 2**	Major abdominal surgery* Stroke* *Severe pneumonia, hematologic malignancy*
Severe **Score 3**	Wt loss >5% in 1 mth (>15% in 3 mths) or BMI <18.5 + impaired general condition or Food intake 0-25% of normal requirement in preceding week in preceding week.	Severe **Score 3**	Head injury* Bone marrow transplantation* *Intensive care patients (APACHE>10).*
Score:	+	**Score:**	**=Total score**
Age	if ≥70 years: add 1 to total score above	**=age-adjusted total score**	

Score ≥3: the patient is nutritionally at-risk and a nutritional care plan is initiated
Score <3: weekly rescreening of the patient. If the patient e.g. is scheduled for a major operation, a preventive nutritional care plan is considered to avoid the associated risk status.

NRS-2002 is based on an interpre-tation of available randomized clinical trials. *indicates that a trial directly supports the categorization of patients with that diagnosis. Diagnoses shown in *italics* are based on the prototypes given below.

Nutritional risk is defined by the present **nutritional status** and risk of impairment of present status, due to **increased requirements** caused by stress metabolism of the clinical condition.

A nutritional care plan is indicated in all patients who are

(1) severely undernourished (score = 3), or (2) severely ill (score = 3), or (3) moderately undernourished + mildly ill (score 2 + 1), or (4) mildly undernourished + moderately ill (score 1 + 2).

Prototypes for severity of disease

Score = 1: a patient with chronic disease, admitted to hospital due to complications. The patient is weak but out of bed regularly. Protein requirement is increased, but can be covered by oral diet or supplements in most cases.

Score = 2: a patient confined to bed due to illness, e.g. following major abdominal surgery. Protein requirement is substantially increased, but can be covered, although artificial feeding is required in many cases.

Score = 3: a patient in intensive care with assisted ventilation etc. Protein requirement is increased and cannot be covered even by artificial feeding. Protein breakdown and nitrogen loss can be significantly attenuated.

FIGURE 14.2 National Risk Screening (NRS 2002).

>10% = 2; acute disease: absent = 0, present = 2. Overall risk of malnutrition is established as follows: 0 = low risk, 1 = medium risk, 2 = high risk. The MUST can be adapted for special circumstances (e.g., when weight and height cannot be measured) using alternative measurements (recalled height or weight, knee height), including subjective criteria. It has a high degree of reliability (low interobserver variation) with = 0.88 to 1.00. Recently several studies have been published showing its successful application in hospital patients.[53] Furthermore, Stratton and coworkers tested it in acutely ill elderly. In this study, all included patients could be screened by the MUST.[54] It was regarded as easy to use and took approximately 3 to 5 min per patients. They found that 58% of their patients were at malnutrition risk and that these individuals had greater mortality and longer hospital stays. They also showed an even higher prevalence rate for malnutrition and an associated poorer outcome in those that could not be weighed (56% of the patients) or whose height could not be measured.

The Nutritional Risk Screening (NRS 2002) was originally designed for application in hospitals.[55] It is based on the concept that nutritional support is indicated in patients who have increased energy requirements as a consequence of severe acute or chronic disease, or who are severely undernourished, or who have certain degrees of acute or chronic disease in combination with certain degrees of undernutrition. The scale for severity of disease and undernutrition is based on the data from a selected number of randomized controlled trials and has been converted to a numeric score. The NRS 2002 is composed of a small screening part consisting of four questions (BMI, loss of weight, oral intake, stress). If one of these questions is answered yes, one is to proceed to the second part, which consists of two components. The first one graduates malnutrition with the help of BMI, weight loss, and oral intake; the second one reflects disease severity. One point is added to the score for age above 70.

In a retrospective evaluation the NRS 2002 was able to distinguish between trials with a positive effect and those with no effect of nutritional support on clinical outcome. This result was clearer for studies involving enteral nutrition than for trials testing the effect of parenteral nutrition. According to the authors, the NRS 2002 can identify patients who are likely to benefit from nutritional support. In a study by Johansen and coworkers, the NRS 2002 could be applied successfully in 99% of patients. The interobserver variability between a physician, a nurse, and a dietitian was tested to have = 0.67. Possibly there may have been some discrepancies with regard to the classification of the severity of the patients' acute or chronic diseases.[56]

The Mini-Nutritional Assessment (MNA) has been assigned to be an ESPEN screening tool for the elderly. It will be a valuable instrument for application in the frail elderly who are on the edge of dependence and can cooperate in the completion of the tool. In nursing home inhabitants and in geriatric hospital patients the MNA often may not be applicable. Problems are obvious with regard to the demented and aphasic elderly. Patients with a PEG are not suitable for screening with the MNA at all. Similiar difficulties are present in severely ill geriatric patients in hospitals. In one study from Germany, the MNA could be completed only in 66.1% of participants.[35] Another large study from a geriatric clinic in Geneva, Switzerland, supports this view.[57] In the Swiss geriatric patients, mortality was significantly higher in those who were not tested by the MNA, probably because sicker patients were not submitted to the MNA.

In another Swiss study, the correlations of the NRS 2002 and the MUST with anthropometric and body composition parameters in geriatric hospital patients were slightly higher than those for the SGA. Furthermore, a significant association between nutritional status according to NRS 2002 or MUST and length of stay could be shown in this population.[53] This association was stronger for the NRS 2002, which therefore may be regarded as superior in the hospital setting.

In summary, the applicability of the MNA may be limited under certain circumstances. The MUST for the community setting or the NRS 2002 for nursing homes and hospitals may be valuable alternatives. The ease of their application supports this view.

With regard to the decision to use a certain malnutrition screening tool it has to be taken into account whether it is to be used for scientific or practical purposes.

Randomized controlled trials that test the effects of screening and assessment on the success of associated care plans in elderly patients with malnutrition are lacking.

In future intervention studies, it will be necessary to characterize the study population by parameters or instruments that are well known and established. Here the restriction to the above-mentioned screening tools may be helpful. The ever-increasing number of new screening instruments will make the comparison of study populations difficult.

Among the technical methods that may be used for the analysis of body composition, bioelectrical impedance analysis is the most widely known in Europe.[58] Bioelectrical impedance analysis (BIA) is considered to be a simple, fast, and noninvasive bedside technique. Nevertheless, it is not routine practice in most institutions or among community practitioners, even for those who are interested in nutrition. Among the data generated by the bioelectrical analysis, the phase angle has been regarded to be the most useful parameter. It has been shown that it is associated with outcome in different chronic diseases with accompanying malnutrition. But still there is some debate about the correct interpretation of data in the elderly. Comorbidity and instability of fluid balance reduce the reliability of BIA, especially in the elderly. Only recently have reference values for the elderly in Europe been published.[59] At present, bioelectrical impedance analysis will be a useful and reliable method only in the hands of experts.

14.4 UNDERNUTRITION AND THE ESPEN GUIDELINES ON ENTERAL NUTRITION: GERIATRICS

In spring 2006, the ESPEN Guidelines on Enteral Nutrition were published.[60] In comparison with the ASPEN guidelines,[61] they address the issues of nutrition in the elderly population in a more detailed fashion. The expert group also commented on the indication of enteral nutrition in patients with undernutrition. For them, undernutrition and the risk of undernutrition represent essential and independent indications for enteral nutrition in geriatric patients. Oral nutritional supplements are recommended in order to increase energy, protein, and micronutrient intake, maintain or improve nutritional status, and improve survival in patients who are undernourished or at risk of undernutrition (Class A recommendation). Oral nutritional supplementation or tube feeding is recommended early in patients at nutritional risk (e.g., insufficient nutritional intake, unintended weight loss of >5% in 3 months or >10% in 6 months, BMI <20 kg/m^2) (Class B recommendation). These recommendations are to a large extent based on the Cochrane analysis of Milne et al. from 2005.[62] In another section the ESPEN expert group also comments on the indication of enteral nutrition in frail elderly. Oral nutritional supplements are recommended in order to improve or maintain nutritional status (Class A recommendation). Furthermore, the elderly may benefit from tube feeding as long as they are not in a terminal phase of illness. Tube feeding is therefore recommended early in case of nutritional risk (Class B recommendation), where normal food intake is insufficient.

Tube feeding is explicitly not recommended in frail elderly who have progressed to an irreversible final stage.

14.5 PERSPECTIVES ON THE AWARENESS OF MALNUTRITION IN THE ELDERLY AND ON NUTRITIONAL INTERVENTION

As far as our experience goes, awareness of nutritional problems in daily routine is generally low. It can be argued that several options in nutritional care are underused, and thus there is a potential for improvement of nutritional care. Guidelines for the special needs of the elderly should be developed and implemented. Nutritional screening and assessment should become routine procedures followed by adequate nutritional interventions.

In some of the European countries special initiatives concentrating on the problem of malnutrition in the elderly have been started. For example, the German Allianz gegen Mangelernährung may be mentioned. Here experts aim to raise public awareness of the problem with the help of public relation networks. In France, the National Nutrition-Health Program deals in part with the diagnosis and treatment of malnutrition in the elderly.

On the expert level, it may be stated that in several studies various interventions to improve the nutritional situation in nursing homes and hospitals have been tested, for example, improvement of meal ambience,[63,64] energy-dense food,[65] or nutritional supplements.[62,66] However, there is still a need for more studies showing whether and which nutritional interventions may improve nutritional status and outcome among the European elderly who have overt malnutrition or are at risk.

REFERENCES

1. European Health Report 2005, http://www.euro.who.int/ehr2005, accessed September 2006.
2. Europäische Kommission, Eurostat Jahrbuch 2004, *Amt für amtliche Veröffentlichungen der Europäischen Gemeinschaft*, 2004.
3. de Groot, L.C.P.G.M., Hautvast, J.G.A.J., and van Staveren, W.A., Euronut-SENECA: nutrition and the elderly in Europe, *Eur. J. Clin. Nutr.*, 45, 1, 1991.
4. de Groot, C.P.G.M. et al., Eds., SENECA: nutrition and the elderly in Europe. Follow-up study and longitudinal analysis, *Eur. J. Clin. Nutr.*, 50 (Suppl. 2), S1, 1996.
5. Moreiras-Varela, O. et al., Euronut-SENECA: nutrition and the elderly in Europe. Intake of energy and nutrients, *Eur. J. Clin. Nutr.*, 45, 105, 1991.
6. Moreiras, O. et al., Longitudinal changes in the intake of energy and macronutrient of elderly Europeans, *Eur. J. Clin. Nutr.*, 50, S67, 1996.
7. Sulander, T. et al., Changes and associations in healthy diet among the Finnish elderly, 1985–2001, *Age Ageing*, 32, 394, 2003.
8. Huijbregts, P.P.C.W. et al., Dietary intake in five ageing cohorts of men in Finland, Italy and the Netherlands, *Eur. J. Clin. Nutr.*, 49, 852, 1995.
9. Volkert, D. et al., Energy and nutrient intake of young-old, old-old and very-old elderly in Germany, *Eur. J. Clin. Nutr.*, 58, 1190, 2004.

10. Bates, C.J., Prentice, A., and Finch, S., Gender differences in food and nutrient intakes and status indices from the National Diet and Nutrition Survey of people aged 65 years and over, *Eur. J. Clin. Nutr.*, 53, 694, 1999.
11. Amorim Cruz, J.A. et al., Euronut-SENECA: intake of vitamins and minerals, *Eur. J. Clin. Nutr.*, 45, 121, 1991.
12. Bates, C.J. et al., Micronutrients: highlights and research challenges from the 1994–5 National Diet and Nutrition Survey of people aged 65 years and over, *Br. J. Nutr.*, 82, 7, 1999.
13. Bianchetti, A. et al., Nutritional intake, socioeconomic conditions and health status in a large elderly population, *J. Am. Geriatr. Soc.*, 38, 521, 1990.
14. Campillo, J.E. et al., Vitamins and mineral intake in elderly people from Extremadura, *J. Nutr. Health Aging*, 6, 55, 2002.
15. Hurson, M., Corish, C., and Sugrue, S., Dietary intakes in Ireland of a healthy elderly population, *Ir. J. Med. Sci.*, 166, 220, 1997.
16. Martins, I. et al., Vitamin and mineral intakes in elderly, *J. Nutr. Health Aging*, 6, 63, 2002.
17. Nydahl, M. et al., Food and nutrient intake in a group of self-managing elderly Swedish women, *J. Nutr. Health Aging*, 7, 67, 2003.
18. Wierzbicka, E., Brzozowska, A., and Roszkowski, W., Energy and nutrients intake of elderly people living in the Warsaw region, Poland, *J. Nutr. Health Aging*, 5, 248, 2001.
19. Löwik, M.R.H. et al., Nutrition and aging: dietary intake of "apparently healthy" elderly (Dutch Nutrition Surveillance System), *J. Am. Coll. Nutr.*, 8, 347, 1989.
20. Nicolas, A.-S. et al., Nutrient adequacy of dietary intake in a healthy elderly French population, *Eur. J. Ger.*, 3, 140, 2001.
21. Schroll, K. et al., Food patterns of elderly Europeans, *Eur. J. Clin. Nutr.*, 50, S86, 1996.
22. Schlettwein-Gsell, D. et al., Fruit and vegetable servings in ten SENECA towns and the impact of the midday meal, *J. Nutr. Health Aging*, 5, 230, 2001.
23. Schlettwein-Gsell, D. et al., Nutrient intake of healthy elderly subjects, in *Malnutrition in the Elderly*, Seiler, W.O. and Stähelin, H.B., Eds., Steinkopf Verlag, Darmstadt, 1999, p. 1.
24. de Groot, C.P.G.M. et al., Euronut-SENECA: nutrition and the elderly in Europe. Nutritional status: anthropometry, *Eur. J. Clin. Nutr.*, 45 (Suppl. 3), 31, 1991.
25. de Groot, C.P. et al., Ten-year changes in anthropometric characteristics of elderly Europeans, *J. Nutr. Health Aging*, 6, 4, 2002.
26. Stehle, P. et al., Ernährung älterer Menschen, in *Ernährungsbericht 2000*, Deutsche Gesellschaft für Ernährung (DGE), Ed., Druckerei Henrich GmbH, Frankfurt am Main, 2000, p. 147.
27. *Aging Nutrition: Comparative Analysis of Existing Data on Nutrition and Lifestyle of the Ageing Population in Europe, Especially in the "New" Baltic, Central and Eastern Regions of the Community*, research project funded by the European Commission, final report, 2006.
28. Dormenval, V. et al., Associations between malnutrition, poor general health and oral dryness in hospitalized elderly patients, *Age Ageing*, 27, 123, 1998.
29. Gariballa, S.E. et al., Nutritional status of hospitalized acute stroke patients, *Br. J. Nutr.*, 79, 481, 1998.
30. Greer, A., McBride, D.H., and Shenkin, A., Comparison of the nutritional state of new and long-term patients in a psychogeriatric unit, *Br. J. Psychiatry*, 149, 738, 1986.
31. Mowé, M. and Bohmer, T., The prevalence of undiagnosed protein-calorie undernutrition in a population of hospitalized elderly patients, *J. Am. Geriatr. Soc.*, 39, 1089, 1991.

32. Mühlethaler, R. et al., The prognostic significance of protein-energy malnutrition in geriatric patients, *Age Ageing*, 24, 193, 1995.
33. Ponzer, S. et al., Nutritional status, insulin-like growth factor-1 and quality of life in elderly women with hip fractures, *Clin. Nutr.*, 18, 241, 1999.
34. Pirlich, M. et al., The German hospital malnutrition study, *Clin. Nutr.*, 25, 563, 2006.
35. Bauer, J.M. et al., Comparison of the Mini Nutritional Assessment, Subjective Global Assessment, and Nutritional Risk Screening (NRS 2002) for nutritional screening and assessment in geriatric hospital patients, *Z. Gerontol. Geriatr.*, 38, 322, 2005.
36. Ek, A.-C. et al., Interrater variability and validity in subjective nutritional assessment of elderly patients, *Scan. J. Caring Sci.*, 10, 163, 1996.
37. Incalzi, R.A. et al., Nutritional assessment: a primary component of multidimensional geriatric assessment in the acute care setting, *J. Am. Geriatr. Soc.*, 44, 166, 1996.
38. Baldelli, M.V. et al., Evaluation of the nutritional status during stay in the subacute care nursing home, *Arch. Gerontol. Geriatr. Suppl.*, 9, 39, 2004.
39. Compan, B. et al., Epidemiological study of malnutrition in elderly patients in acute, sub-acute and long-term care using the MNA, *J. Nutr. Health Aging*, 3, 146, 1999.
40. Gerber, V. et al., Nutritional status using the Mini Nutritional Assessment questionnaire and its relationship with bone quality in a population of institutionalized elderly women, *J. Nutr. Health Aging*, 7, 140, 2003.
41. Griep, M.I. et al., Risk of malnutrition in retirement homes elderly persons measured by the "Mini-Nutritional Assessment," *J. Gerontol.*, 55A, M57, 2000.
42. Lamy, M. et al., Oral status and nutrition in the institutionalized elderly, *J. Dent.*, 27, 443, 1999.
43. Ruiz-Lopez, M.D. et al., Nutritional risk in institutionalized older women determined by the Mini Nutritional Assessment test: what are the main factors? *Nutrition*, 19, 767, 2003.
44. Salva, A., Jose Bleda, M., and Bolibar, I., The Mini Nutritional Assessment in clinical practice, *Nestle Nutr. Workshop Ser. Clin. Perform. Programme*, 1, 123, 1999.
45. Suominen, M. et al., Malnutrition and associated factors among aged residents in all nursing homes in Helsinki, *Eur. J. Clin. Nutr.*, 59, 578, 2005.
46. Saletti, A. et al., Nutritional status according to Mini Nutritional Assessment in an institutionalized elderly population in Sweden, *Gerontology*, 46, 139, 2000.
47. Volkert, D., DGEM and DGG guidelines of enteral nutrition: nutritional status, energy and substrate metabolism in the elderly, *Aktuelle Ernaehrungsmedizin*, 29, 190, 2004.
48. World Health Organization, *Physical Status: The Use and Interpretation of Anthropometry*, Report of a WHO Expert Committee, Geneva, 1995.
49. Rolland, Y. et al., Sarcopenia, calf circumference, and physical function of elderly women: a cross-sectional study, *J Am Geriatr Soc.*, 51, 1120, 2003.
50. Brantervik, A.M. et al., Older hospitalised patients at risk of malnutrition: correlation with quality of life, aid from the social welfare system and length of stay? *Age Aging*, 34, 444, 2005.
51. Kondrup, J. et al., ESPEN guidelines for nutrition screening 2002, *Clin. Nutr.*, 22, 415, 2003.
52. Stratton, R.J. et al., Malnutrition in hospital outpatients and inpatients: prevalence, concurrent validity and ease of use of the "Malnutrition Universal Screening Tool (MUST)" for adults, *Br. J. Nutr.*, 92, 799, 2004.
53. Kyle, U.G. et al., Comparison of tools for nutritional assessment and screening at hospital admission: a population study, *Clin. Nutr.*, 25, 409, 2006.
54. Stratton, R.J. et al., "Malnutrition Universal Screening Tool" predicts mortality and length of stay in acutely ill elderly, *Br. J. Nutr.*, 95, 325, 2006.

55. Kondrup, J. et al., Ad Hoc ESPEN Working Group. Nutritional risk screening (NRS 2002): a new method based on an analysis of controlled clinical trials, *Clin. Nutr.*, 22, 321, 2003.
56. Johansen, N. et al., Effect of nutritional support on clinical outcome in patients at nutritional at risk, *Clin. Nutr.*, 23, 539, 2004.
57. Van Nes, M.C. et al., Does the Mini Nutritional Assessment predict hospitalization outcomes in older people? *Age Aging*, 30, 221, 2001.
58. Kyle, U.G., Bosaeus, I., and De Lorenzo, A.D., Bioelectrical impedance analysis. I. Review of principles and methods, *Clin. Nutr.*, 23, 1226, 2004.
59. Kyle, U.G. et al., Comparison of fat-free mass and body fat in Swiss and American adults, *Nutrition*, 21, 161, 2005.
60. Volkert, D. et al., ESPEN Guidelines on Enteral Nutrition: geriatrics. *Clin. Nutr.*, 25, 330, 2006.
61. A.S.P.E.N. Board of Directors and the Clinical Guidelines Task Force, Geriatrics in guidelines for the use of parenteral and enteral nutrition in adult and pediatric patients, *J. Parent. Enteral Nutr.*, 26 (Suppl.), 51, 2002.
62. Milne, A.C., Potter, J., and Avenell, A., Protein and energy supplementation in elderly people at risk from malnutrition, *Cochrane Database Syst. Rev*, 1, CD003288, 2005.
63. Nijs, K.A. et al., Effect of family style mealtimes on quality of life, physical performance, and body weight of nursing home residents: cluster randomised controlled trial, *Br. Med. J.*, 332, 1180, 2006.
64. Mathey, M.F. et al., Health effect of improved meal ambiance in a Dutch nursing home: a 1-year intervention study, *Prev. Med.*, 32, 416, 2001.
65. Olin, A.Ö. et al., Energy enriched meals improve energy intake in elderly residents in a nursing home, *Clin. Nutr.*, 17 (Suppl. 1), 31, 1998.
66. Potter, J.M., Oral supplements in the elderly, *Curr. Opin. Clin. Nutr. Metab. Care*, 4, 21, 2001.

15 The Oral Cavity and Nutrition

Nathalia Garcia, D.D.S.
D. Douglas Miley, D.M.D., M.S.D.

CONTENTS

15.1 INTRODUCTION

Oral health is an integral part of health, nutrition, and quality of life for the elderly population. The prevalence and severity of oral health problems are assumed to be underestimated among older adults. This is compounded with inadequate oral health care in some institutional settings and lack of dental insurance.[1]

Oral health and nutrition have a synergistic relationship. Oral infectious diseases, as well as acute, chronic, and terminal systemic diseases with oral manifestations, impact the functional ability to eat as well as diet and nutritional status. Oral problems may lead to chronic pain, discomfort, and subsequently poor diet.[2] Likewise, nutrition and diet may affect the development and integrity of the oral cavity as well as the progression of oral diseases.[3]

According to the Surgeon General's report *Oral Health in America*, diet and nutrition are major multifactorial environmental factors in the etiology and pathogenesis of craniofacial diseases and disorders. This report noted that elders are at particularly high risk for oral health problems, and poor oral health in seniors has been linked to general systemic health risks such as cardiovascular disease, stroke, poor nutrition, and respiratory infection.[4]

The possible association between oral conditions and systemic diseases involves different mediator factors, such as infection, chronic inflammation, and genetic predisposition to oral and systemic disease. Nutrition has also been proposed as a mediator. The presence and severity of many oral conditions may correlate to nutrient intake and nutritional status.[5]

Since 1900, the percentage of Americans age 65 and over has more than tripled. A greater number of elderly are also retaining their natural teeth. Older adults report more primary health care provider visits annually than dental visits, which are often not covered by health insurance for seniors. Elderly individuals who have their natural teeth then remain at risk for oral disease and disability.[6]

Numerous studies have found that fewer remaining teeth, edentulism, poorer masticatory function caries, and other oral problems are associated with decreased nutrient intake.[7,8] Selecting foods of lower nutritional quality and avoiding fiber-containing foods are also consequences of these dental problems.[9]

15.2 NORMAL FUNCTION: MOISTENING, MASTICATION, AND TASTING

Taste occurs during mastication and swallowing when chemicals in foods come in contact with taste buds. (The sense of smell also contributes to taste perception.) Taste buds are found on the dorsal surface of the tongue, the soft palate, pharynx, larynx, epiglottis, uvula, and the upper third of the esophagus.[10] Taste cells transmit signals regarding quality (e.g., bitter) and intensity. Like olfactory receptor cells, taste cells constantly reproduce with a life span of approximately 10 to 101 days. Taste receptor cells are replenished continually from a basal cell stem population. Taste receptor cells contain taste pores that are the initial site of signal transduction. Tastants must travel through salivary secretions and mucus to reach the taste buds and interact with the taste receptor cells. Saliva is a necessary component of taste transduction because it plays an essential role in the transport of water-soluble tastants. These tastant molecules may need a soluble carrier protein to reach the taste receptor. All components of the taste signal pathway are vulnerable to disease states and malnutrition that can impair reproduction and taste sensitivity.[11] Taste cells can detect five primary taste sensations: sweet, sour, salty, bitter, and umami (the taste of protein that includes the synergistic combination of glutamates and 50 nucleotides).[12]

Recent reports relating aging to anatomic changes in taste yield conflicting results.[13] In normal healthy aging adults, just a few taste cells are loss; however, changes in taste perception occur in older adults, both in the detection of taste (discriminating a tastant from water) and in the recognition of the type of taste. Older adults have more difficulty detecting salty, bitter, and less so, sweet. These modest changes are amplified among older adults who have chronic medical conditions and are taking multiple medications.[2]

Very few studies have evaluated nutritional changes among people with reduced or altered taste. No real differences have been noted in these subjects with regard to nutrient intake. Patients with taste distortion have been more likely to report altering their intake than people without taste distortion or patients with taste loss. One study evaluated 65 patients with dysgeusia. In this intervention, nutrient intake decreased progressively as dysgeusia severity increased, especially for vitamins A and C and calcium.[5]

Older adults have a decreased ability to identify foods based on taste; this decrease appears to be exacerbated in conditions of malnutrition and cachexia.[14] Oral conditions also may interfere with taste. These conditions may be a result of the aging process or secondary to systemic problems and treatments like medications, radiotherapy, and chemotherapy (Box 15.1).

Box 15.1 Oral Factors Associated with Altered Taste Disorders in the Elderly

Conditions	Therapy
Mucosal trauma	Anesthetic
Soft tissue lesions	Dentures
Caries and periodontal disease	Oral mouth rinses, gels, tooth paste
Xerostomia	Medications
Oral candidiasis	Oral galvanism (dental material interactions)
Oral liquen planus	Chemotherapy
Burning mouth syndrome	Radiation therapy (head and neck)
Dentoalveolar infections	Cancer surgery
Tooth loss	
Impaired chewing	

Tooth loss is a frequent finding in older individuals and may affect diet selection, chewing, and swallowing, which are involved in taste. Replacement of lost teeth with a removable prosthesis may result in decline in masticatory function. Taste cells and dentures that cover the palate have been reported to alter flavor and recognition thresholds.[2]

The number and distribution of teeth influence the ease of chewing, as does the functional capacity of complete or partial dentures. Chewing with conventionally retained dentures can be a very complex action, where the prostheses are controlled by the oral musculature and the forces of adhesion and cohesion holding them in place against the edentulous mucosa. The food itself will act as a destabilizing influence in this process as forces are applied eccentrically to the dentures, unless the bolus can be manipulated such that chewing occurs simultaneously on the right and left sides. These effects are only made worse in someone with impaired salivary output in whom denture stability and tolerance will also be reduced.

Changes in taste carry several nutritional implications. Decreased perception of salty qualities has been associated with an increased preference for salt. For individuals with hypertension, this loss in salt perception may make it difficult to adhere to a low-salt diet.[2] Likewise, changes in sweet taste perception may make older adults with diabetes more prone to consume excess sucrose. Studies in healthy older adults, however, have not shown a clear relationship between a decline in taste sensitivity and food intake. Other influences, such as habit and beliefs about food intake, may mask this relationship.[15]

15.3 ORAL CONDITIONS

15.3.1 Root Caries

Dental caries is a major cause of tooth loss in the U.S. Almost 80% of young adults and approximately 95% of older adults have experienced dental decay.[16]

Nearly one third of adults in the U.S. who are 65 years of age or older have untreated dental caries. Decay in aging is often seen around restorations, at the gingival margin, and on the root following exposure after receding gums (gingival recession).[17] In a 1998 study, it was found that the average 75-year-old had only 15 natural teeth.[18] The most important reason for tooth loss is dental caries, and there is more untreated decay in older adults, particularly in men, than in younger people.[19]

Root caries are progressive lesions limited to the root surface or involving the undermining of the cement–enamel junction (edge between dental crown and root),

TABLE 15.1
Oral Conditions in Older Population

Edentulous	33% of older American are edentulous
Periodontal disease	23% of adults between 65 and 74 years old have periodontitis
Oral and pharyngeal cancer	30,000 cases are diagnosed annually, primarily in the elderly
Mucosal diseases	
Candidiasis	3.6% of full denture wearers have candidiasis (the majority of them are old)
Denture stomatitis	25% of people have two full dentures
	32% of people have one full denture
	26% of people have partial dentures
	(the majority of people who use dentures are old)
Xerostomia	Most old Americans take medications; at least one of the medications has an oral side effect (usually xerostomia)

Source: U.S. Department of Health and Human Services, National Institute of Dental and Craniofacial Research, National Institutes of Health, *Oral Health in America: A Report of the Surgeon General*, Rockville, MD, 2000.

but they are clinically indicated to be initiated on the root surface. Gum recession and other risk factors for root caries, like xerostomia (dry mouth), poor oral hygiene, wearing partial dentures, or cleaning the dentures inappropriately, are more common in old age.[20,21] There is also a strong relationship between past root caries experience and the development of new lesions, and a weaker association between coronal decay history and root caries. Restoring the cavities caused by root caries is often difficult because of the position of the decay at the gingival margin, and extensive root caries can easily result in loss of the tooth.

Diet has a direct influence on the progression of tooth decay. There are strong links between sugars in the diet and caries in younger people. The frequency of intake of sugars, particularly added refined sugars, is most closely linked to decay experience. Among older people, this association remains strong for root caries. One of the risks for root caries is the higher pH for demineralization of enamel (crown) as compared to exposed dentin (root). The same level of sugar exposure that may not cause a problem in younger subjects may do so in older individuals, particularly if compounded by dry mouth or altered levels of salivary function.[21]

Improving dental hygiene through tooth brushing with fluoride toothpaste, flossing, and professional topical application of fluoride gel can have good results in preventing or detaining root caries.

15.3.2 Lesions in Oral Mucosa

Nutritional deficiency in the elderly may result in alterations in oral mucosal integrity, exacerbating age-associated changes in the oral tissue. The micronutrients most commonly associated with mucosal lesions include vitamin B12, iron, and folate, which may cause aphthous stomatitis, characterized by painful recurring ulcerations. Besides their effects on the oral mucosa, such deficiency is also associated with *Candida albicans* infection.

One of the first organs to react to vitamin inadequacies is the oral cavity, possibly because of the rapid rate of cell renewal of the mucous membrane. For example, vitamin C deficiency (scurvy) leads to an increased capillary fragility with bleeding gums, edematous, and ulcerated gingival tissue and delayed wound healing. Folate deficiency may be accompanied by red or pale smooth tongue and vitamin A deficiency by keratosis of the mucosa. Oral lesions like glossitis and glossopyritis (inflammation of or a burning sensation in the tongue) can be from a lack of B-group vitamins. Even though a vitamin deficit has to be severe for oral manifestations to appear, when they occur and persist for a long time, they can affect dental health.[22]

15.3.3 Oral Candidiasis

Candidiasis is a frequent oral mucosal infection in the elderly. This condition is very common in older adults because they are often edentulous and wear partial or complete dentures. In the past, this disease was considered to only be an opportunistic infection, affecting individuals who suffered another disease. Now it is recognized that oral candidiasis may develop in healthy people.

Salivary flow is a local factor that limits proliferation of *C. albicans*. Due to a reduced salivary flow, oral candida infections are seen more frequently in patients with xerostomia (dry mouth). Other predisposing factors, such as mouth breathing, recent use of antibiotics, topical or systemic immunosuppressant drugs, and general debilitation caused by underlying systemic disease, are often present in the elderly.[23]

Candidiasis is often accompanied by symptoms of burning and soreness in the mouth and increased sensitivity to acidic and spicy foods. Several different presentations of oral candidiasis can be encountered. One of the most common forms of this lesion in older patients is **denture stomatitis (chronic atrophic candidiasis)**, which is caused by continuous wearing of ill-fitting or inadequately cleaned dental appliances.[2] This condition is characterized by varying degrees of erythema, sometimes accompanied by petechial hemorrhage localized to the denture-bearing areas of a maxillary removable dental prosthesis.[24] Dentures should not be worn overnight but instead be immersed in a dilute hypochlorite solution. Topical antifungal agents like miconazole 2% in gel may be applied to the fitting surface of the upper denture.

Other presentations of this oral infection may be observed. **Pseudomembranous candidiasis** presents as a whitish plaque that, when removed, leaves a superficially denuded mucosal surface. It may occur anywhere in the oral cavity and it may be asymptomatic. On other occasions, patients may complain of taste alteration or burning sensation. **Erythematous (atrophic) candidiasisis** is characterized by a subtle smooth red patch. This change is often difficult to detect on a mucosal surface that is already somewhat red. **Hyperplastic candidiasis** presents as a thickened white patch that cannot be removed and may be symptomatic or asymptomatic.

Therapy for oral candidiasis may include the use of topical and systemic antifungal medications such as nystatin oral suspension, clotrimazole, amphotericin B oral suspension, and fluconazole tablets. Clorhexidine gluconate has been reported to have some antifungal properties, but this agent is best used for prevention rather than treatment.[24,25]

15.3.4 Angular Cheilitis

Angular cheilitis is a condition characterized by erythema and deep splits at the corners of the mouth. If severe, the splits or cracks may bleed when the mouth is opened and a shallow ulcer or a crust may form. This condition may be seen as a component of chronic candidiasis. Often it occurs alone, typically in elderly patients with a reduced vertical dimension of occlusion and pronounced folds at the corners of the mouth. These areas are usually moist because saliva tends to pool there and promote a micotic infection. Some cases are caused by *C. albicans* alone, but most are associated with both *C. albicans* and *Staphylococcus aureus*. Other common causes of this condition are vitamin B and iron deficiency.[24,26]

Patients exhibiting this condition are usually very symptomatic with local soreness, tenderness, pain, or burning. Treatment depends on the cause and can include lip lubrication, antifungal and antibiotic medications, vitamins, and new dentures for patients using old dentures in which the vertical dimension has been reduced owing to excessive wear of the teeth.

15.3.5 Recurrent Apthous Ulceration

Recurrent apthous ulcers are one of the most common oral mucosal findings. The prevalence of this condition ranges from 10 to 50% depending on the study population.[27]

The hypotheses for the pathogenesis of this lesion are numerous. Different subgroups of patients appear to have different causes for the occurrence of apthae. Trauma, allergies, nutritional deficiencies, hormonal influences, hematologic abnormalities, infectious agents, and stress are the most commons factors associated with these lesions.

This condition has been implicated with ulcerative colitis, Crohn's disease, celiac disease, and numerous vitamin deficiencies that may or may not be associated with a malabsorption disorder.[27] Gastrointestinal disorders should be considered possible etiologic agents in patients with persistent apthae or recurrent apthous ulcerations exhibiting a high rate of recurrence.[28] An increased prevalence of apthous-like ulcerations has been noted with many systemic diseases.[24]

Apthous ulcers appear as shallow and round with a surrounding band of erythema. These lesions often cause inadequate nutrition because patients feel very uncomfortable eating, particularly with spicy, salty, or sour foods. Most apthous ulcers heal without scarring in 10 to 14 days.

In patients with mild ulcerations, the therapy is topical corticosteroids. Major apthous lesions are more resistant to treatment and warrant more potent intralesional corticosteroids, such as triamcinolone 0.025% or clobetasol propionate 0.05% in orabase paste.

15.3.6 Atrophic Glossitis

Atrophic glossitis is characterized by painful burning tongue, inflammation, and defoliation. The loss of filiform papillae produces an erythematous and granular-appearing tongue, and the eventual complete atrophy of papillae produces a smooth tongue.

This condition is common in elderly patients and is considered to be a marker of nutritional deficiency. Atrophic glossitis has been associated with lack of vitamins or folic acid deficiency, but vitamin substitution does not always improve this disease.[23]

In 2000, Bohmer and Mowe conducted a study to examine the relationship between atrophic glossitis and the nutritional status in elderly people. They evaluated 310 patients recently admitted to the hospital and 106 randomly selected subjects at home. It was found that atrophic glossitis occurred in 13.2% of men and 5.6% of women at home and in 26.6% of men and 37% of women in the hospital. The condition was related to weight loss, body mass index, triceps skinfold thickness, arm muscle circumference, muscular strength, and concentrations of ascorbic acid and cholesterol. It was concluded that this condition is common in the elderly and is a marker for malnutrition and reduced muscle function.[29]

In some older patients, more than one nutrient may be deficient. Studies have found that atrophic glossitis has been related to protein-calorie malnutrition and also to low levels of vitamins C and D. Nutrients with a short half-life (e.g., vitamin C and the B vitamins) could be reduced long before the concentration of serum albumin is reduced and before deficiencies of lipid-soluble vitamins as A and D have developed. One or more factors might inhibit normal tongue development.[29]

15.3.7 Burning Mouth Syndrome (Stomatopyrosis)

Burning mouth syndrome is a common dysesthesia, especially in elderly women. It is characterized by a diffuse, dry burning sensation of the tongue, lips, and cheeks in the absence of clinically apparent mucosal alterations. In addition to the burning sensation, some patients may feel pain. Different factors have been associated with the syndrome, but none have been demonstrated. Although it has been believed that progesterone and estrogen deficit can cause this condition, there is not a strong correlation between such substances. Depression and anxiety states have also been linked with burning mouth syndrome.[24]

In stomatopyrosis, the tongue is the most commonly affected area. Mucosal changes are seldom visible, but some patients show a reduced number of filiform papillae. Patients with this condition describe altered taste and discomfort with increasing intensity throughout the day.[30]

Almost no treatment has been proven to be effective against this alteration, but some individuals with idiopathic disease have shown improvement of their symptoms when taking mood-altering drugs such as chlordiazepoxide.[24]

15.3.8 Periodontal Disease

Forty-one percent of adults in the U.S. who are over 65 years suffer from periodontal disease.[31] This condition is an oral infectious disease caused by bacterial plaque, which produces inflammation of the gingiva. If the inflammatory process is allowed to progress to involve the underlying alveolar bone and connective tissue, teeth loosen because of the lack of support from bony and connective tissues.

The pathogenesis of periodontal disease involves the interaction between bacteria and the host response to these bacteria. Numerous microorganisms are present in the subgingival flora (below the gum line). Systemic influences affect the disease and include the immune status of the host, hereditary factors, hormonal factors, smoking, stress, and some diseases such as diabetes. These factors might affect the severity and progression of this condition.[32]

Many reports have shown a possible association between periodontal disease and other chronic disease states, like cardiovascular disease.[33] Although longitudinal studies have indicated that the presence of alveolar bone loss, as a result of periodontitis, increases the risk of death from cardiovascular disease, it cannot be said that a direct relationship exists between these two conditions.[34] To date, much of the evidence has been based on epidemiological and historical data, including the National Health and Nutrition Examination Survey (NHANES) III. Prospective clinical studies in large populations are needed to identify the exact connection in greater detail.[3]

Diet, nutrition, and saliva play significant roles in the formation and maturation of dental plaque. The volume, physiochemical, and antibacterial properties of saliva can be affected in malnutrition states. Likewise, nutritional status has a direct influence on the synthesis and release of pro-inflammatory cytokines and their action. Consequently, malnutrition is associated with increased needs for calories and protein to promote wound healing and an improved immune response.

Nutrient deficiencies, such as vitamin C and calcium, may compromise the systemic response to inflammation and infection and alter nutrient needs. Theoretically, vitamin C could play a role at the level of tissue repair supporting collagen and bone formation or at the level of immune defense involving phagocytosis and chemotaxis.

Even though some studies have demonstrated that certain populations who consume low levels of vitamin C have significantly higher levels of periodontal disease, the role of vitamin C in preventing destructive periodontal disease is controversial, and there are not recommendations for supplemental doses of this vitamin.[35]

Removal of the chronic inflammatory stimuli from dental plaque is indispensable in diminishing the severity of periodontal disease. Good nutrition and dietary practices are also important in mitigating severe inflammatory periodontal lesions and promoting healing.

15.3.9 Osteoporosis and Periodontal Disease

Bone resorption and loss are common denominators for both periodontal disease and osteoporosis. The risk factors for osteoporosis include many of those associated with advanced periodontal disease. Since both osteoporosis and periodontitis are resorptive diseases, it has been hypothesized that osteoporosis could be a risk factor for the progression of periodontal disease.[36]

Many cross-sectional reports using different populations and different methods have discussed the relationship between systemic bone mineral density and oral bone density. The data obtained from most studies appear to indicate a relationship between the two. Findings have supported a positive association between osteoporosis and periodontitis; however, a causal relationship remains to be established. Cross-sectional studies have limitations and additional data from longitudinal studies are needed.[36]

Analysis of the third National Health and Nutrition Examination Survey (NHANES III) data demonstrated a relationship between low dietary calcium and increased risk of periodontal disease.[35] Numerous research studies have shown that calcium and vitamin D deficiencies increase inflammation and bone loss. This suggests that calcium deficiency could be a risk factor for periodontal disease. Although studies have demonstrated associations among tooth loss, low calcium intake, and periodontal disease, there has not been a clinical trial in which randomization and masking were controlled to determine the influence of calcium and vitamin D deficiency on periodontal disease.[37] No evidence supports recommendations for calcium intake beyond what is consistent with the Dietary Reference Intakes (DRIs) and for the treatment of osteoporosis.[3]

15.3.10 Oral Cancer

The most serious oral health conditions include oral and pharyngeal cancers; they are the sixth most common cancers worldwide. Each year in the U.S. approximately 28,900 new cases are diagnosed, and the majority of these are found in older adults. The median age at diagnosis of oral cancer is 64, and the recurrence rate rises with increasing age.[2] The American Cancer Society estimates about 30,900 new cases (20,180 in men and 10,810 in women) of oral cavity and oropharyngeal cancer will be diagnosed in the U.S. in 2006. The overall 5-year relative survival rate is 59%, and the 10-year survival rate is 48%. African Americans have the lowest survival rate at 34%. These survival rates have not changed much in the past 20 years.[38]

Tobacco and alcohol are the most important risk factors for oral and oropharyngeal cancers. Approximately 90% of people with these cancers smoke or chew tobacco. The risk of developing these lesions increases with the amount, frequency, and duration of the habit. Individuals with heavy alcohol consumption have six times more risk of developing these cancers.[30]

The most consistent findings on the role of diet and nutrition in the etiology of oral cancer are the positive effects of high fruit and vegetable consumption on the carcinogenic effect from alcohol consumption. The protective value of a diet rich in fruits and vegetables in reducing the risk of oral and pharyngeal cancers has been demonstrated. Research has demonstrated that vitamin C, carotene, and flavonoids found in citrus fruits and some vegetables have an inverse relationship with the incidence of oral cancer. The American Cancer Society recommends eating a variety of healthful foods, with an emphasis on plant sources. At least five servings of fruits and vegetables are recommended each day, as well as servings of whole grain foods from plant sources such as breads, cereals, and beans. It also suggested to eat fewer red meats and to avoid processed foods or those high in fat.[3]

Because patients with an early stage of the disease rarely have pain or other symptoms, detecting an early lesion is primarily dependent upon the clinician providing a comprehensive examination.[1] Oral cancer is usually treated by surgery, radiation therapy, or a combination of these treatments. The role of adjunctive chemotherapy is not clear yet. Treatment for cancer often produces oral complications that decrease appetite and intake. Radiation therapy of the oropharyngeal area can result in dental caries, loss of teeth, painful osteonecrosis and stomatitis, fibrosis of the muscles of mastication, and taste changes.[2] Common treatment for any type of cancer can also cause inflammation and infection of the oral mucosa and xerostomia, increasing the caries risk caused by a lack of saliva. Dietary management of this condition must include caries risk reduction measures. Surgical treatment increases the nutrient needs for wound healing and causes alterations in masticatory function that may permanently affect chewing and swallowing. Nutrition management should therefore consider functional abilities, appetite, and individual nutrient requirements.[3]

15.4 ORAL FUNCTION IN OLDER ADULTS

15.4.1 Muscles, Bone, and Temporomandibular Joint (TMJ) Function

The influence of age on masticatory muscles results in a reduction of muscle mass, the development of aponeurotic structures, a significant reduction in maximum tension, the loss of isometric and dynamic muscle strength, and a prolongation of the contraction time.[39] The muscle mass reduction directly affects the ability to chew food, which influences the choice of foods. The consumption of meat is often restricted in elderly people and may lead to nutritional deficiencies such as a lack of iron, resulting in anemia.[23]

The effect of tooth loss on masticatory muscles is controversial, although the number of teeth and bite force are considered essential factors for masticatory function.[39] The size and structure of the alveolar process of the jaws are connected to the presence of teeth; reduced mechanical load due to tooth loss reduces the density, stiffness, and strength of bone structure. The difference between dentate and edentulous individuals in terms of morphology and mechanical properties involves bone mass and components of the masticatory system, such as teeth, muscles, and osseous structures.[40] There is evidence that replacement of the natural dentition by dentures reduces the level of masticatory force and chewing efficiency. Nevertheless, many people wearing complete dentures often consider their masticatory function satisfactory.[39]

It is probable that age constitutes the predominant factor associated with degeneration of the TMJ. Temporomandibular disorder (TMD) covers many alterations, including masticatory muscle dysfunctions (such as myositis, muscle spasm, muscle contracture, and myofascial pain syndrome), temporomandibular joint disorders (such as inflammatory lesions and alteration of the condyle–disk complex), and chronic mandibular hypomobility and growth disorders.[41]

According to traditional beliefs, TMD increases concomitant with the loss of natural teeth, but some recent studies have concluded that the risk for TMD at an older age is minimal.[42,43] Loss of teeth and loss of occlusal support seem to have only a minor impact on the signs and symptoms of TMD in older populations. Prosthodontic treatment of the elderly patient should thus be for reasons to maintain masticatory function or aesthetics. For prevention of TMD, treatment does not seem to be warranted.[44] Maintenance of natural dentition or provision and maintenance of dentures improves the quality of life and nutritional intake.

15.4.2 Tooth Loss

Even though there has been a decrease in edentulism (total tooth loss) during the last several years, almost one of every four individuals over 65 has lost all of his or her teeth. This condition has negative esthetic and functional consequences by affecting speech and chewing capacity. It has been shown that individuals who have lost teeth suffer psychological effects; they lose self-confidence and feel more inhibited in their daily life.[45]

In the U.S., a high prevalence of edentulism has been reported for African American individuals, people with lower education levels, those without dental insurance, and current smokers. Edentulous individuals use less dental services than people who still have teeth, which decreases the probability to detect oral conditions and diseases.[4] Rates of edentulism are much higher among institutionalized individuals; 52% of nursing home residents are edentulous.[1,45]

Tooth loss may affect diet selection, chewing, and swallowing, which are involved in smell and taste. It has been reported that retronasal odor perception is improved significantly with mouth movements and that disorders of mastication and deglutition that are exacerbated frequently by tooth loss may lead to chemosensory impairment.[11]

Nutritional deficiency has been associated with tooth loss. Many studies have demonstrated a connection between tooth loss and dietary intake in older people. Some of them suggest that edentulous people are more likely to ingest an unhealthy diet than individuals who have natural teeth. Older people are edentulous or have fewer natural teeth and are vulnerable to dietary restrictions for many reasons, including medical conditions, physical or mental disability, or economic and social conditions. This may lead to less total energy and malnutrition. It has been noted that they consume less fiber and fewer vegetables, fruits, and nutrient-dense foods. Edentulous individuals consume higher amounts of saturated fat, cholesterol, and calorie-rich foods. As a result, they ingest less nutrients, including protein, calcium, iron, and vitamins C and D.[2,46] Unhealthier diets may explain part of the recent findings suggesting a relationship between tooth loss and cardiovascular disease.[2]

15.4.3 Denture Wearing

The preservation of natural teeth is important for eating, speech, tasting food, and maintaining aesthetics. Dental prostheses (dentures), however, can help persons who have lost some or all of their natural teeth and improve their quality of life by restoring lost function and esthetics. In spite of the positive aspects of dentures, some studies have shown that dietary intake is compromised in denture wearers. There is a dramatic difference in occlusal forces when comparing patients with natural dentitions and patients that are completely edentulous. The average occlusal force in the first molar region of a dentate person has been measured at 150 to 250 psi.[47] Patients wearing complete dentures for more than 15 years may have a maximum occlusal force of 5.6 psi.[48] Reports have suggested that individuals with full dentures consume fewer calories, proteins, thiamin, iron, folate, vitamin A, and carotene than those with natural teeth. It has also been reported that people using dentures consume more refined carbohydrates, sugar, and cholesterol.[2] Even though these findings suggest that the presence of dentures contributes to poorer-quality intake of nutrients, this could be associated more with dentures fitting poorly than with the wearing of the prosthesis.

Research has found that people with well-fitting dentures have nutrient intake and scores on dietary quality indexes similar to those of subjects with natural teeth. These data suggest that tooth loss in itself may not represent a nutritional problem, but rather that impaired nutrient intakes arise when teeth are not replaced or when denture fit and stability are inadequate. With age, the oral mucosa loses vascularity, which leads to decreased tissue elasticity. Bone support also diminishes as a result of periodontal disease or tooth loss. These physiological and pathological changes cause dentures to fit poorly, resulting in lesions of the oral mucosa or discomfort for the patient, making it difficult to use the dentures. This is especially critical in the mandible, where the elderly often have minimal ridge support, making it even harder to fabricate a retentive and stable prosthesis.[49] As a consequence, removable dentures have one of the lowest patient acceptance rates in dentistry. One study revealed that only 60% of the patients with free-end partial dentures were still wearing the prosthesis after 4 years.[50]

The use of dental implants to retain and support prostheses for both partially and completely edentulous patients can have a major impact on oral and systemic health. The mechanical retention provided by implants for a prosthesis is dramatically improved over one only retained by the soft tissues. Many treatment options may exist for these patients, and the amount of implant support can vary depending on the number and location of dental implants placed. The end result is that an implant prosthesis patient may exhibit occlusal forces similar to those of a patient with a fixed restoration supported by natural teeth. A 10-year study reported the outcomes of implant-supported overdentures. It found that the prosthetic and implant cumulative survival rates were both in excess of 90%.[51] This confirmed the long-term outcome success of patients treated with an overdenture prosthesis. Another literature review indicated that implants placed in the anterior mandible have a success rate better than 95% and that patients reported a high degree of satisfaction with this treatment.[52] While each patient must be evaluated on an individual basis, it has become well recognized that implant-supported overdentures in the mandible provide predictable results, with improved stability, retention, function, and patient satisfaction, compared with conventional dentures.

Regular dental care to replace missing teeth and preserve denture function may be critical to the maintenance of dietary quality and adequate nutrient intake in the elderly.[8] Health care providers should inquire about dentition status and strategize with patients regarding improving nutritional status in the context of their oral health limitations.[2]

15.4.4 Salivary Flow

Salivary flow naturally decreases with age, because a portion of the secretory acini of salivary gland tissues are replaced by fat and fibrous tissue. However, the reduction of saliva in the elderly is mostly affected by micronutrient deficiencies, dehydration, and medications.[45]

15.4.5 Xerostomia

This condition refers to a dry mouth sensation and is frequently associated with salivary gland hypofunction. Nevertheless, there are a number of other circumstances that may cause xerostomia, such as medications, systemic diseases, and local, developmental, and iatrogenic factors (see Box 15.2). Approximately 25% of older adults have reported this condition, mainly as a result of medications or systemic conditions.

Patients who suffer this problem clinically demonstrate a reduction in salivary secretions, and the residual saliva appears either thick or frothy. The mucosal surface seems dry and the dorsal tongue often looks fissured and lacks filiform papillae.[2] Dry mouth sensation can cause difficulty with taste perception, chewing, speaking, denture wearing, and swallowing, as well as increase the risk of caries and trauma to the soft tissue. Oral candidiasis is prevalent due to a reduction in the antimicrobial activity provided by saliva.

Even though there is not strong evidence, some reports have suggested that xerostomia affects nutrition. It has been shown that older adults with xerostomia are more likely to avoid crunchy vegetables and dry and sticky foods. Lower caloric and nutrient intakes have also been observed in subjects with this condition.[2] Rhodus and Brown (1990) evaluated 84 older patients and noted that energy, protein, fiber, vitamins A, C, and B6, thiamin, riboflavin, calcium, and iron were significantly lower in individuals with xerostomia than in those without.[53] Additionally, reduced salivary flow rates have been associated with a low body mass index.[5]

Box 15.2 Causes of Xerostomia

Systemic Factors	**Local Factors**
Sjögren syndrome	Decreased mastication
Diabetes mellitus	Mouth breathing
Sarcoidosis	Smoking
HIV infection	
Salivary gland aplasia	**Iatrogenic Factors**
Metabolic abnormalities	Head and neck radiotherapy
Bleeding	Medications
Dehydration	
Vomiting/diarrhea	

Source: Modified from Neville, B. et al., *Oral and Maxillofacial Pathology*, 2nd ed., W.B. Saunders, Philadelphia, 2002.

Sometimes the treatment of xerostomia is difficult and only partially successful. Artificial saliva and intake of copious amounts of water throughout the day may help to reduce discomfort. In addition, chewing sugarless gum and snacking on nonadherent food such as celery and carrots can stimulate salivary flow. The utilization of oral hygiene products that contain lactoperoxidase, lactoferrin, and lysozyme may be helpful. Systemic sialogogues such as systemic pilocarpine or cevimeline hydrochloride may be effective promoters of salivary secretion. On the other hand, the condition may be secondary to medications, and discontinuation, medication dose, or a substitute drug may be considered by the physician.[24] Use of topical fluorides and frequent dental visits are recommended in patients with xerostomia because of the increased potential for dental caries.

15.5 CONCLUSIONS

In the elderly population, many physiologic changes occur in the oral cavity. Dental caries, periodontal disease, oral cancer, infectious diseases, tooth loss, and xerostomia are some of the more common conditions that may develop. Several stomatologic disorders can be prevented and treated. The lack of appropriate therapy can have an effect on systemic functions and accordingly on the quality of life. The most important aspect in which oral health is perceived by elderly people as affecting the quality of life is its effect on eating. There are very deep interactions between nutrition and oral health. Dental problems can lead to dietary, nutritional, and systemic illnesses. Also, diet and nutrition are major factors in the etiology and pathogenesis of craniofacial diseases and disorders.

In the geriatric population, there is a decreased ability to identify foods based on taste. Olfactory and gustatory changes, which may be related to both aging and disease, contribute to altered nutritional selections, thereby complicating certain medical conditions.

Dental status is affected by several factors in older individuals. The major causes of tooth loss in this population include severe caries and periodontal disease. Consequently, tooth loss may influence diet selection, chewing, and swallowing, which are involved in taste. Evidence suggests that tooth loss affects dietary quality and nutrient intake, increasing the risk for systemic diseases. Edentulous subjects generally suffer from poor nutrition, but a well-fitting prosthesis can help to restore lost function and esthetics and improve nutrient intake. On the other hand, a poor-fitting denture will most likely result in poor nutrition.

Xerostomia afflicts approximately one third of the elderly and increases their susceptibility to caries, gingivitis, and oral mucosal infections. These patients may experience difficulty with mastication and swallowing. Oral mucosal diseases, such as candidiasis, apthous ulceration, and atrophic glossitis, and neuropathic conditions such as burning mouth syndrome can be uncomfortable and even debilitating for patients. Neoplastic diseases may occur and be life threatening. Indisputably, these disorders affect the nutrition and quality of life in the geriatric population.

Poor oral health is associated with a limited dietary variety and lower nutrient intake. Preventive care to maintain the natural dentition throughout life may decrease the risk of malnutrition in elderly patients. Regular dental care is important to recognize and treat various oral conditions in this population.

REFERENCES

1. Vargas CM, Kramarow EA, Yellowitz JA, *The Oral Health of Older Americans*, Aging Trends 3, National Center for Health Statistics, Hyattsville, MD, 2001.
2. Ritchie CS, Oral health, taste, and olfaction, *Clin Geriatr Med*, 2002;18:709–717.
3. Position of the American Dietetic Association, oral health and nutrition, *J Am Diet Assoc*, 2003;103:615–625.
4. U.S. Department of Health and Human Services, National Institute of Dental and Craniofacial Research, National Institutes of Health, *Oral Health in America: A Report of the Surgeon General*, Executive Summary, Rockville, MD, 2000.
5. Ritchie CS, Kaumudi J, Hsin-Chia H, et al., Nutrition as a mediator in the relation between oral and systemic disease: associations between specific measures of adult oral health and nutrition outcomes, *Crit Rev Oral Biol Med*, 2002;13:291–300.
6. Coleman P, Opportunities for nursing-dental collaboration: addressing oral health needs among the elderly, *Nurs Outlook*, 2005;53:33–39.
7. Krall E, Hayes KC, Garcia R, How dentition status and masticatory function affect nutrient intake, *J Am Dent Assoc*, 1998;129:1261–1269.
8. Marshall RD, Warren JJ, Hand JS, et al., Oral health, nutrient intake and dietary quality in the very old, *J Am Dent Assoc*, 2002;133:1369–1379.
9. Greksa LP, Parraga IM, Clark CA, The dietary adequacy of edentulous older adults, *J Prosthetic Dent*, 1995;73:142–145.
10. Doty RL, Influence of age and age-related diseases on olfactory function, *Ann NY Acad Sci*, 1989;561:76–86.
11. Seiberling KA, Conley DB, Aging and olfactory and taste function, *Otolaryngol Clin North Am*, 2004;37:1209–1228.
12. Rolls ET, The representation of umami taste in the taste cortex, *J Nutr*, 2000;130:960S–965S.

13. Bradley RM, Effects of aging on the anatomy and neurophysiology of taste, *Gerodontics*, 1988;4:244–248.
14. Schiffman SS, Wedral E, Contribution of taste and smell losses of the wasting syndrome, *Age Nutr*, 1996;7:106–120.
15. Rolls BJ, Do chemosensory changes influence food intake in the elderly? *Physiol Behav*, 1999;66:193–197.
16. National Institutes of Health, *Diagnosis and Management of Dental Caries throughout Life*, NIH Consensus Statement, 2001;18:1–30.
17. Beck JD, Hunt RJ, Hand JS, et al., Prevalence of root and coronal caries in a noninstitutionalized older population, *J Am Dent Assoc*, 1985;111:964–967.
18. Steele JG, et al., *National Diet and Nutrition Survey: People Aged 65 Years and Over*, Vol. 2, The Stationery Office, London, 1998.
19. Walls A, et al., Oral health and nutrition in older people, *J Public Health Dent*, 2000;60:304–307.
20. Steele JG, Sheiman A, Wagner M, et al., Clinical and behavioral risk indicators for root caries in older people, *Gerodontology*, 2001;18:95–101.
21. Oral health and older people, *Gerodontology*, 2005;22:12–15, doi:10.1111/j.1741–2358.2005.00095—5.x.
22. Gerster H, Dental health and nutrition in the elderly: a review, *J Nutr Med* 1991;2:293–311.
23. Pathy J, Sinclair A, Morley J, *Principles and Practice of Geriatric Medicine*, 4th ed., Wiley, West Sussex, 2006.
24. Neville B, Damm D, Allen C, et al., *Oral and Maxillofacial Pathology*, 2nd ed., W.B. Saunders, Philadelphia, 2002.
25. Terrell CL, Antifungal agents. II. The azoles, *Mayo Clinic Proc*, 1999;74:78–100.
26. Öhman S, Dahle G, Moller A, et al., Angular cheilitis: a clinical and microbial study, *J Oral Pathol*, 1986;15:213–217.
27. Ship JA, Recurrent aphthous stomatitis: an update, *Oral Surg Oral Med Oral Pathol Oral Radiol Endod*, 996;81:141–147.
28. Parks E, Oral manifestations of systemic diseases, *Dermatol Clin*, 2003;21:171–182.
29. Bohmer T, Mowe M, The association between atrophic glossitis and protein-calorie malnutrition in old age, *Age Ageing*, 2000;29:47–50.
30. Grushka M, Sessle BJ, Burning mouth syndrome, *Dent Clin North Am*, 1991;35:171–184.
31. Brown L, Brunelle JA, Kingman A, Periodontal status in the United States, 1988–1991: prevalence, extent, and demographic variation, *J Dent Res*, 1996;75:672–683.
32. Oral health related to general health in older people, *Gerodontology*, 2005;22:9–11, doi:10.1111/j.1741–2358.2005.00095—4.x
33. Slavkin HC, Baum BJ, Relationship of dental and oral pathology to systemic illness, *JAMA*, 2000;284:1215–1217.
34. Beck JD, Garcia R, Heiss G, et al., Periodontal disease and cardiovascular disease, *J Periodontal*, 1996;67:1123–1137.
35. Krall E, The periodontal-systemic connection: implications for treatment of patients with osteoporosis and periodontal disease, *Ann Periodontol*, 2001;6:209–213.
36. Geurs N, Lewis E, Jeffcoat E, Osteoporosis and periodontal disease progression, *Periodontol 2000*, 2003;3:105–110.
37. Hildebolt C, Effect of vitamin D and calcium on periodontitis, *J Periodontol*, 2005;76:1576–1587.
38. American Cancer Society, Detailed Guide: Oral Cavity and Oropharingeal Cancer, www.cancer.org/CRI/content 2006.

39. Newton JP, Yemm R, Abel RW, et al., Changes in human jaw muscles with age and dental state, *Gerodontology*, 1993;10:16–22.
40. Giesen EB, Ding M, Dalstra M, van Eijden TM, Reduced mechanical load decreases the density, stiffness, and strength of cancellous bone of the mandibular condyle, *Clin Biomech*, 2003;18:358–363.
41. Okeson JP, *Management of Temporomandibular Disorders and Occlusion*, 5th ed., Mosby, St. Louis, 2003.
42. Österberg T, Carlsson GE, Wedel A, Johansson U, A cross-sectional and longitudinal study of craniomandibular dysfunction in an elderly population, *J Craniomandib Disord*, 1992;6:237–246.
43. Pow EH, Leung KC, McMillan AS, Prevalence of symptoms associated with temporomandibular disorders in Hong Kong Chinese, *J Orofac Pain*, 2001;5:228–234.
44. Witter DJ, De Haan AF, Käyser AF, Van Rossum GM, A 6-year follow-up study of oral function in shortened dental arches. II. Craniomandibular dysfunction and oral comfort, *J Oral Rehabil*, 1994;21:353–366.
45. Bayle R, Gueldner S, Ledikwe J, et al., The oral health of older adults, *J Gerodontol Nurs*, 2005;31:11–17.
46. Sheiham A, Steele JG, Marcenes W, et al., The relationship among dental status, nutrient intake, and nutritional status in older people, *J Dent Res*, 2001;80:408–413.
47. Howell AW, Manley RS, An electronic strain gauge for measuring oral forces, *J Dent Res*, 1948;27:705.
48. Carr A, Laney WR, Maximum occlusal force levels in patients with osseointegrated oral implant prostheses and patients with complete dentures, *Int J Oral Maxillofac Implants*, 1987;2:101–110.
49. Shepherd A, The impact of oral health on nutritional status, *Nurs Stand*, 2002;16:20–27.
50. Carlsson GE, Hedegard B, Koivumaa KK, Studies in partial denture prosthesis. IV. A 4-year longitudinal investigation of dentogingivally-supported partial dentures, *Acta Odontol Scand*, 1965;23:443–472.
51. Attard NJ, Zarb GA, Long-term treatment outcomes in edentulous patients with implant overdentures: the Toronto study, *Int J Prosthodont*, 2004;17:425–433.
52. Doundoulakis JH, Eckert SE, Lindquist CC, Jeffcoat MK, The implant-supported overdenture as an alternative to the complete mandibular denture, *J Am Dent Assoc*, 2003;134:1455–1458.
53. Rhodus NL, Brown J. The association of xerostomia and inadequate intake in older adults. *Am Diet Assoc*, 1990;90:1688–1692.

16 Management of Protein-Energy Undernutrition in Older Adults

David R. Thomas, M.D.

CONTENTS

… for wasting which represents old age [sarcopenia] and wasting that is secondary to fever [cachexia] and wasting which is called doalgashi [starvation] …

—Maimonides (1135–1204)

16.1 INTRODUCTION

Undernutrition in older populations is associated with poor clinical outcomes and is an indicator of risk for increased mortality (Table 16.1). Patients with severe malnutrition are at higher risk for a variety of complications (Table 16.2).[1] A number of chronic medical conditions are associated with increased risk of malnutrition (Table 16.3). Identification of malnutrition leads to early intervention, which may correct reversible nutritional deficits.

Body weight is easily measured and a critical first sign of malnutrition in the nursing home. Clearly, a large number of older adults lose weight, particularly in institutionalized settings. Involuntary weight loss, reduced appetite, and cachexia are common in the geriatric population and are often unexplained.[2] Appetite is regulated by a variety of psychological, gastrointestinal, metabolic, and nutritional factors. Appetite regulators in the central feeding and peripheral satiation systems have been extensively reviewed.[3,4]

TABLE 16.1
Nutritional Status of Nursing Home Patients

Author	Year	N	Prevalence	Time	Outcome
Shaver et al.[128]	1980	115	PCM 85% BMI 43%	6 months	48% death rate in anergic residents
Pinchcopy-Devin et al.[129]	1987	227	PCM 52 %		
Silver et al.[130]	1988	130	BMI 23% Low albumin 8%	1 year	Mortality not associated with BMI
Thomas et al.[131]	1991	61	PCM 54%	2 months	Mortality associated with malnutrition Improvement in only 63%
Larsson et al.[132]	1991	501	PCM 29%		
Nelson et al.[133]	1993	100	PCM 39%		
Wright[134]	1993	309	51% had 5% weight loss	6 months	Slightly increased mortality (15% vs. 12%)
Abbasi and Rudman[135]	1993	2811	Underweight 11% Low albumin 27.5%		Recognition by physicians from 7 to 100%
Morley and Kraenzle[136]	1994	185	15% had 5% weight loss	6 months	Depression most common cause of weight loss
Blaum et al.[137]	1995	6832	9.9% had 5% weight loss Low BMI 25%		Poor intake, eating dependency, depression predict malnutrition

TABLE 16.2
Risk Associated with Undernutrition

Author	Year	N	Time	Outcome
Bistrian et al.[138]	1977	12	—	Impaired delayed hypersensitivity skin test
Weinsier et al.[139]	1979	134	2 weeks	Longer hospital stay (20 vs. 12 days) Increased mortality (13% vs. 4%)
Warnold and Lundholm[140]	1984	215	29 days	Increased postoperative complications (31% vs. 9%)
Pinchosky-Devin et al.[141]	1986		—	Undernutrition associated with pressure ulcers
Detsky et al.[142]	1987	202	—	Increased postoperative complications
Dwyer et al.[143]	1987	335	4 years	Loss of 4.5 kg associated with increased death
Windsor and Hill[144]	1988	102	—	Increased sepsis, pneumonia, longer stay
Berlowitz and Wilking[145]	1989		—	Impaired nutritional intake associated with pressure ulcers
Chang et al.[146]	1990	199	5 years	10% weight loss associated with death and functional impairment
Brandeis et al.[147]	1990		—	Difficulty feeding oneself associated with pressure ulcers
Thomas et al.[148]	1991	61	2 months	Increased mortality
Windsor[149]	1993		—	Increased postoperative complications
Murden and Ainslie[150]	1994	146	2 years	10% weight loss predicts death
Kaiser et al.[151]	1994	5	—	Impaired immune dysfunction Decreased CD4 and T lymphocytes
Franzoni et al.[152]	1996	72	28 months	Low triceps skinfold thickness predicts death
Berkhout et al.[153]	1997	264	3 years	Increased death in low BMI or weight loss within 3 months of admission
Flacker and Kiely[154]	1998	780	2 years	Weight loss and low BMI associated with death
Gambassi et al.[155]	1999	9264	23 months	Malnutrition independent predictor of death (relative risk = 1.31)
Perry et al.[156]	1999	400	2 years	Weight loss of 5% predicts mortality at 6 months
Sullivan et al.[157]	1999	102	3 months	Higher-rate mortality (relative risk = 8.0) and 90-day mortality (relative risk = 2.9)

Although body weight is easily measured, the evaluation of unintended weight loss is difficult.[5] Whether anorexia and weight loss are reversible or unavoidable requires a careful clinical evaluation in the individual patient. A structured approach to the differential diagnosis of undernutrition in older persons is therefore mandatory.[6] A consensus panel has recommended an algorithmic approach to the management of involuntary weight loss (Figure 16.1 and 16.2).

TABLE 16.3
Medical Conditions Associated with Protein-Energy Malnutrition in Nursing Home Residents

			Mechanism	
Medical Condition	**Increased Metabolism**	**Anorexia**	**Swallowing Difficulties**	**Malabsorption**
Cardiac disease	X	X		X
Cancer	X	X	X	X
Pulmonary disease	X	X		X
Infections		X		X
AIDS	X	X	X	X
Tuberculosis	X	X		
Esophageal candidiasis		X	X	
Alcoholism	X	X		X
Rheumatoid arthritis	X	X	X	X
Gallbladder disease		X		
Malabsorption syndromes				X
Hyperthyroidism/ hyperparathyroidism	X	X		
Parkinson's disease	X			
Essential tremors	X			

The first step in management should be a careful evaluation for the causes of weight loss (see Chapter 12). Involuntary weight loss in older adults usually occurs for one of three reasons: starvation, sarcopenia, or cachexia.

Starvation results from failure to consume adequate protein and energy. The reasons for starvation include lack of access to food, inability to consume adequate calories because of mechanical limitations, such as inability to swallow, or inability to absorb ingested nutrients.

Weight loss may be due to an age-related loss of skeletal muscle mass, or sarcopenia. Sarcopenia may also occur without a change in total body weight in obese individuals.

Weight loss may also occur in cachexia, a syndrome of muscle wasting and weight loss, resembling marasmus. A number of chronic disease conditions have been associated with muscle wasting and weight loss, including cancer,[7] end-stage renal disease,[8] chronic pulmonary disease,[9] congestive heart failure,[10] rheumatoid arthritis,[11] and AIDS.[12] A common feature of cachexia is the presence of proinflammatory cytokines.[13]

16.2 TRIGGERS FOR NUTRITIONAL INTERVENTION

Three factors can be used to trigger nutritional interventions. These parameters were derived from the Omnibus Budget Reconciliation Act (OBRA) 1987 guidelines: (1) involuntary weight loss of greater than 5% in 30 days or 10% in 180 days; (2) leaving

Clinical Guide to Prevent and Manage Malnutrition in Long-Term Care

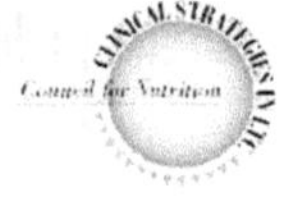

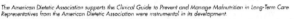

FOR NURSING STAFF AND DIETARY STAFF AND DIETITIANS (EVALUATE, DOCUMENT AND TREAT)

The American Dietetic Association supports the Clinical Guide to Prevent and Manage Malnutrition in Long-Term Care Representatives from the American Dietetic Association were instrumental in its development.

These Guidelines were developed by the Council for Nutrition convened by Programs in Medicine under a grant from Bristol-Myers Squibb. A special committee of The Gerontological Society of America (GSA) served as critical reviewers and provided input and modification of the final Guidelines. While GSA does not endorse specific clinical measures, we support the principles underlying these Guidelines and their potential to improve nutrition in the nursing home.

Trigger Conditions

Involuntary 5% weight loss in 30 days or 10% in 180 days or less
or
BMI ≤ 21
or
Resident leaves 25% or more of food uneaten at two thirds of meals (Assess over 7 days, based on 2000 cal/day)

This is a tool to assist in compliance. This is not an endorsement of the HCFA mandated criteria. It should be noted that because malnutrition in long-term care is multifactorial, any treatment that is initiated should be monitored for efficacy, and nursing interventions should proceed simultaneously with medical interventions.

Put on weekly weight monitoring program/
Proceed with documentation utilizing Nursing Nutritional Checklist

Suggestions for family:

- Visit at meal time
- Help feed
- Discuss alternate food sources
- Review food preferences
- Recommend favorite foods or comfort foods
- Discuss quality of life issues and treatment goals

Quality indicator conditions:
- Fecal impactions, Infection (UTI, URI, pneumonia, GI)
- Tube feeding, decline in ADL's or pressure ulcer on low risk resident

Check hydration status
minimum 1500 cc fluid/day unless contraindicated
(For tube feeding patients, approximately 75% of the total tube feeding volume should be considered free fluid)

Inform physician/dietitian

Checklist for nurse to provide physician/dietitian:

- Temperature
- Constipation
- Fecal impaction
- Drug list
- Mood/behavior
- Food/fluid intake
- Vomiting/nausea
- Indigestion
- Skin condition
- Swallowing problem
- Appetite assessment
- Infection – UTI, URI, GI
- Pain
- Albumin < 3.4 g/dL
- Cholesterol < 160 mg/dL
- Hgb < 12 g/dL
- Serum transferrin < 180*

* Included in MDS

Physician considerations:

- Albumin
- Complete blood count
- Blood urea nitrogen
- Creatinine
- Hemoglobin
- Hematocrit
- Serum transferrin
- Cholesterol
- Consultation by dietitian
- Consult Clinical Guide for Physicians, Pharmacists, and Dietitians

Food/environmental considerations

Food considerations:

- Stop therapeutic diet
- Food preferences (e.g., ethnic)
- Consistency changes based on assessed needs
- Offer meal substitutes
- Snacks (between meals and HS)
- Medications not given at meal time
- Supplements not given at meal time
- Food served at proper temperature
- Food palatability (consider taste enhancers)
- Encourage family involvement in feeding

Other:

- Taste/sensory changes
- Ill-fitting dentures, missing teeth
- Motor agitation, tremors, wandering

Environmental considerations:

- Surroundings quiet and calm, comfortable
- Positive dining room atmosphere
- Well lighted
- Caregivers are friendly and polite
- Residents are happy with the meals and meal service
- Staff directs conversation to resident at meal time
- Dining room service not rushed
- Assistance encouraged
- Prompt service and assistance
- Compatible companions

Needs feeding assistance — Meal time assistance, restorative dining program

Dysphagia/aspiration — Swallowing evaluation/food consistency change, thickened liquids, special feeding program, enteral/parenteral feeding

Caloric-dense foods
Exercise program for appetite stimulation

Between-meal liquid calorically dense supplements

Consider other treatment options, e.g. hospitalize or palliative care — Document reason

While presented for simplicity as a linear guide in two parts, many of the suggestions can be done simultaneously, and the order in which this approach is taken can be varied dependent on individual resident needs.

FIGURE 16.1 To prevent and manage malnutrition in long-term care.

Nursing Nutritional Checklist (for use in Care Planning)

Council for Nutrition — Clinical Strategies in LTC

The American Dietetic Association supports the Nursing Nutritional Checklist (for use in Care Planning). Representatives from the American Dietetic Association were instrumental in its development.

This Nursing Nutritional Checklist (for use in Care Planning) was developed by the Council for Nutrition convened by Programs in Medicine under a grant from Bristol-Myers Squibb. A special committee of The Gerontological Society of America (GSA) served as critical reviewers and provided input and modification of the final Checklist. While GSA does not endorse specific clinical measures, we support the principles underlying this Checklist and its potential to improve nutrition in the nursing home.

Problem List (check all that apply)	**Suggested Action Plan (check when completed)**
1. Patient has ≥ 5% involuntary weight loss in 30 days? 2. Patient has ≥10% involuntary weight loss in 180 days or less. 3. BMI is ≤ 21. (703 x weight in lbs/height in inches² **or** weight in kilograms/height in meters²) 4. Resident leaves 25% or more food on tray? (in last 7 days)	1-4. Monitor weight weekly. Continue to step #5 on problem list
5. Quality Indicators — Does patient have: A. Fecal impaction in last 7 days B. Infection (UTI, URI, Pneumonia, GI) in last 7 days C. Tube feeding D. Functional ADL decline E. Development of pressure ulcer in low risk patient	5. A. Implement bowel program B. Get physician order for U/A C. Contact dietitian for assessment D. Consider OT/PT assessment E. Implement skin program
6. Patient takes in ≤1500cc fluid/day for the last 7 days? Is patient on fluid restriction?	6. Develop systematic plan to ensure adequate fluid intake (e.g., 300 mL with meals and 240 mL between meals)
7. Available labwork completed in the last 30 days: Hgb ______ Albumin ______ Hct ______ Cholesterol ______ Serum WBC ______ U/A: Sodium ______ Urine WBC ______ Potassium ______ Spec. Gravity ______ Glucose ______ Leuk. Esterase ______ BUN ______ Other ______ Creatinine ______	7. Notify physician of values
8. Nursing assessment of physical/psychological problems A. Skin (pressure ulcers and skin tears) B. Presence of fever (2° above baseline) C. Presence of diarrhea D. Presence of constipation E. Takes drugs other than multivitamins/minerals F. Symptoms of depression/anxiety G. Loss of usual appetite H. Presence of nausea/vomiting I. Presence of dysphagia/choking J. Ill-fitting dentures, missing teeth, periodontal disease	8. A. Implement skin program B. Implement facility protocol C. Implement facility protocol D. Implement facility protocol E. Contact pharmacy consultant for drug review F. Evaluate for depression/anxiety (short geriatric mini depression scale) G. Implement care plan to increase appetite H. Implement facility protocol I. Contact dietitian for evaluation J. Contact dentist or dental technician
9. Not satisfied with food currently offered (for example, ethnic preferences)	9. Stop therapeutic diets and provide preferred foods/food substitutions
10. Patient needs meal time assistance	10. Provide timely, polite assistance during dining Provide tray set up Provide partial assistance/supervision (evaluate resident/staff ratio and supervision by licensed professional staff) Provide total assistance (consider resident/staff ratio and supervision by licensed professional staff) Consider training staff to provide meal time assistance
11. Patient has motor agitation, tremors, or wanders	11. Consider OT evaluation Provide meal time assistance Provide self-help feeding devices Offer finger foods
12. Presence of environmental distractions or meal time environment concerns	12. Minimize environmental distractions Provide compatible companions
13. Inadequate lighting in the dining room	13. Evaluate location in dining room
14. Patient needs 30–60 minutes to eat	14. Implement dining program, e.g. special area to eat for impaired residents or two meal time sessions
15. Patient is unable to tolerate current food consistency	15. Contact dietitian for texture screen
16. Supplements are given at meal time	16. Give liquid supplements in a pattern that optimizes nutrient intake
17. Medications are given at meal time	17. Contact pharmacist for appropriate administration time
18. Impaired visual acuity	18. Assure resident is wearing clean glasses at meal time Provide meal time assistance (see #10)
19. Impaired hearing	19. Ensure that hearing aid is in place and working at meal time
20. Patient has a decline in taste and smell	20. Season foods Serve food at proper temperature

When problem list is completed, contact physician, dietitian and pharmacist as appropriate with suggested action plan.

Completed by: ______________________ Date: ______________

FIGURE 16.2 Nutritional checklist for nurses.

more than 25% of food in the past 7 days or two thirds of meals based on a 2000-kcal diet; or (3) a body mass index (BMI; calculated as weight divided by height squared) equal to or less than 19.

Age- and gender-adjusted BMI below the 10th dectile has been used to define undernutrition (<19 in men and <19.4 in women).[20] In hospitalized adults with serious illness, excess mortality within 6 months (risk ratio = 1.23, $p < 0.001$) has been demonstrated when the body mass index is less than 20.[14] The increase in mortality is linear—the lower the BMI, the greater the risk. Increased risk of death has been shown to begin at a body mass index of <23.5 in men and <22.0 in women.[15] Therefore, rather than waiting for the body mass index to reach lower values, a body mass index of less than 21 may result in earlier intervention.[16]

16.3 DIFFERENTIAL DIAGNOSIS

The first focus should be on differential diagnosis. Weekly weight assessments are useful in following the course and rapidity of the weight loss.

16.3.1 Depression and Mood Disorders

Depression is a major cause of weight loss in long-term-care settings, accounting for up to 36% of residents who lost weight.[17] An evaluation for depression, for example, using the Geriatric Depression Scale,[18,19] should be obtained for residents with anorexia. Depression may be reversed in a moderate number of individuals by pharmacological treatment. Electroconvulsive therapy is effective in persons who do not respond to pharmacological treatment. When weight loss is caused by depression, treatment with antidepressant medications may lead to weight gain. However, some antidepressant medications may variably cause weight loss themselves. Careful attention to the choice of a prescribed antidepressant is necessary. Delirium due to acute illness or pain may be a reversible cause of decreased dietary intake. Reversal of delirium may result in resumption of appetite.

16.3.2 Drugs

A number of drugs have been found to be a cause of weight loss or anorexia in long-term-care residents.[20] The association is not intuitive. Consultation with a pharmacologist is often necessary. All drugs potentially aggravating anorexia should be discontinued.[21]

16.3.3 Medical Conditions

Medical conditions that produce decreased food intake or increased metabolic requirements should be assessed. Anorexia may be associated with illness, drugs, dementia, or mood disorders.[22–24] Decreased food intake may result from dysphagia,[25] chewing problems,[26] nausea, vomiting, diarrhea, pain, or fecal impaction. Increased metabolic requirements may be precipitated by fever, infection, or the presence of chronic skin wounds. Treatment of these conditions may restore appetite and body weight. A mnemonic, Meals on Wheels, is useful in considering the potential treatable causes of malnutrition.[27] A useful tool to assess appetite and food intake is the Simplified Nutrition and Appetite Questionaire.[28]

16.3.4 Hydration

Fluid intake and hydration status may affect body weight. An assessment of hydration status may account for weight loss due to low fluid intake. Dehydration may be difficult to detect by clinical signs alone and require the use of biochemical parameters.[29] The recommended amount of fluid consumed by nursing home residents is confusing. Amounts range from 1 ml/kcal,[30] 30 ml/kg body weight,[31] or the sum of 100 ml fluid/kg for the first 10 kg actual body weight, 50 ml fluid/kg for the next 10 kg actual body weight, and 15 ml fluid/kg for the remaining kilograms actual body weight.[32] Direct observations of institutionalized adults indicate a total fluid intake, including fluids derived from meals, of 1783 ± 545 ml.[33] When compared to the standards of 1 ml/kcal and 30 ml/kg, recommended intakes were low, primarily due to low body weight or low caloric intake. The calculated value provides at least 1500 ml daily, even for residents with low weight. A general recommendation suggests that residents should ingest 1500 to 2000 ml fluid/day,[34] though a recent study and accompanying editorial have suggested that community-dwelling adults consume about 1000 ml/day.[35,36]

16.3.5 Laboratory Parameters

Evaluation of available biochemical parameters associated with malnutrition should be considered at this point. Suggested biochemical parameters include serum albumin,[37] cholesterol,[38] hemoglobin, and serum transferrin. While these parameters may be abnormal in several conditions unassociated with undernutrition, they are useful as guides to predicting future mortality or morbidity.[39] However, laboratory parameters are not useful for the serial follow-up of undernourished persons.

16.4 Treatment of Undernutrition

16.4.1 Advanced Directives

In some circumstances, weight loss is an inevitable consequence of cachexia-related disease or a terminal condition. In this circumstance, it is essential that the older person or their proxy have a full discussion of their health care wishes with a health care professional. The decision that they make should be documented and guide how aggressively the management of their nutritional problem is addressed. For example, enteral or parenteral feeding may be lifesaving, but is associated with a considerable burden of treatment.

16.4.2 Environmental Factors

Food and environmental conditions that may affect intake should be considered in a continuing evaluation. Unpalatability due to overly restricted diets may cause decreased intake.[40] Consideration of food preferences, food consistency,[41,42] food temperature, and snacks should be included. Provision of pleasant, well-lighted, unhurried mealtimes in a social environment may increase intake.[43]

Early interventions include family involvement to visit or assist with feeding at mealtimes,[44] exploration of alternate food sources, evaluation of food preferences, and identification of favorite foods. A discussion of the treatment goals and the resident's ongoing quality of life should be initiated at this point.

Dependency in eating is associated with increased mortality.[45] Persons needing feeding assistance require a restorative feeding program.[46] Recognition of feeding problems and proper feeding techniques may improve weight loss in older persons. Dysphagia and swallowing disorders, with or without recurrent aspiration, require swallowing interventions, alteration of food consistency, or consideration of enteral or parenteral feeding.[47]

Assistance with eating by trained personnel over a mean of 16 weeks did not improve markers of nutritional status, Barthel score, grip strength, length of stay, or mortality in acutely ill older adults.[48]

16.4.3 Adequate Food

Simple nutritional calculations can define adequate food intake (see Chapter 7). A simple dietary interview can determine whether community-dwelling older adults are reaching their targeted intake. In hospitalized or long-term-care populations, food is prepared to meet dietary needs. However, assessment of the amount of the offered food should be performed and residents should eat about 75% of the offered food.

16.4.4 Nutritional Supplements

Increased nutrient intake may be achieved by use of calorie-dense foods.[49] Exercise may increase dietary intake.[50–52] Nutritional supplementation can increase dietary intake and produce weight gain.[53,54] Nutritional supplementation must be given between meals in order not to substitute for calorie intake at meals.[55]

A meta-analysis of 55 randomized controlled trials with 9187 older participants evaluated the effect of nutritional supplements across a variety of health care settings.[56] Nutritional supplementation produced a small but significant percentage weight gain of 1.8% (95% confidence interval (CI) = 1.1 to 2.3%) in hospitalized subjects. Percentage weight change for subjects in long-term-care settings was 2.5% (95% CI = 1.7 to 3.2%), and 2.3% (95% CI = 1.7 to 2.7%) for older people living at home. Mortality in the supplemented group was reduced, although the reduction was only borderline statistically significant (odds ratio = 0.9, 95% CI = 0.7 to 1.0).

For short-term hospital stays, mortality was not reduced (odds ratio = 0.9, 95% CI = 0.7 to 1.0). However, a reduction in mortality was seen in trials that only included undernourished subjects (odds ratio = 0.7, 95% CI = 0.5 to 0.9). A reduction in mortality was not seen in supplemented residents in long-term-care settings (odds ratio = 0.7, 95% CI = 0.4 to 1.0) or for people living at home (odds ratio = 1.1, 95% CI = 0.6 to 2.0). Hospitalized patients who were given supplements had a statistically significant decrease in complications (odds ratio = 0.7, 95% CI = 0.5 to 0.9), but supplementation did not have an effect on morbidity or complications in residents in long-term care (odds ratio = 0.9, 95% CI = 0.6 to 1.5) or at home (odds ratio = 1.0, 95% CI = 0.6 to 1.6).

Oral nutritional supplements have been evaluated in subjects with Alzheimer's type dementia. In a prospective controlled study, 91 subjects older than 65 years with dementia of the Alzheimer's type who were at risk of undernutrition by the Mini-Nutritional Assessment instrument and who had lost more that 5% of their body weight were randomized to receive either an oral supplement or usual care. Despite a significant improvement in dietary intakes and body weight in the intervention group, no significant changes were found for biological markers of nutrition, functional status, or cognitive function.[57]

Fiatarone et al. randomized 100 long-term-care residents age 87.1 ± 0.6 years to high-intensity exercise training or to no exercise.[58] The groups were further randomized to receive 240 ml of nutritional supplementation or no supplementation. While muscle strength increased by 113 ± 8% in the training group, the addition of a nutritional supplement did not improve outcome. In a previous study of 11 long-term-care residents, the addition of 560 kcal of a nutritional supplement did not increase muscle strength, but computed tomography of the thigh showed more gain in muscle mass in the supplemented group.[59] The nutritional intervention may have been too small or the observation period too short to detect a difference in outcome.

16.4.5 Orexigenic Drugs

Drugs that stimulate appetite, orexigenic drugs, should be considered to reverse anorexia.[60–63] Corticosteroids in randomized placebo-controlled trials have improved appetite, but have not demonstrated body weight gain.[64–69] Cannabinoids (dronabinol, marinol, and nabilone) have shown promise in improving mood and appetite in cancer patients and in AIDS cachexia, but body weight gain was not seen.[70–72] Dronabinol has shown weight gain in patients with Alzheimer's disease and improvement in disturbed behavior in a small study.[73] Thalidomide, a tumor necrosis factor inhibitor, has produced body weight gain in patients with human immunodeficiency virus-associated wasting syndrome.[74] Recombinant human growth factors have produced weight gain (mean = 1.6 vs. 0.1 kg in the placebo group) in patients with AIDS, but at substantially higher than physiological doses,[75] and in long-term-care residents.[76]

Sex steroids have shown promise in producing weight gain in ill subjects. Testosterone replacement leads to an increase in muscle mass[77] and muscle strength[78,79] and to improved function in a rehabilitation center.[80] An anabolic-androgenic steroid, oxymetholone, has produced body weight gain in advanced HIV-1 infection,[81] but not in cachectic cancer patients.[82] The weight gain has usually occurred only in patients who were hypogonadal.

A systemic review of megestrol acetate in cancer trials has shown increased appetite, weight gain, and assessment of improved health-related quality of life, compared to placebo. Weight gain has also been demonstrated in AIDS patients.[83]

Megestrol acetate has been evaluated in three long-term-care settings. In a prospective trial, weight gain occurred in 68% of treated subjects.[84] In another study of elderly nursing home residents who were losing weight and refused enteral feeding, megestrol acetate produced improvement in food intake, body mass index, and serum albumin.[85] In a noncontrolled trial of feeding assistance, 47% of long-term-care subjects treated with megestrol acetate experienced a mean weight gain of 5.9 ± 4.9 pounds. Appetite was increased in 53% of subjects, and 41% reported an increase in energy during the trial.

Comparisons of nandrolone decanoate, megestrol acetate, or dietary counseling in patients have been evaluated in subjects with human immunodeficiency syndrome-associated weight loss. Weight increased significantly in all treatment arms (dietary counseling, 1.13 ± 0.36 kg; nandrolone, 4.01 ± 1.68 kg; megestrol, 10.20 ± 4.51 kg ($p < 0.05$)). Fat-free mass increased significantly in patients receiving nandrolone (3.54 ± 1.98 kg, $p = 0.001$) and those receiving megestrol acetate (2.76 ± 0.55 kg, $p = 0.002$), but there was no change in subjects receiving dietary counseling alone.[86]

Dronabinol has been directly compared to megestrol acetate in cancer cachexia subjects.[87] Seventy-five percent of megestrol acetate-treated patients reported appetite improvement, compared with 49% of dronabinol-treated patients ($p = 0.0001$), and 11% of megestrol acetate-treated patients reported greater than 10% gain from baseline vs. 3% in the dronabinol-treated subjects ($p = 0.02$). Combination treatment resulted in no significant differences in appetite or weight compared with megestrol acetate alone. Quality of life improved in both the megestrol acetate-treated and combination-treated patients measured by the Functional Assessment of Anorexia/Cachexia Therapy questionnaire ($p = 0.002$).

An eicosapentaenoic acid supplement has been compared to megestrol acetate in cancer subjects with weight loss or caloric intake less than 20 calories/kg/day. Six percent of subjects taking the supplement gained more than 10% of baseline weight compared to 18% of those taking megestrol acetate. Greater than a 10% weight gain occurred in 11% of subjects taking combination therapy with both agents. Subjects receiving megestrol acetate reported greater appetite improvement than with the eicosapentaenoic acid supplement arm.[88]

Although body weight gain has been shown with growth hormone, thalidomide, oxandrolone, and megestrol in cancer cachexia and AIDS cachexia, very little data are available on whether this effect occurs in geriatric anorexia and cachexia syndromes not associated with cancer or immunodeficiency syndrome.[89]

16.4.6 Failure to Improve

Failure to improve nutritional status with these measures requires consideration of enteral or parenteral feeding.[90] The resident's wishes and advanced directives may lead to a decision for palliative care.

16.4.7 Enteral Feeding

The indications for enteral nutrition by feeding tube generally fall into one of three categories.[91,92] First, neuromuscular disease may impair swallowing or gag reflexes. Second, patients may be unable to meet nutritional needs by eating alone, as in hypermetabolic cancer patients or patients with cachexia. Finally, an underlying condition may prevent eating, such as in ventilator-dependent or postoperative patients. The only contraindication to enteral feeding is mechanical obstruction of the gut. Diarrhea, vomiting, fistulae, dysmotility, and aspiration represent problems that complicate feeding, but are not contraindications. Patient preferences factor into the decision to use enteral feeding.

Access to the gut can be achieved by nasogastric, nasointestinal, percutaneous gastric, or percutaneous jejunal (PEJ) routes. Each route is associated with benefits and risks, but the percutaneous gastrostomy (PEG) is the most common, and arguably the preferred route when the enteral feeding is expected to last for more than 30 days. Most oral medications cannot be used with jejunal intubation (PEJ), and long-term nasogastric (NG) intubation may be uncomfortable.

All enteral formulas contain protein, fat, and carbohydrates. In similar categories, there is very little difference between products. In surveys among nutritionists, cost is cited as the most important factor used by formulary committees to pick a product.

Products differ in source of protein and in the degree of digestion required (Table 16.4). The choice of a product depends on the condition of the gut and the expected degree of digestion required. As the degree of digestion required lessens, the cost rises considerably. Intact nutrients (blenderized) and milk-based products are the cheapest and will adequately meet nutritional needs. The most commonly prescribed products, and the largest category, are lactose-free products aimed at preventing lactose-associated diarrhea. Hydrolyzed proteins and crystalline amino acids are used when normal digestive enzymes are not present due to disease or the absorptive surface of the intestine is altered, in conditions such as pancreatitis or malabsorption. Incomplete amino acids are reserved for patients whose protein must be restricted, for example, in such conditions as renal or hepatic failure.

Simple nutritional calculations are necessary to determine the total volume required to deliver adequate protein, calories, and water (Table 16.5). Proteins are the most critical component. Controversy exists over the percent of total caloric requirement derived from protein. Generally, formulas contain about 7 to 16% of total calories from protein. The Recommended Daily Allowance for adults is 0.8 g/kg/day for protein, which is probably too low for older persoons. For most institutionalized patients with underlying disease, protein intake should be 1.2 to

TABLE 16.4
Class of Nutrition Products by Protein Source and Degree of Digestion

Class	Protein Source	Digestion
Intact nutrients	Pureed beef and calcium caseinate	Requires normal pancreatic enzymes
Milk based	Skin or powdered milk, caseinate	Requires normal pancreatic enzymes
Lactose-free	Soybean, caseinates, de-lactosed lacalbumin	Requires normal pancreatic enzymes except lactose
Hydrolyzed proteins	Whey, meat, soy	No digestion; requires intact brush border absorption
Crystalline amino acids	All amino acids	No digestion; no brush border with only passive absorption
Incomplete amino acids	Only branched-chain remains	Hepatic or renal failure

TABLE 16.5
Calculating Enteral Feeding Requirements

	Clinical Condition	Amount
Protein	Maintenance	1.2 to 1.5 g/kg/day
	Stress[a]	1.5 to 2.0 g/kg/day
Calories	Maintenance	25–30 kcal/kg/day
	Stress	30–35 kcal/kg/day
Free water		30–35 ml/kg/day

[a] Stress generally refers to persons with burns, wounds, cancer, infections, and other similar conditions.

1.5 g/kg/day. However, half of chronically ill elderly persons are unable to maintain nitrogen balance at this level.[93] However, increasing the total protein percentage may simply supply calories from protein rather than from carbohydrate sources and may dehydrate the patient.[94]

Caloric requirements range from 25 kcal/kg/day for sedentary adults to 40 kcal/kg/day for stressed adults. Stress generally refers to persons with burns, wounds, cancer, infections, and other similar conditions. In general, caloric requirements can be met at 30 to 35 kcal/kg/day for elderly patients under moderate stress. Various formulas, including the Harris–Benedict equation, can be used to predict caloric requirements, but controversy exists over accuracy in obese or severely malnourished individuals.[95] Other formulas have been adjusted for severely stressed hospitalized subjects.[96] Considerable debate exists over whether to use ideal body weight or an adjusted body weight in calculations.

The chief difference among formulas is whether the source includes milk, and thus includes lactose. The majority of formulas are lactose-free. All products require an intact intestinal brush border for absorption. Most feeding formulas contain approximately 1 kcal/ml. Alternative calories per unit volume are available, ranging from 0.5 to 2.0 kcal/ml. As caloric density increases, gastric motility and emptying decrease. This may increase the risk of aspiration.

Fats are added to formulas for additional calories, to add flavor, and for absorption of fat-soluble vitamins. The amount of fat and source of fat differ from product to product. The percentage of fat should be about 30% of calories, but an exact requirement is not known.

Free water requirement is 30 to 35 ml/kg/day. Each product varies in the amount of free water per unit volume, but in most products it is about 75% of volume. The product free water should be subtracted from the total calculated daily water requirement. Water flushes of the tube can be adjusted to meet free water requirements. Using a low-calorie formula results in a higher volume requirement to meet caloric needs and results in increased fluid intake. When 2.0 kcal/cc density formulas are used, the volume necessary to meet caloric needs decreases and the amount of free water decreases. This can be useful when fluid restriction is necessary in certain clinical conditions, such as the syndrome of inappropriate secretion of antidiuretic hormone or congestive heart failure requiring fluid restriction.

Feedings can be given either intermittently or continuously. The stomach is normally a reservoir for receiving intermittent feedings. For this reason, an intermittent schedule is preferred. There may be several advantages to intermittent feedings. Intermittent feedings are more convenient to nursing staff, do not require infusion pumps, permit more patient mobility, better simulate normal feeding patterns with fasting periods, and may be more physiologic.[97]

If the patient has not been fed in the last 5 days, feedings should begin as low-volume continuous flow, in the range of 25 cc/hour, depending on tolerance. When caloric needs are met, the schedule can be interrupted for intermittent feedings. The average volume of intermittent feedings should be between 240 and 400 ml. The higher the feeding rate, the higher the residual volume. The gastric residual should be checked prior to each feeding. You should be concerned if the residual volume is >200 ml for nasogastric tube or >100 ml for gastrostomy tube, but this does not always necessitate holding feedings. Residual volumes are not reliable if tube is <10 French. Feedings may be given by gravity drainage with a roller clamp or by a constant infusion pump. There are little data to suggest that infusion pumps are superior[98,99]; pumps are more expensive, and intermittant feeding may be superior for the reasons stated above.

Enteral nutritional support in persons diagnosed with undernutrition has shown only modest benefits.[100] In patients who cannot eat for more than 10 to 14 days, nutritional support is indicated to prevent morbidity and mortality from starvation. In patients with major trauma and in severely malnourished patients undergoing major elective surgery, the reduction in major complications has been demonstrated. However, the use of nutritional support is not associated with a reduction in the length of hospital stay.[101] Furthermore, there has been little improvement in specific disease states, such as cancer, AIDS, or hemodialysis patients.[102]

Nutritional parameters were compared among 44 hospitalized, bed-confined subjects over age 65 years, with and without tube feeding, and 41 age-matched free-eating elders in a nursing home. Tube-fed subjects received 26 kcal/kg/day and 1.0 g of protein/day, an amount calculated to equal predicted total energy expenditure. However, the incidence of protein energy undernutrition as evidenced by decreased arm muscle circumference (<80% of normal) and hypoalbuminemia (<35 g/l), was significantly higher in the patients with tube feeding compared to that in the orally fed older persons. Thus, undernutrition was still demonstrable in patients fed energy and protein that approximated calculated predicted values.[103] Survival for 24 months was not different in nursing home residents with progressive dementia than in residents who were and were not enterally fed.[104]

Complications of enteral feeding can be divided into mechanical, gastrointestinal, and metabolic. In the largest study,[105] the overall complication rate was 11.7%. The rates in this study were low: gastrointestinal, 6.2%; mechanical, 3.5%; and metabolic, 2.0%. Diarrhea was reported in only 2.3%. Mechanical clogging has been observed only with premixed formulas.[106] The tube should be flushed tube with at least 30 ml water every 4 hours during continuous feeding, after every medication, after intermittent feeding, and after every check for residual.

Pulmonary complications can be due to improper placement. Of 100 placements of a nasogastric tube, 19% were in neither the stomach nor the duodenum.[107] In the elderly, or in patients without intact gag reflex, pneumothorax, pleural penetration, empyema, and bronchopleural fistula may occur more frequently. Using insufflation over the stomach for tube placement is frequently misleading. Radiological confirmation of placement should be obtained.

Aspiration of gastric contents is the most serious among the pulmonary complications of tube feedings. As many as 40% of deaths associated with tube feedings result directly from aspiration pneumonia.[108] Reported risk factors for aspiration include conditions such as diabetes, pancreatitis, vagotomy, and malnutrition. Formula-associated risks include high-nutrient-density formulas,[109] hypo- and hyperosmolar solutions,[110] and cold formulas.

Aspiration appears to occur equally with nasogastric or PEG intubation.[111] In one study,[112] the only risk factor associated with subsequent aspiration in gastrostomy tubes was previous pneumonia. Age, mental status, or method of feeding (intermittent vs. continuous) was not associated with subsequent risk.

Comparison of PEG and PEJ tubes in another study showed aspiration within 30 days in 5% of PEG patients and 17% of PEJ patients.[113] The high rate of PEJ aspiration may occur because these tubes are used in chronic aspirators. Nevertheless, this strategy is not effective in preventing this serious complication.

Diarrhea is the most frequently reported gastrointestinal complication of tube feeding in most studies. Incidence ranges from 2.3% to as high as 68% in ICU patients.[114] The pathogenesis is poorly understood. Major studies show often conflicting data in identifying causes of diarrhea. The associations for increased diarrhea include osmolarity, rate of delivery, H2 blockers, antibiotics, and fiber content. Other authors conclude that osmolarity, antibiotics, and H2 blockers are *not* associated with incidence of diarrhea.[115] The discrepancy is likely due to study design, population, and definition of diarrhea. Antibiotics have been cited as the most common medications associated with diarrhea. In other studies, there has been no association between diarrhea and antibiotic usage. The association with H2 blockers and diarrhea may be related to bacterial overgrowth in patients whose stomach pH exceeds 4 when receiving H2 blockers.[116] Drugs containing sorbitol are an often overlooked source of diarrhea.

Formulas high in fiber may decrease the cecal bacterial load or translocation of mesenterial bacteria in rats.[117] Whether this is important in humans is not known. Fiber content of formulas probably has little effect on diarrhea related to enteral feeding.

Metabolic complications of enteral feeding include hyperglycemia, hypercapnea, and electrolyte abnormalities. Complications are seen more often with high-caloric-density formulas or in diabetics. Special formulas are available for diabetic patients, but data are limited on effectiveness. Hyperosmolar formulas in diabetics may lead to hyperosmolar nonketotic coma. High carbohydrate concentrations may increase respiratory quotients and increase carbon dioxide production.

Numerous studies have attempted to characterize the benefits of tube feeding. In an analysis of 434 tube-fed residents on the Wisconsin Minimum Data Set sample, Grant et al.[118] found that 51% of the residents had a diagnosis of stroke, 36% of the residents were diagnosed with dementia, only 10% of the residents ambulated independently, and 74% of the residents were incontinent of either urine or feces. Only one third of those residents assessed could communicate adequately. Mitchell et al.,[119] in a study of 1386 nursing home residents with cognitive impairment, found no evidence that tube feeding prolonged survival. The most common reasons for choosing tube feeding were aspiration risk, dysphagia, presence of pressure ulcers, stroke, lack of dementia, younger age, and a lower level of activity of daily living impairment. In a small study of the quality of life in tube-fed patients, Weaver et al.[120] found no improvement in their quality of life. Forty-nine percent of family members responded that they would not have chosen a feeding tube under other circumstances. O'Brien et al.[121] found that 25% of patients surveyed would have refused feeding tubes if they had known that they might be restrained. This study also revealed that males and African Americans were more likely to choose tube feeding than other groups. In another study, tube feeding was associated with better wound healing and a lower rate of late mortality.[122] In this study, 80% of those assessed had cutaneous complications, 39% had pulmonary aspiration, 15% had vomiting, and 20% attempted to withdraw the tube.

16.4.8 Irreversible Causes

Unquestionably, providing nutritional support can prevent the effects of starvation. Death is an inevitable consequence of starvation. Whether nutrition can improve the outcome of a disease remains disputable. Improvements in nutritional markers, such as serum protein concentrations, nitrogen balance, and weight gain, have not usually been accompanied by clinical benefits.[123] Certain causes of malnutrition may be irreversible. Palliative care, including orexigenic drugs and enteral or parenteral feeding, consistent with the resident's wishes, should be considered.[124]

16.4.9 Parenteral Nutrition

Parenteral nutrition has been shown to reduce septic complications in critically ill patients, but not ventilator days, length of hospital stay, or mortality. In critically ill patients, a 20% decline in lean body mass has been demonstrated despite agressive caloric support.[125] In a study of 325 nutritionally at-risk patients receiving total parenteral nutrition, 219 patients were defined as malnourished using improvement in body cell mass with parenteral feedings as the standard for malnutrition. Nonresponders, 106 patients, were defined as nonmalnourished, based on no change in body cell mass with feedings. The outcome in elderly patients was dismal. In the 179 patients over the age of 65 years, no statistically significant improvement in body weight, body fat, lean body mass, extracellular mass, or body cell mass occurred.[126] By necessity, parenteral nutrition is short term. Long-term (approximately 2 weeks) peripheral parenteral nutrition has not been shown to have beneficial effects on prealbumin, CD4 cell count, and functional status compared to untreated controls in a rehabilitation setting.[127]

16.5 SUMMARY

Undernutrition is defined as a state induced by nutrient deficiency that may be improved solely by administration of nutrients. By this definition, provision of adequate protein and energy sources should reverse the clinical presentation and correct the problem. However, a large number of patients who appear to be undernourished fail to respond to refeeding. A developing understanding of the acute phase inflammatory response to illness and the role of cytokines in the pathophysiology of chronic illness has challenged the current diagnostic paradigm of undernutrition.

A structured approach to the management of unintended weight loss or undernutrition in older adults is essential. Understanding the relative role of inadequate nutrient intake assists in targeting the interventions to the individual subject. In the presence of adequate food, weight loss is most often due to cytokine-associated cachexia and anorexia. Failure of appetite, or anorexia, may play a role in involuntary weight loss. Interventions for involuntary weight loss should aim first at the provision of adequate calories and protein, often in the form of high-density nutritional supplements. However, cytokine-mediated cachexia is remarkably resistant to hypercaloric feeding. With continued weight loss, the use of an orexigenic drug should be considered. Consideration of enteral feeding should be based on the individual's condition and goals of care.

REFERENCES

1. Dempsey DT, Mullen JL, Buzby GP. The link between nutritional status and clinical outcome: can nutritional intervention modify it? *Am J Clin Nutr* 1988;47(Suppl):352–356.
2. Thompson MP, Merria LK. Unexplained weight loss in ambulatory elderly. *J Am Geriatr Soc* 1991;39:497–500.
3. Morley JE, Thomas DR. Anorexia and aging: pathophysiology. *Nutrition* 1999;15:499–503.
4. Morley JE. Anorexia in older persons: epidemiology and optimal treatment. *Drugs Aging* 1996;8:134–156.
5. Omran ML, Morley JE. Assessment of protein energy malnutrition in older persons. 1. History, examination, body composition, and screen tools. *Nutrition* 2000;16:50–63.
6. Thomas DR, Ashmen W, Morley JE, Evans JE. Nutritional management in long-term care: Development of a clinical guideline. *J Gerontology: Med Sci* 2000;55:725–734.
7. Shike M, Russell DM, Detsky AS, Harrison JE, McNeill KG, Shepherd FA, et al. Changes in body composition in patients with small-cell cancer. The effect of total parenteral nutrition as an adjunct to chemotherapy. *Ann Intern Med* 1984;101:303–309.
8. Mitch WE. Mechanisms causing loss of lean body mass in kidney disease. *Am J Clin Nutr* 1998;67:359–366.
9. Hedlund J, Hansson LO, Ortqvist A. Short- and long-term prognosis for middle-aged and elderly patients hospitalized with community-acquired pneumonia: impact of nutritional and inflammatory factors. *Scand J Infect Dis* 1995;27:32–37.
10. Toth MJ, Gottlieb SS, Goran MI, Fisher ML, Poehlman ET. Daily energy expenditure in free-living heart failure patients. *Am J Physiol* 1997;272:469–475.
11. Roubenoff R, Roubenoff RA, Cannon JG, Kehayias JJ, Zhuang H, Dawson-Hughes B, et al. Rheumatoid cachexia: cytokine-driven hypermetabolism accompanying reduced body cell mass in chronic inflammation. *J Clin Invest* 1994;93:2379–2386.
12. Kotler DP, Wang J, Pierson RN. Body composition studies in patients with the acquired immunodeficiency syndrome. *Am J Clin Nutr* 1985;42:1255–1265.
13. Morley JE, Thomas DR, Wilson MM. Cachexia: pathophysiology and clinical relevance. *Am J Clin Nutr* 2006;83:735–743.
14. Galanos AN, Pieper CF, Kussin PS, Winchell MR, Fulkerson WJ, Harrell FE Jr, Teno JM, Layde P, Connors AF Jr, Phillips RS, Wenger NS. Relationship of body mass index to subsequent mortality among seriously ill hospitalized patients. *Crit Care Med* 1997;25:1962–1968.

15. Calle EE, Thun MJ, Petrilli JM, Rodriguez C, Heath CW Jr. Body-mass index and mortality in a prospective cohort of U.S. adults. *N Engl J Med* 1999;341:1097–1105.
16. Tayback M, Kumanyika S, Chee E. Body weight as a risk factor in the elderly. *Arch Intern Med* 1990;150:1065–1072.
17. Morley JE, Kraenzle D. Causes of weight loss in a community nursing home. *J Am Geriatr Soc* 1994;42:583–585.
18. Yesavage JA. Geriatric Depression Scale. *Psychopharmacol Bull* 1988;24:709–711.
19. Sheikh J, Yesavage J. Geriatric Depression Scale: recent evidence and development of a shorter version. *Clin Gerontol* 1986;5:165–173.
20. Morley JE, Kraenzle D. Causes of weight loss in a community nursing home. *J Am Geriatr Soc* 1994;42:583–585.
21. Lewis CW, Frongillo EA Jr, Roe DA. Drug-nutrient interactions in three long-term-care facilities. *J Am Diet Assoc* 1995;95:309–315.
22. Chapman KM, Nelson RA. Loss of appetite: managing unwanted weight loss in the older patient. *Geriatrics* 1994;49:54–59.
23. Wright BA. Recent weight loss is related to short-term mortality in nursing homes. *J Gen Intern Med* 1994;9:648–650.
24. Wang SY, Fukagawa N, Hossain M, Ooi WL. Longitudinal weight changes, length of survival, and energy requirements of long-term care residents with dementia. *J Am Geriatr Soc* 1997;45:1189–1195.
25. Keller HH. Malnutrition in institutionalized elderly: how and why? *J Am Geriatric Soc* 1993:41:1212–1218.
26. Blaum CS, Ries BE, Fiatarone MA. Factors associated with low body mass index and weight loss in nursing home residents. *J Gerontol A Biol Sci Med Sci* 1995;50:M162–M168.
27. Morley JE, Silver AJ. Nutritional issues in nursing home care. *Ann Intern Med* 1995;123:850–859.
28. Wilson MM, Thomas DR, Rubenstein LZ, Chibnall JT, Anderson S, Baxi A, Diebold MR, Morley JE. Appetite assessment: simple appetite questionnaire predicts weight loss in community-dwelling adults and nursing home residents. *Am J Clin Nutr* 2005;82:1074–1081.
29. Chidester JC, Spangler AA. Fluid intake in the institutionalized elderly. *J Am Diet Assoc* 1997;97:23–28.
30. Food and Nutrition Board. *Recommended Dietary Allowances*, 10th ed. National Academy Press, Washington, DC, 1989.
31. Chernoff R. Meeting the nutritional needs of the elderly in the institutional setting. *Nutr Rev* 1994;52:132–136.
32. Skipper A. Monitoring and complications of enteral feeding. In *Dietian's Handbook of Enteral and Parenteral Nutrition*, Skipper A, Ed. Aspen Publishers, Rockville, MD, 1993, p. 298.
33. Chidester JC, Spangler AA. Fluid intake in the institutionalized elderly. *J Am Diet Soc* 1997;97:23–28.
34. McGee S, Abernethy W III, Simel DL. Is this patient hypovolemic? *JAMA* 1999;281:1022–1029.
35. Lindeman RD, Romero LJ, Liang HC, Baumgartner RN, Koehler KM, Garry PJ. Do elderly persons need to be encouraged to drink more fluids? *J Gerontol A Biol Sci Med Sci* 2000;55:M361–M365.
36. Morley J. Water, water everywhere and not a drop to drink. *J Gerontol A Biol Sci Med Sci* 2000;55:M359–M360.

37. Rudman D, Feller AG, Nagraj HS, Jackson DL, Rudman IW, Mattson DE. Relation of serum albumin concentration to death rate in nursing home men. *J Parenter Enteral Nutr* 1987;11:360–363.
38. Grant MD, Piotrowski ZH, Miles TP. Declining cholesterol and mortality in a sample of older nursing home residents. *J Am Geriatr Soc* 1996;44:31–36.
39. Frisoni GB, Franzoni S, Rozzini R, Ferrucci L, Boffelli S, Trabucchi M. A nutritional index predicting mortality in the nursing home. *J Am Geriatr Soc* 1994;42:1167–1172.
40. Buckler DA, Kelber ST, Goodwin JS. The use of dietary restrictions in malnourished nursing home patients. *J Am Geriatr Soc* 1994;42:1100–1102.
41. Hotaling DL. Nutritional considerations for the pureed diet texture in dysphagic elderly. *Dysphagia* 1992;7:81–85.
42. Johnson RM, Smiciklas-Wright H, Soucy IM, Rizzo JA. Nutrient intake of nursing home residents receiving pureed foods or a regular diet. *J Am Geriatr Soc* 1995;43:344–348.
43. Kayser-Jones J. Mealtime in nursing homes: the importance of individualized care. *J Gerontol Nurs* 1996;22:26–31.
44. Holzapfel SK, Ramirez RF, Layton MS, Smith IW, Sagl-Massey K, DuBose JZ. Feeder position and food and fluid consumed by nursing home residents. *J Gerontol Nurs* 1996;22:612.
45. Siebens H, Trupe E, Siebens A, Cook F, Anshen S, Hanauer R, Oster G. Correlates and consequences of eating dependency in institutionalized elderly. *J Am Geriatr Soc* 1986;34:192–198.
46. Thomas DR, Verdery RB, Gardner L, Kant A, Lindsay J. A prospective study of outcome from protein-energy malnutrition in nursing home residents. *J Parenter Enteral Nutr* 1991;15:400–404.
47. Pick N, McDonald A, Bennett N, et al. Pulmonary aspiration in a long-term care setting: clinical and laboratory observations and an analysis of risk factors. *J Am Geriatr Soc* 1996;44:763–768.
48. Hickson M, Bulpitt C, Nunes M, Peters R, Cooke J, Nicholl C, Frost G. Does additional feeding support provided by health care assistants improve nutritional status and outcome in acutely ill older in-patients? A randomised control trial. *Clin Nutr* 2004;23:69–77.
49. Gants R. Detection and correction of underweight problems in nursing home residents. *J Gerontol Nurs* 1997;23:26–31.
50. Dawe D, Moore-Orr R. Long-intensity range of motion exercise: invaluable nursing care for elderly patients. *J Adv Nurs* 1995;21:675–681.
51. Ruuskanen JM, Ruoppila I. Physical activity and physiologic well being among people 65–84 years. *Age Ageing* 1995;24:292–296.
52. Fiatarone MA, Marks EC, Ryan ND, et al. High-intensity training in nonagenarians: effects on skeletal muscle. *JAMA* 1990;263:3029–3034.
53. Johnson LE, Dooley PA, Gleick JB. Oral nutritional supplement use in elderly nursing home patients. *J Am Geriatr Soc* 1993;41:947–952.
54. Elmstahl S, Steen B. Hospital nutrition in geriatric long-term care medicine. II. Effects of dietary supplements. *Age Ageing* 1987;16:73–80.
55. Wilson MM, Purushothaman R, Morley JE. Effect of liquid dietary supplements on energy intake in the elderly. *Am J Clin Nutr* 2002;75:944–947.
56. Milne AC, Avenell A, Potter J. Meta-analysis: protein and energy supplementation in older people. *Ann Intern Med* 2006;144:37–48.
57. Lauque S, Arnaud-Battandier F, Gillette S, Plaze JM, Andrieu S, Cantet C, Vellas B. Improvement of weight and fat-free mass with oral nutritional supplementation in patients with Alzheimer's disease at risk of malnutrition: a prospective randomized study. *J Am Geriatr Soc* 2004;52:1702–1707.

58. Fiatarone MA, O'Neill EF, Ryan ND, Clements KM, Solares GR, Nelson ME, Roberts SB, Kehayias JJ, Lipsitz LA, Evans WJ. Exercise training and nutritional supplementation for physical frailty in very elderly people. *N Engl J Med* 1994;330:1769–1775.
59. Meredith CN, Frontera WR, O'Reilly KP, Evans WJ. Body composition in elderly men: effect of dietary modification during strength training. *J Am Geriatr Soc* 1992;40:155–162.
60. Volicer L, Stelly M, Morris J, McLaughlin J, Volicer BJ. Effects of dronabinol on anorexia and disturbed behavior in patients with Alzheimer's disease. *Int J Geriatr Psychiatry* 1997;12:913–919.
61. Kardinal CG, Loprinzi CL, Schaid DJ, Hass AC, Dose AM, Athmann LM, Mailliard JA, McCormack GW, Gerstner JB, Schray MF. Controlled trial of cyproheptadine in cancer patients with anorexia and/or cachexia. *Cancer* 1990;65:2657–2662.
62. Simons JP, Aaronson NK, Vansteenkiste JF, ten Velde GP. Effects of medroxyprogesterone acetate on appetite, weight and quality of life in advance-stage non-hormone-sensitive cancer: a placebo-controlled multicenter study. *J Clin Oncol* 1996;14:1077–1084.
63. Fietau R, Riepl M, Kettner H, et al. Supportive use of megestrol acetate in patients with head and neck cancer during radio/chemotherapy. *Eur J Cancer* 1997;33:75–79.
64. Moertel C, Schutt AG, Reiteneier RJ, et al. Corticosteroid therapy of pre-terminal gastrointestinal cancer. *Cancer* 1974;33:1607–1609.
65. Willox J, Corr J, Shaw J, et al. Prednisolone as an appetite stimulant in patients with cancer. *Br Med J* 1984;288(6410):27.
66. Bruera E, Roca E, Cedaro L, et al. Action of oral methylprednisolone in terminal cancer patients: a prospective randomized double blind study. *Cancer Treat Rep* 1985;69:751–754.
67. Robusteli Della Cuna G, Pellegrini A, Piazzi M. Effect of methylprednisoloone sodium succinate on quality of life in pre-terminal cancer patients: a placebo controlled multicenter study. *Eur J Cancer Clin Oncol* 1989;25:1817–21.
68. Popiela T, Lucchi R, Giongo F. Methylprednisolone as palliative therapy for female terminal cancer patients. The Methylprednisolone Female Preterminal Cancer Study Group. *Eur J Cancer Clin Oncol* 1989;25:1823–1829.
69. Nelson K, Walsh D, Deeter P, et al. A phase II study of delta-nine-tetrahydrocannabinol for appetite stimulation in cancer-associated anorexia. *J Palliative Care* 1994;10:14–18.
70. Plassee TF, Gorter RW, Krasnow SH, et al. Recent clinical experience with dronabinol. *Pharmacol Biochem Behav* 1991;40:695–700.
71. Nelson K, Walsh D, Deeter P, et al. A phase II study of delta-nine-tetrahydrocannabinol for appetite stimulation in cancer-associated anorexia. *J Palliative Care* 1994;10:14–18.
72. Beal JE, Olson R, Lefkowitz L, et al. Long-term efficacy and safety of dronabinol for acquired immunodeficiency syndrom-associated anorexia. *J Pain Symp Manage* 1997;14:7–14.
73. Mantovani G, Maccio A, Bianchi A, et al. Megestrol acetate in neoplastic anorexia/cachexia: clinical evaluation and comparison with cytokine levels in patients with head and neck carcinoma treated with neoadjuvant chemotherapy. *Int J Clin Lab Res* 1995;25:135–141.
74. Reyes-Teran G, Sieira-Madero JG, Martinez del Cerro V, et al. Effects of thalidomide on HIV-associated wasting syndrome: a randomized, double-blind, placebo-controlled clinical trial. *AIDS* 1996;10:1501–1507.
75. Schambelan M, Mulligan K, Grunfeld C, et al. Recombinant human growth hormone in patients with HIV-associated wasting: a randomized, placebo-controlled trial. *Ann Intern Med* 1996;125:873–872.

76. Kaiser FE, Silver AJ, Morley JE. The effect of recombinant human growth hormone on malnourished older individuals. *J Am Geriatr Soc* 1991;39:235–240.
77. Snyder PJ, Peachey H, Berlin JA, et al. Effects of testosterone replacement in hypogonadal men. *J Clin Endocrinol Metab* 2000;85:2670–2677.
78. Morley JE, Perry HM 3rd, Kaiser FE, et al. Effects of testosterone replacement therapy in old hypogonadal males: a preliminary study. *J Am Geriatr Soc* 1993;41:149–152.
79. Sih R, Morley JE, Kaiser FE, et al. Testosterone replacement in older hypogonadal men: a 12-month randomized controlled trial. *J Clin Endocrinol Metab* 1997;82:1661–1667.
80. Bakhshi V, Elliott M, Gentili A, et al. Testosterone improves rehabilitation outcomes in ill older men. *J Am Geriatr Soc* 2000;48:550–553.
81. Hengge UR, Baumann M, Maleba R, et al. Oxymetholone promotes weight gain in patients with advance human immunodeficiency virus (HIV-1) infection. *Br J Nutr* 1996;75:129–138.
82. Pengelly CD. Oxymetholone in the chemotherapy of malignant disease. *Curr Med Res Opin* 1973;1:401–406.
83. Pascual LA, Roque FM, Urrutia CG, et al. Systematic review of megestrol acetate in the treatment of anorexia-cachexia syndrome. *J Pain Symp Manage* 2004;27:360–369.
84. Yeh SS, Wu SY, Lee TP, et al. Improvement in quality-of-life measures and stimulation of weight gain after treatment with megestrol acetate oral suspension in geriatric cachexia: results of a double-blind, placebo-controlled study. *J Am Geriatr Soc* 2000;48:485–492.
85. Karcic E, Philpot C, Morley JE. Treating malnutrition with megestrol acetate: literature review and review of our experience. *J Nutr Health Aging* 2002;6:191–200.
86. Batterham MJ, Garsia R. A comparison of megestrol acetate, nandrolone decanoate and dietary counselling for HIV associated weight loss. *Int J Androl* 2001;24:232–240.
87. Jatoi A, Windschitl HE, Loprinzi CL, et al. Dronabinol versus megestrol acetate versus combination therapy for cancer-associated anorexia: a North Central Cancer Treatment Group Study. *J Clin Oncol* 2002;20:567–573.
88. Jatoi A, Rowland K, Loprinzi CL, et al. An eicosapentaenoic acid supplement versus megestrol acetate versus both for patients with cancer-associated wasting: a North Central Cancer Treatment Group and National Cancer Institute of Canada collaborative effort. *J Clin Oncol* 2004;22:2469–2476.
89. Thomas DR. Guidelines for the use of orexigenic drugs in long-term care. *Nutr Clin Pract* 2006;21:82–87.
90. Mitchell SL, Kiely DK, Lipsitz LA. Does artificial enteral nutrition prolong the survival of institutionalized elders with chewing and swallowing problems? *J Gerontol A Biol Med Sci* 1998;53:M207–M213.
91. Thomas DR. A complete primer on enteral feeding. *Ann Long-Term Care* 2001;9:41–48.
92. Haddad RY, Thomas DR. Enteral nutrition and tube feeding: a review of the evidence. *Geriatr Clin North Am* 2002;18:867–882.
93. Gersovitz M, Motil K, Munro HN, et al. Human protein requirements: assessment of the adequacy of the current recommended dietary allowance for dietary protein in elderly men and women. *Am J Clin Nutr* 1982;35:6–14.
94. Klein CJ, Stanek GS, Wiles CE 3rd. Overfeeding macronutritents to critically ill adults: metabolic complications. *J Am Diet Assoc* 1998;98:795–806.
95. Choban PS, Burge JC, Flanobaum L. Nutrition support of obese hospitalized patients. *Nutr Clin Pract* 1997;12:149–154.

96. Ireton-Jones CS. Evaluation of energy expenditures in obese patients. *Nutr Clin Pract* 1989;4:127–129.
97. Rombeau JL, Caldwell MD, Eds. Nasoenteric tube feeding. In *Clinical Nutrition*, Vol 1. W.B. Saunders, Philadelphia, 1984, p. 261.
98. Kocan MJ, Hickisch SM. A comparison of continuous and intermittent enteral nutrition in NICU patients. *J Neurosci Nurs* 1986;18:333–337.
99. Ciocon JO, Galindo-Ciocon DJ, Tiessen C, Galindo D. Continuous compared with intermittant tube feeding in the elderly. *J Parenter Enteral Nutr* 1992;16:525–528.
100. Haddad RY, Thomas DR. Enteral nutrition and tube feeding: a review of the evidence. *Geriatr Clin North Am* 2002;18:867–882.
101. Montejo JC, Zarazaga A, Lopez-Martinez J, Urrutia G, Roque M, Blesa AL, Celaya S, Conejero R, Galban C, Garcia de Lorenzo A, Grau T, Mesejo A, Ortiz-Leyba C, Planas M, Ordonez J, Jimenez FJ, Spanish Society of Intensive Care Medicine and Coronary Units. Immunonutrition in the intensive care unit. A systematic review and consensus statement. *Clin Nutr* 2003;22(3):221–233.
102. Souba WW. Drug therapy: nutritional support. *N Engl J Med* 1997;336:41–48.
103. Okada K, Yamagami H, Sawada S, Nakanishi M, Tamaki M, Ohnaka M, Sakamoto S, Niwa Y, Nakaya Y. The nutritional status of elderly bed-ridden patients receiving tube feeding. *J Nutr Sci Vitaminol* 2001;47:236–241.
104. Mitchell SL, Kiely DK, Lipsitz LA. The risk factors and impact on survival of feeding tube placement in nursing home residents with severe cognitive impairment. *Arch Intern Med* 1997;157:327–332.
105. Cataldi-Betcher EL, Seltzer MH, Slocum BA, Jones KW. Complications occurring during enteral nutrition support: a prospective study. *J Parenter Enteral Nutr* 1983;7:546–552.
106. Mancuard RP, Perkins AM. Clogging of feeding tubes. *J Parenter Enteral Nutr* 1988;12:403–405.
107. Benya R, Langer S, Mobarhan S. Flexible nasogastric feeding tube tip malposition immediately after placement. *J Parenter Enteral Nutr* 1990;14:108.
108. Ciocon JO, Silverstone FA, Graver LM, Foley CJ. Tube feedings in elderly patients: indications, benefits, and complications. *Arch Intern Med* 1988;148:429.
109. Hunt JN, Stubbs DF. The volume and energy content of meals as determinations of gastric emptying. *J Physiol* 1974;245:209.
110. Davenport HW. *Physiology of the Digestive Tract*, 4th ed. Year Book Medical Publishers, Chicago, 1977.
111. Gustke R, Varme R, Soergel K. Gastric reflux during perfusion of the proximal small bowel. *Gastroenterology* 1970;59:890–895.
112. Cogen R, Weinryb J. Aspiration pneumonia in nursing home patients fed via gastrostomy tubes. *Am J Gastroenterol* 1989;84:1509–1512.
113. Wolfsen HC, Kozarek RA, Ball TJ, Patterson DJ, Botoman VA. Tube dysfunction following percutaneous endoscopic gastrostomy and jejunostomy. *Gastointest Endosc* 1990;36:261–263.
114. Kelly TWJ, Patrick MR, Hillman KM. Study of diarrhea in critically ill patients. *Crit Care Med* 1983;11:7–9.
115. Benya R, Mobarhan S. Enteral alimentation: administration and complications. *J Am Coll Nutr* 1991;10:209–219.
116. Hillman KM, Riordan T, O'Farrell SM, Tabaqchali S. Colonization of the gastric contents in critically ill patients. *Crit Care Med* 1982;10:444–447.
117. Alverdy JC, Aoys E, Moss GS. Effect of commercially available chemically defined liquid diets on the intestinal microflora and bacterial translocation from the gut. *J Parenter Enteral Nutr* 1990;14:1–6.

118. Grant MD, Rudberg M, Brody JA. Life on the slippery slope: tube-fed in the nursing home. *Gerontologist* 1996;36:47.
119. Mitchell SI, Keely DL, Lipitz LA. The risk factors and impact on survival of feeding tube placement in nursing home residents with severe cognitive impairment. *Arch Intern Med* 1997;157:327–332.
120. Weaver JP, Odell P, Nelson C. Evaluation of the benefits of gastric tube feeding in an elderly population. *Arch Fam Med* 1993;2:953–956.
121. O'Brien LA, Siegert EA, Grisso JA, et al. Tube feeding preferences among nursing home residents. *J Gen Intern Med* 1997;12:364–371.
122. Bourdel-Marchasson I, Dumas F, Finganaud G, et al. Audit of percutaneous endoscopic gastrostomy in long-term enteral feeding in a nursing home. *Int J Qual Health Care* 1997;8:297.
123. Souba WW. Nutritional support, *N Engl J Med.* 1997;336(1):41–8.
124. McCann RM, Hall WJ, Groth-Juncker A. Comfort care for terminally ill patients. The appropriate use of nutrition and hydration. *JAMA* 1994;272:1263–1266.
125. Plank LK, Connolly AB, Hill GI. Sequential changes in the metabolic response in severely septic patients during the first 23 days after the onset of peritonitis. *Ann Surg* 1998;228:146–158.
126. Shizgal HM, Martin MF, Gimmon Z. The effect of age on the caloric requirement of malnourished individuals. *Am J Clin Nutr* 1992;55:783–789.
127. Thomas DR. A prospective, randomized clinical study of adjunctive peripheral parenteral nutrition in adult subacute care patients. *J Nutr Health Aging* 2005;9:321–325.
128. Shaver HJ, Loper JA, Lutes RA. Nutritional status of nursing home patients. *J Parenter Enteral Nutr* 1980;4:367–370.
129. Pinchocofsky-Devin GD, Kaminski MV. Incidence of protein calorie malnutrition in the nursing home population. *J Am Coll Nutr* 1987;6:109–112.
130. Sliver AJ, Morley JE, Strome LS, Jones D, Vickers L. Nutritional status in an academic nursing home. *J Am Geriatr Soc* 1988;36:487–491.
131. Thomas DR, Verdery RB, Gardner L, Kant AK, Lindsay J. A prospective study of outcome from protein-energy malnutrition in nursing home residents. *J Parenter Enteral Nutr* 1991;15:400–404.
132. Larsson J, Unosson M, Ek A-C, Nilsson L, Thorslund S, Bjurulf P. Effect of dietary supplement on nutritional status and clinical outcome in 501 geriatric patients: a randomized study. *Clin Nutr* 1990;9:179–184.
133. Nelson KJ, Coulston AM, Sucher KP, Tseng RY. Prevalence of malnutrition in the elderly admitted to long-term-care facilities. *J Am Diet Assoc* 1993;93:459–461.
134. Wright BA. Weight loss and weight gain in a nursing home: a prospective study. *Geriatr Nurs* 1993;14:156–159.
135. Abbasi AA, Rudman D. Observations on the prevalence of protein-calorie undernutrition in VA nursing homes. *J Am Geriatr Soc* 1993;41:117–121.
136. Morley JE, Kraenzle D. Causes of weight loss in a community nursing home. *J Am Geriatr Soc* 1994;42:583–585.
137. Blaum CS, Fries BE, Fiatarone MA. Factors associated with low body mass index and weight loss in nursing home residents. *J Gerontol A Biol Sci Med Sci* 1995;50:M162–M168.
138. Bistrian BR, Sherman M, Blackburn GL, Marshall R, Shaw C. Cellular immunity in adult marasmus. *Arch Intern Med* 1977;137:1408–1411.
139. Weinsier RL, Hunker EM, Krumdieck CL, Butterworth CE Jr. Hospital malnutrition. A prospective evaluation of general medical patients during the course of hospitalization. *Am J Clin Nutr* 1979;32:418–426.

140. Warnold I, Lundholm K. Clinical significance of preoperative nutritional status in 215 noncancer patients. *Ann Surg* 1984;199:299–305.
141. Pinchcofsky-Devin GD, Kaminski MV Jr. Correlation of pressure sores and nutritional status. *J Am Geriatr Soc* 1986;34:435–440.
142. Detsky AS, Baker JP, O'Rourke K, Johnston N, Whitwell J, Mendelson RA, Jeejeebhoy KN. Predicting nutrition-associated complications for patients undergoing gastrointestinal surgery. *J Parenter Enteral Nutr* 1987;11:440–446.
143. Dwyer JT, Coleman KA, Krall E, Yang GA, Scanlan M, Galper L, Winthrop E, Sullivan P. Changes in relative weight among institutionalized elderly adults. *J Gerontol* 1987;42:246–251.
144. Windsor JA, Hill GL. Weight loss with physiologic impairment. A basic indicator of surgical risk. *Ann Surg* 1988;207:290–296.
145. Berlowitz DR, Wilking SVB. Risk factors for pressure sore: a comparison of cross-sectional and cohort-derived data. *J Am Geriatr Soc* 1989;37:1043–1050.
146. Chang JI, Katz PR, Ambrose P. Weight loss in nursing home patients: prognostic implications. *J Fam Pract* 1990;30:671–674.
147. Brandeis GH, Morris JN, Nash DJ, Lipsitz LA. Epidemiology and natural history of pressure ulcers in elderly nursing home residents. *JAMA* 1990;264;2905–2909.
148. Thomas DR, Verdery RB, Gardner L, Kant AK, Lindsay J. A prospective study of outcome from protein-energy malnutrition in nursing home residents. *J Parenter Enteral Nutr* 1991;15:400–404.
149. Windsor JA. Underweight patients and the risk of major surgery. *World J Surg* 1993;17:165–172.
150. Murden RA, Ainslie NK. Recent weight loss is related to short-term mortality in nursing homes. *J Gen Intern Med* 1994;9:648–650.
151. Kaiser FE, Morley JE. Idiopathic CD4+ T lymphopenia in older persons. *J Am Geriatr Soc* 1994;42:1291–1294.
152. Franzoni S, Frisoni GB, Boffelli S, Rozzini R, Trabucchi M. Good nutritional oral intake is associated with equal survival in demented and nondemented very old patients. *J Am Geriatr Soc* 1996;44:1366–1370.
153. Berkhout AM, van Houwelingen JC, Cools HJ. Increased chance of dying among nursing home patients with lower body weight. *Nederlands Tijdschrift Geneeskunde* 1997;141:2184–2188.
154. Flacker JM, Kiely DK. A practical approach to identifying mortality-related factors in established long-term care residents. *J Am Geriatr Soc* 1998;46:1012–1015.
155. Gambassi G, Landi F, Lapane KL, Sgadari A, Mor V, Bernabei R. Predictors of mortality in patients with Alzheimer's disease living in nursing homes. *J Neurol Neurosurg Psychiatry* 1999;67:59–65.
156. Perry HM III, Ali AS, Morley JE. The effect of weight loss on outcomes in a nursing home. *J Invest Med* 1999;47:225A.
157. Sullivan DH, Sun S, Walls RC. Protein-energy undernutrition among elderly hospitalized patients: a prospective study. *JAMA* 1999;281;2013–2019.

17 Prescription for Enteral Nutrition

Zareen Syed, M.D.
Syed H. Tariq, M.D.

CONTENTS

17.1 INTRODUCTION

As the population is aging and individuals live longer, enteral feeding is becoming a common medical intervention. As with any medical intervention, enteral nutrition carries with it benefits and risks. Enteral nutrition has been a hot topic in the media due to the ethical issues involved with it. These ethical issues become more important when dealing with the geriatric population. Enteral nutrition is the provision of nutrients to the stomach or intestine via a tube to individuals who are unable to eat or do not eat enough.

17.2 PREVALENCE OF ENTERAL FEEDING

With the advent of percutaneous endoscopic gastrostomy (PEG) tubes in the 1980s, there has been an increase in the number of patients with feeding tubes. From 1988 to 1995, the number of gastrostomies increased from 61,000[1] to 121,000.[2] According to the National Center for Health Statistics in 2003, there were 146,000 feeding tubes placed in patients.

In 1991, in a retrospective cohort study on Medicare beneficiaries 65 and older and discharged from the hospital with gastrostomies, a total of 59,969 were PEG placements and 21,136 were placed surgically. The most common indication was cerebrovascular accidents (CVA) followed by neoplasms (Table 17.1). It was also noted that a higher percentage of patients were older and black.[3] The disparity may be due to different risk factors for stroke[4] or cultural differences regarding enteral feeding.[5] In this study dementia was a secondary diagnosis in 10% of the patients. In another study with 186,635 cognitively impaired residents in a nursing home, 34% had feeding tubes.[6]

TABLE 17.1
Discharge Diagnoses Post Gastrostomies in Medicare Beneficiaries 65 Years Old or Older in 1991

Diagnoses	Women (%)	Men (%)	Total (%)
CVA	30.2	29.4	29.9
Neoplasms	17.2	28.9	21.9
Malnutrition	28.7	25.1	27.3
Dementia	12.2	8.3	10.7
Swallowing disorder	10.4	10.6	10.5
Aspiration pneumonia	6.8	10.5	8.3

17.3 INDICATIONS FOR TUBE FEEDING

Tube feeding should be considered in a patient who will not be able to have adequate nutritional intake for over 2 to 3 weeks. Prior to insertion of enteral tubes, several things need to be taken into consideration: the medical illness, diagnosis, prognosis, patient's wishes, and quality of life. It should not be considered in patients with a poor prognosis or terminal disease. It is important to take a thorough history regarding oral intake and medication use, and to look for reversible causes of poor oral intake. Oral supplements should be tried along with a swallow evaluation. If this fails, an enteral tube should be inserted early in the disease to prevent further decline in nutritional status. Prospective clinical trials have shown that insertion of enteral tubes in a timely fashion can halt further deterioration of nutritional status, but rarely will the patient gain the lost weight completely even in benign conditions.[7]

There are three main indications for enteral feeding (Table 17.2). The first is neurological disorder with impaired swallowing, accounting for 19% of patients on enteral feeds.[3] The second group of patients are unable to meet the nutritional demands by oral intake secondary to increased catabolic states, like in chemotherapy or radiation treatment for cancers or cachexia. The third groups of patients are those who are unable to eat. One study estimated 11% of tube feeders belonged to this group.[3]

TABLE 17.2
Indications for Enteral Nutrition

Neurological Disorders
CVA
Motor neuron disorder
Multiple sclerosis
Gullian–Barre
Parkinson's disease
Unable to Meet Nutritional Demands
Cystic fibrosis
Extensive burns
Perioperative
Decreased Desire to Eat
Severe depression
Chronic medical illnesses
Dementia
Anorexia nervosa
Post chemotherapy/radiation
Unable to Eat
GI obstruction—strictures, cancer, intestinal failure
Ventilated patients
Trauma

Dementia is one of the most controversial areas in regard to enteral feeding. In elderly patients the most common reason is dysphagia and frequent aspirations.[8] To date, no studies confirm that PEG tubes prevent aspiration.

Enteral tubes could be placed temporarily or permanently depending on the indication.

17.4 CONTRAINDICATIONS

Serious coagulation disorders (INR > 1.5, PTT > 50 sec, platelets < 50,000/mm^3), mechanical obstruction of the GI tract, severe ascites, peritonitis, severe psychosis, and limited life expectancy are contraindications for a G tube and J tube placement.[9] Relative contraindications are enterocutaneous fistula, severe pancreatitis, and gastrointestinal ischemia.[10]

17.5 ENTERAL FEEDING SYSTEMS

Enteral tube systems can be placed via a nasal route, percutaneously, or surgically. Patients can receive enteral feeding for a short period (less than 4 weeks) via the nose to the stomach or the small bowel. Patients who have gastroparesis or have had their stomach surgically removed would be candidates for small bowel feeding with a nasojejunal (NJ) tube. Nasogastric (NG) tubes are usually 8 to 12 French tubes passed in the stomach. Auscultation with abdominal radiograph is recommended for confirmation of placement. Around 12% of the patients will have complications with an NG tube placement. Examples include nasal mucosal ulceration, ear infection, pharyngitis, sinusitis, tracheoesophageal fistula, tube migration, aspiration pneumonia, and tube obstruction.[11]

If patients require enteral feeding for more than a month, endoscopic percutaneous routes are preferred. This procedure requires sedation. Enteral feeds could be provided by a percutaneous endoscopic gastrostomy (PEG) tube, percutaneous endoscopic gastojejunostomy (PEG/J), and direct percutaneous jejunostomy. PEG tubes are currently the preferred route, mostly because of safety, cost, and comfort. When compared with an NG tube, they were more socially acceptable. Regarding nutritional efficacy, PEGs were better than NG tube feeding.[12] PEG tubes range from 15 to 28 French. With appropriate care, they can last 1 to 2 years. Procedure-related complication rates ranged from 0 to 2%.[13–15]

Percutaneously, a jejunostomy can be placed via either a gastrostomy or a direct jejunostomy. A 20 French gastrostomy tube is placed and a second 8 to 12 French jejunostomy tube is passed through the gastrostomy tube. The jejunostomy tubes often become clogged or displaced in the stomach.[16] A PEG/J would last 3 to 6 months. Due to the small bore of the J tubes, the PEG/J becomes clogged easily and needs aggressive flushing. The clogging rates vary from 3.5 to 35%.[17,18,19] Tube migration can also occur during vomiting.

Prior to the advent of percutaneous endoscopic procedures, the enteral tubes were introduced surgically. Gastrostomy, gastojejunostomy, and jejunostomy were procedures performed via open technique or laproscopically. Studies have shown that percutaneous gastrostomy is cost effective, saves operative time, and decreases morbidity compared to surgical gastrostomies.[20]

Patients who are intolerable to gastric feeds, high-risk aspiration, gastroparesis, gastric resection, severe gastroesophageal reflux, gastric or duodenal fistula, or gastric outlet obstruction are candidates for surgical or percutaneous jejunostomy. Surgical jejunostomes have been associated with a mortality rate of 10%. Common complications are intestinal obstruction, necrosis, and fistulas.[21]

17.6 JEJUNAL VERSUS GASTRIC FEEDING

It had been believed that if a jejunal tube was placed there was less of a chance of aspiration. Vanek[22] reported that there was more aspiration pneumonia with percutaneous endoscopic gastrostomy/jejunostomy then with a PEG. They also concluded that the patients with the PEG/J were sicker and more prone to aspiration. Intestinal tube feeds still stimulate gastric acid secretion, and hence the risk of aspiration persists. It has been noted that when the feeding tube was 60 cm away from the ligament of Trietz, the pancreatic secretions decreased to 50% compared to the feeding tube in the jejunum.[23]

17.7 FORMULA SELECTION

Enteral formula selection is patient specific. Various factors have to be taken into account, like medical illness, nutritional status, digestive and absorptive capacity, renal, cardiac, or hepatic diseases, route of administration, and cost. All formulas contain carbohydrates, fats, and proteins. Table 17.3 gives an example of different classes of products. The amount of enteral formula that a patient needs can be calculated by nutritional calculations, as shown in Table 17.4. The protein content of a formula should be between 7 and 16% of the total calories. The recommended daily requirement of proteins is 0.8 g/kg/day, but in elderly patients the requirement may go up to 1.2 to 1.5g/kg/day.[24]

Proteins could be intact, partially hydrolyzed, or free amino acid. Patients with abnormal digestive enzymes would benefit from hydrolyzed proteins and crystalline amino acids. Formulas for renal disease patients contain essential amino acids, while formulas for hepatic failure patients contain branched-chain amino acids.

TABLE 17.3
Class of Nutrition Products and Degree of Digestion

Class	Degree of Digestion
Intact nutrients	Requires normal pancreatic enzymes
Milk based	Requires normal pancreatic enzymes
Lactose-free	Requires normal pancreatic enzymes, except lactose
Hydrolyzed proteins	No digestion; requires intact brush border for absorption
Crystalline amino acids	No digestion; no brush border absorption; uses passive absorption
Incomplete amino acids	Hepatic or renal failure

TABLE 17.4
Calculating Enteral Feeding Requirements

Proteins	Maintenance	1.2–1.5 g/kg/day
	Stress	1.5–2.0 g/kg/day
Calories	Maintenance	25–30 kcal/kg/day
	Stress	30–40 kcal/kg/day
	Sepsis	40–50 kcal/kg/day
	Free water	30–35 ml/kg/day

Carbohydrates are the primary source of calories in an enteral formula and a major determinant of osmolarity. The carbohydrate content may be in the form of polysaccharides, oligosaccharides, or saccharides. The smaller molecules are sweeter and more osmolar than the bigger molecules. For lactose-intolerant individuals, there are many formulas that are lactose-free. Formulas can contain up to 0.5 to 2 kcal/ml. In patients with fluid restriction, a high-calorie formula can be used. High-calorie formulas can clog tubes, decrease gastric motility and emptying, and may increase the risk of aspiration.

Lipids are a concentrated source of energy and should constitute 30% of the total calories of a formula. Higher concentrations lead to diarrhea.[25] There are specialized formulas in which lipids are the major source of calories (lipid content up to 55%). These formulas are used for patients who have problems of CO_2 retention and go into respiratory failure.[26]

The usual free water requirement is 30 to 35 ml/kg/day. Most of the formulas are 75% free water. The amount and frequency of water flushes can be adjusted to meet the daily requirement. Commonly used enteral formulas are shown in Table 17.5.

17.8 ENTERAL NUTRITION IN DIABETICS

Fluctuation in blood sugars, lipid abnormalities, and dehydration are concerns in diabetic patients on enteral nutrition. Standard enteral formulas are high in carbohydrates, low in fat, and low in fiber. These formulas may lead to loss of glycemic control secondary to rapid gastric emptying and rapid nutrient absorption.[27] A meta-analysis showed that diabetic-specific formulas have better glycemic control.[28] Special diabetic formulas are higher in fat (40 to 50% of the total caloric requirement, with more of the monosaturated fatty acids) and lower in carbohydrates (30 to 40% of the calories and 15% from fructose). This composition of the enteral formula helps improve glycemic control. The combination of fats and fiber reduce gastric emptying; the fiber content helps in slowing intestinal absorption of the carbohydrates, and fructose causes less glycemic fluctuations. A meta-analysis of increased fat content in the formula did not find any drastic effects on the lipid panel.[28] One study done in long-term-care patients with type 2 diabetes found that a diabetes-specific formula was associated with less pneumonia, fever, and urinary tract infections.[29]

TABLE 17.5
Commonly Used Enteral Formulas

Formula	Features	Comments
Ensure Plus	High calorie, high protein, MCTs, fortified with mineral and vitamins	Complete and balanced
Jevity	Isotonic, fiber	Complete and balanced
Jevity Plus	High nitrogen, prebiotics FOSs, fiber and beta-carotene	FOSs are undigested CHO that are fermented in colon to produce SCFAs; helps in absorption of H_2O and electrolytes, reducing diarrhea
Glucerna	Reduced CHO, modified MUFAs, has fiber	Glycemic control in diabetics and stress-induced hyperglycemia
Nepro	Mod protein, fortified vitamins and minerals, high Ca, low phosphorus, contains FOSs	In renal failure
Perative	For metabolically stressed patients (burns, wounds)	No data to support healing
Pulmocare	Low CHO for COPD patients	Doubtful clinical use
Two Cal	Condensed formula with fluid restriction	CHF, SIADH

Note: FOSs = fructooligosaccharides; SCFAs = short-chain fatty acids; MCTs = medium-chain triglycerides; MUFA = monounsaturated fatty acids; CHO = carbohydrates.

17.8.1 Initiating Feeds

Isotonic formulas can be started at full strength, while hypertonic formulas may need to be diluted. To determine the rate of feeding, a volume of water equivalent to the amount of desired feeding is infused in the stomach. The tube is clamped and residuals are checked in 30 min. If the residual volume is less than 50% of the volume infused, it is appropriate to start the tube feeding at that rate.[30]

17.8.1.1 Stomach

The stomach is a reservoir, and gastric secretions can dilute the feeding formula, so they can be started at full strength without a starter regime.[31] Feedings should be started at 15 to 25 ml/h and advanced by 20 ml/h every 4 to 8 h until the goal rate is achieved.

17.8.1.2 Jejunum

The jejunum does not have reservoir ability and cannot dilute the formula, so a starter regime is usually needed. The strength of the feeding formula is diluted by one fourth to one third and started at a rate of 15 to 25 ml/h, and the rate is increased every couple of days until the target rate is achieved. Once the target is reached, the strength of the formula can be increased as tolerated by the patient.[32]

17.8.2 Intermittent versus Continuous

Enteral feeding could be intermittent or continuous. With a gastrostomy tube, intermittent feeding schedules are used and are usually preferred due to convenience of staff, more mobility of the patient, no need for infusion pump, and it is more physiologic.[33] Residual volumes checked prior to every feeding, if greater than 200 ml for nasogastric tube or 100 ml for gastrostomy tube, should raise concern.

Continuous feeding may be better in patients who experience nausea and early satiety with intermittent feeding, e.g., patients with severe gastroparesis. Patients receiving enteral nutrition directly in the duodenum or jejunum should be on a continuous feeding regime to avoid abdominal distention, pain, and dumping syndrome. The volume can be titrated every 6 to 8 h as the patient tolerates it. Residual volume should be checked every 2 to 4 h, and if greater than 1.5 times the hourly rate, the tube feeds should be stopped.[34]

17.9 DRUG ADMINISTRATION AND ENTERAL NUTRITION

When patients are on enteral feeding, the medication should be reviewed and all unnecessary medications should be stopped. Medications should be given via other routes (transdermal or intravenous) if possible. Once-a-day dosing is preferred. Dosage might need adjustment when changed from tablets to liquid forms. The liquid formulations may have sorbitol, which is a laxative and can cause diarrhea.[35] Liquid medications should be diluted with 30 cc of water to decrease the osmolality.[36] Medication should be given separately with water flushes in between them.

As a general rule, if medication absorption is altered with food or antacids, it will be affected with enteral feeds as well. Dilantin, ciprofloxacin, theophylline, digoxin, tetracycline, and rifampin are good examples. Potassium- and calcium-containing medications cause precipitation. Some medications should never be crushed. Long-acting medications should not be crushed; they may lead to variable levels in the plasma and side effects. Not all liquid preparations are appropriate for administration via PEG tubes. Augmentin and lansoprazole suspensions form clumps, carbemeazpine adheres to the plastic tube,[37] and temazepam makes the tube green.

If the patient is on continuous feeding via nasogastric tube or gastrostomy, the feeding should be held for 15 to 20 min prior to the medication. If the patient has jejunostomy, there is no need to stop the feedings until the drug is actually administered. The medications are directly absorbed from the small bowel. If the patients are on intermittent feeding, medications should be administered at least 2 h after feeding.[38] If the patient is pregnant, avoid crushing finaseteride, because it can be absorbed from the skin and affect the genitalia of a male fetus.[39] Table 17.6 shows the list of oral medications that should not be crushed.

17.9.1 Removal of a PEG Tube

It is recommended to remove the PEG endoscopically because there have been cases of ileus requiring surgery,[40,41] but some tubes could be cut externally and the distal

TABLE 17.6
Oral Medications That Should Not Be Crushed[a]

Request a Substitute Drug
Cannot be crushed and not available in another oral form
Bisacodyl (Dulcolax)
Diclofenac (Voltaren)
Diltiazem (Cardizem SR)
Omeprazole (Prilosec)
Pentoxyphylline (Trental)
Piroxicam (Feldene)
Change Administration
Can open the capsules and administer these via the tubes
Ferrous Fumarate (Ferro-Sequels)
Indomethacin (Indocin SR)
Nifedipine (Procardia)
Nitroglycerin SR (Nitro-Bid)
Phenytoin (Dilantin Capseals)
Theophylline (Slo-Phyllin Gyrocaps, Theo-Dur Sprinkle)
Use Alternate Dosage Forms
A liquid dose or oral form that can be crushed can be used in place of these drugs—most are sustained release. Adjustment in the dose and frequency will be needed.
Acetazolmide (Diamoz sequels)
Morphine sulfate (MS contin)
Albuterol (Proventil repetabs)
Potassium chloride (slow K)
Asa enteric coated (Ecotrin)
Propanolol (Inderal LA)
Carbidopa and levodopa (Sinemet CR)
Theophylline (Theo-Dur)
Lithium carbonate (Eskalith CR)
Methylphenidate (Ritalin SR)
Divalproex (Depakote)
Erythomycin base (E-mycin)
Ferrous sulfate, enteric coated (Feosol)
Isosorbide dinitrate (Isordil Tembids)

[a] Pertains only to the brand names listed.

part passes through the rectum.[40] Most of the newer PEG systems can be pulled out without any endoscopy.

17.10 COMPLICATIONS

Chances of major complications after a percutaneous endoscopic placement of a tube range from 0.4 to 8.4%. These complications include wound infections, necrotizing fasciitis, aspiration, bleeding, perforation, ileus, tumor seeding, and death.[13,42–44] Procedure-related complication chances range from 0 to 2%.[13–15] Minor complications include stomal soreness and minor infection, stomal leakage, tube blockage, and gastrointestinal upset related to onset of tube feeding.

The most common complication is local wound infection (15%). Prophylactic use of antibiotics has reduced the rate of wound infections.[45,46] Most of the time it is less than 5 mm of the surrounding area of the stoma, usually due to movement. Most of the local infections are treatable with local wound care. If the infection persists, antibiotics should be used. Pnemoperitoneum is found in 50% of patients after having a PEG placed. The patient should be monitored; there is no clinical evidence that it leads to adverse events. Patients may initially complain of pain in the stomal site, fever, or leakage of gastric secretions. A hydrocolloid dressing can be used to protect the skin.

If the tube is pulled out, it cannot be replaced prior to 3 weeks, because that is the time needed for the tract to mature. An attempt to reinsert the tube should be made within 6 to 12 h; otherwise, the patient needs to be referred to a specialist.

Long-term complications include clogging, dislodging, aspiration pneumonia, and diarrhea. Tube clogging is one of the most common problems in patients on enteral nutrition. Blockage of the tube results from smaller tubes, hypertonic formulas, inadequate flushing, and inappropriate administrations of medications. Evidence suggests that flushing tubes with water and pancreatic enzyme solution is better than with cranberry juice, colas, or meat tenderizer.

Diarrhea is found in 30% of patients receiving enteral nutrition; mostly the etiology is not the formula. Medications are the most common reason for the diarrhea in 61% of the cases. Some examples are antibiotics, H-2 blockers, laxatives, antacids, sorbitol or fructose-based elixirs, and antineoplastic agents.[47] Fifty percent of patients on antibiotics get diarrhea.[48] The high osmolar formulas can cause diarrhea if delivered to the small intestine, especially in patients with recent intestinal surgeries or diseases involving the small intestine.[49] The composition of the enteral formula alters the bowel flora and may increase the risk of antibiotic-associated diarrhea. *Lactobacillus* can be used to reduce the risk on *Clostridium difficile* diarrhea.

Enteral feeding does not prevent aspiration. Aspiration pneumonia is found in about 23 to 58% of patients with a gastrostomy tube.[50,51] The risk of aspiration can be decreased if patients are tube-fed with the head of the bed elevated to 30°. One study reported that 40% of patients had some elevation of liver enzymes.[52] In elderly demented patients, a feeding tube might necessitate restraints and make them more agitated. In one study, 71% of patients with tube feeds were restrained.[53]

17.11 EFFICACY OF ENTERAL NUTRITION

17.11.1 Malnutrition

The feeding tubes are inserted in elderly demented patients to improve nutrition. Observational studies have failed to show increase in weight or improvement in parameters related to malnutrition like serum albumin.[54] In one study, 40 enterally fed patients in a nursing home continued to lose weight despite adequate calories and proteins.[55] In severe Alzheimer dementia, malnutrition may represent end-stage disease rather than a reversible problem. In trials with cancer patients there was no survival benefit of enteral feeding.[56]

17.11.2 Life Prolongation

Feeding tubes are supposed to prolong life; however, that is not true. One study involving elderly demented patients with PEG tubes showed a 30-day mortality rate of 24 to 27% and a 1-year mortality rate of 50 to 63%.[57,58] Another study with VA patients 75 and older showed a median survival of 5.7 month.[44] A study with 5266 nursing home residents found that tube-fed patients were 1.44 times more at risk of dying after a year than orally fed patients.[59] A study with orally fed demented and nondemented elderly in nursing homes showed the same survival rate.[60] A 2-year retrospective chart review of elderly demented patients who received the PEG and those without it showed no survival benefit between the two groups.[61,62]

17.11.3 Aspiration

Feeding tubes are inserted in elderly patients to prevent aspiration. Contaminated oral secretions play a role in aspiration. Studies have shown that mechanically ventilated patients who received subglottic suctioning had less incidence of pneumonia than the ones who did not.[63]

To date, there are no studies to prove that tube feedings prevent aspiration. However, the most common cause of death in tube feeders in nursing homes is aspiration pneumonia.[64] Aspiration occurs with oral and pharyngeal secretions, which cannot be reduced by an enteral feeding. Good oral care reduces the risk of aspiration.[65] The risk factors for aspiration with a PEG tube include a previous history of aspiration, being elderly, and dementia.[50]

One nonrandomized study showed that orally fed patients had less aspiration pneumonia than tube-fed patients.[66] Jejunostomy is also not associated with lower risk of aspiration.[67,68] One of the studies found similar rates of aspiration between enteral feeds delivered to the stomach and the jejunum. It was also noted that patients in the first group gained more weight than those in the second group.[69]

17.11.4 Wound Healing

It is believed that good nutritional status improves wound healing. Studies suggest that tube feedings do not heal preexisting wounds[70] or prevent new ones.[71]

17.11.5 Comfort

Comfort is the important thing families want for their loved one. In advanced dementia, when elderly stop eating, the topic of tube feeding comes up. Families do not want their loved ones to die of hunger and thirst. When deciding about enteral feeding, families should be informed that patients usually do not feel hungry or thirsty at the end of life. Data support that patients who do not want to eat or cannot eat (terminal cancer) deny feeling hungry or thirsty and are relieved with just moist lips or ice chips.[72]

A hospice nurse survey found that patients with voluntary dehydration died more peacefully and usually within 2 weeks.[73] It has been reported that people who fast for spiritual reasons have intact mental capacity and no suffering.[74] Hunger and nausea are thought to be increased by tube feeding. Patients had less social interaction (no one-to-one feeding) once placed on feeding tubes.[75] The American Academy of Hospice and Palliative Medicine (AAHPM)[76] position statement asserts:

> When a person is approaching death, the provision of artificial hydration and nutrition is potentially harmful and may provide little or no benefit to the patient and at times may make the period of dying more uncomfortable for both patient and family. For this reason, the AAHPM believes that the withholding of artificial hydration and nutrition near the end of life may be appropriate and beneficial medical care.

17.12 MORTALITY

According to one study, the mortality of patients with PEG for 7 days is 48%; risk factors included prior aspiration, UTI, and being greater than 75 years old, vs. mortality of 4% in patients without these risk factors.[77]

17.13 DISEASE-SPECIFIC DATA ON EFFICACY

17.13.1 Stroke

Neurological disorders are the most common indication for a gastrostomy tube. Approximately 25 to 29% of the patients are able to swallow again, and the tube can be removed in 2 to 3 years.[78,79]

17.13.2 Motor Neuron Disease

Motor neuron disease is a progressive degenerative disorder involving the loss of motor neurons in the cortex, brainstem, and spinal cord. Bulbar dysfunction leads to weakness of the pharyngeal, respiratory, and limb muscles. These patients are prone to malnutrition and aspiration and have a higher requirement for energy secondary to spasms and fasciculations. Malnutrition is a negative prognostic factor[80] when weight loss of 5% or bulbar signs appear; a gastrostomy tube should be discussed with the patient.[81] One study showed that patients on enteral feeding increased survival by 6 months.[82]

17.13.3 Parkinson's Disease

Oropharyngeal dysphagia is common in Parkinson's disease. In many patients it is unrecognized. With weight loss, a swallow evaluation should be the next step. No study shows the effect of enteral nutrition in Parkinson's patients.

17.13.4 Cancer

Head and neck cancer patients tend to do better when they have a PEG placed prior to radiation and chemotherapy. They had less weight loss than those without the PEG (3.1 vs. 7 kg). They also had less hospitalizations and less interruption in their chemotherapy and radiation.[83]

Esophageal cancers are associated with a great amount of weight loss, and the treatment leads to further nutritional deterioration. The bilateral vagotomy with the esophagectomy leads to delayed gastric emptying. These patients benefit from a PEG or PEJ tube. In one study of patients with complications of espophagectomy, 84% had successful placement of a direct PEJ and were weaned off the total parenteral nutrition (TPN) and discharged home early.[84] It has been shown that around 30% of cancer patients are able to resume oral intake and do not need enteral feeds in the first year.[85]

17.13.5 Enteral Feeds and Hip Fracture

Bastow et al. showed that patients with hip fracture who were undernourished, when provided with nightly enteral feeds along with their normal oral intake in the daytime, required shorter rehabilitation time and had decreased mortality.[86] In a meta-analysis, 943 patients showed that protein-energy supplementation decreased the mortality and complications in patients with hip fracture.[87]

17.14 DECISION-MAKING CAPACITY AND ENTERAL NUTRITION

About 10% of patients with enteral nutrition have dementia and are living in a nursing home. For patients with advanced dementia, the decision about artificial nutrition falls upon the surrogate decision maker. It is usually very helpful if patients have advanced directives regarding artificial nutrition. In a discussion about enteral tube feeding, the risks and benefits and alternative methods should be offered to the surrogate decision maker. Forty-five percent of surrogate decision makers stated that no alternative was offered, and 2% were offered spoon feeding.[88] In a study from Boston and Ottawa, 54% of the proxies stated they were given adequate information, 49% understood the benefit of tube feeding, and 83% said they understood the benefits to be life prolongation and decreased risk of aspiration.[89] Another survey of proxies' decisions regarding enteral nutrition was based on the following reasons: better nutrition (70%), comfort (22%), life prolongation (18%), increase in strength (14%), and help in overcoming the acute illness (10%).[90]

17.15 RELIGION AND ENTERAL NUTRITION

Religion and faith are an important part in how we make decisions regarding life and death. Sanctity of life is an important principle in all religions. *Jewish law halacha* states that life-sustaining treatment can be withheld if the person dying is suffering or the treatment would produce suffering. In advanced dementia, when patients stop eating the median survival is 6 months, with or without feeding tubes.[91] Dementia itself does not cause pain, but other problems associated with dementia, like pressure ulcers or contractors, can lead to suffering. Enteral feeding may add to the suffering; it may increase urinary and fecal incontinence, and many patients need restraints.[92] Rav Moshe Feinstein states that for patients with a life expectancy of several weeks to months, their quality of life should be the concern.[93] According to the *halacha*, patients with advanced dementia are dying and suffering, and tube feeding would add to their suffering, so withholding enteral feeding is appropriate.

Among Catholics it is believed that euthanasia is an act or omission of a procedure leading to the death of a patient. Withdrawal of artificial nutrition may not always be an act of omission leading to death of the patient.[94] It is also believed that all patients should get normal care. It is not clear if artificial nutrition is part of basic care or medical treatment. In March 2004, in a speech regarding the Terri Schiavo case, Pope John Paul II stated that withdrawal of artificial nutrition was part of basic care and withdrawal is equivalent to euthanasia.[95] It is thought that this means it is morally obligatory in patients who are not actively dying. In demented patients, where it is more burdensome to the patient, it may be morally optional.[96]

Medical treatment that is burdensome is defined as "too painful, too damaging to the patient's bodily self and functioning, psychologically repugnant to the patient, restrictive of the patient's liberty and preferred activities, suppressive of the patient's mental life, or too expensive."[97] Decisions regarding benefit and burden should be discussed with the patient directly, and if the patient cannot make the decision, health care proxies and families should be involved.

Like in all religions, in Islam there are two main principles: sanctity of life and duty to feed. According to the Quran and Hadith, it is recommended to feed the sick and eradicate hunger by providing food, financial assistance, and food preparation. Islam suggests that if enteral nutrition prolongs life, it should be done, and if it hastens death, it is not recommended. In advanced dementia it does neither. So the duty-to-feed principle comes in play. Like in Catholicism, enteral nutrition is considered basic care and should be instituted in advanced dementia patients. Even though it is not clearly mentioned in the Quran and Hadith regarding dementia and enteral nutrition, it is still debatable.[98]

17.15.1 State Laws

State laws regarding enteral nutrition vary. In most of the states, a surrogate can make the decision if the patient specifically addressed artificial nutrition with him or her. If there is no surrogate, the state has a hierarchy for default surrogate decision makers.

In New York and Missouri, surrogates cannot make the decision regarding artificial nutrition, as it was in the Nancy Cruzan case. Nursing homes in these states require adequate documentation that it was the patient's wish to withhold artificial nutrition.

17.16 COST OF ENTERAL NUTRITION IN A NURSING HOME

Nursing homes are reimbursed more if a patient is on tube feeding. Less staff is needed to help with tube feeding than with hand feeding. In a study done by Mitchell et al. in 2004, it was noted that the cost for tube-feeding patients was $2379 ± 1032, vs. $4219 ± 1545 for a manual feeding, with the staff time being 25.2 ± 12.9 min for a tube feeding vs. 72.8 ± 16.5 min for a manual feeding. Tube-fed patients followed for 6 months were found to be more expensive, secondary to hospitalizations for placement and complications related to the tube. [99]

17.17 CONSERVATIVE ALTERNATIVES

As mentioned earlier, a thorough review of medications may help improve the nutritional status. In one study, education of the nursing staff, medication adjustment, environmental changes, dental care, swallowing evaluation, and increased nutritional intake with illness led to a 4.5-kg increase in weight in 50% of the residents.[100] Other useful methods include finger foods, strong flavors, hot and cold food, frequent reminders to swallow, liquid supplements, bolus sizes less than a teaspoon, facilitation techniques like vibration and stroking of the cheek, assistance with meals, and frequent small snacks.[101–104]

17.18 CONCLUSION

Enteral feeding has become a common medical intervention. It carries with it several ethical, social, and medical issues. Patients and families should be made aware of the benefits and risks of enteral nutrition. To date, no studies show benefits in end-stage dementia patients. It does not prolong life, does not prevent aspiration, and has no effect on pressure sores. Patients in nursing homes with enteral nutrition have a higher mortality. It is the physician's responsibility to discuss in detail and help the family understand the risks and current literature on benefits of feeding tubes.

REFERENCES

1. Graves EJ. Detailed diagnoses and procedures: national hospital discharge survey, 1988. *Vital Health Stat 13* 1991;107:116.
2. Graves EJ. Detailed diagnoses and procedures: national hospital discharge survey, 1995. *Vital Health Stat 13* 1997;130:124.
3. Grant M. Gastrostomy and mortality among hospitalized Medicare beneficiaries. *JAMA* 1998;279:1973–1976.
4. Gaines K, Burk G. Ethnic differences in stroke: black–white differences in the United States population. *Neuroepidemiology* 1995;14:209–239.
5. Caralis PV, Davis B, Wright K, Marcial E. The influence of ethnicity and race on attitudes toward advanced directives, life-prolonging treatments, and euthanasia. *J Clin Ethics* 1993;4:155–165.

6. Mitchell SL, Buchanan JL, Littlehale S, Hamel MB. Tube feeding versus hand-feeding nursing home residents with advanced dementia: a cost comparison. *J Am Med Dir Assoc* 2004;5(Suppl.):S22–S29.
7. Loser C, et al. Enteral long-term nutrition via percutaneous endoscopic gastrostomy in 210 patients: a four year prospective study. *Dig Dis Sci* 1998;43:2549–2557.
8. Cicon JO. Indications for tube feedings in elderly patients. *Dysphagia* 1990;5:1–5.
9. American Society for Gastrointestinal Endoscopy. Role of PEG/PEJ in enteral feeding. *Gastroint Endosc* 1998;48:699–701.
10. ASPEN Board of Directors. Guidelines for the use of parental and enteral nutrition in adults and pediatrics. *J Parenter Enteral Nutr* 1993:17(Suppl. 4):7–9.
11. Cataldi-Belcher EL, Selzer MH, Sloccumb BA, Jones KW. Complications during enteral nutrition therapy: a prospective study. *Pract.* 1994;9:101–103.
12. Norton B, et al. A randomized prospective comparison of percutaneous gastrostomy and nasogastric tube feeding after acute dysphagic stroke. *BMJ* 1996;312:13–16.
13. Foutch PG, Haynes WC, Bellapravalu S, Sanowski RA. Percutaneous endoscopic gastrostomy (PEG). A new procedure comes of age. *J Clin Gastroenterol* 1986;8:10–15.
14. Wolfden HC, Kozarek RA, Ball TJ, et al. Long term outcomes of patients receiving percutaneous endoscopic gastrostomy and jejunostomy. *Am J Gastroenterol* 1990;85:1120–1122.
15. Hull MA, Rawlings J, Murray FE, et al. Audit of outcome of long term enteral nutrition by percutaneous endoscopic gastrostomy. *Lancet* 1993;341:869–872.
16. Shike M, Latkany L. Direct percutaneous endoscopic jejunostomy. *Gastrointest Endosc Clin North Am* 1998;8:569–580.
17. Myers JG, Page CP, Stewart RM, Schweisinger WH, Sirinek KR, Aust JB. Complications of needle catheter jejunostomy in 2022 consecutive applications. *Am J Surg* 1995;170:547–550.
18. Holmes JH, Brundage SI, Yeun PC, Hall RA, Maier RV, Jurk-ovrich GJ. Complications of surgical feeding jejunostomy in trauma patients. *J Trauma Infect Crit Care* 1997;47:1009–1012.
19. Maple JT, Peterson BT, Baron TH, Gostout CJ, Wong Kee Song LM, Buttar NS. Direct percutaneous endoscopic jejunostomy: outcomes in 307 consecutive attempts. *Am J Gastroenterol* 2005;100:2681–2688.
20. Scott JS, De La torre RA, Unger SW. Comparison of operative versus direct percutaneous endoscopic gastrostomy placement in the elderly. *Am Surg* 1991;57:338–340.
21. Tapia J, Murguia R, Garcia G, et al. Jejunostomy: techniques, indications, and complications. *World J Surg* 1999;23:596–602.
22. Vanek VW. In and outs of enteral access. 3. Long-term-access jejunostomy. *Nutr Clin Pract* 2003;18:201–220.
23. Vu MK, van der Veek PP, Frolich M, et al. Does jejunal feeding activate exocrine pancreatic secretion? *Eur J Clin Invest* 1999;29:1053–1059.
24. Gersovitz M, Motil K, Munro HN, et al. Human protein requirements: assessment of adequacy of the current recommended dietary allowance for dietary protein in the elderly men and women. *Am J Clin Nutr* 1982;35:6–15.
25. Marino PL. *The ICU Book.* Williams & Wilkins, New York, 1998.
26. Al Saady NM, Balckmore CM, Bennett ED. High fat, low carbohydrate, enteral feeding lowers PaCO2 and reduces the period of ventilation in artificially ventilated patients. *Intensive Care Med* 1989;15:290–295.
27. Campbell S, Schiller M. Consideration for enteral nutrition support for patients with diabetes. *Top Clin Nutr* 1998;7:23–32.

28. Elia M, Ceriello A, Laube H, Sinclair AJ, Engfer M, Stratton RJ. Enteral nutritional support and use of diabetic specific formulas for patients with diabetes. A systematic review and meta-analysis. *Diabetes Care* 2005;28:2267–2279.
29. Craig LD, Nicholson S, Silverstone FA, Kennedy RD. Use of reduced carbohydrate, modified enteral formula for improving metabolic control and clinical outcomes in long term care residents with type 2 diabetes: results of a pilot trial. *Nutrition* 1998;14:529–534.
30. Delmi M, Rapin CH, Bengoa JM, Delmas PD, Vasey H, Bonjour JP. Dietary supplementation in elderly patients with fractured neck or femur. *Lancet* 1990;335:1013–1016.
31. Rees RG, Keohane PP, Grimble GK, Frost PG, Attrill H, Silk DB. Elemental diet administered nasogastrically without a starter regime to patients with inflammatory bowel disesase. *J Parenter Enteral Nutr* 1986;10:258–262.
32. Collier P, Kudsk KA, Glezer J, Brown RO. Fiber containing formula and needle catheter jejunostomies: a clinical evaluation. *Nutr Clin Pract* 1994;9:101–103.
33. Breslow RA, Hallfrisch J, Guy DG, et al. The importance of dietary protein in healing pressure ulcers. *J Am Geriatr Soc* 1993;41:357–362.
34. Ciocon JO, Galindo-Ciocon DJ, Tiessen C, et al. Continuous compared with intermittent tube feeding in the elderly. *J Parenter Enteral Nutr* 1992;16:525–528.
35. British Association for Parenteral and Enteral Nutrition (BAPEN). *Administering Drugs via Enteral Feeding Tubes: A Practical Guide*. London, 2003.
36. Cynthia A, Padula AK, Planchon C, Lamourex C. Enteral feedings: what the evidence says. *Am J Nurs* 2004;104:62–69.
37. Naysmith M, Nicholson J, Nasogastric drug administration. *Prof Nurse* 1998;13:424–451.
38. *United States Pharmacopeial Drug Index*, 14th ed. Rand McNally, Taunton, MA, 1994.
39. Miller D, Miller HW. A nurse's guide to tube feeding: giving meds through the tube. *RN* 1995;58:44–48.
40. Coentry BJ, Karatassas A, Gower L, Wilson P. Intestinal passage of the PEG end piece: is it safe? *J Gastroenterol Hepatol* 1994;9:311–313.
41. Korula J, Harma C. A simple and inexpensive method of removal or replacement of gastrostomy tubes. *JAMA* 1991;265:1426–1428.
42. Waxman I, Al-Kawas F, Bass B, Glouderman M. PEG ileus. A new case of small bowel obstruction. *Dig Dis Sci* 1991;36:251–254.
43. Dranoff JA, Angood PJ, Topazian M. Transnasal endoscopy for enteral feeding tube placement in critically ill patients. *Am J Gastroenterol* 1999;94:2902–2904.
44. Amann W, Mischinger HJ, Berger A, et al. Percutaneous endoscopic gastrostomy (PEG): 8 years of clinical experience in 232 patients. *Surg Endosc* 1997;11:741–744.
45. Rabeneck L, Wray NP, Peterson NJ. Long term outcomes of patients receiving percutaneous endoscopic gastrostomy tubes. *J Gen Intern Med* 1996;11:287–293.
46. Grossner L, Keymling J, Hahn EG, Ell C. Antibiotic prophylaxis in percutaneous endoscopic gastrostomy. *Lancet* 1993;341:869–872.
47. Preclik G, Grune S, Leser HG, et al. Prospective, randomized double blind trial of prophylaxis with single dose of co-amoxiclav before percutaneous endoscopic gastrostomy. *BMJ* 1999;319:881–884.
48. Edes TE, Walk BE, Austin JL. Diarrhea in the tube fed patients: feeding formula not necessarily the cause. *Am J Med* 1990;88:91–93.
49. Keohane PP, Attrill H, Love M. Relationship between osmolality of diet and gastrointestinal side effects in enteral nutrition. *BMJ* 1984;288:678–681.

50. Silk DBA, Payne-James JJ. Complications of enteral nutrition. In *Enteral and Tube Feeding*, 2nd ed., Rombeau JL, Caldwell MD, Eds. W.B. Sanders, Philadelphia, 1990, pp. 510–531.
51. Cogen R, Weinryb J. Aspiration pneumonia in nursing home patients fed via gastrostomy tubes. *Am J Gastroenterol* 1989;84:1509–1512.
52. Hassett JM, Sunby C, Flint LM. No elimination of aspiration pneumonia in neurologically disabled patients with feeding gastrostomy. *Surg Gynecol Obstet* 1988;167:383–388.
53. Zarchy TM, Lipman TO, Finkelstein JP. Elevated transaminase with an elemental diet. *Ann Intern Med* 1978;89:221–222.
54. Peck A, Cohen C, Mulivihill M. Long-term enteral feeding of aged demented nursing home patients. *J Am Geriatr Soc* 1990;38:1195–1198.
55. Kaw M, Sekas G. Long-term follow-up of consequences of percutaneous endoscopic gastrostomy (PEG) tubes in nursing home patients. *Dig Dis Sci* 1994;39:738–743.
56. Henderson CT, Trumbore LS, Mobarhan S, Benya R, Miles TP. Prolonged tube feeding in long term care patients: nutritional status and clinical outcomes. *J Am Coll Nutr* 1992;11:309–325.
57. Koretz RL. Nutritional support: how much for how much? (review). *Gut* 1986;27(Suppl.):85–95.
58. Reisberg B, Ferris S, Anard R, et al. Functional staging of dementia of the Alzheimer's type. *Ann NY Acad Sci* 1984;435:481–484.
59. Cowen ME, Simpson SL, Vettese TE. Survival estimates for patients with abnormal swallowing studies. *J Gen Intern Med* 1997;12:88–94.
60. Mitchell SL, Kiely DK, Lipsitz LA. Does artificial enteral nutrition prolong the survival of institutionalized elders with chewing and swallowing problems? *J Gerontol* 1998;53A:M1–M7.
61. Franzoni S, Frisoni GB, Boffelli S, Rozzini R, Trabucchi M. Good nutritional oral intake is associated with equal survival in demented and nondemented very old patients. *J Am Geriatr Soc* 1996;44:1366–1370.
62. Murphy LM, Lipman TO. Percutaneous endoscopic gastrostomy does not prolong survival in patients with dementia. *Arch Intern Med* 2003;163:1351–1353.
63. Groher M, Gonzalez E. Mechanical disorders of swallowing. In *Dysphagia: Diagnosis and Management*, Groher M, Ed. Butterworth-Heinemann, Boston, 1992, pp. 53–84.
64. Valles J, Artigas A, Rello J, et al. Continuous aspiration of subglottic secretions in preventing ventilator associated pneumonia. *Ann Intern Med* 1995;122:179–186.
65. Kaw M, Sekas G. Long-term follow-up of consequences of percutaneous endoscopic gastrostomy (PEG) tubes in nursing home patients. *Dig Dis Sci* 1994;39:738–743.
66. Terpenning MS, Taylor GW, Lopatin DE, Kerr CK, Dominguez BL, Loesche WJ. Aspiration pneumia: dental and oral risk factors in older veteran population. *J Am Geriatr Soc* 2001;49:557–563.
67. Feinberg MJ, Knebl J, Tully J. Prandial aspiration and pneumonia in an elderly population followed over 3 years. *Dysphagia* 1996;11:104–109.
68. Lazarus BA, Murphy JB, Culpeper L. Aspiration associated with long term gastric versus jejunal feeding: a critical analysis of the literature. *Arch Phys Med Rehab* 1990;71:46–53.
69. Fox KA, Mularski RA, Sarfati MR, et al. Aspiration pneumonia following surgically placed feeding tubes. *Am J Surg* 1995;170:564–566.

70. Strong RM, Condon SC, Solinger MR, et al. Equal aspiration rates from post pyloric and intragastric placed small-bore nasoenteric feeding tubes: a randomized, prospective study. *J Parenter Enteral Nutr* 1992;16:59–63.
71. Berlowitz D, Brandeis G, Anderson J, Brand H. Predictors of pressure ulcer healing among long-term care residents. *J Am Geriatr Soc* 1997;45:30–34.
72. Berlowitz DR, Ash AS, Brandeis GH, Brand HK, Halpern JL, Moskowitz MA. Rating long term care facilities on pressure sore development: importance of case-mix adjustment. *Ann Intern Med* 1996;124:557–563.
73. McCann R, Hall W, Groth-Juncker A. Comfort care for the terminally ill patients. *JAMA* 1994;272:1263–1266.
74. Ganzini L, Goy ER, Miller LL, Harvath TA, Jackson A, Delorit MA. Nurses' experiences with hospice patients who refuse food and fluids to hasten death. *N Engl J Med* 2003;349:359–365.
75. Kerndt PR, Naughton JL, Driscoll CE, Loxterkamp DA. Fasting: the history, pathophysiology and complications. *West J Med* 1982;137:379–399.
76. Scott AG, Austin HE. Nasogastric feeding in the management of severe dysphagia in motor neurone disease. *Palliat Med* 1994;8:45–49.
77. American Academy of Hospice and Palliative Medicine (AAHPM). Position statement on artificial nutrition and hydration near end of life. www.aahpm/org/position/nutrition.html. Accessed 2/28/07.
78. Light VL, Siezak FA, Porter JA. Predictive factors for early mortality after percutaneous endoscopic gastrostomy. *Gastrointest Endosc* 1995;42:330–335.
79. James A, Kapur K, Hawthorne AB. Long-term outcome of percutaneous endoscopic gastrostomy (PEG) in patients with dysphagic stroke. *Age Ageing* 1998;27:671–676.
80. Skelly R, Terry H, Millar E, Cohen D. Outcomes of percutaneous endoscopic gastrostomy feeding. *Age Ageing* 1999;28:416.
81. Wijdicks EF, McMahon MM. Percutaneous endoscopic gastrostomy after acute stroke: complication and outcome. *Cerbrovasc Dis* 1999;9:109–111.
82. Desport JC, Preux PM, Truont TC, Vallat JM, Santerean D, Couratier P. Nutritional status is a prognostic factor for survival in ALS patients. *Neurology* 1999;53:1059–1063.
83. Kasarskis EJ, Neville HE. Management of ALS: nutritional care. *Neurology* 1996;47(Suppl. 2):S118–S120.
84. Mazzini L, Corra T, Zaccala M, Mora G, Del Piano M, Galante L. Percutaneous endoscopic gastrostomy and enteral nutrition in amyotrophic lateral sclerosis. *J Neurol* 1995;242:695–698.
85. Lee JH, Machtay M, Unger L, et al. Prophylactic gastrostomy tubes in patients undergoing intensive irradiation for cancer of the head and neck. *Arch Otolaryngol Head Neck Surg* 1998;124:871–875.
86. Bueno JS, Barrera R, Gerdes H, et al. Placement of direct percutaneous endoscopic jejunostomy in patients with complications following esophageal resection. *Gastrointest Endosc* 2001;53:AB209.
87. Howard L, Patton L, Dahl RS. Outcome of long-term enteral feeding. *Gastrointest Endosc Clin North Am* 1998;8:705–722.
88. Bastow MD, Rawlings J, Allison SP. Benefits of supplementary tube feeding after fractured neck of femur: a randomised controlled trial. *BMJ* 1983;287:1589–1592.
89. Avenell A, Handoll HH. Nutritional supplementation for hip fracture aftercare in the elderly. *Cochrane Database Syst Rev* 2004;1:CD001880.

90. Callahan C, Haag K, Buchanan N, Nisi R. Decision making for percutaneous endoscopic gastrostomy among older adults in a community setting. *J Am Geriatr Soc* 1999;47:1105–1109.
91. Mitchell S, Berkowitz R, Lawson F, Lipsitz L. A cross-national survey of tube feeding decisions in cognitively impaired older persons. *J Am Geriatr Soc* 2000;48:391–397.
92. Callahan CM, Haag KM, Weinberger M, et al. Outcomes of percutaneous endoscopic gastrostomy among older adults in a community setting. *J Am Geriatr Soc* 2000;48:1048–1054.
93. Mitchell S, Kiely D, Lipsitz L. The risk factors and impact on survival of patients with feeding tube placement in nursing home residents with severe cognitive impairment. *Arch Intern Med* 1997;157:327–332.
94. Peck A, Cohen C, Mulivihill M. Long-term enteral feeding of aged demented nursing home patients. *J Am Geriatr Soc* 1990;38:1195–1198.
95. Tendler M. Responsa of Rav Moshe Feinstein: Translation and Commentary, Vol. 1, Care of the Critically Ill. KTAV Publishing House, Hoboken, NJ, 1996.
96. Roach J. Life-Support Removal: No Easy Answers. *Catholic Bulletin*, March 7, 1991. (Citing Bio/medical Ethics Commission of the Archdiocese of St. Paul–Minneapolis.)
97. www.natcath.com/NCR_Online/archives2/2004b/041604/041604i.php.
98. Sulmasy DP. *Are Feeding Tubes Morally Obligatory?* St. Anthony Messenger, January 2006.
99. May WE, et al. Feeding and hydrating the permanently unconscious other vulnerable persons. *Issues Law Med* 1987;3:208.
100. Alibhai SMH. Artificial Nutrition and Hydration in Advanced Dementia: Scientific Challenges and a Proposed Islamic Ethic Response. Islam and Bioethics: Concerns, Challenges and Responses. Paper presented at Nittany Lion Inn, Penn State University, March 27–28, 2006.
101. Mitchell SL, Buchanan JL, Littlehale S, Hammel MB. Tube-feeding versus hand-feeding nursing home residents with advanced dementia: a cost comparison. *J Am Med Dir* 2004;5(2):S23–S29.
102. Abbasi AA, Rudman D. Under nutrition in the nursing home: prevalence, consequence, causes and prevention. *Nutr Rev* 1994;52:113–122.
103. Torres A, Serra-Batlles J, Ros E, et al. Pulmonary aspiration of gastric contents in patients receiving mechanical ventilation: the effect of body composition. *Ann Intern Med* 1992;116:540–543.
104. Morley JE. Dementia is not necessarily a cause of undernutrition. *J Am Geriatr Soc* 1996;44:1403–1404.
105. Boylston E, Ryan C, Brown C, Westfall B. Preventing precipitous weight loss in demented patients by altering food texture. *J Nutr Elder* 1996;15:43–48.
106. Horner J, Massey EW, Riski JE, Lathrop DL, Chase KN. Aspiration following stroke: clinical correlates and outcome. *Neurology* 1998;38:1359–1362.

18 Prescription for Parenteral Nutrition

David R. Thomas, M.D.

CONTENTS

18.1 INTRODUCTION

Dramatic weight loss and hypoalbuminemia often follow acute hospitalization. Both concurrent illness and undernutrition present prior to hospital admission account for these changes. Forty to sixty percent of hospitalized patients are undernourished, at least by traditional diagnostic criteria.[1] Sixty percent of elderly adults are undernourished on the day of admission to the hospital.[2] Hospital nutritional status is poorly monitored,[3–6] and patients often subsist on inadequate intake for days at a time.[7–9] Despite the high prevalence of undernutrition, nutrition is rarely addressed during hospital stays.[10]

Undernutrition is associated with patient outcome. A four-fold increase in complications and a six-fold increase in mortality have been reported among hospitalized patients with a serum albumin less than 35 g/l.[11] A significantly higher mortality among surgical patients with greater than 20% weight loss preoperatively has been shown.[12] Protein-energy undernutrition is a strong independent risk factor for 1-year mortality after discharge from a geriatric rehabilitation ward.[13] The severity of undernutrition is a strong independent risk factor for life-threatening morbidity, even when controlling for illness severity.[14] It is not clear whether diagnosis of undernutrition by traditional laboratory parameters correctly predicts response to feeding, or whether these acute phase markers simply select sicker individuals (see Chapter 12).

Undernutrition as a result of acute illness or poorly addressed nutritional status in hospitals persists after discharge. In a subacute facility, over 90% of subjects were undernourished or at risk for undernutrition.[15] The high prevalence of malnutrition in long-term-care facilities may reflect, in part, transfer of undernourished patients from acute-care hospitals to long-term-care facilities following an acute illness.[16]

After an illness, a number of patients are unable to maintain adequate oral intake to meet protein-calorie needs, even when high-density nutritional supplements are added.[17,18] For these patients, enteral feeding by tube or parenteral intravenous feeding must be considered.

18.2 ENTERAL VERSUS PARENTERAL FEEDING ROUTE

Enteral nutrition has advantages over parenteral nutrition, including more effective nutrient utilization and preservation of gastrointestinal mucosa integrity and function.[19–21] Enteral feeding has also been shown to play a significant role in preventing bacterial translocation and maintaining immune function.[22,23]

In critically ill subjects with an intact gastrointestinal tract, the use of enteral nutrition compared with parenteral nutrition demonstrates a reduction in infections (relative risk, 0.64; 95% confidence interval (CI), 0.47 to 0.87), although no effect on mortality or length of stay was observed.[24] Therefore, in patients with an intact gastrointestinal tract, enteral nutrition is strongly recommended over parenteral nutrition.[25]

In elective-surgery patients with cancer of the stomach or esophagus prospectively randomized to receive either enteral feeding or total parenteral nutrition, no differences were found in nutritional, immunologic, and inflammatory variables between patients. Infectious or noninfectious complications, length of hospital stay, and mortality were not different between groups. A similar overall complication rate was observed in the two groups (36% for enteral and 40% for parenteral nutrition). These outcomes were similar despite the fact that only 79% of the enterally fed group reached nutritional goals, compared to 98% of the parenterally fed group. Hyperglycemia or electrolyte abnormalities were higher in the parenterally fed group. Parenteral nutrition was four-fold more expensive than enteral nutrition.[26]

In other studies, increases in infective complications (8%), noninfectious complications (5%), catheter-related sepsis (4%), and length of hospital stay (1.2 days) have been observed with total parenteral nutrition. Enteral nutrition was associated with an increase in diarrhea (9%).[27] The in-hospital mortality rate was not higher with parenteral nutrition in this study, although enteral nutrition has been associated with a lower mortality rate in other studies.

Some frail, older, undernourished patients are unable to accept or tolerate adequate enteral nutrition. Tolerance to enteral nutrition by gastric tube is poor in this group of patients. Enteral nutrition frequently fails to meet nutritional goals due to interruptions of feeding, intolerance to feeding volume, high gastric residuals, or clinical status of the patient.[28] Parenteral nutrition may be an effective method of administering nutritional support to patients with mild to moderate nutritional deficiencies who are unable to receive enteral nutrition or for whom enteral nutrition alone cannot meet energy needs. Whether resorting to parenteral feedings can improve outcome is controversial.

18.3 INDICATIONS FOR PARENTERAL NUTRITION

The indications for parenteral nutrition have evolved over time. A number of randomized controlled clinical trials have reported the effect of parenteral nutrition. Parenteral nutrition also has been widely applied to a number of conditions, despite a lack of clinical trials to determine the efficacy of parenteral nutrition.

The current recommendations for parenteral nutrition are shown in Table 18.1. Unfortunately, the risk–benefit ratio for a large number of conditions suggests that routine use of parenteral nutrition should be limited. In most circumstances, the decision to initiate parenteral nutrition must be made on an individual patient basis.

The published benefits of total parenteral nutrition depend on the methodological quality of the clinical trial and the year of publication (Table 18.2). In a meta-analysis of the use of total parenteral nutrition in surgical patients, higher quality and more recent trials showed no benefit compared to standard care or no total parenteral nutrition. In patients with malnutrition at baseline, a reduction in major complications was seen, but no difference in mortality was observed.[29]

18.4 SPECIAL GROUPS FOR PARENTERAL NUTRITION

18.4.1 Intensive Care Unit

Parenteral nutrition is most commonly used in critically ill patients in intensive care settings. A meta-analysis of 26 controlled trials involving 2211 patients compared total parenteral nutrition with standard care. No reduction in mortality or overall morbidity was observed in persons in the intensive care unit, persons undergoing surgery, persons with burns, or persons with pancreatitis.[30] In a subgroup analysis, there was a reduction in morbidy in subjects who received total parenteral nutrition and who were undernourished at baseline (risk ratio, 0.52; 95% CI, 0.3 to 0.91).

In a randomized trial comparing parenteral nutrition to enteral nutrition in trauma patients, an increased incidence of sepsis was observed in the TPN subjects.[31] In another trial, increased sepsis with TPN compared to enteral feeding was also observed.[32]

18.4.2 Pancreatitis

A meta-analysis of six randomized controlled trials found that enteral nutrition was associated with a lower incidence of infections (relative risk, 0.45; 95% CI, 0.26 to 0.78; $p = 0.004$), a reduced length of hospital stay (mean reduction, 2.9 days; 95% CI, 1.6 to 4.3 days; $p < 0.001$), and a trend toward reduced surgical interventions

TABLE 18.1
Summary of Guidelines for Parenteral Nutrition

Condition	Recommendation	Rationale
Cancer patients undergoing chemotherapy or radiation therapy	Should not be routinely used	Increased risk of complications; impaired response to treatment
Bone marrow transplantation	No clear direction	Conflicting data regarding mortality
Liver disease, alcoholic hepatitis	Should not be routinely used	Does not alter morbidity or mortality
Hepatic encephalopathy, cirrhosis	Branched-chain amino acid-enriched solutions are beneficial	Expense (compared with alternative therapies) limits utility
Other liver diseases	No recommendation	No RCT
Acute pancreatitis, mild	Should not be given	Increased cost and duration of hospitalization; may increase risk of infectious complications
Acute pancreatitis, severe	No recommendation	No RCT
Inflammatory bowel disease, acute colitis	Should not be routinely used	No increase in rate of remission or decrease in need for surgery
Inflammatory bowel disease, Crohn's disease	Should not be routinely used	Parenteral nutrition less effective than steroid therapy
Inflammatory bowel disease	Should not be routinely used	Bowel rest not necessary for clinical remission
Acquired immunodeficiency syndrome	Should not be routinely used	Expense and potential for infection
Pulmonary disease	Should not be routinely used	Parenteral nutrition not effective in mechanical ventilation or remission
Renal disease	No recommendation	No RCT
Burn injury	Contraindicated unless enteral route unavailable	Higher mortality than enteral nutrition
Trauma	Should not be routinely used	No clinical benefit; does not shorten duration of mechanical ventilation
Protein-sparing therapy, hypocaloric nitrogen-containing intravenous infusions	Not recommended	No clinical benefit
Home parenteral therapy	Indicated for patients with prolonged gastrointestinal tract failure that prevents absorption of adequate nutrients to sustain life	Should not be provided to patients with limited life expectancies (less than 3 months)
Prolonged inadequate nutrient intake	Should not be provided to patients who are expected to receive adequate oral or enteral feeding within 1 week	Patients who are not severely malnourished can likely tolerate at least 1 week of starvation without adverse effects

Note: Should not be routinely used = must be determined on a case-by-case basis, considering alternatives and risk; RCT = randomized controlled trial.

Source: Adapted from the American Gastroenterological Association Medical Position Statement: Parenteral Nutrition, approved by the Clinical Practice and Practice Committee on April 13, 2001, and by the AGA Governing Board on May 18, 2001. Koretz, R.L. et al., *Gastroenterology*, 121, 970–1001, 2001.

TABLE 18.2
Comparison of Published Benefits for Total Parenteral Nutrition in Surgical Patients: A Meta-Analysis of 27 Randomized Controlled Trials Comparing TPN to Standard Care or No TPN

Outcome	1988 or Prior	1989 or After
Risk of complications	0.42 95% CI = 0.26–0.68	1.09 95% CI = 0.91–1.31
Mortality rate	0.68 95% CI = 0.43–1.10	1.11 95% CI = 0.83–1.48
	Quality Score Less Than 7	**Quality Score at Least 7**
Risk of complications	0.75 95% CI = 0.47–1.19	1.08 95% CI = 0.81–1.43
Mortality rate	0.50 95% CI = 0.32–0.76	1.07 95% CI = 0.86–1.32
	Malnourished at Baseline	**Not Malnourished**
Risk of complications	0.52 95% CI = 0.30–0.91	0.95 95% CI = 0.75–1.21
Mortality rate	1.13 95% CI = 0.75–1.71	0.90 95% CI = 0.66–1.21

Note: Risk, 95% confidence interval (CI); quality score, author-derived 14-point scale.

Source: Heyland, D.K. et al., *Can. J. Surg.*, 44, 102–111, 2001.

to control pancreatitis (relative risk, 0.48; 95% CI, 0.22 to 1.0; $p = 0.05$) compared to parenteral nutrition. No difference was observed for mortality (relative risk, 0.66; 95% CI, 0.32 to 1.37; $p = 0.3$) or noninfectious complications (relative risk, 0.61; 95% CI, 0.31 to 1.22; $p = 0.16$) between the two groups of patients.[33]

18.4.3 Abdominal Surgery

Enteral feeding following major abdominal surgery does not reduce postoperative complications and mortality when compared with parenteral nutrition. In a randomized controlled trial, no difference in major postoperative complications following major elective abdominal surgery (38% in the enteral nutrition group and 39% in the total parenteral nutrition group), or overall postoperative mortality rate (5.9 and 2.5%, respectively), was observed between enterally fed and parenterally fed groups.[34]

18.4.4 Long-Term Total Parenteral Nutrition

In persons who are unable to ingest food for considerable periods, total parenteral nutrition has been used for longer times. In a retrospective review of home parenteral nutrition therapy, the overall probability of 5-year survival was 60%. Only 20 deaths (9%) were directly attributable to complications of parenteral nutrition. Survival was best predicted by the underlying disease. A distinct age-related survival effect was observed, with the probability of 5-year survival by age at initiation of parenteral therapy being 80% for persons younger than 40 years, 62% for persons 40 to 60 years old, and 30% for persons older than 60 years.[35]

18.4.5 Parenteral Access

Parenteral nutrition requires a catheter located in the superior vena cava or right atrium. Access into the superior vena cava can be made through the internal jugular vein, the subclavian vein, or peripheral veins in the arm. Catheters inserted through other sites, such as the femoral vein, have a higher rate of complications. Placement of a catheter should be verified by radiological means to avoid mechanical complications.

Complications of parenteral nutrition include catheter-related infections and mechanical complications such as misplacement. Catheter-related sepsis occurs in five to eight subjects per 1000 insertions.[36] Various methods have been recommended to decrease the risk of sepsis, including strict aseptic insertion technique, skin preparation with chlohexidine,[37] antibiotic-impregnanted catheters,[38] and special catheter care teams. Interventions that have not been effective include antibiotic ointment at the insertion site, transparent skin dressings, prophylactic antibiotics, and prophylactic catheter exchange.[39] Risk of catheter-related infection increases with use of the catheter for infusion of non-nutrition-related fluids, failure to disinfect the catheter hub before administration of nutrition, and bathing or showering.

18.4.6 Peripheral Parenteral Nutrition

Peripheral parenteral nutrition (PPN) has advantages over total parenteral nutrition. PPN can be administered more easily without a central venous line, does not require mixing, and is less costly. Peripheral parenteral nutrition (PPN) may be an effective method of administering nutritional support to patients with mild to moderate nutritional deficiencies who are unable to receive enteral nutrition or for whom enteral nutrition alone cannot meet energy needs.

Peripheral parenteral nutrition (PPN) accounted for almost 20% of all parenteral nutrition administered in a U.K. study. Effective PPN is possible in about 50% of inpatients requiring parenteral nutrition.[40]

Most studies of PPN have been not been longer than 2 weeks. Positive nitrogen balance has been observed after 5 days of PPN infusion.[41] In a longer-duration study of PPN in undernourished subjects transferred to a subacute facility, little change in nutritional parameters was observed.[42] However, a trend toward improvement in prealbumin and CD4 count were observed in the PPN group. Mid-arm circumference and functional status (measured by a timed 6-m walk) also trended toward improvement in the PPN group. The magnitude of the effect may have been smaller in this study due to the severity of malnutrition, older age, and poor functional status in these patients. Despite a longer duration of intravenous therapy, the rate of complications, including phlebitis, in this study was low (22%).

18.5 NUTRITIONAL PRESCRIPTION FOR TOTAL PARENTERAL NUTRITION

Since total parenteral nutrition serves as the only source of nutrients, the preparations used must provide total nutritional support. The normal nutritional requirements must be met in terms of energy, protein, and water (see Chapter 7). Protein estimates must be individualized, considering the person's comorbid condition. Metabolic complications increase when more than 7 g/kg/day of carbohydrates and 2.5 g/kg/day of lipids are administered. In critically ill subjects, the maximum of 1 g/kg/day of lipids may be appropriate.[43] Essential fatty acid deficiency should be prevented by including 1 to 2% of total fatty acids from linoleic acid and 0.5% of energy from alpha-linoleic acid.[44] Parenteral feedings must include vitamins and trace elements. Multivitamin preparations do not usually contain vitamin K, which should be supplemented.

A variety of nutrients have been added to formulas in attempts to improve nutritional status or clinical outcome. The term *immunonutrition* has been used to define a variety of enteral and parenteral nutrients such as arginine, glutamine, omega-3 fatty acids, and nucleotides. Recommendations for nutrients in critically ill adults are given in Table 18.3.

18.5.1 Arginine

Formulas containing arginine and other selective nutrients have been compared to an isocaloric, nonisonitrogenous standard enteral formula in critically ill subjects. In those patients who were fed for more than 48 hours by an intention-to-treat analysis, no difference in hospital mortality, infectious complications, intensive care

TABLE 18.3
Recommendations for Parenteral Nutrition in Critically Ill Patients in the ICU

Comparison	Outcome, Risk (95% Confidence Interval)	Recommendation
Early vs. delayed feeding	Infections, 0.78 (0.6–1.02) Mortality, 0.65 (0.41–1.01)	Feed enterally within 24 to 48 hours
Parenteral nutrition vs. standard care	Infections, not done Mortality, 0.82 (0.41–1.61)	Do not use parenteral route routinely in patients with intact GI tract
Formula supplemented with arginine and other select nutrients	Infections, 0.97 (0.81–1.15)	Do not use
Formula containing glutamine	Infections, 0.69 (0.46–1.04) Mortality, 0.67 (0.48–0.92)	Glutamine should be included
Formula containing probiotics		Insufficient data to recommend

Source: Dhaliwal, R. and Heyland, D.K., *Curr. Opin. Crit. Care*, 11, 461–467, 2005.

unit length of stay, or duration of mechanical ventilation was observed between the two groups in both the overall analysis and several subgroup analyses.[45]

In patients with severe sepsis, the use of enteral immunonutrition when compared with total parenteral nutrition was found to be associated with higher mortality (44.4% vs. 14.3%; $p = 0.039$).[46] In critically ill subjects, an increase in mortality has also been observed with the use of arginine-containing formulas.[47,48] Other trials of enteral immunonutrition have shown a lack of treatment effect when compared to an isocaloric, isonitrogenous standard enteral formula.[49–51] Because of the lack of treatment effect on mortality and infectious complications, several guidelines recommend that diets containing arginine with or without other select nutrients not be used in critically ill patients.[52]

18.5.2 Glutamine

In a meta-analysis of randomized trials of glutamine supplementation in surgical and critically ill patients, no difference in mortality was observed (risk ratio, 0.78; 95% CI, 0.58 to 1.04). A shorter length of hospital stay was found (–2.6 days; 95% CI, –4.5 to –0.7), but no lower rate of infectious complications (relative risk, 0.81; 95% CI, 0.64 to 1.00). The greatest benefit was observed in patients receiving high-dose parenteral glutamine. In subgroup analysis, the shorter length of hospital stay was confined to surgical patients, but not in critically ill patients.[53] Glutamine should be considered an addition to total parenteral nutrition in critically ill patients.

There is no gold standard for nutritional repletion. Nitrogen balance studies have been used most often to assess nutritional efficacy, but may not reflect nutritional status accurately because of comorbid illness.

18.6 COMPLICATIONS OF PARENTERAL NUTRITION

In severely undernourished persons, rapid introduction of carbohydrates can lead to hypophosphatemia, hypokalemia, and hypomagnesemia, known as the refeeding syndrome. Close monitoring of these parameters and overall volume status is required. Hyperglycemia is frequent, particularly in diabetic subjects, and may lead to hyperosmolar states. Hypertriglyceridemia may occur in persons receiving fat emulsions and can lead to pancreatitis and affect pulmonary function. Excessive production of carbon dioxide may occur and complicate ventilatory support. A syndrome of fat accumulation in the liver may occur and is reversible with discontinuation of parenteral nutrition. Cholestasis of the liver occurs later, is irreversible, and may lead to progressive liver disease and death.

Centrally placed catheters have been associated with major complications, such as septic shock, suppurative phlebitis, metastatic infection, endocarditis, or arteritis in 32% of cases.[54] The incidence of phlebitis seems to be related to the nutrition solution, rather than to bacteria or particulate matter. The point prevalence of phlebitis was 65% in patients receiving peripheral intravenous hyperalimentation compared to 18% in nonhyperalimentation patients. When standard in-living particulate filters were added, the rate of phlebitis was 74% compared to 64% with a sham filter. When the glucose-based solution was replaced with a glycerol-based solution, the incidence of phlebitis decreased from 68% to 27% ($p = 0.001$).[55]

In other studies, using an infusion of an amino acid and dextrose solution, grade 2 or greater phlebitis was observed in 71 to 86% of sites during a 3-day period. The rate of phlebitis in this study was 76% even when 5% dextrose alone was infused.[56] Intravenous antibiotics have been associated with high rates of phlebitis, ranging from 41% with intravenous push antibiotics to 47% using intravenous piggyback administration. Intravenous bolus infusion may be superior to intravenous piggyback continuous infusion, with a time to phlebitis of 45 ± 20.5 hours with an intravenous bolus, compared to 36.2 ± 17.6 hours with an intravenous piggyback infusion.[57]

Several strategies have been studied to reduce the incidence of postinfusion phlebitis. Antiseptic dressings have not been effective, with 3-day phlebitis rates of 60% with povidone-iodine dressing vs. 59% with gauze control dressings.[58] Coated intravenous catheters have not been effective, with phlebitis rates of 17% compared to 23% in uncoated catheters ($p = 0.32$).[59] The type of catheter seems to make little difference, with reported rates of 31 to 33% phlebitis in 3 days with two different types of catheters.[60] Catheter length may have a role, at least in preventing high rates of phlebitis associated with antibiotic infusion. Phlebitis occurred in 53% of patients using a 51-mm catheter in a mean of 3 days, 41% of patients using a 28-cm catheter in a mean of 5 days, and 10% of patients using a 71-cm catheter in a mean of 9 days.[61]

18.7 SUMMARY

Total parental nutrition is lifesaving in persons who have no functioning gastrointestinal tract. Maintenance of total parental nutrition is feasible in this group over long periods, but is affected by the underlying comorbid condition and the person's age. In persons who have a functional gastrointestinal tract, enteral nutrition should be the route of choice and should be begun early rather than later in the clinical course.

Total parenteral nutrition must deliver complete nutrition requirements. Supplementation of select nutrients, or immunonutrition, has not been shown to be beneficial and may be harmful, with the possible exception of glutamine in burn and trauma patients.

Total parenteral nutrition must be carefully monitored to prevent the refeeding syndrome or development of nutritional deficiencies not included in the feeding formula. The predominant complications of total parenteral nutrition are sepsis and catheter-related infections.

REFERENCES

1. Mowe M, Bohmer T. The prevalence of undiagnosed protein-calorie undernutrition in a population of hospitalized elderly patients. *J Am Geriatr Soc* 1991;39:1089–1092.
2. Mowe M, Bohmer T, Kindt E. Reduced nutritional status in an elderly population (<70y) is probable before disease and possibly contributes to the development of disease. *Am J Clin Nutr* 1994;59:317–324.

3. Prevost EA, Butterworth CE. Nutritional care of hospitalized patients. *Am J Clin Nutr* 1974;27:432.
4. Sullivan DH, Moriarty MS, Chernoff R, et al. Patterns of care: an analysis of the quality of nutritional care routinely provided to elderly hospitalized veterans. *J Parenter Enteral Nutr* 1989;13:249–254.
5. McNab H, Restivo R, Ber L, et al. Dietetic quality assurance practices in Chicago area hospitals. *J Am Diet Assoc* 1987;85:635–637.
6. Kamath SK, Lawler M, Smith AE, et al. Hospital malnutrition: a 33-hospital screening study. *J Am Diet Assoc* 1986;86:203–206.
7. Tobias AL, Van Itallie TB. Nutritional problems of hospitalized patients. *J Am Diet Assoc* 1977;71:253–257.
8. Riffer J. Malnourished patients feeding rising costs. *Hospitals* 1986;60:86.
9. Sullivan DH, Sun S, Walls RC. Protein-energy undernutrition among elderly hospitalized patients: a prospective study. *JAMA* 1999;281:2013–2019.
10. Morley JE. Why do physicians fail to recognize and treat malnutrition in older persons? *J Am Geriatr Soc* 1991;39:1139–1140.
11. Seltzer MH, Bastidas JA, Cooper DM, Engler P, Slocum B, Fletcher HS. Instant nutritional assessment. *J Parenter Enteral Nutr* 1979;3:157–159.
12. Studly HO. Percentage of weight loss: a basic indicator of surgical risk in patients with chronic peptic ulcer. *JAMA* 1936;106:458–460.
13. Sullivan DH, Walls RC, Bopp MM. Protein-energy undernutrition and the risk of mortality within one year of hospital discharge: a follow-up study. *J Am Geriatr Soc* 1995;43:507–512.
14. Sullivan DH, Walls RC. The risk of life-threatening complications in a select population of geriatric patients: the impact of nutritional status. *J Am Coll Nutr* 1995;14:29–36.
15. Thomas DR, Zdrowski CD, Wilson MM, Conright KC, Lewis C, Tariq S, Morley JE. Malnutrition in subacute care. *Am J Clin Nutr* 2002;75:308–313.
16. Thomas DR, Verdery RB, Gardner L, Kant AK, Lindsay J. A prospective study of outcome from protein-energy malnutrition in nursing home residents. *J Parenter Enteral Nutr* 1991;15:400–404.
17. Ofman J, Koretz RL. Clinical economics review: nutritional support. *Aliment Pharmacol Ther* 1997;11:453–471.
18. Potter J, Langhome P, Roberts M. Routine protein energy supplementation in adults: systematic review. *BMJ* 1998;317:495–501.
19. Kripke SA, Fox AD, Berman JM, Settle RG, Rombeau JL. Stimulation of intestinal mucosal growth with intracolonic infusion of short chain fatty acids. *J Parenter Enteral Nutr* 1989;13:109–116.
20. Zaloga GP, Ward KA, Prielipp RC. Effect of enteral diet on whole body and gut growth in unstressed rats. *J Parenter Enteral Nutr* 1991;1542–1547.
21. Adams S, Dellinger EP, Wertz MJ, Dreskovich MR, Simonwitz D, Johansen K. Enteral versus parenteral nutritional support following laparotomy for trauma: a randomized prospective trial. *J Trauma* 1986;26:882–891.
22. Souba W, Klimberg S, Plumley D. The role of glutamine in maintaining a healthy gut and supporting the metabolic responses to injury and infection. *J Surg Res* 1990;48:383–391.
23. Barbul A. Arginine: biochemistry, physiology, and therapeutic implications. *J Parenter Enteral Nutr* 1986;10:227–228.
24. Gramlich L, Kichian K, Pinilla J, et al. Does enteral nutrition compared to parenteral nutrition result in better outcomes in critically ill adult patients? A systematic review of the literature. *Nutrition* 2004;20:843–848.

25. Heyland DK, Dhaliwal R, Drover JW, Gramlich L, Dodek P, Canadian Critical Care Clinical Practice Guidelines Committee. Canadian clinical practice guidelines for nutrition support in mechanically ventilated, critically ill adult patients. *J Parenter Enteral Nutr* 2003;27:355–373.
26. Braga M, Gianotti L, Gentilini O, Parisi V, Salis C, Di Carlo V. Early postoperative enteral nutrition improves gut oxygenation and reduces costs compared with total parenteral nutrition. *Crit Care Med* 2001;29:242–248.
27. Peter JV, Moran JL, Phillips-Hughes J. A metaanalysis of treatment outcomes of early enteral versus early parenteral nutrition in hospitalized patients. *Crit Care Med* 2005;33:213–220.
28. Hammarqvist F. Can it all be done by enteral nutrition? *Curr Opin Clin Nutr Metab Care* 2004;7:183–187.
29. Heyland DK, Montalvo M, MacDonald S, Keefe L, Su XY, Drover JW. Total parenteral nutrition in the surgical patient: a meta-analysis. *Can J Surg* 2001;44:102–111.
30. Heyland DK, MacDonald S, Keefe L, Drover JW. Total parenteral nutrition in the critically ill patient. A meta-analysis. *JAMA* 1998;280:2013–2019.
31. Moore FA, Moore EE, Jones TN, McCroskey BL, Peterson VM. TEN versus TPN following major abdominal trauma reduced septic morbidity. *J Trauma* 1989;29:916–923.
32. Kudsk KA, Croce MA, Fabian TC, Minard G, Tolley EA, Poret A, Kuhl MR, Brown RO. Enteral versus parenteral feeding. *Ann Surg* 1992;215:503–513.
33. Marik PE, Zaloga GP. Meta-analysis of parenteral nutrition versus enteral nutrition in patients with acute pancreatitis. *BMJ* 2004;328:1407.
34. Pacelli F, Bossola M, Papa V, Malerba M, Modesti C, Sgadari A, Bellantone R, Doglietto GB, Modesti C. EN-TPN Study Group. Enteral vs. parenteral nutrition after major abdominal surgery: an even match. *Arch Surg* 2001;136:933–936.
35. Scolapio JS, Fleming CR, Kelly DG, Wick DM, Zinsmeister AR. Survival of home parenteral nutrition-treated patients: 20 years of experience at the Mayo Clinic. *Mayo Clinic Proc* 1999;74:217–222.
36. Sitges-Serra A, Girvent M. Catheter-related bloodstream infections. *World J Surg* 1999;23:589–595.
37. Maki DG, Riger M, Alvarodo CJ. Prospective randomized trial of povidone iodine, alcohol, and chlorhexideine for prevention of infection associated with central venous and arterial catheters. *Lancet* 1991;338:339–343.
38. Mermel LA. Prevention of intravascular catheter-related infections. *Ann Intern Med* 2000;132:391–402.
39. Attar A, Messing B. Evidence-based prevention of catheter infection during parenteral nutrition. *Curr Opin Clin Nutr Metab* 2001;4:211–218.
40. Anderson AD, Palmer D, MacFie J. Peripheral parenteral nutrition. *Br J Surg* 2003;90:1048–1054.
41. Freeman JB, Fairfull-Smith R, Rodman GH, Bernstein DM, Gazzaniga AB, Gersovitz M. Safety and efficacy of a new peripheral intravenously administered amino acid solution containing glycerol and electrolytes. *Surg Gynecol Obstetr* 1983;156:625–631.
42. Thomas DR. A prospective, randomized clinical study of adjunctive peripheral parenteral nutrition in adult subacute care patients. *J Nutr Health Aging* 2005;9:321–325.
43. Battistella FD, Widergren JT, Anderson JT, et al. A prospecitve, randomized trial of intravenous fat emulsion administration in trauma victims requiring total parenteral nturition. *J Trauma* 1997;43:52–60.
44. Kris-Etherton PM, Taylor DS, Yu-Poth S, et al. Polyunsaturated fatty acids in the food chain in the United States. *Am J Clin Nutr* 2000;71:179S–188S.

45. Kieft H, Roos AN, van Drunen JD, et al. Clinical outcome of immunonutrition in a heterogeneous intensive care population. *Intensive Care Med* 2005;31:524–532.
46. Bertolini G, Iapichino G, Radrizzani D, et al. Early enteral immunonutrition in patients with severe sepsis: results of an interim analysis of a randomized multicentre clinical trial. *Intensive Care Med* 2003;29:834–840.
47. Dent DL, Heyland DK, Levy H, et al. Immunonutrition may increase mortality in critically ill patients with pneumonia: results of a randomized trial. *Crit Care Med* 2003;30:A17.
48. Bower RH, Cerra FB, Bershadsky B, et al. Early enteral administration of a formula (Impact) supplemented with arginine, nucleotides, and fish oil in intensive care unit patients: results of a multicenter, prospective, randomized, clinical trial. *Crit Care Med* 1995; 23:436–449.
49. Kieft H, Roos AN, van Drunen JD, et al. Clinical outcome of immunonutrition in a heterogeneous intensive care population. *Intensive Care Med* 2005;31:524–532.
50. Tsuei BJ, Bernard AC, Barksdale AR, et al. Supplemental enteral arginine is metabolized to ornithine in injured patients. *J Surg Res* 2005;123:17–24.
51. Chuntrasakul C, Siltham S, Sarasombath S, et al. Comparison of an immunonutrition formula enriched arginine, glutamine and omega-3 fatty acid, with a currently high-enriched enteral nutrition for trauma patients. *J Med Assoc Thai* 2003;86:552–561.
52. Heyland DK, Dhaliwal R, Drover JW, Gramlich L. Dodek P, Canadian Critical Care Clinical Practice Guidelines Committee. Canadian clinical practice guidelines for nutrition support in mechanically ventilated, critically ill adult patients. *J Parenter Enteral Nutr* 2003;27:355–373.
53. Novak F, Heyland DK, Avenell A, Drover JW, Su X. Glutamine supplementation in serious illness: a systematic review of the evidence. *Critl Care Med* 2002;30:2022–2029.
54. Arnow PM, Quimosing Em, Beach M. Consequences of intravascular catheter sepsis. *Clin Infect Dis* 1993;16:778–784.
55. Rypins EB, Johnson BH, Reder B, Sarfeh IJ, Shimoda K. Three-phase study of phlebitis in patients receiving peripheral intravenous hyperalimentation. *Am J Surg* 1990;159:222–225.
56. Massar EL, Daly JM, Copeland EM 3d, Johnson DE, Von Eshenbach AC, Johnston D, Rundell B, Dudrick SJ. Peripheral vein complications in patients receiving amino acid/dextrose solutions. *J Parenter Enteral Nutr* 1983;7:159–162.
57. Garrelts JC, Ast D, LaRocca J, Smith DF Jr, Peterie JD. Postinfusion phlebitis after intravenous push versus intravenous piggyback administration of antimicrobial agents. *Clin Pharmacy* 1988;7:760–5.
58. Leibovici L. Daily change of an antiseptic dressing does not prevent infusion phlebitis: a controlled trial. *Am J Infect Control* 1989;17:23–25.
59. Sheretz RJ, Stephens JL, Marosok RD, Carruth WA, Rich HA, Hampton KD, Motsinger SM, Harris LC, Scuderi PE, Pappas JG, Felton SC, Solomon DD. The risk of peripheral vein phlebitis associated with chlorhexidene-coated catheters: a randomized, double-blind trial. *Infect Control Hosp Epidemiol* 1997;18:230–236.
60. Russell WJ, Micik S, Gourd S, Mackay H, Wright S. A prospective clinical comparison of two intravenous polyurethane cannulas. *Anaesth Intensive Care* 1997;25:42–47.
61. Monreal M, Quilez F, Rey-Joly C, Rodriguez S, Sopena N, Neira C, Roca J. Infusion phlebitis in patients with acute pneumonia: a prospective study. *Chest* 1999;115:1576–1580.

19 Nutrition Management in Nursing Homes

Devaraj Munikrishnappa, M.D.

CONTENTS

Individuals aged 65 years or older continue to increase in America—for instance, an increase of 3.1 million since 1994 was noted in 2004.[1] In the same age group, although a relatively small number of about 1.56 million, or 4.5%, lived in nursing homes in 2000, the percentage increased strikingly with age, varying from 1.1% for persons 65 to 74 years to 4.7% for persons 75 to 84 years and 18.2% for persons 85+.[1] Women in nursing homes are typically older (83 years) than men (80 years) and are three times more in number than men.[2,3] In addition to these trends, older adults tended to live longer.[4] Nevertheless, the average length of stay (current resident) in nursing homes was reduced from 1026 days in 1985 to 892 days according to the data from the 1999 National Nursing Home Survey.[2,3] This is still a significant length of time spent in nursing homes, especially in the latter part of one's life, when the dependent's needs are more, and are unlikely to be unmet regardless of the location. About 96% of nursing home patients needed help with their activities of daily living (ADLs), with the mean number of ADLs for which help was needed being 4.4 in 1997, implying that a greater number of more functionally impaired individuals resided in the nursing homes.[3] While bathing is often the first ADL to be lost, eating, fortunately, is generally the last. Yet, in 1997, 45% of nursing home residents needed help with this ADL compared to 40% in 1985.[3] This may not necessarily reflect an increase in the number of people needing assistance with eating; rather, it may simply reflect that the staff are more aware today to recognize the need and intervene. However, what could be stated without doubt is that malnutrition is widespread in nursing homes, ranging from 52 to 85%, and a decades-old scourge with dreadful impact on almost every aspect of the afflicted individual's life.[5,6] The elements of nutrition management in nursing homes therefore merit a vigorously renewed attention and application of well-studied corrective actions at different levels, including the patient, the staff, and the physician.

Three key elements that play a vital role in nursing home nutrition management—food service system, nutritional status, and medical nutritional therapy—will be discussed in this chapter, with additional insights into some of the aspects that the studies in the last decade or so have revealed to be important.

19.1 FOOD SERVICE MANAGEMENT

A review of the food service system and its management gives information about the meal service and nutritive quality of the food provided in nursing homes. Federal guidelines regulate the majority of food service programs in nursing homes. Interpretive guidelines and regulations are then specified by each state to meet these federal guidelines. Nursing home facilities must provide food service meeting these guidelines. Governmental financial reimbursement for care in nursing homes is determined by a formula, which is adjusted periodically to reflect increased costs. However, the allocation of funds to various services, such as nursing, housekeeping, supplies, and dietary, is left to the discretion of the facility. Because most nursing homes are operated for profit, any increase in costs that exceeds the increase in reimbursement usually must be offset by reductions in other expenses, such as food budgets. Inadequate food budgets may result in food of lesser quality and potentially marginal nutritional adequacy. But given the fact that malnutrition is still a bane in nursing homes and bodes such devastating consequences as pressure ulcers, cognitive impairment, postural hypotension, infections, and anemia in this inherently vulnerable population with usually numerous other chronic medical diseases, it may well be economically and ethically wiser to rank nutrition a high priority in budget allocations to meet the federal guidelines.[7]

Federal guidelines require nursing homes to provide each resident with a nourishing, palatable, well-balanced diet that meets his or her daily nutritional and special dietary needs.[8] The other pertinent dietary services-related federal guidelines requirements from the electronic Code of Federal Regulations[8] are detailed below.

A qualified dietitian or a designated food service director who receives scheduled consultations from a qualified dietitian should be on staff at the nursing home as part of the team to ensure appropriate nutrition to the residents. The dietitian must be supported by sufficient support personnel to carry out the functions of the dietary services. Food in nursing homes should be procured from sources approved or considered satisfactory by federal, state, or local authorities. It should be stored, prepared, distributed, and served under sanitary conditions. The food menus must meet nutritional needs of residents as per the Recommended Dietary Allowances of the Food and Nutrition Board of the National Research Council, National Academy of Sciences. The menus must be prepared in advance and be followed. The food served to each resident should be prepared by methods that conserve nutritive value, flavor, and appearance of the food. Food should be palatable, attractive, at the appropriate temperature, and served in a form according to an individual's requirements. If residents refuse such food served, substitutes of similar nutritive value to the particular resident should be offered. Therapeutic diets require an attending physician's prescription. Each resident must be provided at least three meals daily at regular times comparable to normal mealtimes in the community. No more than 14 hours should lapse between a substantial evening meal and breakfast next day, except if a nourishing snack has been provided at bedtime, when up to 16 hours may elapse, and a resident group agrees to this exceptional meal span. However, the snacks must be offered to all residents at bedtime daily. The guidelines also require nursing homes to provide residents with special eating equipment and utensils if they need them. Effective October 27, 2003, the guidelines allowed for a facility to use paid feeding assistants who could be other than nurses or trained nursing aides to feed nursing home residents, if it is also consistent with state laws to use them.[9,10] The paid feeding assistants must have completed a state-approved training course (that meets federal guidelines requirements) before feeding residents and should be under direct supervision of a registered nurse (RN) or a licensed practical nurse (LPN). The resident selection for paid assistants to feed must be based on the charge nurse's assessment and the resident's latest assessment and plan of care. They can only feed residents who do not have feeding complications, including, but not limited to, difficulty swallowing, recurrent lung aspirations, and tube or parenteral/IV feedings.

Food service sections in nursing homes have made some innovative strides toward improvement in the recent past, including in the organizational aspects, dining styles and standards, ethnonutrition, social aspects, and individualization. Feeding assistance is an important organizational factor that influences nutritional status of many residents. Introduction of paid feeding assistants, as mentioned above, is a step in this direction. A Centers for Medicare and Medicaid (CMS) study revealed that in 2000, over 91% of nursing homes were noted to have nurse's aide staffing levels less than those required to provide adequate services for their specific resident populations.[11] As pointed out by Jackson in *Health Care Food & Nutrition*, Phase II of the CMS study also revealed that weight loss was more with less staffing and with less work hours of the RN and LPN combined (although the nurse's aides, not RNs or LPNs, usually provide feeding assistance), and that the inadequate staffing affected nutritional status more than cleanliness or appearance of the residents.[10] These findings emphasize the utmost importance of team effort required to thwart nutritional problems in nursing homes. While the nurse's aides primarily help with feeding assistance, the RNs and LPNs are vital for overseeing them, monitoring weight loss, providing resident assessment and accurate care plans, and effectively communicating to other interdisciplinary members, including physicians, in a timely manner.[10] These findings also suggest that feeding assistance, compared to some other chores in nursing homes, is perhaps more demanding on staff, in terms of time and effort. Simmons and Schnelle showed in their study that irrespective of level of physical dependency of residents, all residents responsive to assistance required an average of 35 to 40 minutes for enabling adequate oral intake, which was considerably more time than that spent under usual nursing home care by the nursing home staff helping with feeding assistance.[12] Of importance in the same study is the finding that the less physically dependent residents, who needed just supervision and verbal cuing, required as much staff time as more physically dependent ones.[12] Both allocation of resources by nursing home management and reimbursement provisions to them could therefore be erroneous if they are not based on these considerations.

In another study by Simmons and Schnelle, an increase in daily oral food and fluid intake in about 90% of the participant nursing home residents was noted as a response to one or both of the two interventions implemented by a trained research staff—mealtime feeding assistance and between-meal snack.[13] These interventions may help to improve as well as individualize feeding assistance without having to increase the staff number.[13] The key, however, is to be selective of those residents who need and are likely to respond to the interventions, as well as organizing, training, and supervising the available staff.[12–20] Paid feeding assistants and certified nursing assistants (CNAs) could assume responsibility of feeding residents in small groups while other nursing home personnel from other departments could help with such mealtime tasks as transport of residents and intake documentation.[13] With strategies like snacks between meals, volunteers or social activity personnel can assume responsibility and relieve the other staff not only at mealtime, but the entire day.[13] Even among those with poor intake at mealtime with assistance, significant oral intake gains were noted by offering snacks between meals.[13] Dietary supplements may also result in more energy consumption if administered between meals instead of with meals.[21] Family members, however, prefer that nutritional interventions other than oral supplements or pharmacological remedies be tried first to improve food intake, and they perceive the need for such interventions upon observation that their resident's intake is, on average, half of that provided during mealtime.[22] It is important that both the resident and family members are happy with the food quality, service, and dining area, as these obviously impact on the resident's desire to eat. Crogan and colleagues describe a tool called food and food service questionnaire (FoodEx-LTC) in an effort to create instruments to accurately assess resident satisfaction with the food and food service.[23] Nursing homes today are making efforts to make dining a more pleasurable, personalized, and social experience based on studies that this helps to increase the appetite and food intake in residents. A net result from many studies is what is becoming a common, welcome adornment in today's nursing home dining rooms—well-lit, spacious, restaurant-style dining arrangements, wall murals, soothing music, aroma therapies, better food presentation, flavor enhancers, colorful food, food cart, buffet-style food choices, and provision for family members to join in at mealtimes.[19,24–34] Some recent studies, however, dispute that enhancing flavor increases intake in the elderly.[35,36]

The nursing home population could be expected to become more racially and ethnically diverse with time as a truer reflection of the population mix in the U.S. In 1997, in fact, data found that there was more racial diversity in this population than that of previous data. Racial and ethnic preferences, if not addressed where appropriate, could pose a nutritional risk to these residents, as was noted in one study.[37] Ethnonutrition therefore needs an increased focus in the future.[38] Apart from all this, keeping residents active through physical exercise, recreational activities, and compassionate social interaction at all times, especially by the staff who become an extension of family to the residents over time, could contribute to a healthier and happier stay at nursing homes.

Although clear and conclusive data specific to this incredibly heterogeneous nursing home population is either insufficient or completely lacking in many aspects of nutrition-related recommendations, certain reasonable extrapolations can be drawn and applied from the now emerging data specific to the elderly in the general population. For instance, the Modified Food Pyramid for 70+ Adults can be used as a guide in choosing quality nutritive food for elderly residents in nursing homes.[39] The general dietary principles remain the same as for adults, i.e., plenty of variety; diets high in grain products, vegetables, and fruits; diets low in saturated fatty acids and cholesterol; low to moderate use of sugar, salt, and alcohol; and physical activity in balance with energy intake.[39]

With aging, however, there is a decrease in energy need, and consequently a decrease in food intake, but the need for micronutrients taken with food either remain the same or increase, potentially making the elderly prone for micronutrient malnutrition. Physiological changes associated with aging, such as physiological anorexia of aging, altered taste and smell, slower gastric emptying time, decreased basal metabolic rate, and other factors, may contribute to the decline in food intake in the elderly by as much as 1000 to 1200 kcal in men and 600 to 800 kcal in women.[40,41] This will lead to a concomitant decrease in most nutrients, including calcium, B vitamins, iron, zinc, and vitamin E, even though the need for some nutrients, as mentioned before, may actually remain the same or even increase with aging (calcium, vitamin D, and vitamin B6).[41–43]

Providing nutrient-dense (high nutrient/calorie ratio) food, as per the Modified Food Pyramid for 70+ Adults, could circumvent this potential for micronutrient malnutrition in the elderly. Examples of nutrient-dense foods are fortified or enriched whole-grain breads, rice, cereals, and pasta; deeply colored dark green, orange, or yellow fresh, frozen, or canned vegetables (rich in vitamin C, folic acid, and vitamin A); cruciferous vegetables, including beets, kale, cabbage, and broccoli (contribute antioxidant phytochemicals such as indoles, flavones, and isothiocyanates); beans and yellow, orange, or red whole fruits (not juices). Sweet foods that are high in sugar, such as donuts and cookies, are comparatively less nutrient dense. In addition, the pyramid guidelines emphasize fiber and fluid intake at recommended levels and allow for supplements, especially calcium, vitamin D, and vitamin B12 for optimal health.[39]

Recently, a review of studies related to vitamins in health and aging by Thomas revealed that the strong association of dietary intake of vitamins and *disease* in epidemiological studies has not been borne out in clinical trials.[41] However, a healthy diet should contain adequate amounts of these essential nutrients, as research has shown that there are substances in food that are vital for *metabolic* functions.[41] Thomas, in his review, recommends that the most prudent approach is to have a daily intake of fruits and vegetables, failing which vitamin supplements should be encouraged. Another large recent systematic review by Huang and colleagues for a National Institutes of Health State-of-the-Science Statement for health care providers and the general public concluded:

> The strength of evidence is insufficient to support the presence or the absence of a benefit from routine use of multivitamin and mineral supplements by adults in the United States for primary prevention of cancer, cardiovascular disease, hypertension, cataracts, or age-related macular degeneration, and that there are no data from randomized, controlled trials on the efficacy of multivitamin and mineral supplement use for preventing type 2 diabetes mellitus, Parkinson disease, dementia, hearing loss, osteoporosis, osteopenia, rheumatoid arthritis, osteoarthritis, nonalcoholic steatohepatitis, chronic renal insufficiency, chronic nephrolithiasis, HIV infection, hepatitis C, tuberculosis, or chronic obstructive pulmonary.[44]

A few micronutrients and cholesterol data relevant to the elderly are detailed below. Vitamin A acts on osteoblast and osteoclast activity and increases the effect of parathyroid hormone on bone, causing bone resorption.[5,6] While some studies have noted osteoporosis with vitamin A consumed in excess of 1500 μg/day, a review by Crandall recently revealed that it is not yet possible to determine a specific level of retinol intake above which bone health is compromised.[45–47] In the same review, increasing retinol intake, attributable primarily to retinol (from either diet or supplements), but not beta-carotene intake, was noted to have a graded increase in relative risk of hip fracture; however, of the 20 clinical studies, the 3 randomized controlled studies reviewed involved serum markers of bone metabolism but not bone density or fracture outcomes.[47]

Vitamin D deficiency is likely in nursing home residents due to multiple factors, including lack of sunlight exposure, decreased skin synthesis of cholecalciferol, decreased vitamin D intake, decreased 1-alpha hydroxylation of vitamin D in the kidney, and altered binding capacity for vitamin D metabolites in the serum.[48] While Chapuy and colleagues showed that calcium and vitamin D supplement reduced hip fractures in elderly women, Bischoff and colleagues showed that vitamin D and calcium supplement reduced the rate of falls in long-term-care residents.[49,50] There has been an increasing focus on secondary hyperparathyroidism caused by even mild vitamin D deficiency with resultant high bone turnover and cortical loss.[51,52] There is consensus to evaluate vitamin D status with serum 25-hydroxyvitamin D [25(OH)D], but none regarding what level of its serum level should define deficiency.[52] The current practice in the literature, however, is shown in Table 19.1.[51–55] Complications noted with different levels of vitamin D deficiency are as follows: osteoporosis and increased risk of fractures can occur at all levels of deficiency, secondary hyperparathyroidism is seen with mild and moderate levels, and only in severe levels of deficiency are rickets and osteomalacia seen.[51–55] One recent study

TABLE 19.1
Vitamin D Deficiency Based on Serum 25(OH)D Level

Vitamin D Deficiency Level	25(OH)D Level in ng/ml	25(OH)D Level in nmol/l
Severe	<5–8	<12.5–20
Moderate	<15	<37.5
Mild insufficiency	<20	<50

concluded that decreased serum 25(OH)D concentrations in older persons are associated with a greater risk of future admission into nursing homes.[56] Secondary hyperparathyroidism is increasingly noted in nursing homes in emerging data with various factors as possible contributing factors, including vitamin D, diuretic use, phosphate, and weight.[57,58] The occult mild vitamin D deficiency state is more widespread than once realized, and with vitamin D supplements, parathyroid hormone levels and bone resorption markers decline in this condition.[52] Chronic vitamin D deficiency may have extra-skeletal manifestations, which is gaining more focus of late. Supplemental doses of both vitamin D and calcium for individual residents should be decided after taking into account the estimated contributions from dietary and other sources and, where feasible, 25(OH) levels. Innovative ways of administering vitamin D, such as vitamin D3 orally once every 3 months, are also currently being explored.[59]

Antioxidant therapy (vitamin E, 600 mg; vitamin C, 250 mg; and beta-carotene, 20 mg daily) was evaluated by the Heart Protection Study group in about 5806 participants who were 70 years or older, with primary outcomes being major coronary events or vascular events. No difference was found between this group and the placebo group.[60]

Epidemiological data suggest that low levels of vitamins B2, B6, B12, and C and folate in older adults are frequently associated with cognitive decline. Similarly, studies also suggest a relation between vitamins E and C, and zinc intake in maintenance of cognitive function.[61] High fish consumption also seems to protect against cognitive impairment.[62]

Evidence has not been conclusive for lowering cholesterol in the elderly; in fact, increased mortality has been noted to be associated with low cholesterol levels in this population.[63] A more recent prospective study also cautions against aggressively lowering cholesterol in the elderly.[64]

Some studies indicate that diets rich in lutein plus zeaxanthin may protect against age-related macular degeneration in healthy women younger than 75 years.[61]

The Dietary Reference Intakes (DRIs) for various nutrients for older adults and the general population can be found at the following links:

http://www.fiu.edu/~nutreldr/SubjectList/D/DRI_RDA.htm
http://www.iom.edu/Object.File/Master/21/372/0.pdf

19.2 NUTRITIONAL STATUS

Despite seemingly appropriate food service standards and regulations, patients in nursing homes remain at risk for malnutrition. This is usually attributable to multiple factors, including the complex medical condition of the patient at the nursing home both at admission and after, various factors intrinsic to the nursing home itself, including financial and staffing issues, and medical care.

The two most common perilous consequences of nutritional problems in nursing homes are weight loss and protein-energy malnutrition (PEM). Several studies have now clearly established that weight loss in the elderly increases mortality. The common error in dealing successfully with reversible nutritional problems is the delay in recognizing of them. It is important to identify the patients when they are at risk for weight loss rather than wait until it occurs. The Simplified Nutritional Appetite Questionnaire (SNAQ) is an efficient, yet simple appetite assessment tool that is reliable and valid.[65] It could be used (by any staff) in nursing homes to identify residents at risk for anorexia-related weight loss and to intervene early.[65]

Causes of weight loss include many that are potentially treatable and others that are inevitable, as in cancer-related or cardiac cachexia. The mnemonic for treatable causes of weight loss, Meals on Wheels, created by Dr. John E. Morley at St. Louis University and VMAC, St. Louis, Missouri, is useful in its evaluation (see Table 19.2 for elaboration).

A potential cause could be identified in most patients in nursing homes.[66] Depression and adverse drug effects are the most common reversible causes of PEM. Medications commonly used in the elderly could directly or indirectly lead to weight loss. For instance, digitalis causes anorexia, aspirin causes gastric irritation, and calcium channel blockers cause constipation. Depression affects about 8 to 38% of nursing home populations and is more likely to manifest as weight loss and anorexia in the elderly than in younger patients.[67] Depression-related loss of weight responds to treatment of depression.[68] Anorexia could occur for the first time in the elderly and is then called anorexia tardive.[48] These patients may avoid eating when they are hungry, trying to display oral control patterns.[69] Older patients may refuse to eat, fearing being poisoned. Swallowing difficulty could result from stroke, Parkinson's disease, or dementia. Oral factors are generally an issue in nursing homes, as most of the residents have tooth loss or ill-fitting dentures or have lost their dentures. Financial constraints in nursing homes, as mentioned above, could impact food service and lead to weight loss. *Helicobacter pylori* infection can cause gastritis and dyspepsia, while other nosocomial infections can also result in decreased food intake. Increased energy expenditure coupled with decreased intake in cognitively impaired patients who constantly wander or have other forms of constant increased activity could lead to weight loss. Similarly, metabolic disorders like hyperthryroidism (weight loss with preserved appetite) and

TABLE 19.2
Mnemonic for Treatable Causes of Weight Loss

M	Medications
E	Emotional (depression)
A	Anorexia tardive (nervosa), alcoholism abuse
L	Late-life paranoia
S	Swallowing problems
O	Oral problems
N	Nosocomial infections, no money
W	Wandering and other dementia-related problems
H	Hyperthyroidism, hypoadrenalism, hyperglycemia, hypercalcemia, hypertension (pheochromocytoma)
E	Enteral problems
E	Eating problems
L	Low-salt, low-cholesterol diet
S	Social problems

pheochromocytoma (weight loss with hypertension); malabsorption, tremors, or posture-related problems causing eating problems; restrictive or unpalatable diets; and social factors like loneliness, family issues, or fellow-resident problems could result in weight loss. Chronic infections leading to weight loss, as in rheumatoid arthritis or tuberculosis, could be related to cytokines.[48]

The irreversible causes of weight loss, like cancer-related or cardiac cachexia, should also be kept in mind as causes while evaluating weight loss in this population, and palliative therapy could be offered to them.

Evaluation involves an interdisciplinary team approach with a detailed history from nursing home staff as well as family caregivers to assess the intake and recent changes in the condition of the patient and to note concerns. A detailed medical history with attention to medications, gastro-intestinal symptoms including oral condition, and mental and functional status should be taken. Likely diseases that could be associated with weight loss, such as anemia, depression, and cancer, should be borne in mind during evaluation. On physical examination, signs of malnutrition such as alopecia, chielitis, desquamation, glossitis, angular stomatitis, and dependent edema should be specifically looked for besides careful attention to the rest of the systemic examination.[48]

Drug–nutrient interactions are potentially reversible causes that should be sought. When food interferes with drug, it is more readily recognized due to the suspicion raised by either lack of therapeutic effect of the given drug or low serum levels of it. On the contrary, when drug interferes with nutrients and nutritional state, it is not so readily recognized.[70] Cancer drugs, for instance, affect food intake by altering the taste or appetite and by causing nausea and vomiting.[70] Similarly, anticonvulsants and nutritional state can interact with each other. For instance, low protein levels tend to predispose residents to have toxicity of the drug due to decreased clearance, whereas high protein intake may induce CYP activity and cause rapid clearance.[70–73] Diuretics causing loss of electrolytes other than potassium and water-soluble vitamins are grossly underrecognized. Thiamine is vital for maintenance of the cardiac muscle and adequate heart function.[74–76] As cited by Brady, Kwok and colleagues found poor appetite to be associated with thiamin status in elderly individuals with congestive heart failure treated with diuretics.[76,77] Therefore, if a resident becomes anorexic on diuretics, a thiamin supplementation trial along with usual medical treatment is reasonable.[70] From being solely a site for digestion and absorption previously, intestinal mucosa has become a major site for drug metabolism for some drugs (e.g., cyclosporine, nifedipine) currently.[78] At times of even short-term malnutrition, intestinal cell integrity declines, which in turn could affect drug absorption and metabolism.[70] Grapefruit juice and other foods have forancoumarins that inhibit the human CYP3A enzymes, but many drugs with potential to interact with this juice do not result in any clinically significant event.[79] Drugs may have a warning to avoid fortified foods, such as calcium-fortified orange juice, to prevent chelation and adsorption that reduce the efficacy of the drug.[70] Antimicrobials are most susceptible to such an interaction, potentially leading to antibiotic resistance.[80] Folate fortification can affect hypercoagulation.[81] Thus, numerous drug–nutrient interactions are possible, which we need to watch for and prevent, before they precipitate an adverse clinical event.

Under investigations for evaluating weight loss, serum albumin of <35 g/l, once considered the gold standard for identifying malnutrition residents, is no longer the sole important test. There are a few important reasons for this. First, albumin has a long half-life. Therefore, residents who arrive at a nursing home with hypoalbuminemia, possibly have had it for a while before they came in. It does not necessarily reflect the nutrition care at the current nursing home. Inadequate attention to this fact could potentially set up a nursing home for citation erroneously, especially with the literature indicating that hypoalbuminemia of <35 g/l is associated with such adverse outcomes as higher risk of infection, decubitus ulcers, and mortality. Second, some data suggest that patients with albumin levels of 35 to 39 g/l carry the same risk for mortality as the ones with levels of <35 g/l. Therefore, nutrition interventions may be needed earlier if they are based on this level. Third, some patients present with normal levels of albumin but have calorie-deprived weight loss, i.e., marasmus. Fourth, the albumin is an acute-phase reactant, and hypoalbuminemia may reflect inflammatory extravasation from damaged endothelium due to cytokines.[48]

Weight trends along with albumin may be a better guide in identifying residents at higher risk for malnutrition.[48] One study showed that residents who lost 10% of their weight in 6 months carried a significantly higher mortality, irrespective of diagnoses or causes, while another showed that those who lost 5% of their weight in 1 month carried a four times higher risk of mortality.[82,83] So, it is essential to weigh all the residents periodically and those at risk more frequently.

Low cholesterol (<4 mmol), particularly in frail residents, could be an ominous marker of malnutrition. Since elderly residents could develop hypocholesterolemia during their hospital stay, the cholesterol level in residents returning from the hospital should be checked.[48] The other methods of nutritional evaluation have not been evaluated. The rest of the investigative evaluation should be based on clinical suspicion of the most likely cause. An initial panel of tests could include a complete blood count (for anemia, hematological cancer, infection), chemistry panel (for renal status, dehydration, electrolyte imbalance), thyroid hormone, urine analysis, and fecal occult blood. Chest x-ray in long-standing smokers is a reasonable initial investigation. If nutritional supplementation is considered, the serum prealbumin, transferrin, or albumin level can be obtained for guidance of progress.[84]

Interdisciplinary and individualized approaches combined are fruitful in the management of nutritional problems in nursing homes. Separate algorithms for nurses and physicians to routinely monitor residents at nutritional risk and intervene are available for use from the Council for Nutritional Clinical Strategies in Long-Term Care.[85] The treatment approach should essentially be directed at stopping further weight loss and finding the cause.

19.2.1 Prevention of Further Weight Loss and Maintenance of Nutrition

Proper feeding assistance, making as much calories as possible available, innovations to improve intake, applying the principles of the dining-with-dignity program, and other strategies discussed earlier may be attempted.[34]

Oral supplements (OSs) are often used as initial interventions in residents with weight loss. They have not been studied extensively regarding their prescription and benefit. Most recently, Simmons and Patel found that the physician orders were not followed by staff in delivering the OSs, often delivering on an average of less than once a day when it was ordered for multiple times, and staff spent as minimal as less than a minute in assisting residents to consume them when providing OSs between meals.[86] The result was that residents consumed less calories. So, further research is needed to determine when OSs are most appropriate, at what dose or strength, how often without having counterproductive effects like decreased appetite for the main food, whether they improve resident's nutrition, and who should ideally get them.[87] OSs should still be offered to the at-risk as well as weight loss residents, as some European studies have shown that residents find them acceptable and do respond with an increase in weight.[87–90]

Medications such as mirtazipine (weight loss with depression), dronabinol (for palliation in cancer–cachexia patients), megestrol acetate (weight loss in ambulatory patients), and reglan (weight loss secondary to nausea-related anorexia) have been used with varying successes in weight loss management.

A feeding tube is considered if weight loss is relentless.

19.2.2 Treatment of Underlying Cause Should Be Based on Cause Found

19.3 MEDICAL NUTRITION THERAPY FOR CHRONIC CONDITIONS

This term is meant for special or therapeutic diets that are frequently ordered in nursing homes following the return of residents from the hospital. These residents generally have chronic diseases such as diabetes, hypertension, or cardiovascular disease (CVD). It is usually ordered by a physician as part of a treatment of a disease or a clinical condition. Examples include "no concentrated sweets diet," "no added salt diet," "low cholesterol diet," "mechanical soft diet," and "2 g sodium diet." These diets are often not palatable and are associated with weight loss, low albumin, and orthostasis in these residents.[66,91] Changing dietary consistency, for example, from pureed to mechanical soft diet has not been shown to increase nutrient intake.[92]

Two characteristics stand out for these type of diets: (1) it is unlikely that the dietary approach instituted will have been shown under experimental conditions to be clinically useful in the nursing home setting, and (2) the initiation of a special diet will restrict the variety of foods available to the patient.

19.3.1 Diabetes

Both the American Dietetic Association and the American Diabetes Association (ADA) take the position that residents in nursing homes should no longer be prescribed restrictive diets.[93,94] The ADA also takes the position that medication changes to control any increase in blood sugar is preferable to food restrictions in this group.[94]

Tariq and colleagues found no difference in mean fasting blood glucose level or glycated hemoglobin level at 6 months between a group that received a regular diet and another that received a no concentrated sweets diet. Although insulin was required in both groups, the magnitude of increase in insulin dose was small, implying that the change in diet was easily manageable.[95] This study supports the above-mentioned stance taken by the ADA.

Coulston and colleagues also showed no advantage in glycemic control of nursing home diabetic patients who were given the calorie-restrictive diabetic diet compared to those who were given a regular diet.[96]

Advantages of using a regular diet are that it is cheaper, more homely, palatable, and provides for more consistent intake.

Carbohydrate intolerance could be exacerbated by deficiencies of minerals such as potassium and possibly zinc and chromium in diabetics.[94] The deficiency of the latter two minerals is more difficult to recognize. However, a benefit from chromium supplementation has not been clearly demonstrated from well-designed studies. Zinc has been linked to poor wound healing and impaired immune function.[97]

19.3.2 Hypercholesterolemia

Many epidemiological studies have shown that with aging, cholesterol association as a cardiovascular risk factor declines.[98–101] Rudman and colleagues in their study of 129 nursing home men found that those with cholesterol less than 150 mg/dl had a death rate of 63% during the 14 months after the cholesterol analysis, compared to a death rate of 9% in men with cholesterol greater than 150 mg/dl.[102] Therefore, a low-cholesterol diet is not justifiable in nursing home residents who are already predisposed to nutritional risk unless clear randomized controlled data emerge to show that it is prudent to do otherwise.

19.3.3 Hypertension and Congestive Heart Failure

Restriction of sodium intake has been the primary intervention in treating volume overload patients. Although a sodium-restricted diet is reasonable with severe heart failure, its benefit for mild disease in a group of patients for whom transfer to acute hospitals is frequently due to dehydration is questionable. Considering that their thirst threshold is impaired and they are commonly on a diuretic or an antihypertensive, it is even more irrational.

A 6-month trial of a less restrictive sodium diet in a 220-bed nursing home by Hadler found no significant change in body weight, blood pressure, electrolytes, serum creatinine, blood urea nitrogen, or general clinical status.[103] Nursing home residents differ from acute-care patients in that they are more compliant with diet and drug therapy by the nature of the nursing home routine. If there is no clinical benefit to be gained from restrictive sodium diets, then these patients can be spared less palatable meals and the loss of preferred foods.

19.4 CONCLUSION

When the moment of leaving behind one's home comes, perhaps the first fears of a permanent separation also accompany. Transitioning into a nursing home may be very stressful and difficult during this time. Residents could be expected to be apprehensive and anxious, irrespective of their cognitive status. Therefore, the overall goal of the entire team at the nursing home should be to simulate a home for the residents. Key is to interact pleasantly and effectively. Basic needs like eating and bathing should be facilitated. Frequent family interactions, pleasant dining experiences, adequate nutrition with variety, and recreational activities should be allowed for. Residents must eat nutrient-dense food adequately, do physical exercise, take calcium and vitamin D, and maintain their weight and cholesterol level. The staff should use the screening questionnaires and algorithms mentioned above to identify, assess, and intervene with residents at risk for weight loss at their level. Physicians should watch for the subtle signs of malnutrition, recognize it early, and intervene as well. Liberalized diets should be prescribed and compassionate care should be rendered.

REFERENCES

1. A Statistical Profile of Older Americans Aged 65+, U.S. Administration on Aging, U.S. Department of Health and Human Services, accessed at http://www.aoa.gov/PRESS/fact/pdf/Attachment_1304.pdf.
2. Nursing Home Care, U.S. Department of Health and Human Services, Centers for Disease Control and Prevention, National Center for Health Statistics, accessed at http://www.cdc.gov/nchs/fastats/nursingh.htm.
3. Sahyoun, R.N., Pratt, A.L., Lentzner, H., et al., The Changing Profile of Nursing Home Residents: 1985–1997, U.S. Department of Health and Human Services, Centers for Disease Control and Prevention, National Center for Health Statistics, accessed at http://www.cdc.gov/nchs/data/ahcd/agingtrends/04nursin.pdf.
4. Trends in Health and Aging, U.S. Department of Health and Human Services, Centers for Disease Control and Prevention, National Center for Health Statistics, accessed at http://www.cdc.gov/nchs/agingact.htm.
5. Flood, K.L. and Carr, D.B., Nutrition in the elderly, *Curr. Opin. Gastroenterol.*, 420, 125, 2004.
6. Johnson, K.A., Bernard, M.A., and Funderburg, K., Vitamin nutrition in older adults, *Clin. Geriatr. Med.*, 18, 773, 2002.
7. Morley, J.E., Nutritional status of the elderly, *Am. J. Med.*, 81, 679, 1986.
8. Requirements for States and Long Term Care Facilities: Dietary Services, Electronic Code of Federal Regulations (e-CFR) Title 42, Part 483.35, Subpart B, accessed at http://ecfr.gpoaccess.gov/cgi/t/text/text-idx?c=ecfr&sid=691a5f8fd66cce9187de087cd4be0e89&rgn=div8&view=text&node=42:3.0.1.5.22.2.199.10&idno=42.
9. Requirements for States and Long Term Care Facilities: Dietary Services, Code of Federal Regulations Title 42, Part 483.35, 2003 ed., accessed at:http://www.gpo.gov/nara/cfr/waisidx_03/42cfr483_03.html.

10. Nursing home quality: current issues and CMS's plans for improvement, *Health Care Food Nutr. Focus*, 22, 1, 2005.
11. Jackson R. Appropriateness of Minimum Nurse Staffing Ratios in Nursing Homes, Overview of the Phase II Report: Background Study Approach, Findings, and Conclusions. A Time-Motion Approach to Setting Nurse Staffing Standards, Centers for Medicare and Medicaid Services, U.S. Department of Health and Human Services, accessed at http://www.frontlinepub.com/pdf/OverviewStaffingStudy.pdf.
12. Simmons, S.F. and Schnelle, J.F., Feeding assistance needs of long-stay nursing home residents and staff time to provide care, *J. Am. Geriatr. Soc.*, 54, 919, 2006.
13. Simmons, S.F. and Schnelle, J.F., Individualized feeding assistance care for nursing home residents: staffing requirements to implement two interventions, *J. Gerontol. A Biol. Sci. Med. Sci.*, 59, M966, 2004.
14. Simmons, S.F., Osterweil, D., and Schnelle, J.F., Improving food intake in nursing home residents with feeding assistance: a staffing analysis, *J. Gerontol. A Biol. Sci. Med. Sci.*, 56, M790, 2001.
15. Simmons, S.F., Babineau, S., Garcia, E., et al., Quality assessment in nursing homes by systematic direct observation: feeding assistance, *J. Gerontol. A Biol. Sci. Med. Sci.*, 57, M665, 2002.
16. Simmons, S.F. and Schnelle, J.F., Translating psychosocial research into practice. Selected topics in Alzheimer's disease. Assessment of nutritional care in the nursing home, *Alz. Care Q.*, 4, 286, 2003.
17. Kayser-Jones, J. and Schell, E., The effect of staffing on the quality of care at mealtime, *Nurs. Outlook*, 45, 64, 1997.
18. Kayser-Jones, J., Schell, E.S., Porter, C., et al., Factors contributing to dehydration in nursing homes: inadequate staffing and lack of professional supervision, *J. Am. Geriatr. Soc.*, 47, 1187, 1999.
19. Evans, B.C. and Crogan, N.L., Quality improvement practices: enhancing quality of life during mealtimes, *J. Nurses Staff Dev.*, 17, 131, 2001.
20. Crogan, N.L. and Shultz, J.A., Nursing assistants' perceptions of barriers to nutrition care for residents in long-term care facilities, *J. Nurses Staff Dev.*, 16, 216, 2000.
21. Wilson, M.M., Purushothaman, R., and Morley, J.E., Effect of liquid dietary supplements on energy intake in the elderly, *Am. J. Clin. Nutr.*, 75, 944, 2002.
22. Simmons, S.F., Lam, H.Y., Rao, G., et al., Family members' preferences for nutrition interventions to improve nursing home residents' oral food and fluid intake, *J. Am. Geriatr. Soc.*, 51, 69, 2003.
23. Crogan, N.L., Evans, B., and Velasquez, D., Measuring nursing home resident satisfaction with food and food service: initial testing of the FoodEx-LTC, *J. Gerontol. A Biol. Sci. Med. Sci.*, 59, 370, 2004.
24. Schiffman, S.S., Intensification of sensory properties of foods for the elderly, *J. Nutr.*, 130, 927S, 2000.
25. Remsburg, R.E., Luking, A., Bara, P., et al., Impact of a buffet-style dining program on weight and biochemical indicators of nutritional status in nursing home residents: a pilot study, *J. Am. Diet. Assoc.*, 101, 1460, 2001.
26. Evans, B.C., Crogan, N.L., and Shultz, J.A., The meaning of mealtimes: connection to the social world of the nursing home, *J. Gerontol. Nurs.*, 31, 11, 2005.
27. Nijs, K.A., de, G.C., Kok, F.J., et al., Effect of family style mealtimes on quality of life, physical performance, and body weight of nursing home residents: cluster randomised controlled trial, *Br. Med. J.*, 332, 1180, 2006.
28. Pearson, A., Fitzgerald, M., and Nay, R., Mealtimes in nursing homes. The role of nursing staff, *J. Gerontol. Nurs.*, 29, 40, 2003.

29. Ragneskog, H., Brane, G., Karlsson, I., et al., Influence of dinner music on food intake and symptoms common in dementia, *Scand. J. Caring Sci.*, 10, 11, 1996.
30. Mathey, M.F., Siebelink, E., de, G.C., et al., Flavor enhancement of food improves dietary intake and nutritional status of elderly nursing home residents, *J. Gerontol. A Biol. Sci. Med. Sci.*, 56, M200, 2001.
31. Clydesdale, F.M., Changes in color and flavor and their effect on sensory perception in the elderly, *Nutr. Rev.*, 52, S19, 1994.
32. Pfeiffer, N.A., Rogers, D.A., Roseman, M.R., et al., What's new in long-term care dining? *N.C. Med. J.*, 66, 287, 2005.
33. Simmons, S.F. and Levy-Storms, L., The effect of dining location on nutritional care quality in nursing homes, *J. Nutr. Health Aging*, 9, 434, 2005.
34. Marken, D., Enhancing the dining experience in long-term care: dining with dignity program, *J. Nutr. Elder.*, 23, 99, 2004.
35. Essed, N.H., van Staveren, W.A., Kok, F.J., et al., No effect of 16 weeks flavor enhancement on dietary intake and nutritional status of nursing home elderly, *Appetite*, 48(1), 29–36, 2006.
36. Kremer, S., Bult, J.H., Mojet, J., et al., Compensation for age-associated chemosensory losses and its effect on the pleasantness of a custard dessert and a tomato drink, *Appetite*, 48(1), 96–103, 2006.
37. Chan, J. and Kayser-Jones, J., The experience of dying for Chinese nursing home residents: cultural considerations, *J. Gerontol. Nurs.*, 31, 26, 2005.
38. Tanabe, M.K. and Jasper, C., Ethnonutrition: those home-sweet-home foods, *J. Am. Geriatr. Soc.*, 54, 1010, 2006.
39. Russell, R.M., Rasmussen, H., and Lichtenstein, A.H., Modified Food Guide Pyramid for people over seventy years of age, *J. Nutr.*, 129, 751, 1999.
40. Morley, J.E., Decreased food intake with aging, *J. Gerontol. A Biol. Sci. Med. Sci.*, 56, 81, 2001.
41. Thomas, D.R., Vitamins in health and aging, *Clin. Geriatr. Med.*, 20, 259, 2004.
42. Fralic, J. and Griffin, C., Nutrition and the elderly: a case manager's guide, *Lippincotts Case Manage.*, 6, 177, 2001.
43. Drewnowski, A. and Shultz, J.M., Impact of aging on eating behaviors, food choices, nutrition, and health status, *J. Nutr. Health Aging*, 5, 75, 2001.
44. Huang, H.Y., Caballero, B., Chang, S., et al., The efficacy and safety of multivitamin and mineral supplement use to prevent cancer and chronic disease in adults: a systematic review for a National Institutes of Health state-of-the-science conference, *Ann. Intern. Med.*, 145, 372, 2006.
45. Melhus, H., Michaelsson, K., Kindmark, A., et al., Excessive dietary intake of vitamin A is associated with reduced bone mineral density and increased risk for hip fracture, *Ann. Intern. Med.*, 129, 770, 1998.
46. Feskanich, D., Singh, V., Willett, W.C., et al., Vitamin A intake and hip fractures among postmenopausal women, *JAMA*, 287, 47, 2002.
47. Crandall, C., Vitamin A intake and osteoporosis: a clinical review, *J. Womens Health*, 13, 939, 2004.
48. Morley, J.E. and Silver, A.J., Nutritional issues in nursing home care, *Ann. Intern. Med.*, 123, 850, 1995.
49. Chapuy, M.C., Arlot, M.E., Duboeuf, F., et al., Vitamin D3 and calcium to prevent hip fractures in the elderly women, *N. Engl. J. Med.*, 327, 1637, 1992.
50. Bischoff, H.A., Stahelin, H.B., Dick, W., et al., Effects of vitamin D and calcium supplementation on falls: a randomized controlled trial, *J. Bone Miner. Res.*, 18, 343, 2003.

51. Lips, P., Vitamin D deficiency and secondary hyperparathyroidism in the elderly: consequences for bone loss and fractures and therapeutic implications, *Endocr. Rev.*, 22, 477, 2001.
52. Hickey, L. and Gordon, C.M., Vitamin D deficiency: new perspectives on an old disease, *Curr. Opin. Endocrinol. Diabetes*, 11, 18, 2004.
53. Malabanan, A., Veronikis, I.E., and Holick, M.F., Redefining vitamin D insufficiency, *Lancet*, 351, 805, 1998.
54. Gordon, C.M., DePeter, K., and Grace, E., Hypovitaminosis D in healthy adolescents, *J. Bone Miner. Res.*, 18, 57, 2003.
55. Arya, V., Bhambri, R., Godbole, M.M., et al., Vitamin D status and its relationship with bone mineral density in healthy Asian Indians, *Osteoporos. Int.*, 15, 56, 2004.
56. Visser, M., Deeg, D.J., Puts, M.T., et al., Low serum concentrations of 25-hydroxyvitamin D in older persons and the risk of nursing home admission, *Am. J. Clin. Nutr.*, 84, 616, 2006.
57. Stein, M.S., Scherer, S.C., Walton, S.L., et al., Risk factors for secondary hyperparathyroidism in a nursing home population, *Clin. Endocrinol.*, 44, 375, 1996.
58. Stein, M.S., Flicker, L., Scherer, S.C., et al., Relationships with serum parathyroid hormone in old institutionalized subjects, *Clin. Endocrinol.*, 54, 583, 2001.
59. Wigg, A.E., Prest, C., Slobodian, P., et al., A system for improving vitamin D nutrition in residential care, *Med. J. Aust.*, 185, 195, 2006.
60. MRC/BHF Heart Protection Study of antioxidant vitamin supplementation in 20,536 high-risk individuals: a randomised placebo-controlled trial, *Lancet,* 360, 23, 2002.
61. Moeller, S.M., Parekh, N., Tinker, L., et al., Associations between intermediate age-related macular degeneration and lutein and zeaxanthin in the Carotenoids in Age-Related Eye Disease Study (CAREDS): ancillary study of the Women's Health Initiative, *Arch. Ophthalmol.*, 124, 1151, 2006.
62. Solfrizzi, V., Panza, F., and Capurso, A., The role of diet in cognitive decline, *J. Neural Transm.*, 110, 95, 2003.
63. Schatz, I.J., Masaki, K., Yano, K., et al., Cholesterol and all-cause mortality in elderly people from the Honolulu Heart Program: a cohort study, *Lancet*, 358, 351, 2001.
64. Curb, J.D., Abbott, R.D., Rodriguez, B.L., et al., Prospective association between low and high total and low-density lipoprotein cholesterol and coronary heart disease in elderly men, *J. Am. Geriatr. Soc.*, 52, 1975, 2004.
65. Wilson, M.M., Thomas, D.R., Rubenstein, L.Z., et al., Appetite assessment: simple appetite questionnaire predicts weight loss in community-dwelling adults and nursing home residents, *Am. J. Clin. Nutr.*, 82, 1074, 2005.
66. Morley, J.E. and Kraenzle, D., Causes of weight loss in a community nursing home, *J. Am. Geriatr. Soc.*, 42, 583, 1994.
67. Fitten, L.J., Morley, J.E., Gross, P.L., et al., Depression, *J. Am. Geriatr. Soc.*, 37, 459, 1989.
68. Kahn, R., Weight loss and depression in a community nursing home, *J. Am. Geriatr. Soc.*, 43, 83, 1995.
69. Miller, D.K., Perry, H.M., III, and Morley, J.E., Associations among the Mini Nutritional Assessment instrument, dehydration, and functional status among older African Americans in St. Louis, Mo., USA, *Nestle Nutr. Workshop Ser. Clin. Perform. Programme*, 1, 79, 1999.
70. McCabe, B.J., Prevention of food-drug interactions with special emphasis on older adults, *Curr. Opin. Clin. Nutr. Metab. Care*, 4, 21, 2004.

71. McCabe, B.J., Frankel, E.H., and Wolfe, J.J., Monitoring nutritional status in drug regimens, in *Handbook of Food-Drug Interactions*, McCabe, B.J., Frankel, E.H., and Wolfe, J.J., Eds., CRC Press, Boca Raton, FL, 2003, p. 73.
72. Anderson, K.E., Effects of macronutrients and micronutrients on drug metabolism, *J. Am. Pharm. Assoc.*, 42, S28, 2002.
73. Anderson, K.E. and Kappas, A., Dietary regulation of cytochrome P450, *Annu. Rev. Nutr.*, 11, 141, 1991.
74. Zanger, A. and Shainberg, A., Thiamine deficiency in cardiac cells in culture, *Biochem. Pharmacol.*, 7, 575, 1997.
75. Djoenaidi, W., Notermans, S.L., and Dunda, G., Beriberi cardiomyopathy, *Eur. J. Clin. Nutr.*, 46, 227, 1992.
76. Brady, J.A., Rock, C.L., and Horneffer, M.R., Thiamin status, diuretic medications, and the management of congestive heart failure, *J. Am. Diet. Assoc.*, 95, 541, 1995.
77. Kwok, T., Falconer-Smith, J.F., Potter, J.F., et al., Thiamine status of elderly patients with cardiac failure, *Age Ageing*, 21, 67, 1992.
78. Doherty, M.M. and Charman, W.N., The mucosa of the small intestine: how clinically relevant as an organ of drug metabolism? *Clin. Pharmacokinet.*, 41, 235, 2002.
79. Greenblatt, D.J., Understanding drug interactions with grapefruit juice, *J. Am. Pharm. Assoc.*, 42, S29, 2002.
80. Wallace, A.W., Victory, J.M., and Amsden, G.W., Lack of bioequivalence when levofloxacin and calcium-fortified orange juice are coadministered to healthy volunteers, *J. Clin. Pharmacol.*, 43, 539, 2003.
81. Mayer, O., Jr., Simon, J., Rosolova, H., et al., The effects of folate supplementation on some coagulation parameters and oxidative status surrogates, *Eur. J. Clin. Pharmacol.*, 58, 1, 2002.
82. Murden, R.A. and Ainslie, N.K., Recent weight loss is related to short-term mortality in nursing homes, *J. Gen. Intern. Med.*, 9, 648, 1994.
83. Ryan, C., Bryant, E., Eleazer, P., et al., Unintentional weight loss in long-term care: predictor of mortality in the elderly, *South. Med. J.*, 88, 721, 1995.
84. Huffman, G.B., Evaluating and treating unintentional weight loss in the elderly, *Am. Fam. Physician*, 65, 640, 2002.
85. Thomas, D.R., Ashmen, W., Morley, J.E., et al., Nutritional management in long-term care: development of a clinical guideline. Council for Nutritional Strategies in Long-Term Care, *J. Gerontol. A Biol. Sci. Med. Sci.*, 55, M725, 2000.
86. Simmons, S.F. and Patel, A.V., Nursing home staff delivery of oral liquid nutritional supplements to residents at risk for unintentional weight loss, *J. Am. Geriatr. Soc.*, 54, 1372, 2006.
87. Kayser-Jones, J.S., Use of oral supplements in nursing homes: remaining questions, *J. Am. Geriatr. Soc.*, 54, 1002, 2006.
88. Lauque, S., Arnaud-Battandier, F., Mansourian, R., et al., Protein-energy oral supplementation in malnourished nursing-home residents. A controlled trial, *Age Ageing*, 29, 51, 2000.
89. Wouters-Wesseling, W., Wouters, A.E., Kleijer, C.N., et al., Study of the effect of a liquid nutrition supplement on the nutritional status of psycho-geriatric nursing home patients, *Eur. J. Clin. Nutr.*, 56, 245, 2002.
90. Faxen-Irving, G., Andren-Olsson, B., Geijerstam, A., et al., The effect of nutritional intervention in elderly subjects residing in group-living for the demented, *Eur. J. Clin. Nutr.*, 56, 221, 2002.

91. Kamel, H.K., Thomas, D.R., and Morley, J.E., Nutritional deficiencies in long-term care: management of protein energy malnutrition and dehydration, *Ann. Long-Term Care*, 6, 250, 1998.
92. Johnson, R.M., Smiciklas-Wright, H., Soucy, I.M., et al., Nutrient intake of nursing-home residents receiving pureed foods or a regular diet, *J. Am. Geriatr. Soc.*, 43, 344, 1995.
93. Niedert, K.C., Position of the American Dietetic Association: liberalization of the diet prescription improves quality of life for older adults in long-term care, *J. Am. Diet. Assoc.*, 105, 1955, 2005.
94. American Diabetes Association position statement: evidence-based nutrition principles and recommendations for the treatment and prevention of diabetes and related complications, *J. Am. Diet. Assoc.*, 102, 109, 2002.
95. Tariq, S.H., Karcic, E., Thomas, D.R., et al., The use of a no-concentrated-sweets diet in the management of type 2 diabetes in nursing homes, *J. Am. Diet. Assoc.*, 101, 1463, 2001.
96. Coulston, A.M., Mandelbaum, D., and Reaven, G.M., Dietary management of nursing home residents with non-insulin-dependent diabetes mellitus, *Am. J. Clin. Nutr.*, 51, 67, 1990.
97. Niewoehner, C.B., Allen, J.I., Boosalis, M., et al., Role of zinc supplementation in type II diabetes mellitus, *Am. J. Med.*, 81, 63, 1986.
98. Allred, J.B., Gallagher-Allred, C.R., and Bowers, D.F., Elevated blood cholesterol: a risk factor for heart disease that decreases with advanced age, *J. Am. Diet. Assoc.*, 90, 574, 1990.
99. Schatz, I.J., Masaki, K., Yano, K., et al., Cholesterol and all-cause mortality in elderly people from the Honolulu Heart Program: a cohort study, *Lancet*, 358, 351, 2001.
100. Simons, L.A., Simons, J., Friedlander, Y., et al., Cholesterol and other lipids predict coronary heart disease and ischaemic stroke in the elderly, but only in those below 70 years, *Atherosclerosis*, 159, 201, 2001.
101. Krumholz, H.M., Seeman, T.E., Merrill, S.S., et al., Lack of association between cholesterol and coronary heart disease mortality and morbidity and all-cause mortality in persons older than 70 years, *JAMA*, 272, 1335, 1994.
102. Rudman, D., Mattson, D.E., Nagraj, H.S., et al., Prognostic significance of serum cholesterol in nursing home men, *J. Parenter. Enteral Nutr.*, 12, 155, 1988.
103. Hadler, M.H., The lack of benefit of modest sodium restriction in the institutionalized elderly, *J. Am. Geriatr. Soc.*, 32, 235, 1984.

20 Providing Optimal Nutrition in the Assisted Living Environment

Connie W. Bales, Ph.D., R.D., C.N.S., L.D.N.
Gwendolen T. Buhr, M.D.
Victoria H. Hawk, M.P.H., R.D., L.D.N.
Linda S. Evanko, R.D., L.D.N.
Heidi K. White, M.D.

CONTENTS

20.1 INTRODUCTION

Optimal nutritional status plays a critical role in successful aging, contributing to both health and quality of life.[1] One key determinant of dietary intake and thus nutritional status in the later years of life is living situation, since living environment influences the availability, cost, nutritional value, aesthetic quality, and convenience of the daily diet. With the growing number and heterogeneity of choices in living situations for older adults, it is becoming increasingly important that the impact of the residential setting on nutritional status be assessed and accounted for when choosing a living location. In this chapter, we focus on a new and increasingly popular residential environment—assisted living—and the important nutritional risk factors that need to be considered in this type of living situation.

20.2 ASSISTED LIVING FACILITIES AND THEIR RESIDENTS

Assisted living (AL) is a marketing term for a supportive group residential setting that provides help with personal care for those who need some assistance because of physical or mental limitations, but who do not require the 24-hour skilled care found in traditional nursing homes (NHs). Some of the basic parameters of AL facilities are listed in Table 20.1. AL goes by many different names, including adult care home, family care home, rest home, residential care setting, domiciliary, or

TABLE 20.1
Characterization of Typical Assisted Living Services and Activities

Services include:
24-hour supervision
Three meals a day in a group dining room
Other assistive services for daily activities may include:
Personal care services (help with bathing, dressing, toileting, etc.)
Medication management or assistance with self-administration of medicine
Social services
Supervision and assistance for persons with Alzheimer's or other dementias and disabilities
Exercise and wellness programs
Housekeeping and maintenance
Arrangements for transportation

Source: American Health Care Association, Nation Center for Assisted Living, http://www.longtermcareliving.com/planning_ahead/assisted/assisted1.htm.

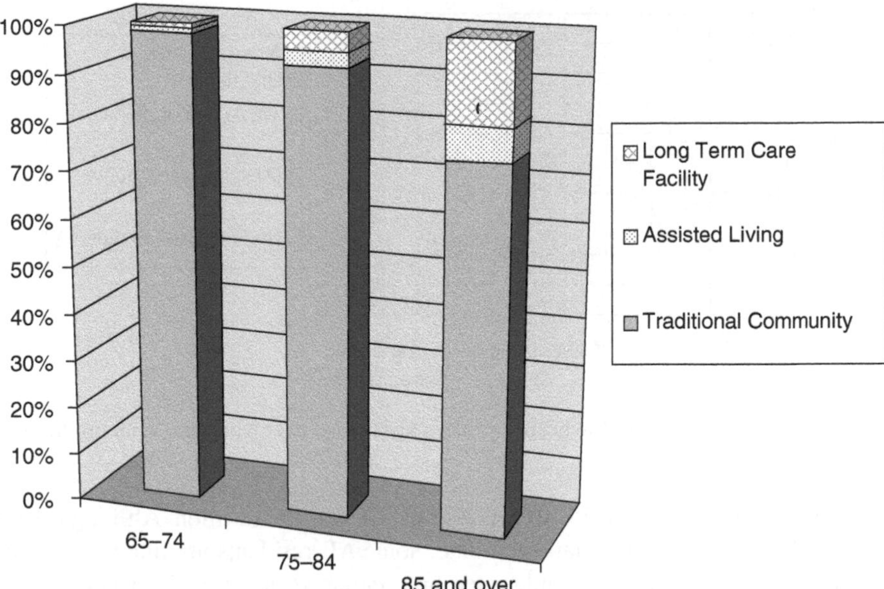

FIGURE 20.1 Percentage of Medicare enrollees age 65 and over residing in selected residential settings, by age group, 2004.

board and care.[2] AL facilities can range from a small house with one or more residents to a large apartment-style complex, with most having 25 to 125 units.[3] In 2004, 36,451 licensed AL facilities with 937,601 units/beds were reported. While the growth in AL facilities has been flat in recent years, this follows a period of dramatic growth in the 1990s. The number of AL beds increased by 33% from 1998 to 2000 and by 13% from 2000 to 2002, slowing to an increase of 3% from 2002 to 2004. As illustrated in Figure 20.1, the percentage of Medicare enrollees living in AL facilities increases with age, from 1% for those 65 to 74 to 7% for those 85 and over in 2004.[4]

Residents of AL facilities often have significant limitations in function (Figure 20.2). In 2004, of those AL residents 65 years of age or older, 12% had limitations in three or more activities of daily living (ADLs), 33% had one or two ADL limitations, 18% had one limitation in only the instrumental activities of daily living (IADLs), and 37% had no limitations. This is compared to the traditional community, where 58% of respondents had no limitations, and the skilled nursing home, where only 6% had no functional limitations.[4] Also indicative of increased health risks for AL residents is the fact that 61% of AL facilities provide dementia care.[5]

20.3 NUTRITIONAL CONCERNS FOR AL RESIDENTS

Overall, the characteristics of residents in AL facilities and NHs are becoming increasingly similar, e.g., in terms of the prevalence of behavioral and depressive symptoms, the number of medications and chronic illnesses, and the prevalence of dementia.[6] Because declining functional status, depressive symptoms, polypharmacy, and more chronic illnesses have all been associated with poor nutritional health, in

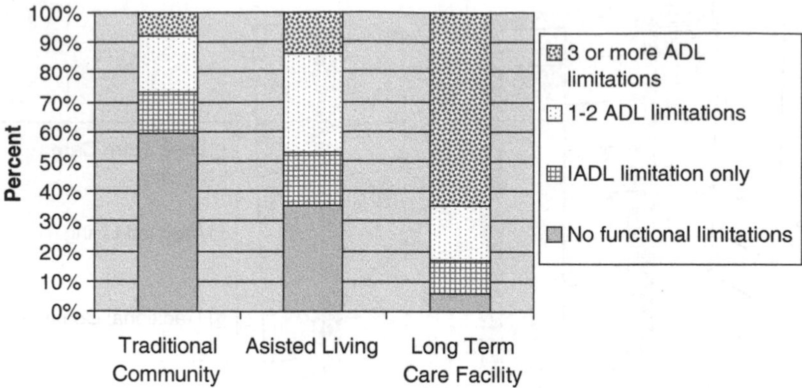

FIGURE 20.2 Percentage of Medicare enrollees age 65 and over with functional limitations, by residential setting, 2004.

NHs, it is likely that AL residents are also at risk for malnutrition. Although there is limited scientific documentation to date, some AL residents are likely at risk of having malnutrition that goes undetected and untreated. Reed et al.[7] examined the cognitively impaired residents in 35 AL facilities and 10 NHs. They studied problems with food and fluid intake and found rates for low food intake of 54.1% and for low fluid intake of 51.3% in AL residents. These rates were only slightly lower than in the NH residents, whose corresponding prevalences were 61.8 and 63.4%. Despite these relatively high rates of nutritional problems, these AL facilities were much less likely than NHs to provide nutritional assessment or treatment for eating and drinking difficulties. Likewise, in their 2003 survey of state regulations governing nutrition in AL facilities, Chao et al.[8] found that nutritional assessments were rarely required (in only 8 of 45 states). Undetected malnutrition can contribute to further functional decline and increase medical risk. Rosenberg et al.[9] followed 198 randomly selected AL residents for 36 months, examining risk factors for transition to a skilled nursing facility. Along with several other significant risk factors, they found that changes in appetite (measured using the Neuropsychiatric Inventory) were linked with an increased risk of needing skilled nursing care.

It should be noted that a distinct type of AL exists when a person living at home receives services that create a type of assisted living. Assistance from home health care, Meals on Wheels programs, adult day services, senior centers, or short-term respite programs in nursing homes can provide some meal supervision and a limited number of meals. Funding for such meal programs is provided to state agencies by the Administration on Aging. As per the federal guidelines, the meals offered at senior centers and by Meals on Wheels are substantial, with each meal offered providing an equivalent of at least one third of the estimated daily needs for calories and nutrients. The meals served in a congregate setting also provide social stimulation and, in some cases, education and other services for the elderly. This type of meal program has been shown to reduce nutritional risk in vulnerable elderly individuals.[10]

20.3.1 Determinants of Nutritional Well-Being

Undernutrition occurs when the intake of energy and other nutrients is inadequate to meet nutritional needs. A review of cohort and cross-sectional studies reveals that food intake declines with age, leading to a decrease in the intake of most nutrients.[11] Several factors may contribute to a decline in dietary intake with age, including impaired appetite and early satiety, also termed the anorexia of aging.[12,13] Underlying causes recognized to influence this process include hormonal changes, physiological changes in the GI system (motility, dry mouth, early satiety), and sensory changes such as decreased sense of taste and smell.[14] These and other determinants of the anorexia of aging are addressed in more detail in Chapter 13.

Chronic inadequate dietary intake (undernutrition) may result in malnutrition and contribute to a multitude of undesirable health concerns, including unplanned weight loss, dehydration, nutritional anemia, and increased functional and cognitive impairment. More specifically, unplanned weight loss is associated with increased incidence of frailty, pressure ulcers, hip fractures, and an overall increased rate of mortality.[15] While a host of factors are known to influence dietary behaviors, the concerns discussed below are particularly important potential determinants of nutritional status of AL residents.

20.3.1.1 Nutritional Adequacy of Foods Offered

Most adults consume a generally adequate diet, abundant in calories, protein, and essential vitamins and minerals. Supplements of vitamins and minerals are also commonly taken; 35% of adults report taking a multivitamin/mineral at least once a month.[16] But for elderly adults living in long-term-care facilities, age-related increases in nutritional risk and the disadvantages and unfamiliarity of institutional food service can combine to contribute to nutritional shortfalls and subsequent undernutrition. This concern is well known in the NH setting, and for this reason, there are strict requirements that stipulate standards of nutritional adequacy for meals served to NH residents. Menus and the corresponding meals served are less rigid in the AL setting for obvious reasons—residents primarily eat in dining rooms where they have free choice from a variety of menu items. A consequence of this freedom of choice is that residents can make adequate or less than adequate meal selections. And while consumption of an inadequate diet may be less common in AL residents, there is also less likelihood that when poor dietary status occurs it will be detected in a timely manner.

20.3.1.2 Food Acceptability: Actual and Perceived Influences

The quality of the food and food presentation are important determinants of the amount of food eaten for subjects of any age. These factors are particularly important for older adults experiencing some degree of sensory impairment (e.g., taste, smell, vision). Many, although not all, older adults have decrements in the chemical senses that affect the acceptability of foods offered.[17] These decrements may lead to a perceived tastelessness of foods and contribute to excessive use of salt, sweeteners, and table fats to enhance their appeal. In search of a healthier way to enhance food intake, studies conducted by Schiffman[18] have shown that adding additional flavors to enhance existing food flavors can improve food intakes in elderly individuals.

But even for seniors with no sensory impairments related to eating, the quality and ambiance of the individual foods and the meal service can be critical determinants of food acceptability and thus nutrient intake. Nijs et al.[19] found that NH residents had improved energy intakes and Mini-Nutritional Assessment scores when meals were served family style, rather than the usual buffet style on trays. Personal food preferences also play an important role in determining the acceptability of meals offered and need to be taken into consideration whenever possible.

20.3.1.3 Psychosocial and Cultural Considerations

20.3.1.3.1 Loss of Independence

One of the most common reasons for older persons to reject the idea of living in a long-term-care facility has to do with the loss of independence and control of their daily lives, including their opportunities to enjoy familiar foods. While having meals prepared for them in the nursing home can meet critical nutritional needs of residents who are unable to shop for food and prepare their own meals, the disadvantages of institutionally prepared meals and the loss of freedom of choice about meal composition must also be recognized. AL facilities that offer kitchenettes in resident rooms or more restaurant-style food services provide a wider range of food choices and thus could help to counteract this problem.

20.3.1.3.2 Loss of Cultural Identity

A related concern is the loss of cultural identity that residents of nursing homes experience when they lose free choice of meal composition. Studies of dietary patterns in multiethnic cohorts show that these patterns differ by ethnicity, as well as age and gender.[20] Some AL settings have the potential to provide greater flexibility for special food choices; others do not.

20.3.1.3.3 Social Isolation and Logistics

While the NH environment provides more social contact than living alone, there is still considerable social isolation (from persons of other ages, activities, and interests) as well as other social disadvantages in this setting. AL arrangements offer the potential for a more real-world type of environment and could partially offset feelings of isolation.

As noted above, the ambiance of the food service and the location for eating can be important determinants of food enjoyment. Timing of meals can also have an important advantage; residents are very likely to benefit from the more flexible AL environment, where they have more freedom of choice about the timing and amount of meals and snacks.

20.4 MEETING SPECIAL NUTRITIONAL NEEDS

20.4.1 Therapeutic Diets That Limit Food Intake

Mealtime should be a positive experience, with the goal of promoting adequate nutritional intake. Thus, the use of restrictive or therapeutic diets in AL needs to be carefully considered on an individualized basis. A therapeutic diet is a meal plan that controls or restricts the intake of one or more nutrients as part of the medical management of a disease. Examples of such diets include a dialysis diet, which limits sodium, potassium, and fluid intake while providing additional protein, a no concentrated sweets or carbohydrate-balanced diet to promote control of diabetes, a sodium-restricted diet to control hypertension or congestive heart failure, and a low-fat/low-cholesterol diet to counteract hyperlipidemia. For the elderly in structured living situations, the use of dietary restrictions to manage various disease states may decrease enjoyment at meals, and thus further compromise intake and health status because of the limited or undesirable food offerings.[15] For example, the use of a sodium-restricted diet has been linked to an overall decrease in energy intake as well as lower intakes of macro- and micronutrients,[21] therefore increasing the risk of undernutrition. Thus, it may be useful to liberalize the diet as tolerated and consider management of chronic conditions with medication rather than through the use of dietary restrictions.[15] There needs to be an overall goal of promoting good health through adequate nutrition with a balance between the physician's therapeutic goals and the resident's quality of life.

20.4.2 Difficulties with Oral Food Intake

20.4.2.1 Dysphagia

For AL clients with dysphagia who need viscosity-adjusted liquids, these liquids need to be available at meals, at medication passes, at bedside, and at social events. Based on the recommendations of the speech language pathologist, commercially prepared liquids can be obtained from major institutional food service providers or from the manufacturer directly. These prepared liquids are available in both nectar and honey consistencies. Alternatively, facilities may choose to prepare their own thickened liquids using commercially available thickening agents. This method is time consuming and the end product may be inconsistent due to variable staff ability, experience, and length of time from preparation to consumption by the patient.

20.4.2.2 Need for Adaptation of Food Texture and Consistency

Due to changes in dentition, involuntary tongue movements, and dysphagia, some residents will need adaptations of food consistency and texture. Use of a blender, food chopper or food processor (Robot Coupe USA, Jackson, MS) allows the facility to accommodate varieties in consistency. Consistencies may need to vary from chopped to ground to puree. Commercially prepared puree items are available from major institutional food service providers or directly from the manufacturers. AL facilities will vary in their ability to provide residents with foods modified in texture or consistency.

20.4.2.3 Eating Dependency

Changes in ability to self-feed are often due to changes in the grip strength, involuntary hand movements, or the loss of use of an individual's dominant hand. Use of a finger food diet and adaptive feeding equipment can often improve the client's ability to maintain independence at meals. Adaptive feeding equipment (including built handles, grip handles, weighted handles, and curved handles) is available commercially, and consultation with an occupational therapist will provide the facility with information about the necessary equipment based on the individual client's needs. The use of a washcloth, wrapped around and taped to the handle of the utensil, can work well. In addition to the adaptive utensils available, high-side plates, plate guards, sticky placemats, and divided/sectional plates allow clients to maintain their feeding independence. When considering an Al facility, it is important to evaluate the availability of appropriate assessment and monitoring of oral intake problems at meals. Compared to the residents of NHs, those residing in AL may be less likely to receive this type of assessment and treatment, and the AL staff are less likely to be qualified to provide these services.[7] AL residents who have difficulties with oral food and fluid intake may need to have extra support. The ability to provide compensatory assistance and adaptive equipment at meals will vary among AL facilities.

20.4.3 Alternate Nutrition via Tube Feedings

Patients who receive an enteral tube (i.e., nasogastric, gastrostomy, or jejunostomy) for an acute, potentially reversible illness are managed in a hospital or rehabilitation setting such as skilled-care facilities. However, more patients are receiving feeding tubes for chronic progressive diseases without a clear endpoint. This may provide an impetus for more AL facilities to attempt to manage patients with well-established feeding tubes and well-tolerated feeding regimens.

In general, enteral feeding tubes such as percutaneous endoscopic gastrostomy tubes and jejunostomy tubes are not managed in AL environments unless the patient can manage the tube feeding independently. However, based on the complexity of the clients that the AL staff are qualified to support, an AL client's tube feedings may be accommodated. It is mandatory that facility personnel monitor the ability of clients to self-administer their feeding, confirm their ability to feed and flush the tube adequately, confirm compliance with feeding regimen, ensure that the surrounding skin remains in good condition, and confirm that the tube is functional.

20.5 SPECIAL MEDICAL CONCERNS THAT INFLUENCE NUTRITIONAL STATUS

In the AL environment, nutritional monitoring and assessment are the responsibilities of the physician. The physician should not assume that the nutritional health of the residents will be monitored as it would be in a NH. Such parameters as weight and nutritional intake may be collected, but unlike in the NH, in the AL environment the monitoring and interpretation of these parameters are the responsibility of the physician. Fewer licensed health professionals such as licensed practical nurses, registered nurses, registered dietitians, and occupational therapists are associated with AL facilities, and in most cases the licensed health professionals function only in a supervisory role and are present only periodically. Additionally, no medical director is required, and rarely is a physician on site. Instead, residents generally receive medical care outside of the facility in medical offices. The communication between physician and facility staff may be minimal, unless initiated by the physician. Medications, injections, glucose monitoring, and tube feeding are more often performed by medication aides or the residents themselves as opposed to licensed health professionals. Although some training for such duties is required, in most cases the training consists of a short course, and therefore, the knowledge base of these personnel is not extensive. In comparison to NHs, it may be difficult for a physician to handle medical symptoms and acute problems over the phone, since a licensed health professional may not be present to make nursing assessments.

Physicians and other clinicians should not assume that patients with special nutritional needs can be accommodated in an AL setting. A facility's ability to provide special diets, feeding assistance, tube feedings, glucose monitoring, and other types of monitoring, such as frequent weigh-ins and monitoring of amount of oral intake, should be clearly established prior to admission. As the resident's condition changes after admission, additional discussions may be needed to determine whether the resident can remain in the AL facility. It is often up to the physician to recommend a higher level of care to the patient and family when the needs of the patient can no longer be adequately met.

20.5.1 Medications

The population living in AL is medically frail and disabled, much like the population in NHs. Data from the 1998 Medicare Current Beneficiary Survey showed that the mean number of medications per month was 8 for both AL and NH populations. Further, 69% of residents in AL compared with 70% in the NH setting received psychotropic medications. In this survey, 39% of AL residents had hypertension, 31% heart disease, 29% dementia, 17% arthritis, and 16% diabetes.[22] Medication review becomes particularly important when malnutrition is present in this frail and highly medicated population. Many medications commonly used in older adults can lead to malnutrition. Nonsteroidal anti-inflammatory drugs such as ibuprofen and even the newer cox-2 inhibitors such as celecoxib can cause dyspepsia, ulceration, bleeding, and diarrhea, which may decrease oral food intake. Acetylcholinesterase inhibitors such as donepezil and galantamine used in the treatment of Alzheimer's disease may cause nausea, vomiting, diarrhea, anorexia, and weight loss. Even the short-term use of antibiotics can lead to nausea, anorexia, or loss of taste sensation that impact nutritional status. Medication-related symptoms that may affect nutritional status include nausea/vomiting, anorexia, altered taste and smell, dry mouth, dysphagia, early satiety, reduced feeding ability through sedation, diarrhea, and hypermetabolism.[23] The list of offending medications is long and also includes commonly prescribed medications such as antidepressants and bisphophonates.

The primary care physician is the individual most likely to monitor for adverse drug events. In contrast to NHs, pharmacists do not review patient charts in AL. The facility may have a specific pharmacy through which they ask patients and families to fill their prescriptions, but many facilities allow patients and families to fill prescriptions using unaffiliated pharmacies in the community or through mail order, thus decreasing the ready availability of a pharmacist for consultation when questions or problems arise. In many facilities, medications are administered by medication aides rather than licensed nurses. Nonadherence to drug regimens or medications errors may contribute to adverse nutritional effects of medications. Some AL environments do not assume responsibility for medication administration, but may provide prompts and allow for the use of pill boxes that simplify medication administration for the patient. The physician should know how much assistance with medication administration is provided. If medications are administered by facility staff, the physicians should always review the medication administration record. This can help to avoid medication errors, especially when more than one physician is involved in the care of the patient.

20.5.2 Dementia

At least half of all AL residents have some form of dementia. A national random sample of AL facilities in 1998 revealed a 32 to 36% prevalence of moderate to severe dementia.[24] Similarly, a four-state survey conducted in 1997 to 1998 found 55% of residents with any degree of dementia, with 27% having moderate to severe dementia.[25] Weight loss and subsequent malnutrition may be an unavoidable part of the natural history of Alzheimer's disease (AD) and other dementias.[26] Whether nutritional intervention can delay functional decline and morbidity is largely untested. However, observational data from subjects with AD indicate that weight gain is associated with a reduced risk of mortality.[27] An understanding of the nutritional consequences of AD along with appropriate assessment and a thoughtful approach to intervention may help to avoid the complications associated with malnutrition, thus preserving a better quality of life up until death. The causes of weight loss and malnutrition in the early stages of AD may range from simple food unavailability and abnormal eating behaviors to taste and smell dysfunction, the effects of inflammatory mediators, and disregulation of the delicate balance between energy intake and energy expenditure.[28] In the later stages of the disease, feeding dependence and dysphagia become more prominent factors in the occurrence of malnutrition.

Patients in the mild to moderate stages of AD usually benefit greatly from the prepared meals and social interactions that accompany mealtime in an AL environment. Facility staff should ensure that patients attend meals and encourage them to stay until the end of the meal. For the most part, getting patients with dementia to eat is a process of trial and error. It is important to make sure that food is available, not just at mealtimes, but whenever the patient is inclined to eat. Many patients need supervision, constant reminders, and simple directions to complete a meal. Providing finger foods can be helpful for patients who are challenged by the use of utensils.[29] Appetite and alertness may be better early in the day, so breakfast becomes the most important meal and should be calorie and nutrient rich. Providing preferred foods can also increase intake.[30] Simplifying the environment so that there are fewer distractions during mealtime may be helpful. Researchers have demonstrated that improving the ambiance during mealtime by manipulating social and environmental aspects improves food consumption and nutritional status.[31] Studies that have implemented soothing dinner music for dementia patients demonstrate that this intervention can improve mealtime agitation and food intake.[32] Taken together, these studies—although few in number and scope of intervention—suggest that a nutritional intervention that seeks to enhance the hedonic reward during mealtime may significantly benefit AD patients who are at risk for nutritional decline. AL facilities may vary in their attention to such factors and their willingness or ability to make changes, but in general, much attention is paid to the quality of the dining experience, which is a readily observed and appreciated aspect of the care that is provided. As AD becomes more advanced and patients require more assistance with eating, including hand feeding and altering food consistencies to minimize aspiration due to dysphagia, the AL facility may not be able to provide the degree of assistance necessary to maintain adequate nutrition.

20.5.3 Depression

Depression in the elderly is common and frequently results in unintentional weight loss. The four-state sample of AL residents in 1997 to 1998 found that the prevalence of depression was 13%, while 18 to 37% of residents displayed symptoms of depression without meeting criteria for depression.[25] Therefore, clinicians should consider depression as a cause of malnutrition and weight loss. Brief depression screens such as the Geriatrics Depression Scale[33] or the Koenig Depression Scale[34] can help identify symptoms of depression, which may be otherwise unnoticed.

In typical NH, the hospital-like atmosphere and advanced medical and cognitive problems of the patient population can contribute to poor outlook and depression in some residents; the right type of AL environment might provide a more upbeat environment and encourage improved food consumption. However, there is generally less medical supervision in the AL setting; it would not be an appropriate living situation for a resident with severe depression.

20.5.4 Chronic Medical Illness

Many patients with chronic stable medical illness do well both medically and nutritionally in an AL environment. The predictability of the food quantity and nutritional quality can be very advantageous for patients with heart failure or hypertension if their condition is particularly sensitive to dietary changes in salt, fluid, and fat content. Patients with diabetes may also benefit from consistent meal schedules and the ability of staff to reliably provide insulin and glucose monitoring at appropriate times. However, for AL residents who have been hospitalized for an acute illness, especially if they have been ill for more than a few days, it may not be appropriate for them to return directly to their AL home. A period of rehabilitation in a skilled nursing facility may be necessary to stabilize their medical and nutritional condition in a more supervised setting where speech language pathologists, occupational therapists, and registered dietitians are available on site for assessments and interventions.

20.6 REACHING THE GOAL OF OPTIMAL NUTRITION FOR AL RESIDENTS

It should be apparent from the foregoing discussion that although there are many potential benefits of the AL environment, there is also substantial risk for nutritional decline in some AL residents. This is particularly true for individuals with nutritional or medical risk factors. Identifying and addressing these concerns requires input from the primary care physician and other appropriate health care professionals (e.g., registered dietitians, speech language pathologists, occupational therapists) and is also subject to the influences of governmental regulation and oversight.

20.6.1 Government Oversight and Licensure Regulations

The complexity of addressing the diverse needs of AL residents can be potentially exacerbated by inconsistencies in governmental oversight. There are no federal government licensing criteria or other mandatory standards for AL; rather, the standards are established on a state-by-state basis.[35] Most states, though not all, provide licensure and other regulations for AL facilities, but their extent and scope differ considerably by state. Moreover, the regulations are in a high degree of flux at present; most states have recently revised their regulations or report that they are currently working on revisions. In general, AL environments, compared to NHs, are not highly regulated. The philosophy of AL begins with the key principle of maximizing autonomy for the residents, with this autonomy extending to the individuals and corporations that operate the facilities. This lack of regulation helps to keep the costs affordable and seems to promote a homelike environment, but the lack of professional staff and minimal attention to patient assessment may not be readily appreciated by community physicians. In particular, state regulations for food and nutrition services are highly variable. In North Carolina, in order to be licensed as an adult care home, an AL facility must serve each resident "three nutritionally adequate, palatable meals a day at regular hours with at least 10 hours between the breakfast and evening meals." There are specific requirements for the number of servings of milk, fruit, vegetables, eggs, protein, cereal and bread, fats, and water, and menus for therapeutic diets need to be planned or reviewed by a registered dietitian.[36]

While these guidelines might seem fundamental and even simplistic for facilities housing residents at recognized nutritional risk, they are more complete than in some other states. In fact, a survey in 2001 by the National Academy for State Health Policy found that five states did not have any specific regulations for food or nutrition services at all.[8] More recently, we characterized (Bales et al., unpublished data) nutritional regulations in a subset of states (n = 11) for which detailed information about foods/nutrition was available for public access and used preestablished criteria to categorize the types of regulations related to foods and nutrition. As shown in Table 20.2, the major categories we evaluated were (1) food service and presentation, (2) nutritional adequacy, and (3) medical/functional requirements. The majority of states had one or more regulations regarding safe food handling. Requirements about the number and nutritional content and standard composition of meals served and the availability of therapeutic diets were stipulated by the majority of states. In contrast, allowances for tube feedings or textural changes in foods were not commonly delineated. In agreement with previous findings of Chao et al.[8] the AL regulations we reviewed did not include any requirements for nutritional assessment, and it was uncommon for food intake monitoring to be required.

TABLE 20.2
Foods and Nutrition-Related Regulations[a] for a Sample of 11 States

Regulation Category	Explanation	Selected States											% States Meeting Standard
		Alaska	Arizona	California	Florida	Iowa	North Carolina	North Dakota	Pennsylvania	Texas	Utah	West Virginia	
Food Service and Presentation													
Food safety	Food temperatures, employee health, personal hygiene, HACCP requirements	—	X	X	X	X	X	X	X	X	X	—	82%
Qualification of FS personnel	FS personnel have appropriate training	—	X	X	X	X	X	—	—	—	X	—	55%
Food handling	Meat inspection, food preparation, serving, receiving and storage standards	—	—	X	—	X	X	—	X	T	X	—	55%
Patient preferences, customs	Menu planning considers personal, cultural, and religious food preferences	X	X	—	X	—	X	—	X	—	—	X	55%
Palatability, presentation	Assess quality of food prepared	—	X	—	X	—	X	X	—	—	X	—	45%
Health department inspections	Regular inspections required	—	X	—	X	X	X	—	—	T	X	—	55%
Nutrition-Related Criteria[b]													
Nutritional adequacy	Nutritional content of meals considered	X	—	—	X	X	X	X	X	X	—	X	73%
Numbers of meals specified	Documents number of meals, snacks, and maximum amount of time between dinner and breakfast	X	X	—	X	X	X	X	X	X	X	X	91%
Meal consumption monitored	Staff document resident's intake at meals	—	—	—	—	—	—	—	X	—	—	—	9%
Menu standards	Facility follows guidelines for recipes, posting of menus, and documentation	X	X	—	X	X	X	X	—	X	—	X	73%

(continued)

TABLE 20.2
Foods and Nutrition-Related Regulations[a] for a Sample of 11 States (continued)

Regulation Category	Explanation	Selected States											% States Meeting Standard
		Alaska	Arizona	California	Florida	Iowa	North Carolina	North Dakota	Pennsylvania	Texas	Utah	West Virginia	
Nutrition assessment by RD or other health professional	Qualified nutrition professional assess the nutritional status of residents	—	—	—	—	—	—	—	—	—	—	—	0%
RD reviews menus		—	X	—	X	—	—	X	—	X*	X	—	45%
Other nutrition professional (not RD) reviews menus	Diet technician, dietary manager, CNS	—	—	X	X	—	—	X	—	—	—	—	27%
Medical/Functional Considerations													
Emergency food supplies	Specification about availability of rations on site	—	X	X	X	—	X	—	—	X	X	—	55%
Therapeutic diets available	Facility offers modified meals as per medical order	—	X	X	X	X	X	X	X	X	X	X	91%
Supervision of therapeutic diets by RD or LD	Dietitian reviews therapeutic menus	—	X	X	X	X	X	X	—	X*	X	—	73%
Food texture adjustments available	Consistency adjustments such as soft, chopped, pureed	—	X	—	X	—	—	—	—	—	—	—	18%
Tube feedings	Allowed (if independently administered)	—	X	—	X	—	X	—	—	—	—	—	27%

Note: HACCP = hazard analysis and critical control point; FS = food service; RD = registered dietitian; CNS = certified nutrition specialist; LD = licensed dietitian; T = facilities that house 17 or more residents; * = therapeutic diet that cannot customarily be prepared by layperson must be reviewed by RD.

[a] This table summarizes the information contained in selected state regulations for AL and adult-care homes that was available for public access in August 2006.

[b] We assessed requirements concerning nutrition education for residents, but none of the states surveyed indicated a requirement for nutrition education.

The scarcity of requirements for nutritional assessment and treatment/intervention in the AL setting underscores the substantial risk of underdiagnosis of malnutrition in the AL setting.

In an attempt to establish more uniform standards, the Joint Commission Accreditation of Health Care Organization (JCAHO) has set regulations for accreditation of AL facilities that require (1) "nutritionally balanced and varied meals" be provided twice a day, (2) a registered dietitian review menus for nutritional adequacy, and (3) the average daily number of servings of food correspond to the recommended number of servings and food categories in the USDA Food Guide Pyramid. In addition, the Assisted Living Federation of America offers a consumer guide that includes a checklist for evaluating nutrition services in AL facilities.[37]

20.7 CONCERNS, RECOMMENDATIONS, AND AGING IN PLACE

The AL living environment offers a number of potential advantages for enhancing nutritional status and quality of life. But pitfalls may exist for high-risk residents with special nutritional or medical needs. Some of the many considerations that influence the nutritional outcomes of residents living in AL are illustrated in Figure 20.3. Physicians and other health care providers must assume the responsibility of monitoring AL residents for signs of nutritional decline, provide the plan of intervention, and monitor the results.

When choosing a new AL environment, residents and their families can benefit from collecting detailed information regarding the food and nutrition services at the facility. They can ask current residents about the quality of the food and the dining experience and talk to administrators about the ability to meet the specific needs that the prospective resident has or anticipates. It may be helpful for family members to ask to eat a meal in the facility with the prospective resident and current residents to experience firsthand not only the nutritional quality of the food, but also the broader quality of the dining experience. If patients or families encounter nutrition-related issues that need to be addressed within the AL facility, they should first approach the nursing supervisor or administrator. If this approach is unsuccessful at reaching a solution, the patient or family member may contact an ombudsman (every state is required to have an ombudsman program). Ombudsmen serve as advocates for NH and AL residents and work to solve problems between residents and these facilities.

In some cases, changes in medical or nutritional needs may necessitate a move from the AL environment to a skilled NH. But for some patients and their families, it is not desirable to leave the AL environment as care needs increase. Rather, many patients and families are interested in finding ways to allow the individual to age in place. Home health services, hospice services, and additional services paid for by the individual can sometimes make this scenario possible. Under these circumstances, even greater communication between the physician and other care providers may be necessary to maintain nutritional well-being.

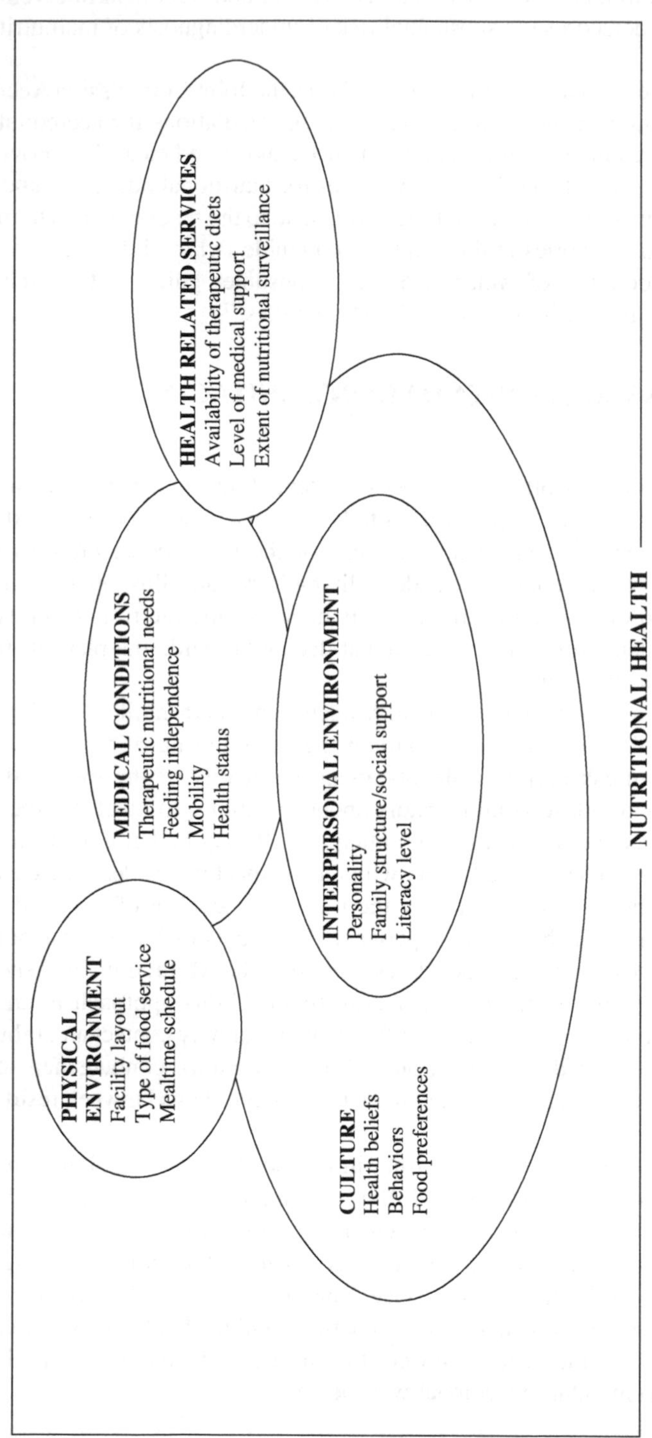

FIGURE 20.3 Determinants of nutritional health for assisted living residents. The major headings shown in bold indicate primary determinants, which will vary in importance for each individual. The factors are interrelated, as shown by the extent of overlapping circles. For example, **CULTURE** will strongly influence the interpersonal environment, to a lesser extent it will influence the medical conditions (through health beliefs or the acceptance of medical treatments), and to a small degree influence the physical environment.

REFERENCES

1. Welsh, P.G., Nutrition and the dining experience in long-term care: critical indicators of nursing home quality care, *N.C. Med. J.*, 66, 278, 2005.
2. Mollica, R. and Johnson-Lamarche, H., State Residential Care and Assisted Living Policy: 2004, National Academy for State Health Policy, 2005, retrieved from www.nashp.org.
3. Metlife website 1: "Assisted living in the U.S. costs an average of $2,524 per month, or $30,288 per year, according to Metlife market survey of assisted living costs," General News: 2004 Press Releases, retrieved from www.metlife.com/Applications/Corporate/WPS/CDA/PageGenerator/0,1674,P7328%257ES600,00.html.
4. Agingstats website: Federal Interagency Forum on Aging-Related Statistics, Older Americans 2004: Key Indicators of Well-Being Appendix A, retrieved from www.Agingstats.gov.
5. Metlife website 2: "More and More Assisted Living Facilities, Nursing Homes Providing Alzheimer's Care, Some with Additional Costs according to Metlife Mature Market Institute Study," General News: 2006 and 2005 Press Releases, retrieved from www.metlife.com/Applications/Corporate/WPS/CDA/PageGenerator/0,1674,P250%257ES794,00.html.
6. Zimmerman S. et al., Assisted living and nursing homes: apples and oranges, *Gerontologist*, 43, 107, 2003.
7. Reed, P. et al., Characteristics associated with low food and fluid intake in long-term care residents with dementia, *Gerontologist*, 45, 74, 2005.
8. Chao, S. et al., Time for assessment of nutrition services in assisted living facilities, *J. Nutr. Elder.*, 23, 41, 2003.
9. Rosenberg, P.B. et al., Transition to nursing home from assisted living is not associated with dementia or dementia-related problem behaviors, *J. Am. Med Dir. Assoc.*, 7, 73, 2006.
10. Keller, H.H., Meal programs improve nutritional risk: a longitudinal analysis of community-living seniors, *J. Am. Diet. Assoc.*, 106, 1042, 2006.
11. Wakimoto, P. and Block, G., Dietary intake, dietary patterns, and changes with age: an epidemiological perspective, *J. Gerontol. A Biol. Med. Sci.*, 56, 65, 2001.
12. Chapman, I.M. et al., The anorexia of aging, *Biogerontology*, 3, 67, 2002.
13. Hays, N.P. and Roberts, S.B., The anorexia of aging in humans, *Physiol. Behav.*, 88, 257, 2006.
14. Morley, J.E., Decreased food intake with aging, *J. Gerontol. A Biol. Med. Sci.*, 56, 81, 2001.
15. Niedert, K.C., Position of the American Dietetic Association: liberalization of the diet prescription improves quality of life for older adults in long-term care, *J. Am. Diet. Assoc.*, 105, 1955, 2005.
16. Radimer, K. et al., Dietary supplement use by US adults: data from the National Health and Nutrition Examination Survey, 1999–2000, *Am. J. Epidemiol.*, 160, 339, 2004.
17. Mattes, R.D., The chemical senses and nutrition in aging: challenging old assumptions, *J. Am. Diet. Assoc.*, 102, 192, 2002.
18. Schiffman, S.S., Intensification of sensory properties of foods for the elderly, *J. Nutr.*, 130, 927S, 2000.
19. Nijs, K.A.N.D. et al., Effect of family-style meals on energy intake and risk of malnutrition in Dutch nursing home residents: a randomized controlled trial, *J. Gerontol. A Biol. Med. Sci.*, 61, 935, 2006.

20. Park, S. et al., Dietary patterns using the Food Guide Pyramid groups are associated with sociodemographic and lifestyle factors: the multiethnic cohort, *J. Nutr.*, 135, 843, 2005.
21. Morris, C.D., Effect of dietary sodium restriction on overall nutrient intake, *Am. J. Clin. Nutr.*, 65, 687S, 1997.
22. ASPE website: Briesacher, B., Stuart, B., and Doshi, J., Medication Use by Medicare Beneficiaries Living in Nursing Homes and Assisted Living Facilities, University of Maryland, Peter Lamy Center, 2002, retrieved from aspe.hhs.gov/daltcp/reports/meduse.htm.
23. Wilson, M.G. and Morley J.E., Nutritional assessment and support in chronic disease management, in *Handbook of Clinical Nutrition and Aging*, Bales, C.W. and Ritchie, S.C., Eds., Humana Press, Totowa, NJ, 2004, p. 77.
24. Hawes, C. et al., A national survey of assisted living facilities, *Gerontologist,* 43, 875, 2003.
25. Watson, L.C. et al., Depression in assisted living: results from a four-state study, *Am. J. Geriatr. Psychiatry*, 11, 534, 2003.
26. White, H.K. et al., Weight change in Alzheimer's disease, *J. Am. Geriatr. Soc.*, 44, 265, 1996.
27. White, H., Pieper, C., and Schmader, K., The association of weight change in Alzheimer's disease with severity of disease and mortality: a longitudinal analysis, *J. Am. Geriatr. Soc.*, 46, 1223, 1998.
28. White, H.K., Dementia, in *Handbook of Clinical Nutrition and Aging*, Bales, C.W. and Ritchie, S.C., Eds., Humana Press, Totowa, NJ, 2004, p. 349.
29. Soltesz, K.S. and Dayton, J.H., Finger foods help those with Alzheimer's maintain weight, *J. Am. Diet. Assoc.*, 93, 1106, 1993.
30. Winograd, C.H. and Brown, E.M., Aggressive oral refeeding in hosptitalized patients, *Am. J. Clin. Nutr.*, 52, 967,1990.
31. Mathey, M.A.M. et al., Health effects of improved meal ambiance in a Dutch nursing home: a 1-year intervention study, *Prev. Med.*, 32, 416, 2001.
32. Ragneskog, H. et al., Influence of dinner music on food intake and symptoms common in dementia, *Scand. J. Caring Sci.*, 10, 11, 1996.
33. Montorio, I. and Izal, M., The Geriatric Depression Scale: a review of its development and utility, *Int. Psychogeriatr.*, 8, 103, 1996.
34. Koenig, H.G. et al., A brief depression scale for use in the medically ill, *Int. J. Psychiatry Med.*, 22, 83, 1992.
35. Grieger, L., Golden opportunity: the demand for RDs in assisted living, *Today's Regist. Dietitian, 8, 40, 2006.*
36. *Website:* http://ncrules.state.nc.us/ncac/title%2010a%20%20health%20and%20human%20services/chapter%2013%20%20nc%20medical%20care%20commission/subchapter%20f/subchapter%20f%20rules.html, *accessed May 2006.*
37. Website: www.alfa.org, accessed October 2006.

21 Nutritional Factors in Dementia

Seema Joshi, M.D.

CONTENTS

Evidence suggests that oxidative stress may be important in the pathogenesis of Alzheimer's disease (AD). Beta-amyloid (A), which is found abundantly in the brains of Alzheimer's disease patients, is thought to be toxic in neuronal cell cultures through a mechanism involving free radicals.[1] This has generated an interest in the potential role of antioxidants for the prevention of AD. The clinical course of dementia represents the challenges this disease presents. AD presents an enormous burden to individuals and society. So far, there are no truly effective therapies for treating dementia. The mainstay of treatment is still symptomatic. Therefore, the identification and treatment of risk factors for dementia may represent an important strategy for prevention of dementia. Evidence linking diet to AD comes from epidemiological data. However, observational data are only useful for generation of hypotheses and not for establishing a causal relationship. Data from clinical trials are needed for dietary recommendations for the prevention of AD. This review provides an overview of the literature as it pertains to dietary factors and AD.

21.1 NUTRITIONAL FACTORS

There has been an increased interest in the role of antioxidants from foods and supplements in reducing the risk of AD by lowering oxidative stress. AD has not been definitely linked to any environmental risk factors. It has been associated with depressive illness, smoking, cardiovascular diseases, and diabetes.[2–7] Some of nutritional factors that will be discussed include:

- Fish and omega-3 fatty acids
- Antioxidant vitamins
- Alcohol
- B vitamins
- Aluminum

21.1.1 Fish and Omega-3 Fatty Acids

Epidemiological data support an association between dietary fish intake and slowing of cognitive decline with age. Fish consumption and intake of omega-3 polyunsaturated fatty acids may be associated with a reduced risk for cognitive impairment. Diets with a higher daily intake of cholesterol and saturated fat may increase the risk of impaired cognitive function.[8–12] However, the Rotterdam Study found no association between intake of fats, cholesterol, and n-3 polyunsaturated fatty acids and risk of dementia.[13] The possible mechanisms by which omega-3 polyunsaturated fatty acids reduce the risk of cognitive decline may include a reduction of inflammation and cardiovascular protection.[10] These associations may be confounded by established links between poverty, poor diet, and failing health, especially in old age.

21.1.2 Antioxidants

Laboratory findings have suggested that oxidative stress may contribute to the pathogenesis of Alzheimer's disease. Antioxidants have therefore been postulated to reduce the risk of AD by lowering oxidative stress. Data from observational studies have suggested that increased dietary intake of vitamin E may have a protective effect against the development of Alzheimer's disease.[14,15] A longitudinal cohort study found that both vitamin E and C supplementation protected against the development of vascular dementia and improved cognitive function late in life.[16] In another prospective study, vitamin E from food, but not other antioxidants, was associated with a reduced risk of AD among individuals without the APOE epsilon 4 allele.[15] In both of these studies, only antioxidant intake from food affected outcomes, and neither study found an association between antioxidant supplements and AD risk. In the Age-Related Eye Disease Study, participants were randomly assigned to receive daily antioxidants or placebo. Daily antioxidant supplements did not show any beneficial effect on cognition in older adults.[17] In another randomized trial of selegiline, vitamin E, both, or placebo among patients with Alzheimer's disease, both selegiline and vitamin E were independently associated with significant reductions in several outcomes, including functional decline.[18] A recent meta-analysis that examined the dose–response relationship between vitamin E and overall mortality in a total of 19 randomized clinical trials found that vitamin E supplementation with a dose of ≥400 IU/day was associated with a significantly increased risk of all-cause mortality.[19] Observational studies have shown that diets rich in fruits and vegetables may decrease the risk of cognitive decline.[20,21]

21.1.3 Alcohol

Excessive alcohol consumption can result in impaired cognitive processing. Also, excessive alcohol consumption has been associated with Wernicke–Korsakoff syndrome and dementia.[22–24] There is growing evidence suggesting that a chronic pattern of light to moderate drinking may have a protective effect against dementia, paralleling the reports of the beneficial effects of moderate alcohol use on cardiovascular health.[25–28] In a longitudinal study of a representative elderly cohort over an average of 7 years, a pattern of mild to moderate drinking, compared to not drinking, was associated with less average decline in cognitive domains.[29] The Nurses' Health Study indicates that older women who consumed up to one drink a day had better mean cognitive test scores and less risk of cognitive decline than nondrinkers.[30] Most of the data suggesting protective effects of alcohol on cognition come from observational studies. There are no randomized control trials studying the effects of alcohol consumption on cognitive function. Thus, recommendations cannot be made based on the current evidence available.

21.1.4 Vitamins

Elevated serum homocysteine levels have been found to be an independent risk factor for Alzheimer's disease. Homocysteine levels are inversely related to cognitive function in people with dementia.[31–34] In a recent study by Miller et al., elevated homocysteine levels were found to be more common among patients with vascular disease than among those with Alzheimer's disease.[35] Studies have shown that the plasma concentration of homocysteine is inversely related to hippocampal and cortical volume in nondemented elderly.[36,37] Results from the Nun Study show that low serum concentrations of folate, but not vitamins B12 and B6, are associated with atrophy of the cerebral cortex.[38] The possible mechanisms by which homocysteine contributes to AD could be secondary to an induction of vascular changes[39] or secondary to its direct neurotoxic effects.[40] Animal studies suggest that homocysteine and folic acid deficiency may impair DNA repair in hippocampal neurons, making them susceptible to toxicity from AD.[41]

Current evidence relating vitamins B12, B6, and folate to cognitive decline and AD is inconsistent. In a case-control study of 164 patients with a clinical diagnosis of dementia of the Alzheimer's type, low blood levels of folate and vitamin B12 and elevated total homocysteine levels were associated with AD.[33] In a prospective study by Wang et al., low concentrations of B12 or folate were associated with doubling of AD risk when compared to normal concentrations of these vitamins.[42] However, the Bronx Longitudinal Aging Study found no association between low serum B12 concentrations and AD risk.[43] In the Framingham Study there was no relation of the concentrations of folate, vitamin B6, or B12 to the risk of AD.[31]

Studies assessing the impact of supplementation of B vitamins on cognition are also inconsistent. In a case series of patients with dementia, oral B12 and folate supplementation in 17 patients with high homocysteine concentrations resulted in improvement of cognitive scores.[44] However, in a study by Kwok et al., intramuscular B12 supplementation in patients with cobalamin deficiency showed no change in cognitive scores.[45] In another study, no improvement in neuropsychological test scores was seen with B12 replacement in patients with dementia and vitamin B12 deficiency; however, there was an improvement in verbal fluency in patients with cognitive impairment without dementia.[46]

21.1.5 Aluminum

Evidence linking AD to aluminum has been based on reports of neurotoxic concentrations of aluminum in the brains of AD patients by Crapper et al.[47,48] The role of aluminum in potentiating oxidative and inflammatory events in the brain, resulting in tissue damage, has also been suggested.[49] Neuropathologic studies demonstrate aluminosilicates at the center of senile plaque cores, suggesting that they may be involved in the initiation or early stages of senile plaque formation.[50] However, no direct link has been established to AD. The results from a case-control study suggest that lifetime occupational exposure to solvents and aluminum is not likely to be an important risk factor for Alzheimer's disease.[51] Data from epidemiologic studies examining the possible link between exposure to aluminum in drinking water and AD have been conflicting. In a study by Martyn et al., the risk of AD was increased by 1.5 times in districts with mean aluminum levels in tap water exceeding 0.11 mg/l.[52] However, a population survey examining 800 residents age 81 to 85 consuming drinking water with aluminum concentration up to 98 mg/l found no association with AD.[53] Clinical data linking aluminum to AD comes from dialysis encephalopathy secondary to aluminum accumulation through hemodialysis fluids and aluminum-containing pharmaceutical agents.[54–56] Studies evaluating the role of aluminum ingestion via antacids have shown no association with AD.[57,58] In a single-blind clinical trial of 48 patients with probable AD, a trivalent ion chelator, desferrioxamine, was shown to reduce the rate of decline in the activities of daily living in AD patients treated with desferrioxamine.[59]

The pathogenic role of aluminum in Alzheimer's disease remains to be defined. Current data do not support a causative role for aluminum in AD. The major dietary sources of aluminum are food and food ingredients. Aluminum utensils increase the aluminum content of food. Aluminum-containing food ingredients include preservatives, coloring agents, leavening agents, and anticaking agents. These ingredients have been evaluated for safety and have been approved by the Food and Drug Administration.[54]

21.2 SUMMARY

The role of antioxidant supplements in the prevention of dementia remains controversial. There is no conclusive evidence of reduced risk for AD for the antioxidant vitamins E and C. A recent meta-analysis suggesting a significant risk of all-cause mortality with high-dose vitamin E supplementation has heightened the controversy.[19] Similarly, evidence relating B vitamins to cognitive decline is controversial. Based on current evidence, individuals with low levels of vitamin B12 and folate should be treated. Epidemiologic data support the protective effects of fish and omega-3 polyunsaturated fats on cognition. Similar effects seem to be seen with moderate alcohol intake; however, it may not be reasonable to recommend alcohol to individuals who do not consume alcohol. Table 21.1 summarizes the current evidence available.

The clinical course of dementia represents the challenges this disease presents. AD presents an enormous burden to individuals and society. So far, there are no truly effective therapies for treating dementia. The mainstay of treatment is still

TABLE 21.1
Summary of the Evidence of Dementia

Study	Population	Design	Association	Results
Morris et al.[9]	815 community residents age 65–94 years unaffected by AD	Prospective study	Food frequency questionnaire to assess dietary fat intake	Dietary intake of n-3 fatty acids and weekly consumption of fish may reduce the risk of incident AD by 60% vs. those who rarely or never consume fish (RR = 0.4, 95% CI = 0.2–0.9)
Huang et al.[10]	CHS Cognition Study participants age 65 years or older	Prospective	Fish intake was assessed by food frequency questionnaires	Consumption of fatty fish more than twice per week was associated with a reduction in risk of dementia by 28% (95% CI = 0.51–1.02) and AD by 41% (95% CI = 0.36–0.95)
Kalmijn et al.[8]	1613 subjects ranging from 45–70 years old	Cross sectional, population based	Food frequency questionnaire was used to assess habitual food consumption	Marine omega-3 polyunsaturated fatty acids (PUFAs) were inversely related to the risk of impaired overall cognitive function and speed (per SD increase, OR = 0.81, 95% CI 0.66–1.00; OR = 0.72, 95% CI = 0.57–0.9); higher cholesterol and saturated fat were associated with an increased risk of impaired memory and flexibility (per SD increase, OR = 1.27, 95% CI = 1.02–1.57; OR = 1.26, 95% CI = 1.01–1.57)
Engelhart et al.[13]	5395 elderly subjects with normal cognition	Prospective cohort study	Fat intake and incident dementia	High intake of total, saturated, and trans fat and cholesterol and low intake of MUFA, PUFA, n-6 PUFA, and n-3 PUFA were not associated with increased risk of dementia or its subtype; rate ratios of dementia per standard deviation increase in intake were for total fat 0.93 (95% CI = 0.81–1.07), for saturated fat 0.91 (95% CI = 0.79–1.05), for trans fat 0.90 (95% CI = 0.77–1.06), for cholesterol 0.93 (95% CI = 0.80–1.08), for MUFA 0.96 (95% CI = 0.84–1.10), for PUFA 1.05 (95% CI = 0.80–1.38), for n-6 PUFA 1.03 (95% CI = 0.77–1.36), and for n-3 PUFA 1.07 (95% CI = 0.94–1.22)

(continued)

TABLE 21.1
Summary of the Evidence of Dementia (continued)

Study	Population	Design	Association	Results
Morris et al.[12]	2560 participants of the Chicago Health and Aging Project, ages 65 and older	Prospective study	Food frequency questionnaires	Higher intakes of saturated fat (p for trend = 0.04) and trans-unsaturated fat (p for trend = 0.07) were linearly associated with greater decline in cognitive score over 6 years
Engelhart et al.[16]	5395 participants at least 55 years in age, community dwelling, and free of dementia	Prospective cohort study	Dietary intake of beta-carotene, flavonoids, vitamins C and E	High intake of vitamins C and E was associated with lower risk of Alzheimer's disease; rate ratios (RRs) per 1 SD increase in intake were 0.82 (95% confidence interval (CI) = 0.68–0.99) and 0.82 (95% CI = 0.66–1.00), respectively
Yaffe et al.[17]	2166 elderly participants	Randomized clinical trial	Daily antioxidants (vitamin C, 500 mg; vitamin E, 400 IU; beta-carotene, 15 mg), zinc and copper (zinc, 80 mg; cupric oxide, 2 mg), antioxidants plus zinc and copper, or placebo	No association with any effect on cognitive function compared with placebo; treatment groups did not differ on any of the six cognitive tests ($p > 0.05$ for all)
Sano et al.[18]	341 patients with Alzheimer's disease of moderate severity	Double-blind, placebo-controlled, randomized, multicenter trial	Selegiline (10 mg a day), alpha-tocopherol (vitamin E, 2000 IU a day), both selegiline and alpha-tocopherol, or placebo for 2 years	The primary outcome was the time to the occurrence of any of the following: death, institutionalization, loss of the ability to perform basic activities of daily living, or severe dementia; in the unadjusted analyses, there was no statistically significant difference in the outcomes; in analyses that included the baseline score on the Mini-Mental State Examination as a covariate there were significant delays in the time to the primary outcome for the patients treated with selegiline (median time = 655 days, $p = 0.012$), alpha-tocopherol (670 days, $p = 0.001$). or combination therapy (585 days, $p = 0.049$), as compared with the placebo group (440 days)

Miller et al.[19]	135,967 participants in 19 clinical trials	Meta-analysis	Dose–response relationship between vitamin E supplementation and total mortality	High-dosage (≥400 IU/day) vitamin E supplements may increase all-cause mortality; the pooled all-cause mortality risk difference in high-dosage vitamin E trials was 39 per 10,000 persons (95% CI = 3–74 per 10,000 persons, $p = 0.035$); for low-dosage vitamin E trials, the risk difference was –16 per 10,000 persons (95% CI = –41 to 10 per 10,000 persons, $p > 0.2$)
Mukamal et al.[26]	373 cases with incident dementia and 373 controls among 5888 adults age 65 years and older who participated in the Cardiovascular Health Study	Nested case-control study	Self-reported alcohol consumption and risk of dementia	Adjusted odds for dementia among those whose weekly alcohol consumption was less than 1 drink were 0.65 (95% CI = 0.41–1.02); 1–6 drinks, 0.46 (95% CI = 0.27–0.77); 7–13 drinks, 0.69 (95% CI = 0.37–1.31); and 14 or more drinks, 1.22 (95% CI = 0.60–2.49, *p* for quadratic term = .001); consumption of 1–6 drinks weekly is associated with a lower risk of incident dementia among older adults
Ganguli et al.[29]	1681 community-dwelling individuals age 65 years or older	Longitudinal study	Self-reported drinking habits and cognitive functions	Mild to moderate drinking, compared to not drinking, was associated with less average decline in cognitive domains over the same period
Stampfer et al.[30]	12,480 participants in the Nurses' Health Study who were 70–81 years old	Prospective cohort study	Alcohol intake assessed by food frequency questionnaire	Relative risk (RR) of a substantial cognitive decline over a 2-year period was 0.85 (95% CI = 0.74–0.98) among moderate drinkers, as compared with nondrinkers; up to 1 drink per day may actually decrease the risk of cognitive decline
Seshadri et al.[31]	1092 subjects without dementia with a mean age of 76 years	Prospective	Plasma total homocysteine level measured at baseline and that measured 8 years earlier to the risk of newly diagnosed dementia on follow-up	The multivariable-adjusted relative risk of dementia was 1.4 (95 % CI = 1.1–1.9) for each increase of 1 SD in the log-transformed homocysteine value either at baseline or 8 years earlier; the relative risk of Alzheimer's disease was 1.8 (95% CI = 1.3–2.5) per increase of 1 SD at baseline and 1.6 (95% CI = 1.2–2.1) per increase of 1 SD 8 years before baseline; with a plasma homocysteine level greater than 14 μmol/l, the risk of Alzheimer's disease nearly doubled

(continued)

TABLE 21.1
Summary of the Evidence of Dementia (continued)

Study	Population	Design	Association	Results
Clarke et al.[33]	164 patients, age 55 years or older, with a clinical diagnosis of dementia of the Alzheimer's type	Case-control	Serum total homocysteine (tHcy), folate, and vitamin B12 levels in patients and controls at entry; the odds ratio (OR) of DAT or confirmed AD with elevated tHcy or low vitamin levels, and the rate of disease progression in relation to tHcy levels at entry	The odds ratio of confirmed AD associated with a tHcy level in the top third (14 μmol/l) compared with the bottom third (11 μmol/l) of the control distribution was 4.5 (95% CI = 2.2–9.2), after adjustment for age, sex, social class, cigarette smoking, and apolipoprotein E epsilon4; the odds ratio for the lower third compared with the upper third of serum folate distribution was 3.3 (95% CI = 1.8–6.3), and for vitamin B12 distribution 4.3 (95% CI = 2.1–8.8)
Wang et al.[42]	370 nondemented persons, age 75 years and older	Longitudinal study	Serum levels of B12 or folate	Subjects with low levels of B12 or folate had two times higher risks of developing AD (RR = 2.1, 95% CI = 1.2–3.5)
Kwok et al.[45]	50 patients older than 60 years with B12 deficiency	Randomized controlled trial	Supplement with intramuscular B12	No association with cognitive scores
Eastley et al.[46]	125 patients with low serum B12	Retrospective study	Treatment with parenteral B12	Vitamin B12 treatment may improve frontal lobe and language function in patients with cognitive impairment, but no improvement in dementia

Crystal et al.[43]	410 nondemented subjects age 75–85 years	Longitudinal cohort study	Annual serum B12 determinations and neuropsychological assessments	Incidence of Alzheimer's disease among the low B12 group was 4.5% compared with 7.5% in the higher B12 group; no association between risk of dementia and low levels of B12
Graves et al.[51]	89 subjects diagnosed with probable AD matched to 89 controls	Case-control study	Occupational history for aluminum exposure	Nonsignificant associations were found between AD and ever having been occupationally exposed to solvents (OR = 1.77, 95% CI = 0.81–3.90) and aluminum (OR = 1.46, 95% CI = 0.62–3.42)
Wettstein et al.[53]	800 residents age 81–85 years	Population survey	Aluminum concentrations [Al] in the drinking water	No association with AD risk
Martyn et al.[52]	Survey of people under 70 years in 88 county districts within England and Wales	Population survey	Aluminum concentrations in water over the past 10 years	The risk of Alzheimer's disease was 1.5 times higher in districts where the mean aluminum concentration exceeded 0.11 mg/l than in districts where concentrations were less than 0.01 mg/l
Flaten et al.[57]	Patient data from 4179 patient records	Retrospective study	High intake of aluminum-containing antacids	Standardized mortality ratio for dementia was 1.10 (95% CI = 0.85–1.40, n = 64) for all patients, while for patients operated on in the period 1967–1978 it was 1.25 (95% CI = 0.66–2.13, n = 13); no association with increased AD risk
Canadian Study of Health and Aging[58]	258 cases with probable AD and 535 controls	Population-based case-control study	History of antacid use	Odds ratio for antacid use was 1.19 (95% CI = 0.72–1.96); no association between the use of aluminum-containing antacids and AD

symptomatic. Therefore, the identification and treatment of risk factors for dementia may represent an important strategy for prevention of dementia. However, the role of dietary factors in the prevention of dementia still remains elusive. Epidemiologic studies have provided conflicting results. The links between diet and dementia appear to be rather complex. Based on current evidence, dietary recommendations for the prevention of dementia cannot be made. A prudent approach would be to recommend a balanced diet rich in fruits and vegetables.

REFERENCES

1. Grundman M. Vitamin E and Alzheimer disease: the basis for additional clinical trials. *Am J Clin Nutr* 2000;71:630S.
2. Devi G, Williamson J, Massoud F, et al. A comparison of family history of psychiatric disorders among patients with early- and late-onset Alzheimer's disease. *J Neuropsychiatry Clin Neurosci* 2004;16:57.
3. Ott A, Slooter AJ, Hofman A, et al. Smoking and risk of dementia and Alzheimer's disease in a population-based cohort study: the Rotterdam Study. *Lancet* 1998;351:1840.
4. Merchant C, Tang M-X, Albert S, Manly J, Stern Y, Mayeux R. The influence of smoking on the risk of Alzheimer's disease. *Neurology* 1999;52:1408.
5. Luchsinger, JA, Reitz, C, Honig, LS, et al. Aggregation of vascular risk factors and risk of incident Alzheimer disease. *Neurology* 2005;65:545.
6. Schnaider Beeri M, Goldbourt U, Silverman JM, et al. Diabetes mellitus in midlife and the risk of dementia three decades later. *Neurology* 2004;63:1902.
7. Ott A, Stolk RP, van Harskamp F, Pols HA, Hofman A, Breteler MM. Diabetes mellitus and the risk of dementia: the Rotterdam Study. *Neurology* 1999;53:1937.
8. Kalmijn S, Van Boxtel MPJ, Ocke M, et al. Dietary intake of fatty acids and fish in relation to cognitive performance at middle age. *Neurology* 2004;62:275
9. Morris MC, Evans DA, Bienias JL, et al. Consumption of fish and n-3 fatty acids and risk of incident Alzheimer disease. *Arch Neurol* 2003;60:940.
10. Huang TL, Zandi PP, Tucker KL, et al. Benefits of fatty fish on dementia risk are stronger for those without APOE epsilon4. *Neurology* 2005;65:1409.
11. Morris MC, Evans DA, Tangney CC, et al. Fish consumption and cognitive decline with age in a large community study. *Arch Neurol* 2005;62:1849.
12. Morris MC, Evans DA, Bienias JL, et al. Dietary fat intake and 6-year cognitive change in an older biracial community population. *Neurology* 2004;62:1573.
13. Engelhart MJ, Geerlings MI, Ruitenberg A, et al. Diet and risk of dementia: does fat matter? The Rotterdam Study. *Neurology* 2002;59:1915.
14. Masaki KH, Losonczy KG, Izmirlian G, et al. Association of vitamin E and C supplement use with cognitive function and dementia in elderly men. *Neurology* 2000;54:1265.
15. Morris MC, Evans DA, Bienias JL, et al. Dietary intake of antioxidant nutrients and the risk of incident Alzheimer disease in a biracial community study. *JAMA* 2002;287:3230.
16. Engelhart MJ, Geerlings MI, Ruitenberg A, et al. Dietary intake of antioxidants and risk of Alzheimer disease. *JAMA* 2002;287:3223.
17. Yaffe K, Clemons TE, McBee WL, Lindblad AS. Impact of antioxidants, zinc, and copper on cognition in the elderly: a randomized, controlled trial. *Neurology* 2004;63:1705.

18. Sano M, Ernesto C, Thomas RG, et al. A controlled trial of selegiline, alpha tocopherol, or both as treatment for Alzheimer's disease. The Alzheimer's Disease Cooperative Study. *N Engl J Med* 1997;336:1216.
19. Miller ER 3rd, Pastor-Barriuso R, Dalal D, et al. Meta-analysis: high-dosage vitamin E supplementation may increase all-cause mortality. *Ann Intern Med* 2005;142:37.
20. Kang JH, Ascherio A, Grodstein F. Fruit and vegetable consumption and cognitive decline in aging women. *Ann Neurol* 2005;57:713.
21. Ortega RM, Requejo AM, Andres P, et al. Dietary intake and cognitive function in a group of elderly people. *Am J Clin Nutr* 1997;66:803.
22. Nutt D. Alcohol and the brain. Pharmacological insights for psychiatrists. *Br J Psychiatry* 1999;175:114.
23. Butters N. Alcoholic Korsakoff's syndrome: some unresolved issues concerning etiology, neuropathology, and cognitive deficits. *J Clin Exp Neuropsychol* 1985;7:181.
24. Edelstein SL, Kritz-Silverstein D, Barrett-Connor E. Prospective association of smoking and alcohol use with cognitive function in an elderly cohort. *J Womens Health* 1998;7:1271.
25. Letenneur L, Dartigues JF, Orgogozo JM. Wine consumption in the elderly. *Ann Intern Med* 1993;118:317.
26. Mukamal KJ, Kuller LH, Fitzpatrick AL, Longstreth WT Jr, Mittleman MA, Siscovick DS. Prospective study of alcohol consumption and risk of dementia in older adults. *JAMA* 2003;289:1405.
27. Espeland MA, Gu L, Masaki KH, et al. Association between reported alcohol intake and cognition: results from the women's health initiative memory study. *Am J Epidemiol* 2005;161:228.
28. Knoops KT, de Groot LC, Kromhout D, et al. Mediterranean diet, lifestyle factors, and 10-year mortality in elderly European men and women: the HALE project. *JAMA* 2004;292:1433.
29. Ganguli M, Vander Bilt J, Saxton JA, Shen C, Dodge HH. Alcohol consumption and cognitive function in late life: a longitudinal community study. *Neurology* 2005;65:1210.
30. Stampfer MJ, Kang JH, Chen J, et al. Effects of moderate alcohol consumption on cognitive function in women. *N Engl J Med* 2005;352:245.
31. Seshadri S, Beiser A, Selhub J, Jacques PF, Rosenberg IH, D'Agostino RB, et al. Plasma homocysteine as a risk factor for dementia and Alzheimer's disease. *N Engl J Med* 2002;346:476.
32. Stewart R, Asonganyi B, Sherwood R. Plasma homocysteine and cognitive impariment in an older British African-Caribbean population. *J Am Geriatr Soc* 2002;50:1227.
33. Clarke R, Smith D, Jobst K, Refsum H, Sutton L, Ueland PM. Folate, vitamin B-12, and serum total homocysteine levels in confirmed Alzheimer's disease. *Arch Neurol* 1998;55:1449.
34. McCaddon A, Davies G, Hudson P, Tandy S, Cattell H. Total serum homocysteine in senile dementia of Alzheimer type. *Int J Geriatr Psychol* 1998;13:235.
35. Miller JW, Green R, Mungas DM, Reed BR, Jagust WJ. Homocysteine, vitamin B6, and vascular disease in AD patients. *Neurology* 2002;58:1471.
36. Williams JH, Pereira EA, Budge MM, Bradley KM. Minimal hippocampal width relates to plasma homocysteine in community-dwelling older people. *Age Ageing* 2002;31:440.
37. den Heijer T, Vermeer SE, Clarke R, et al. Homocysteine and brain atrophy on MRI of non-demented elderly. *Brain* 2003;126:170.

38. Snowdon DA, Tully CL, Smith CD, Riley KP, Markesbery WR. Serum folate and the severity of atrophy of the neocortex in Alzheimer disease: findings from the Nun Study. *Am J Clin Nutr* 2000;71:993.
39. Snowdon DA, Greiner LH, Mortimer JA, Riley KP, Greiner PA, Markesbery WR. Brain infarction and the clinical expression of Alzheimer disease: the Nun Study. *JAMA* 1997;277:813.
40. Ho PI, Ortiz, Rogers E, Shea TB. Multiple aspects of homocysteine neurotoxicity: glutamate excitotoxicity, kinase hyperactivation and DNA damage. *J Neurosci Res* 2002;70:694.
41. Kruman II, Kumaravel TS, Lohani A, et al. Folic acid deficiency and homocysteine impair DNA repair in hippocampal neurons and sensitize them to amyloid toxicity in experimental models of Alzheimer's disease. *J Neurosci* 2002;22:1752.
42. Wang HX, Wahlin A, Basun H, Fastbom J, Winblad B, Fratiglioni L. Vitamin B(12) and folate in relation to the development of Alzheimer's disease. *Neurology* 2001;56:1188.
43. Crystal HA, Ortof E, Frishman WH, Gruber A, Hershman D, Aronson M. Serum vitamin B12 levels and incidence of dementia in a healthy elderly population: a report from the Bronx Longitudinal Aging Study. *J Am Geriatr Soc* 1994;42:933.
44. Nilsson K, Gustafson L, Hultberg B. Improvement of cognitive functions after cobalamin/folate supplementation in elderly patients with dementia and elevated plasma homocysteine. *Int J Geriatr Psychol* 2001;16:609.
45. Kwok T, Tang C, Woo J, Lai WK, Law LK, Pang CP. Randomized trial of the effect of supplementation on the cognitive function of older people with subnormal cobalamin levels. *Int J Geriatr Psychol* 1998;13:611.
46. Eastley R, Wilcock GK, Bucks RS. Vitamin B12 deficiency in dementia and cognitive impairment: the effects of treatment on neuropsychological function. *Int J Geriatr Psychol* 2000;15:226.
47. Crapper DR, Krishnan SS, Dalton AJ. Brain aluminum distribution in Alzheimer's disease and experimental neurofibrillary degeneration. *Trans Am Neurol Assoc* 1973;98:17.
48. Crapper DR, Krishnan SS, Quittkat S. Aluminum, neurofibrillary degeneration and Alzheimer's disease. *Brain* 1976;99:67.
49. Campbell A. The potential role of aluminum in Alzheimer's disease. *Nephrol Dial Transplant* 2002;17:S17.
50. Candy JM, Oakley AE, Klinowski J. Aluminosilicates and senile plaque formation in Alzheimer's disease. *Lancet* 1986;1:354.
51. Graves AB, Rosner D, Echeverria D. Occupational exposure to solvents and aluminum and estimated risk of Alzheimer's disease. *Occup Environ Med* 1998;55:627.
52. Martyn CN, Barker DJ, Osmond C. Geographical relation between Alzheimer's disease and aluminum in drinking water. *Lancet* 1989;14:59.
53. Wettstein A, Aeppli J, Gautschi K. Failure to find a relationship between mnestic skills of octogenarians and aluminum in drinking water. *Int Arch Occup Environ Health* 1991;63:97.
54. Soni MG, White SM, Flamm WG. Safety evaluation of dietary aluminum. *Regul Toxicol Pharmacol* 2001;33:66.
55. Harrington CR, Wishlik CM, McArthur FK. Alzheimer's-disease-like changes in tau protein processing: association with aluminum accumulation in brains of renal dialysis patients. *Lancet* 1994;343:993.
56. Altmann P, Shanesha U, Hamon C. Disturbance of cerebral function by aluminum in haemodialysis patients without overt aluminum toxicity. *Lancet* 1989;2:7.

57. Flaten TP, Glattre E, Viste A. Mortality from dementia among gastroduodenal ulcer patients. *Epidemiol Commun Health* 1991;45:203.
58. The Canadian study of health and aging: risk factors for Alzheimer's disease in Canada. *Neurology* 1994;44:2073.
59. McLachlan DR, Dalton AJ, Kruck TP. Intramuscular desferrioxamine in patients with Alzheimer's disease. *Lancet* 1991;337:1304.

22 Nutrition and Depression

Mehret Gebretsadik, M.D.
George T. Grossberg, M.D.

CONTENTS

22.1 THE DEPRESSION–NUTRITION CONNECTION: CURRENT CONCEPTS

Understanding the neuropathophysiology of depression helps in understanding the nutrition–depression connection. Depression has biological underpinnings that medical research has been unraveling in the past few decades, in addition to its psychosocial bases. Several neurotransmitters and brain regions are implicated in mood regulation and control of emotional behavior. The noradrenergic and serotonergic systems are the major ones associated with depression, while other neurotransmitters, such as dopamine, gamma acetyl butyric acid (GABA), glutamate, glycine, and neuroactive peptides, may also be implicated. Involvement of the hypothalamus, the basal ganglia, and the limbic system in depression is supported by biological research and symptoms of mood disorders. The neurobiogenic inputs to these structures play a significant role in mood regulation and the pathogenesis of depression.[1]

The major concentration of noradrenergic neurons is in the locus ceruleus in the mid-brain. Its neurons are projected upward through the forebrain to the cerebral cortex, limbic system, thalamus, and hippocampus. Norepinephrine is a key neurotransmitter involved in the control of mood and emotional behavior. Serotonin is another key neurotransmitter that is involved in the control of mood. The axons of serotonergic neurons originate in the raphe nuclei of the brain stem and project to the cerebral cortex, limbic system, cerebellum, and spinal cord. Serotonin is involved in the regulation of pain, pleasure, anxiety, panic, arousal, and sleep behavior.[1]

The limbic system has a major role in the production of emotions causing the psychological symptoms of depression. Depressed people's deregulation of sleep, libido, appetite, and biological changes in immunoendocrine functions suggest hypothalamic dysfunction. The typical stooped posture, motor slowness, and minor cognitive impairment often seen with late-life depression are thought to be related to the involvement of the basal ganglia. Dysregulation of multiple neuroendocrine pathways has been reported in depression. While adrenal and thyroid abnormalities are well studied, abnormalities in growth hormone, testosterone (in men), somatostatin, and prolactine malfunction may also be implicated in depression. The correlation between hypersecretion of cortisol and depression is well established, and 5 to 10% of people with depression are diagnosed with thyroid problems.[1]

Most neurotransmitters are manufactured in the body from amino acids using trace elements and vitamins as cofactors. Serotonin is produced from the dietary amino acids tryptophan and 5-hydroxy tryptophan, while norepinephrine is synthesized from the dietary amino acids tyrosine and phenylalanine. The synthesis of both serotonin and norepinephrine requires vitamins B, C, folic acid, and essential minerals, including zinc, magnesium, manganese, iron, and copper. Depletion of these nutrients has been shown to potentially worsen or induce depression.[1,2]

Inositol, a naturally occurring isomer of glucose, is a key intermediate of the phosphatidyl–inositol (PI) cycle, a second messenger system used by several noradrenergic, serotonergic, and cholinergic receptors.[3,4] The role of certain fatty acids such as omega-3 fatty acids in mood regulation is also a focus for investigative inquiry. Omega-3 fatty acids, crucial components of synaptic cell membranes, maintain the stability of serotonin receptors and their functions and have been shown to have a mood-stabilizing and antidepressant effect in unipolar and bipolar depression.[16–19,25,74,75]

Research has shown that excessive sugar and stimulant intake and lack of amino acids, B vitamins (B12, folic acid, B6), and essential fatty acids (omega-3) are strongly associated with depressive symptoms.[2,12,13] Older adults with poor dietary habits, comorbid medical conditions, and who chronically abuse alcohol are prone to have malnutrition that may result in depressive symptoms. Replacement of deficient nutrients and healthy eating habits are associated with faster response to depression treatment, longer periods of remission, and can be the key for effective treatment of depression where they are the primary cause. The cycle of depression and malnutrition may be vicious. Depression can cause or worsen nutritional problems, and nutritionally compromised patients are prone to depression because of the intricate link between the depression and nutrition.[12,14–16] The understanding and application of the nutrition–depression connection is of paramount importance, especially with the elderly population, where both are more prevalent and often coexist.[12,16,18]

The other important connection point of clinical relevance in older adults is the impact of depression and malnutrition on the immune system. The immune system shows a general decline in the elderly, especially cell-mediated vs. humoral immunity. Nutritional factors play a major role in the immune responses of aged individuals, and nutritional influences on immune responses are of great consequence in aged individuals, even in the healthy elderly. Different studies have shown that both protein-energy malnutrition and micronutrient deficiencies are strongly associated with immune dysfunction.[19–22] Malnutrition, especially severe protein-energy malnutrition, can affect all lines of immunity.[20] In addition to general undernutrition, reduced intake of iron, zinc, and vitamins may also contribute to the decline in immune response.

The effect of depression on the immune system is shown with changes in several immunological assays. Findings of immune changes accompanying depression have included decreased lymphocyte count, increased neutrophil number, decreased mitogen responses of peripheral blood lymphocytes, and decreased natural killer (NK) cell activity.[23–26] Elderly patients who are severely depressed and malnourished are at a greatest risk of suffering disease processes secondary to their frail immunity. Infections are the most common manifestations.[27] These patients often represent a true psychiatric/medical emergency. Aggressive treatment of depression and malnutrition can be lifesaving.

22.2 EPIDEMIOLOGY AND CLINICAL FEATURES

22.2.1 Epidemiology

Depression is not a normal part of aging. However, it is widespread, often undiagnosed, and usually inadequately treated in older patients for various reasons. There is wide variability in the estimated prevalence of late-life depression depending on the setting of the sample, diagnostic criteria used, method of assessment, and rater experience. Some of the methodological problems in prevalence studies include the tendency of elderly persons to express psychiatric symptoms in somatic terms, their reluctance to recall and report psychiatric symptoms, and the use of diagnostic criteria that may be unsuitable for elderly individuals. Because of the many physical illnesses and psychosocial problems of the elderly, clinicians often conclude that depression is a normal consequence of these problems, an attitude often seen among older patients as well. All of these factors contribute to make the illness underdiagnosed and, more importantly, left untreated.

According to the Epidemiologic Catchment Area Study, approximately 15% of community residents over 65 years of age experience depressive symptoms at any one time, with an estimated prevalence of less than 3% for major depression. The 5% rate of major or minor depression among elderly people in primary care clinics sharply increases to 15 to 25% in nursing homes. While 13% of residents of nursing homes develop a new episode of major depression over a 1-year period, another 18% develop new depressive symptoms.[28] Major depression is more common in the medically ill, those older than 70 years of age, and among hospitalized patients.[29,30] Medical conditions associated with higher rates of depression include coronary artery disease, stroke, Parkinson's disease, cancer, and dementia.[29,30]

Major depressive disorders (MDDs) in the elderly are often categorized as being early-life onset (before the age of 65) or late-life onset (after the age of 65).[31] A specific cause for either type of depression has not been isolated and is multifactorial. No single gene or single biological event has been associated with late-life depression. Cerebrovascular disease appears to play a role in some late-onset depression and has led to the vascular depression hypothesis.[32,33] Magnetic resonance imaging (MRI) of the brain shows extensive microvascular ischemic changes that are believed to disrupt circuits involved in regulation of mood.[34] Depression also has a high correlation with stroke, especially if the insult is closer to the frontal pole and if the left cerebral cortex is affected.[35,36] Myocardial infarctions (MIs) and cancers are also associated with depression.[37] The highest risk is with pancreatic cancer, carrying a 50% risk of developing depression. It is also common for depression to present in patients with neuropsychiatric disorders such as Alzheimer's disease or Parkinson's disease.[38–40]

Psychosocial factors also may increase the risk of depression. Loss is a frequent theme in the elderly and can be a strong stressor. Transition from active work or play to retirement, the death of friends and loved ones, widowhood and divorce, low socioeconomic level, and other adverse life changes can predispose an elderly individual to depression. Suicide may be an outcome. Identifying risk factors early and providing biological, psychological, or social support can help curb the incidence of suicide among the elderly (Table 22.1 lists risk factors for suicide in the elderly).

Risk factors for depression include female sex, previous and family history of depression, being single or divorced, substance abuse, use of certain medications,

TABLE 22.1
Risk Factors for Suicide in the Elderly

Male, white
Recent loss (e.g., death of spouse, divorce, illness)
Depression
Alcohol/substance abuse (including prescribed medications)
Alone/socially isolated
Lack of confidant/family resources
Multiple medical comorbidities
Past history or family history of depression/suicide

medical and central nervous system illnesses, poor support system, and stressful life events (Table 22.2 lists a variety of risk factors for late-onset depression).[31,40–44] Protein-energy malnutrition and micronutrient deficiency have a significant association with depression. This especially holds true for older patients, where malnutrition is common. Older patients with depression often have poor nutritional status and suppressed immunity, and hence enhanced vulnerability for certain illnesses, especially infections.

As indicated above, malnutrition and depression have a complex interdependent association.[12] Both are common, potentially serious, and frequently underdiagnosed conditions among elderly individuals. Age-related changes in combination with medical and psychiatric illnesses may contribute to the development of malnutrition in the elderly. The estimated prevalence for malnutrition among the elderly varies from 15% in community-dwelling ambulatory elderly persons to 5 to 44% in homebound elders and 20 to 65% in hospitalized patients. The prevalence further increases to 23 to 85% in nursing homes.[18]

Anorexia and weight loss are caused by multiple physiological and pathological factors (Table 22.3).[45–51] Physiological anorexia of aging is thought to be caused by

TABLE 22.2
Risk Factors for Late-Onset Depression

Risk Factors
General Factors
Female sex (female–male ratio, 2.5:1)
Past history of depression
Family history of depression
Medical Illnesses (Selected)
Hypothyroidism (50%)
Myocardial infarction (45%)
Macular degeneration (33%)
Diabetes (8–28%)
Cancer (24%)
Coronary artery disease (20%)
Central Nervous System Disorders (Selected)
Parkinson's disease (25–70%)
Alzheimer's disease (15–57%)
Multiple sclerosis (27–54%)
Stroke (26—54%)
Huntington's disease (9–44%)
Medications
Beta-blockers
Interferon alpha
Many antineoplastic agents
Corticosteroids

Source: Adapted from Raj, A., *Postgrad. Med.*, 115, 26–42, 2004.

TABLE 22.3
Causes of Anorexia and Weight Loss in the Elderly

Physiologic
Decreased central feeding drive
Decreased chemosensory function
Alteration of neuroendocrine functions
Social Factors
Poverty
Poor support system
Bereavement
Elderly abuse
Psychiatric/Neuropsychiatric
Depression
Dementia
Anorexia nervosa/tardive
Late-life paranoia
Late-life mania
Substance abuse/alcoholism
Anxiety disorders
Parkinson's disease
Medical Illnesses
Infections
Oral/denture problems
Swallowing problems
Autoimmune/connective tissue diseases
Hyperthyroidism/hyperparathyroidism
Hypoadrenalism
Stroke
Cardiopulmonary illnesses
Chronic renal failure
Iatrogenic/Medications
Strict therapeutic diet, e.g., low fat, diabetic
Polypharmacy
Digoxin
NSAIDs
Theophylline
Psychotropics

decrease in taste and smell as well as several neuroendocrine changes in both the central feeding system and the peripheral satiety system. Pathological causes include social (poverty, elderly abuse, inability to shop, cook, or feed oneself), psychiatric (depression, dementia, late-life paranoia, later-life mania and anorexia tardive), and physical (infections, cancer, medication side effects, stroke, neuroendocrine illnesses, cardiopulmonary disorders).[45–58] In addition to protein-energy malnutrition

(PEM), deficiency of micronutrients is widely prevalent in the elderly with significant psychiatric manifestations, including depression.[12,46,59]

22.2.2 Clinical Features

Depression is not a single diagnosis but rather a manifestation of multiple psychiatric and medical conditions. Patients who present with depressive symptoms can be diagnosed with major depressive disorder, dysthymia, bipolar disorder, adjustment disorder with depressed mood, schizoaffective disorder, depression secondary to a general medical condition, or substance-induced mood disorder/depressive type. The *Diagnostic and Statistical Manual IV, Text Revision* (DSM-IV TR) of the American Psychiatric Association details the diagnostic criteria for each of these disorders.[60] However, a greater number of older adults may have subsyndromal depressive symptoms that do not fulfill the criteria for any of these disorders. Weight loss and anorexia are very common in all these depressive syndromes.

The criteria for diagnosing major depressive disorder (MDD) according to DSM-IV TR requires that five or more of the following symptoms be present on a day-to-day basis for at least 2 weeks with at least one of the symptoms being depressed mood or loss of interest or pleasure: (1) depressed mood, (2) loss of interest or pleasure in activities, (3) change in weight or appetite, (4) insomnia or hypersomnia, (5) psychomotor agitation or retardation, (6) low energy, (7) feelings of worthlessness, (8) poor concentration, and (9) recurrent suicidal ideation or suicide attempt.[105] A score of more than 10 on the Beck Depression Inventory or 10 or more on the 15-item Geriatric Depression Scale also supports the diagnosis of depression in elderly patients. Although the criteria for MDD are similar for both early-onset and late-onset depression, the latter may have more prominent comorbid conditions or symptoms.

22.2.3 Special Presentation of Depression in the Elderly

In the elderly, MDD may present with anxiety, multiple somatic complaints, or cognitive impairment as the chief presentation. The patient may present with predominantly somatic symptoms that may be particularly prominent, making it difficult to diagnose depression. The patient may focus his complaints on physical problems rather than openly address his depression or may admit to feeling depressed but only as a result of his physical complaints. Anxiety symptoms may accompany depression in the elderly. Comorbid psychotic symptoms, which often involve delusions that are persecutory, guilty, nihilistic, or somatic in nature, are common among the elderly. Elderly patients may present with cognitive impairment that resembles dementia. This is referred to as pseudodementia or the dementia syndrome of depression, where a patient with a clinically significant depression may show objective evidence of memory and cognitive changes secondary to his mood disorder. Unlike other dementias, once the mood disorder is treated, the cognitive changes should disappear, if they were solely secondary to depression.

Understanding the clinical presentation of depression and associated medical comorbidities in the elderly is critical to properly treating it and appreciating its overlap and intricate relationship with nutrition. Clinically depressed elderly are often malnourished, and severely malnourished older adults are invariably depressed. At times, it is difficult to identify the cause of malnutrition. This is partly because the causes for anorexia and weight loss in the elderly are multifactorial and rarely due to one disorder. Thorough clinical evaluation is essential in treating and preventing this potentially serious problem. Fortunately, most causes are reversible if treated promptly and properly. Depressed patients have many symptoms that can lead to weight loss, including weakness (61%), stomach pains (37%), nausea (27%), anorexia (22%), and diarrhea (20%).[51] See Table 22.3 for causes of weight loss/anorexia.[61]

On the other hand, identifying clinical signs and symptoms of different nutritional deficiencies is vital to treating both the underlying causes and disorders, such as depression, which may be the direct outcome of malnutrition. Clinical data and research show that deficiencies of B vitamins (thiamin, niacin, pantothenic acid, pyridoxine, B12, and folic acid) and vitamin C and minerals (magnesium, calcium, zinc, manganese, iron, and potassium) are linked with depressive symptoms.[2,10,49,59,62–65] Clinical screening of depressed older adults for these deficiencies should be considered.[51,57,66] Clinical evaluation also needs to include the amount of food per meal, number of meals per day, and the nutritional content of the patient's dietary routine.

22.3 DIFFERENTIAL DIAGNOSIS AND WORKUP

The assessment of a depressed older adult requires a thorough evaluation of multiple biopsychosocial elements that may be predisposing, precipitating, and perpetuating factors. History taking and physical/mental status examination are the most important parts of the diagnostic process. In addition to current presentation, past psychiatric and medical history, a history of substance abuse including alcohol and prescription drugs, comorbid medical and psychiatric illnesses, a detailed history of compliance and lists of past and present natural remedies, prescription and over-the-counter medications, functional capacity and support systems, a comprehensive dietary history, and cultural and religious practices are essential in the formulation of a reasonable differential diagnosis. A thorough physical examination may reveal important data. A complete mental status exam gives useful information for diagnosis, severity of illness, and future follow-up.

Screening tools are widely used in the assessment of malnutrition and depression in the elderly. Commonly used nutrition screening tools include Instant Nutritional Assessment (INA), the Subjective Global Assessment (SGA) and the Mini-Nutritional Assessment (MNA).[53] The Geriatric Depression Scale and Beck's Depression Scale are commonly used to screen for depression.

All medically ill older patients need to be screened for depression, and most severely depressed patients may have one or more comorbid medical conditions. Among the medically ill, those with acute MI and stroke, cancer, Parkinson's disease, multiple sclerosis, dementia, and autoimmune and most of the neuroendocrine illnesses are especially prone to depressive illnesses. Several medications, including cardiovascular drugs such as beta-blockers, interferon alpha, corticosteroids, antibiotics, anti-Parkinson's, anticonvulsants, and some psychotropics, may contribute to depression symptoms. Some features that suggest depression in the elderly include frequent office visits or use of medical services; persistent reports of pain, fatigue, insomnia, headache, changes in sleep or appetite, unexplained gastrointestinal symptoms; and signs of social isolation and increased dependency. Delayed recovery from a medical or surgical condition such as failure to rehabilitate after stroke or a hip fracture, refusal of treatment, and resistance to discharge from a hospital may also be signs of depression.

Micronutrient deficiencies may cause nonspecific constitutional and cognitive symptoms. Whenever there is a suspicion, patients should be screened. Depression can be part of the presentation and may become treatment resistant until the underlying cause is treated. Causes could be either dietary deficiency or medical comorbidities, which cause anorexia, swallowing problems, malabsorption, or increased or faulty metabolism/excretion.[51,53,54]

Involuntary weight loss, otherwise termed as failure to thrive, in the elderly also needs careful evaluation and workup. Weight loss can be due to decreased food intake, accelerated metabolism, or increased loss of calories, which are caused by factors related to age, social, psychiatric, or medical conditions. History should include if the patient has an adequate support system, income level, and nutritional knowledge. Psychiatric evaluation for dementia, depression, bereavement, anorexia tardive, and alcoholism is vital. Medical conditions such as major organ system diseases, cancer, medication side effects, dentition and swallowing problems, and functional disability are not uncommon. Age-related sensory changes and appetite suppression may also play a role. Once weight loss is confirmed and a complete history and physical examination is done, the differential diagnosis will be narrowed. However, in most instances further laboratory workup is required to reach to a more specific diagnosis, determine the severity of the problem, and for follow-up purposes.

The basic laboratory workup for depression and anorexia/involuntary weight loss is mainly guided by the findings of the initial evaluation and the differential diagnosis considered. Initial or screening laboratory tests include an electrolyte panel, fasting serum glucose level, liver function tests, creatinine level, complete blood count, thyroid-stimulating hormone level, vitamin B12 and folic acid levels, homocystiene level, electrocardiography, chest radiography, and urinalysis. Consider further neurological testing or imaging if warranted by the neurological exam. However, an MRI may prove useful in visualizing changes secondary to vascular depression, dementia, or other neuropsychiatric causes. Where drug and alcohol abuse are thought to be possible causes, a urine and serum drug screen may help. Albumin and total protein levels may be checked to assess severity of malnutrition in the absence of other chronic disease processes that can explain it. In anorexia of undetermined cause, a workup for underlying malignancy should be completed and a follow-up evaluation scheduled before settling on a diagnosis such as anorexia tardive (otherwise known as late-onset anorexia nervosa where investigation reveals no abnormality apart from changes that are consistent with malnutrition, and when typical behavioral and psychological factors with suspected psychodynamic issues are evident).[66–68]

22.4 TREATMENT OF DEPRESSION AND RELATED ANOREXIA/WEIGHT LOSS

The management of depression and related symptoms is individualized, multidisciplinary, and should be systematic. Underlying causes and complications need to be addressed. Treatment of depression is crucial, as are supportive measures and symptomatic relief. A management plan may consist of treatment of depression, addressing underlying reversible causes, supportive/replacement measures, and symptomatic relief (Table 22.4). The biopsychosocial model of understanding the disease process and the diagnostic approach should also be utilized in the treatment process. In addition to the patient, involvement of the family and other caregivers and providers in an integrated manner is crucial for successful treatment outcomes.

22.4.1 Treatment of Depression

Depression is diverse in its presentation, course, and severity. Choice of treatment needs to be individualized and continually tailored. An accurate diagnosis is vital for success of treatment, as is selecting the appropriate treatment modality. Pharmacotherapy is the mainstay of treatment for major depression, and recent advances have made it highly effective with minimal adverse effects.[38,40,44,69–72] Other therapeutic modalities such as psychotherapy and neuromodulation have been useful in combination with medication or as a sole treatment. There is an increasing interest in natural remedies and alternative medicines in the treatment of depression and other psychiatric illnesses. Nutritional, herbal, hormonal, circadian rhythm regulation, and exercise are some of the approaches that are reported to be variably effective in treating depression.

22.4.1.1 Pharmacotherapy

There are several classes of antidepressant medications with variable mechanisms of action, side effects and safety profiles, costs, and limitations of use. Monoamine oxidase inhibitors (MAOIs) and tricyclic antidepressants (TCAs) are among the earliest groups of antidepressants, while selective serotonin reuptake inhibitors (SSRIs) and dual-uptake inhibitors are among the newer generation of antidepressants. Other miscellaneous antidepressants are also available. Mood stabilizers and antipsychotics are indicated where a bipolar or psychotic depression is diagnosed. Response to treatment, safety, proper dosing, length of treatment, and compliance are main issues when considering antidepressant therapy.

22.4.1.1.1 MAOIs

MAOIs are the first group of medications that were developed to treat depression. Their side effect profile, drug–drug interaction, and need for dietary restriction are the main reasons for limited use in the elderly. Otherwise, they are efficacious agents in treating depression. Hypertensive crisis is the feared complication when they are mixed with high-tyramine-containing foods, including some alcoholic beverages, cheeses, and fermented foods. Drug–drug reactions are another common problem, including with other antidepressants. When properly used, hypotension is another adverse effect that may limit their usage in the older population. A

TABLE 22.4
Therapeutics Used for the Treatment of Depression and Comorbid Symptoms

Antidepressants
Monoamine oxidase inhibitors
Trycyclic antidepressants
Selective serotonin reuptake inhibitors
Serotonin norepinephrine dual reuptake inhibitors
Dopamine norepinephrine dual reuptake inhibitors
Miscellaneous classes of antidepressants
Mood Stabilizers
Lithium and anticonvulsants
Antipsychotics
Typical antipsychotics
Atypical antipsychotics
Stimulants
Dextroamphetamine/methylphenidate, madafanil
Orexigenic/Appetite Stimulants
Megestrol acetate
Dronabinol
Ciproheptadine
Thalidomide
Growth hormone
Anabolic steroids
Prokinetic agents
Mirtazepine
Natural/Herbal Remedies
Omega-3 fatty acids
St. John's wort
SAMe
Tryptophan
Vitamins
Inositol
Hormonal Supplements
Testosterone, estrogen, DHEA
Psychotherapy
Neuromodulation
Electroconvulsive therapy (ECT)
Vagus nerve stimulation (VNS)
Repetitive transcranial magnetic stimulation (rTMS)
Deep brain stimulation (DBS)

recently FDA-approved selegiline transdermal patch may be safer and require no or less dietary restriction. It may also improve compliance in older adults. MAOIs are mainly indicated for treatment-resistant depression.

22.4.1.1.2 TCAs

TCAs are also an older group of antidepressants. Once extensively used in the treatment of depression, they are now used less frequently because of their low tolerability and high toxicity profile. Their anticholinergic, orthostatic, and sedative side effects make them poorly tolerated by older adults. Intentional or accidental overdose carries a high risk for cardiotoxicity, convulsions, coma, and death. However, when used properly and if tolerated, they are highly effective for treating depression, neuropathic pain, and headaches. They improve sleep and most patients gain weight on them, which could be an advantage for severely depressed elderly patients.

22.4.1.1.3 SSRIs

SSRIs are the newest class of antidepressants and are often used as a first line of treatment of depression in the elderly.[69,72] The most significant reasons are their side effects and safety profile. Since antidepressants are almost all equally effective, the selection is often based on side effect profile and potential interaction with other medications. An adequate trial is at least 8 weeks at the recommended dosage, and none of the individual SSRIs are proven to be more safe or effective than the other. It is generally recommended to start with half to one third of the recommended dosage for younger adults and to titrate up slowly. When minor side effects occur, decreasing the dose may help, but switching to another agent may be needed if side effects persist. If the side effect is severe, consider switching to a different class of antidepressant. Treatment of comorbid psychiatric illnesses with proper psychotropics is crucial. Where symptoms resolve with treatment, continuation for 12 months is recommended to prevent relapse. However, in patients who have had two or more episodes of MDD in later life, long-term indefinite treatment is recommended at the same dose which got them well.

22.4.1.1.4 Other Agents

There are several newer antidepressants that work differently than SSRIs. They are used interchangeably with SSRIs when patients cannot tolerate or show poor response to one group. These are serotonin–noradrenaline reuptake inhibitors (SNRIs) like duloxetine and venlafaxine; dopamine–noradrenaline reuptake inhibitors (DNRIs) like bupropion, and others such as mirtazepine, nefazodone, and trazodone, which work through a slightly different mechanism. These medications are not superior or more tolerable than SSRIs. However, mirtazepine has an additional advantage of improving appetite and insomnia if given for patients who have poor sleep and decreased appetite. Nefazodone is no longer used because of reported rare hepatotoxicity. Trazodone is often used in low doses for mild irritability and at bedtime as a sedative–hypnotic.

22.4.1.1.5 Stimulants

Stimulants are used where rapid onset is needed and apathy/psychomotor retardation, concurrent medical illness, and intolerance for antidepressants are concerns.[73,74] Effect is variable but can be lasting, and they may enhance appetite as well. Methylphenidate and dextroamphetamine are some of the commonly used stimulants.

Modafinil, a newer agent developed for conditions causing excessive daytime sleepiness, is also beginning to be used.

22.4.1.2 Psychotherapy

Psychotherapy is the oldest modality of treatment for many psychiatric disorders, including depression. It still has high efficacy as a mono- and combination treatment when used in properly selected patients. It is underutilized and less recognized by patients and providers alike in this age group. Moreover, physical limitations such as mobility and transportation problems, hearing/vision loss, and physical frailty may impact on the suitability of psychotherapy. The high prevalence of cognitive problems and older patients' perceptions of aging as an unchanging stage of life make therapy less appealing. Reimbursement issues are also another challenge. However, there is adequate theoretical and practice-based evidence for the effectiveness of psychotherapy in the elderly.[75,76] Depending on the severity and nature of the illness and patient characteristics, psychotherapy can be used alone or in combination with other treatment options.

Among the many options of psychotherapy modalities, interpersonal psychotherapy (IPT), family therapy, brief psychodynamic therapy, cognitive behavioral therapy (CBT), problem-solving therapy, and psychoeducation are proven to be of great benefit.[75] The duration and choice of therapy may vary based on several factors, including disease severity, presence of a support system, individual patient variability, and use of combination treatment modalities. CBT focuses on the environment, behavior, and cognition, in a structured, goal-directed, problem-focused, and time-limited approach. It teaches patients how their thoughts may contribute to symptoms of their affect and how to change these thoughts. It combines increased cognitive awareness with specific behavioral techniques. It is the form of psychotherapy most often used with older adults that is highly effective with depressed patients in both hospital and community settings as well as in individual and group formats.[76–79]

Interpersonal therapy is a practical, focused, brief, and manual-based therapy applicable in the treatment of depression in older adults both in the acute phase and in relapse prevention. It works on dysfunctional current relationships with key themes such as role transition/dispute, abnormal grief, and interpersonal deficit. Its aim is improving communication, expressing affect, and facilitating renegotiated roles in relationships to eventually reduce the impact of symptoms and improve functionality.[5,75,76] Interpersonal therapy has shown clear benefits in depressed older adults.[80,81] Patients with personality disorders and past traumatic experiences, or those living in highly dysfunctional relationships or isolation may benefit from a psychodynamic therapeutic approach.[75,76,80]

In family therapy, the focus is on improving difficulties in communication and relationships and helping the whole family, including the patient. If some of the crucial members of the family can be engaged, it may help relieve the patient's depression and prevent future relapse. Controlled outcome studies support its positive effect in the process of patient recovery and improved family function.[76] Psychoeducation provides patients and families with information about their diagnosis, treatment, how to recognize signs of relapse, relapse prevention, and strategies to cope with the reality of depression. It is widely used in many psychiatric illnesses with the goal of reducing distress, confusion, and facilitating treatment compliance.[76,79] Problems with anorexia, weight loss, and nutritional deficiencies can be addressed in these various modes of therapies by involving families, other caretakers, and the patient.

22.4.1.3 Neuromodulation

Modulating the brain's neurocircuitry using a device-based treatment is another approach in the treatment of many psychiatric illnesses, especially mood disorders, including depression. Electroconvulsive therapy (ECT) had been the sole method in this class for many decades until the recent FDA approval of vagal nerve stimulation (VNS) for treatment-resistant depression. Other options used extensively in clinical trials with promising results are repetitive transcranial magnetic stimulation (rTMS), deep brain stimulation (DBS), and magnetic seizure therapy.[82,83] In addition to opening a new paradigm in the understanding of mental illnesses, these treatments have created a potentially effective therapeutic alternative for adults who are not responding to or who are unable to tolerate pharmacotherapy.

ECT has become an important and effective treatment for selected serious neuropsychiatric illnesses, including severe depression. In the past seven decades since its advent, ECT has evolved into a sophisticated procedure with an excellent safety profile. In severely depressed older adults, typically where there is a failure to respond to or tolerate antidepressant medications, ECT is the treatment of choice. When we do not have the luxury of time for the antidepressants to work, as in agitated, psychotic, or actively suicidal patients or patients whose medical condition is seriously compromised due to severe depression, ECT is used earlier and with greater efficacy. Because of frequent medication side effects, severe comorbidities, severity of illness, and poor response to treatment, elderly patients often will receive ECT earlier than their younger counterparts.[84] Cachexia due to depression with severe anorexia is a true psychiatric emergency where ECT may be the first line of treatment. ECT as a first-line treatment has response rates in the 80 to 90% range, while medication-resistant depression may respond in the range of 50 to 60%.[84] Treatment is given under general anesthesia as unilateral or bilateral scalp electric stimulation to obtain therapeutic seizures. The only absolute contraindications are increased intracranial pressure and recent myocardial infarction. ECT has a very low mortality rate and its main side effects are acute confusion and antero- and retrograde amnesia, which mostly resolve in a few weeks, or more in the case of retrograde amnesia.[84] Patients are maintained on their medications after ECT to prevent relapse.

Among the other options, only VNS is FDA approved for the treatment of treatment-resistant depression in conjunction with medications.[82] Under general anesthesia, a pulse generator is implanted in the left chest wall and a wire threaded into the neck and around the left vagus nerve. The stimulator, similar to a cardiac pacemaker, is programmed through an external handheld device.[83] So far, there are minimal data in the geriatric population. However, it is a potentially beneficial treatment option with a low side effect profile.[85–87] rTMS is another noninvasive technique that uses an electric coil to generate a magnetic field that stimulates the cerebral cortex.[82,83,88] Unlike ECT, it does not require the use of anesthesia, and cognitive impairment does not seem to be a concern. Some geriatric data support potential benefits which can be accepted as an alternative where pharmacotherapy is not tolerated.[89–91] Randomized, controlled, and meta-analytic studies of rTMS have produced conflicting results.[89,92,93] DBS and transcranial magnetic seizure therapy are other modalities with limited data, especially in the geriatric population. However, the treatment outcomes in adult patients are encouraging for patients where all therapeutic options have failed.[82,94]

22.4.1.4 Natural Remedies: Alternative Treatments for Depression

Natural remedies have always been available for a variety of illnesses, including psychiatric disorders. In recent years, there has been a surge in the popularity of natural or alternative medications. Despite this growing popularity, there is limited evidence for the effectiveness of many of these natural treatments. Most natural remedies are herbal, dietary, or hormonally synthesized, mainly from plant or animal products. Depression is one area where these alternative treatments are widely used. It is crucial to note that some recent studies revealed potentially fatal interactions between herbal remedies and traditional drugs.[95]

Extracts of *Hypericum perforatum* (St. John's wort) are widely used for the treatment of depression of varying severity. Their efficacy in major depressive disorder, however, has not been conclusively demonstrated.[96,97] Several studies have shown equivalent results compared to other antidepressants for mild to moderate depression, while some studies could not support its effectiveness in moderate to severe depression.[97,98] Its minimal side effect profile makes it appealing, especially in the elderly population, while substantial drug–drug interactions and potential hepatic enzyme induction are drawbacks. More data are needed to clearly set dosage and indications as well as determine the extent of drug interaction and adverse effects in the geriatric population.

S-adenosyl-L-methionine (SAMe) is one of the better studied natural remedies.[99,100] It is a methyl donor and is involved in the synthesis of various neurotransmitters in the brain.[101,102] A derivative of the amino acid L-methionine, SAMe has been postulated to have antidepressant properties. Several double-blind studies have shown that SAMe is effective, with few side effects.[103–105] Its main drawbacks are that it is very expensive, unstable, and most SAMe preparations sold in health food shops are low potency or impure, and thus ineffective. Overall, SAMe appears to be safe and effective in the treatment of depression, but more research is needed, especially in the elderly, to determine optimal doses, and head-to-head comparisons with newer antidepressants are lacking.[102,103] Another amino acid that is highly linked with depression is 5-hydroxy tryptophan (5-HT), which is a precursor of serotonin. Its depletion is clearly associated with worsening of depression, and tryptophan replacement has been seen to alleviate depression.[2] Studies show that tryptophan treatment may hasten response and prevent future relapse in patients who are on other antidepressants.[64,104] However, care should be taken not to induce a serotonin syndrome in using it with SSRIs. Tyrosine and phenylalanine are precursors of dopamine, noradrenaline, and adrenaline. Supplements of these amino acids have shown improvement in selected depressed patients, but controlled trials and geriatric dosing guidelines are lacking.[2]

Micronutirients are known to be cofactors in the synthesis of essential neurotransmitters. The B vitamins and minerals such as zinc, iron, magnesium, thiamine, manganese, and copper also take part in this process.[2,63] Depressed elderly, specifically those who are treatment resistant, can be deficient in these nutrients. Screening for deficiency and supplementing low levels may be the key to treatment.[105,106] Serum homocysteine and methylmalonic acid levels are more sensitive in detecting clinical significant deficiencies of folate and B12 in depressed patients.[59,65,106–109] One study has shown no association between vitamin E levels and depression.[110] Inositol, a naturally occurring isomer of glucose, is a key intermediate of the phosphatidyl–inositol (PI) cycle, a second messenger system used by several noradrenergic, serotonergic, and cholinergic receptors. Its cerebral spinal fluid (CSF) level was found to be low in depression, and some studies have suggested its beneficial effect in depression treatment.[3,4]

Other important nutritional treatment in depression is the use of polyunsaturated fatty acids (PUFAs).[5–8] Several studies have shown their benefit in depressed patients who failed standard antidepressant treatment.[8,9] Omega-3 fatty acids have been used at various doses and forms with or without other antidepressant medications. They may improve mood and hasten remission of symptoms even in severe depression.[6,11] Omega-3 fatty acids additionally show little evidence of adverse effects, toxicity, or drug interactions. Fish oil is a rich source of these fatty acids. Hormonal therapies have been used in the elderly with variable success and significant limitations.[111–113] Thyroid hormone treatment has been shown to enhance response in treatment-resistant depression as an augmenting agent.[62] Other hormonal therapies that have shown promise in the treatment of depression in the elderly are melatonin, dehydroepiandrosterone (DHEA), estrogen (in perimenopausal women), and testosterone.[111–113] However, there are insufficient data to recommend such treatments at this stage in routine practice apart from clear deficiency states.

22.4.2 Treatment-Resistant Depression (TRD)

TRD has been variously defined as failure to respond to adequate trials of antidepressants, two or more trials of monotherapy with different antidepressants, or failure to respond to four or more trials of different antidepressant therapies, including augmentation, combination, and ECT.[114,115] Patients who do not respond to TCAs, MAOIs, or ECT after adequate trials of other classes of antidepressants are classified as treatment refractory depressives. Partial response and recurrence of depression while on treatment are also possible. Several factors, however, must be considered before diagnosing TRD, including undiagnosed hypothyroidism and anemia, medications that can cause or exacerbate depression (e.g., methyldopa, beta-blockers, and reserpine), poor compliance, and comorbid conditions such as substance abuse. Depression subtypes such as bipolar depression, psychotic depression, or atypical depression, which may require concurrent pharmacotherapy with mood stabilizers or antipsychotics, also need to be ruled out.[116]

The five commonly used strategies for treating TRD are optimization, drug substitution, combination therapy, augmentation therapy, and neuromodulation. Optimization of both the dose and duration of the antidepressant should be the first step before considering other strategies. Inadequate antidepressant dosage and duration are particularly common in elderly patients.[116] Nonresponders can be switched to a different medication, preferably a different class relative to mechanism of action. Improved compliance, fewer side effects, and cost effectiveness are advantages, while possible withdrawal symptoms, reluctance to take new medication, and delayed response are disadvantages. While switching to a different class is optimal for patients who fail to respond to first-line therapy, targeting both noradrenergic and serotonergic systems is one of the most effective combination strategies.[117] One study comparing switching and augmentation failed to find significant differences in efficacy between the two approaches.[118]

In augmentation, a nonantidepressant drug is added to boost the effect of the currently used antidepressant. While the most studied is lithium, other agents used include buspirone, lamotrigine, bupropion, pindolol, thyroid hormone, S-adenosyl-L-methionine (SAMe), omega-3 fatty acids, L-methyfolate, and L-tryptophan.[62,114,118] Atypical antipsychotics are used mostly in psychotic depression, while preliminary data suggest their augmenting benefit even in nonpsychotic TRD.[119] Benefits are rapid onset of action, no withdrawal symptoms, and maintaining the already achieved partial response. Drug interactions, increased cost, and noncompliance are limitations. Combination therapy is the concurrent use of at least two antidepressants. It has similar pros and cons to augmentation. Nonpharmacological options include ECT, psychotherapy, VNS, rTMS, and DBS.[114] Psychotherapy is a good augmentation strategy in selected patients, as is VNS in the maintenance treatment of TRD. Though its efficacy decreases in treatment-resistant depression, ECT often remains the last resort in this group of patients.[119] Patients who are refractory to these options may be good candidates for DBS from the preliminary data available.[82] It is important to keep in mind that all the current, controlled studies looking at combination/augmentation strategies in depressive illness are nongeriatric.

22.4.2.1 Treatment of Underlying Causes

Most elderly depressed patients have underlying medical comorbidities and complicating psychosocial problems. Identifying and treating these predisposing, precipitating, and perpetuating factors is part and parcel of the treatment. This requires a multidisciplinary and systematic approach. The role of nutrition in geriatric depression cannot be overemphasized. A full nutritional evaluation and appropriate treatment are crucial. Often, the underlying cause of depression and nutritional problems is substance abuse or dependence, including alcohol and prescription medications, rarely illicit drugs. Assessing and addressing the elderly patient's support system, living arrangements, financial condition, and physical capacity is vital. Elderly abuse can be an indolent yet serious factor. Malnutrition may present with protein-energy malnutrition (PEM), micronutrient deficiency, or obesity, all of which need to be addressed accordingly.

22.4.2.2 Symptomatic Treatments

Patients with depression have complex symptomatologies that may be related to either the depression or underlying medical comorbidities. Pain, insomnia, weight loss, anorexia, fatigue, psychosis, cognitive difficulties, and suicidality are some symptoms that need prompt attention. Pain is very common and needs to be addressed as it can worsen depression and anorexia. The use of narcotics should be reserved for uncontrolled pain or terminal patients. Proper use of hypnotics and other interventions is part of the treatment of depression. Trazodone and zolpidem can be used safely in insomnia patients. Newly released eszopiclone and rameleton are other options that can be used in this age group. Antipsychotic agents may be helpful in treating patients who refuse to eat because of delusions or other psychotic symptoms.

Management of weight loss and anorexia is beyond the scope of this chapter.[45–55] However, boosting appetite using different medications may be crucial in patients who remain anorexic and cachetic. This is important especially where underlying causes are irreversible or protracted time is needed to treat them. Some of these orexigenic agents are megestrol acetate, dronabinol (a cannabis derivative), ciproheptadine (an antiserotonergic agent), thalidomide, growth hormone, anabolic steroids (like oxandrolone), prokinetic agents (like metoclopramide), and some antidepressants (such as mirtazepine).[120–123] Each of these agents has its own risks and benefits and needs to be used with care. Aggressive use of high-protein supplements, enteral tube feeding, and peripheral parenteral nutrition may have a role in the concommitant management of anorexia in depressed older adults.

22.5 CONCLUSION

Depression and malnutrition are common in geriatric patients. Often, they are interdependent and demand aggressive evaluation and treatment. Older adults can benefit from a range of pharmacologic and psychotherapeutic options for the treatment of depressive syndromes. Often, these are used in combination. A range of treatment options, including ECT, may be useful for treatment-resistant or treatment-intolerant scenarios in late-life depression. Neuromodulation also appears to be a promising treatment modality in selected geriatric depressives.

REFERENCES

1. Mood disorders. In *Kaplan and Sadock's Synopsis of Psychiatry*, 9th ed., Sadock BJ, Sadock VA, Eds., Philadelphia: Lippincott, Williams & Wilkins, 2003, pp. 534–590.
2. Holford B. Depression: the nutrition connection. *Primary Care Mental Health* 2003;1:9–16.
3. Benjamin J, Agam G, Levine J, Bersudsky Y, Kofman O, Belmaker RH. Inositol treatment in psychiatry. *Psychopharmacol Bull* 1995;31:167–175.
4. Palatnik A, Frolov K, Fux M, Benjamin J. Double-blind, controlled, crossover trial of inositol versus fluvoxamine for the treatment of panic disorder. *J Clin Psychopharmacol* 2001;21:335–339.

5. Sontrop J, Campbell MK. Omega-3 polyunsaturated fatty acids and depression: a review of the evidence and a methodological critique. *Prev Med* 2006;42:4–13.
6. Freeman MP. Omega-3 fatty acids in psychiatry: a review. *Ann Clin Psychiatry* 2000;12:159–165.
7. Teimeier H, van Tuijl HR, Hofman A, Kiliaan AJ, Breteler MM. Plasma fatty acid composition and depression are associated in the elderly: the Rotterdam Study. *Am J Clin Nutr* 2003;78:40–46.
8. Nemets B, Stahl Z, Belmaker RH. Addition of omega-3 fatty acid to maintenance medication treatment for recurrent unipolar depressive disorder. *Am J Psychiatry* 2002;159:477–479.
9. Horrobin DF, Manku M. Treatment of Depression with Ethyl-Eicosapentaenoate. Paper presented at International Society for the Study of Fatty Acids and Lipids (ISSFAL), 5th Congress, Montreal, Canada, May 8–11, 2002.
10. Mischoulon D, Fava M. Docosahexanoic acid and omega-3 fatty acids in depression. *Psychiatr Clin North Am* 2000;23:785–794.
11. Peet M, Horrobin DF. A dose-ranging study of the effects of ethyl-eicosapentaenoate in patients with ongoing depression despite apparently adequate treatment with standard drugs. *Arch Gen Psychiatry* 2002;59:913–919.
12. Bhat RS, Chiu E, Jeste DV. Nutrition and geriatric psychiatry: a neglected field. *Curr Opin Psychiatry* 2005;18:609–614.
13. Benton D. Carbohydrate ingestion, blood glucose and mood. *Neurosci Biobehav Rev* 2002;26:293–308.
14. Chen CC, Chang CK, Chynn DA, McCorkle R. Dynamics of nutritional health in a community sample of American elders: a multidimensional approach using Roy adaptation model. *ANS Adv Nurs Sci* 2005;28:376–389.
15. Benton D, Donohoe RT. The effects of nutrients on mood. *Public Health Nutr* 1999;2:403–409.
16. Alpert JE, Fava M. Nutrition and depression: the role of folate. *Nutr Rev* 2003;55:145–149.
17. Bermudez OI, Dwyer J. Identifying elders at risk of malnutrition: a universal challenge. *SCN News* 1999;19:15–17.
18. Hajjar R, Kamel H, Denson K. Malnutrition in aging. *Internet J Geriatr Gerontol* 2004;1.
19. Kawakami K, Kadota J, Iida K, Shirai R, Abe K, Kohno S. Reduced immune function and malnutrition in the elderly. *Tohoku J Exp Med* 1999;187:157–171.
20. Lesourd B. Nutrition: a major factor influencing immunity in the elderly. *J Nutr Health Aging* 2004;8:28–37.
21. Lesourd B. Immune response during disease and recovery in the elderly. *Proc Nutr Soc* 1999;58:85–98.
22. Lesourd B, Mazari L. Nutrition and immunity in the elderly. *Proc Nutr Soc* 1999;58:685–695.
23. Irwin M. Immune correlates of depression. *Adv Exp Med Biol* 1999;461:1–24.
24. Evans DL, Pedersen CA, Folds JD. Major depression and immunity: preliminary evidence of decreased natural killer cell populations. *Prog Neuropsychopharmacol Biol Psychiatry* 1988;12:739–748.
25. Irwin M, Patterson T, Smith TL, Caldwell C, Brown SA, Gillin JC, et al. Reeducation of immune function in life stress and depression. *Biol Psychiatry* 1990;27:22–30.
26. Miller GE, Cohen S, Herbert TB. Pathways linking major depression and immunity in ambulatory female patients. *Psychosom Med* 1999;61:850–860.
27. Buchanan CK, High KP. Nutrition, aging and infection. *Clin Geriatr* 2004;12:44–53.

28. Rovner BW, German PS, Brant LJ, Clark R, Burton L, Folstein MF. Depression and mortality in nursing homes. *JAMA* 1991;265:993–996.
29. Hybels CF, Blazer DG. Epidemiology of late life mental disorders. *Clin Geriatr Med* 2003;19(4):663–96.
30. Burke WJ, Wengel SP. Late life mood disorders. *Clin Geriatr Med* 2003;19:777–797.
31. Reynolds CF 3rd, Dew MA, Frank E, Begley AE, Miller MD, Cornes C, et al. Effects of age at onset of first lifetime episode of recurrent major depression on treatment response and illness course in elderly patients. *Am J Psychiatry* 1998;155:795–799.
32. Conway CR, Steffens DC. Geriatric depression: further evidence for the 'vascular depression' hypothesis. *Curr Opin Psychiatry* 1999;12:463–470.
33. Alexopoulos GS, Meyers BS, Young RC, Campbell S, Silbersweig D, Charlson M. 'Vascular depression' hypothesis. *Arch Gen Psychiatry* 1997;54:915–922.
34. Steffens C, Krishnan R. Structural neuroimaging and mood disorders: recent findings, implications for classification, and future directions. *Soc Biol Psychiatry* 1998;43:705–712.
35. Pohjasvaara T, Leppavuori A, Siira I, et al. Frequency and clinical determinants of poststroke depression. *Stroke* 1998;29:2311–2317.
36. Morris PL, Robinson RG, Raphael B. Prevalence and course of depressive disorders in hospitalized stroke patients. *Int J Psychiatry Med* 1990;20:349–364.
37. Frasure-Smith N, Lesperance F, Juneau M, Talajic M, Bourassa MG. Gender, depression, and one-year prognosis after myocardial infarction. *Psychosom Med* 1999;61:26–37.
38. Birrer RB, Vemuri SP. Depression in later life: a diagnostic and therapeutic challenge. *Am Fam Physician* 2004;69(10):2375–82.
39. Cole MG, Dendukuri N. Risk factors for depression among elderly community subjects: a systematic review and meta-analysis. *Am J Psychiatry* 2003;160:1147–1156.
40. Boswell EB, Stoudemire A. Major depression in the primary care setting. *Am J Med* 1996;101:3S–9S.
41. von Ammon Cavanaugh S, Furlanetto LM, Creech SD, Powell LH. Medical illness, past depression, and present depression: a predictive triad for in-hospital mortality. *Am J Psychiatry* 2001;158:43–48.
42. Holly C, Murrell SA, Mast BT. Psychosocial and vascular risk factors for depression in the elderly. *Am J Geriatr Psychiatry* 2006;14:84–90.
43. Alexopoulos GS. Late life mood disorders. In *Comprehesive Textbook of Geriatric Psychiatry*, 3rd ed., Sadavoy J, Jarvik LF, Grossberg GT, Meyers BS, Eds. W.W. Norton and Company, New York, 2004, pp. 609–653.
44. Lapid MI, Rummans TA. Evaluation and management of geriatric depression in primary care. *Mayo Clinic Proc* 2003;78:1423–1429.
45. Huffman JB. Evaluating and treating unintentional weight loss in the elderly. *Am Fam Physician* 2002;65:640–650.
46. Splett PL, Roth-Yousey LL, Vogelzang JL. Medical nutrition therapy for the prevention and treatment of unintentional weight loss in residential healthcare facilities. *J Am Diet Assoc* 2003;103:352–362.
47. Gazewood JD, Mehr DR. Diagnosis and management of weight loss in the elderly. *J Fam Pract* 1998;47:19–25.
48. Reife CM. Involuntary weight loss. *Med Clin North Am* 1995;79:299–313.
49. Ryan C, Bryant E, Eleazer P, Rhodes A, Guest K. Unintentional weight loss in long-term care: predictor of mortality in the elderly. *South Med J* 1995;88:721–724.
50. Robertson RG, Montagnini M. Geriatric failure to thrive. *Am Fam Physician* 2004;70:343–350.

51. Alibahi SMH, Greenwood C, Payette H. An approach to the management of unintentional weight loss in elderly people. *CMAJ* 2005;172:773–780.
52. Fischer J, Johnson MA. Low body weight and weight loss in the aged. *J Am Diet Assoc* 1990;90:1697–1706.
53. Moriguti JC, Moriguti EKU, Ferriolli E, Cacao JDC, Junior NI, Marchini JS. Involuntary weight loss in elderly individuals: assessment and treatment. *Sao Paulo Med J* 2001;119:72–77.
54. Olsen-Noll CG, Bosworth MF. Anorexia and weight loss in the elderly. Causes range from loose dentures to debilitating illness. *Postgrad Med* 1989;85:140–144.
55. Chapman KM, Nelson RA. Loss of appetite: managing unwanted weight loss in the older patient. *Geriatrics* 1994;49:54–59.
56. van Staveren WA, de graaf C, de Groot LC. Regulation of appetite in frail persons. *Clin Geriatr Med* 2002;18:675–684.
57. Lankisch PG, Gerzmann M, Gerzmann J-F, Lehnick D. Unintentional weight loss: diagnosis and prognosis. The first prospective follow-up study from a secondary referral centre. *J Intern Med* 2001;249:41–46.
58. Lankisch P, Gerzmann M, Gerzmann JF, Lehnick D. Anorexia in older patients: its meaning and management. *Geriatrics* 1990;45:59–62, 65–66.
59. Fava M, Borus JS, Alpert JE, Nierenberg AA, Rosenbaum JF, Bottiglieri T. Folate, vitamin B12, and homocysteine in major depressive disorder. *Am J Psychiatry* 1997;154:426–428.
60. American Psychiatric Association. *Diagnositic Criteria from Diagnostic and Statistical Manual of Mental Disorders*, fourth edition, *Text Revision*. Washington, DC, 2000, pp. 168–171.
61. Fischer J, Johnson MA. Low body weight and weight loss in the aged. *J Am Diet Assoc* 1990;90:1697–1706.
62. Joffe RT, Sokolov ST. Thyroid hormone treatment of primary unipolar depression: a review. *Int J Neuropsychopharmacol* 2000;3:143–147.
63. Benton D, Griffiths R, Haller J. Thiamine supplementation mood and cognitive functioning. *Psychopharmacology* 1997;129:66–71.
64. Moreno FA, Heninger GR, McGahuey CA, Delgado PL. Tryptophan depletion and risk of depression relapse: a prospective study of tryptophan depletion as a potential predictor of depressive episodes. *Biol Psychiatry* 2000;48:327–329.
65. Tiemeier H, Tuijl H, Hofman A, Meijer A, Kiliaan A, Breteler M. Vitamin B12, folate, and homocysteine in depression: the Rotterdam Study. *Am J Psychiatry* 2002;159:2099–2101.
66. Morley JE. Anorexia in older persons: epidemiology and optimal treatment. *Drugs Aging* 1996;8:134–155.
67. Russel JD, Berg J, Lawrence JR. Anorexia tardive: a diagnosis of exclusion? *Med J Aust* 1988;148:199–201.
68. Joughin NA, Crisp AH, Gowers SG, Bhat AV. The clinical features of late onset anorexia nervosa. *Postgrad Med J* 1991;67:973–977.
69. Barbier D. Depression in the elderly. Principles of treatment. *Presse Med* 2001;30:341–344.
70. Raj A. Depression in the elderly: tailoring medical therapy to their special needs. *Postgrad Med* 2004;115:26–42.
71. Lebowitz BD, Pearson JL, Schneider LS, et al. Diagnosis and treatment of depression in late life: consensus statement update. *JAMA* 1997;278:1186–1190.
72. Mulsant BH, Alexopoulos GS, Reynolds CF 3rd, Katz IR, Abrams R, Oslin D, Schulberg HC. PROSPECT Study Group. Pharmacological treatment of depression. *Int J Geriatr Psychiatry* 2001;Jun;16(6):558–92.

73. Masand P, Murray Gb, Pickett P. Psychostimulants in post-stroke depression. *J Neuropsychiatry Clin Neurosci* 1991;3:23–27.
74. Pickett P, Masand P, Murray GB. Psychostimulant treatment of geriatric depressive disorders secondary to medical illness. *J Geriatr Psychiatry Neurol* 1990;3:146–151.
75. Hollon SD. Psychotherapy research with older populations. *Am J Geriatr Psychiatry* 2003;11:7–8.
76. Hepple J. Psychotherapies with older people: an overview. *Adv Psychiatr Treat* 2004;10:371–377.
77. Dobson KS. A meta analysis of the efficacy of cognitive behavioral therapy in depression. *J Consult Clin Psychol* 1989;57:414–419.
78. Lam DH, Watkins ER, Hayward P, Bright J, Wright K, Kerr N, Parr-Davis G, Sham P. A randomized controlled study of cognitive therapy for relapse prevention for bipolar affective disorder: outcome of the first year. *Arch Gen Psychiatry* 2003;60:145–152.
79. Seltzer A, Roncari I, Garfinkel P. Effect of patient education on medication compliance. *Can J Psychiatry* 1980;25:638–645.
80. Hollon SD, Thase ME, Markowitz JC. Treatment and prevention of depression. *Psychol Sci Public Interest* 2002;3:39–77.
81. Mark D, Miller EF, Cornes C, Houck PR, Reynolds CF III. The value of maintenance interpersonal psychotherapy (IPT) in older adults with different IPT foci. *Am J Geriatr Psychiatry* 2003;11:97–102.
82. Brown WA. Brain stimulation methods for treating depression. http://www.appneurology.com/article/printableArticle.jhtml?articleId=181500920&printableArticle=true, *Appl Neurol* 2006;2.
83. Schlaeper T, Kosel M. Novel physical treatments for major depression: vagus nerve stimulation, transcranial magnetic stimulation and magnetic seizure therapy. *Curr Opin Psychiatry* 2004;17:15–20.
84. Greenberg RM, Keller CH. Electroconvulsive therapy: a selected review. *Am J Geriatr Psychiatry* 2005;13:268–281.
85. Bender KJ. Study expands on vagus nerve stimulation for depression. *Psychiatr Times* 2001;18. http://psychiatrictimes.com/p0104vagus.html.
86. Rush AJ, George MS, Sackeim HA, et al. Vagus nerve stimulation (VNS) for treatment-resistant depression: a multicenter study. *Biol Psychiatry* 2000;47:276–286.
87. Rush AJ, Marangell LB, Sackeim HA, George MS, Brannan SK, Davis SM, et al. Vagus nerve stimulation for treatment-resistant depression: a randomized, controlled acute phase trial. *Biol Psychiatry* 2005;58:347–354.
88. O'Reardon JP, Peshek AD, Romero R, Cristancho P. Neuromodulation and transcranial magnetic stimulation. *Psychiatry* 2006;3:30–40.
89. Fitzgerald PB, Brown TL, Marston NA, Daskalakis ZJ, De Castella A, Kulkarni J. Transcranial magnetic stimulation in the treatment of depression: a double blind, placebo-controlled trial. *Arch Gen Psychiatry* 2003;60:1002–1008.
90. Mosimann UP, Schmitt W, Greenberg BD, Kosel M, Muri RM, Berkhoff M, et al. Repetitive transcranial magnetic stimulation: a putative add-on treatment for major depression in elderly patients. *Psychiatry Res* 2004;126:123–133.
91. Fabre I, Galinowski A, Oppenheim C, Gallarda T, Meder JF, De Montigny C, et al. Antidepressant efficacy and cognitive effects of repetitive transcranial magnetic stimulation in vascular depression: an open trial. *Int J Geriatr Psychiatry* 2004;19:833–842.
92. Ebmeier KP, Lappin JM. Electromagnetic stimulation in psychiatry. *Adv Psychiatr Treat* 2001;7:181–188.

93. Couturier JL. Efficacy of rapid-rate repetitive transcranial magnetic stimulation in the treatment of depression: a systematic review and meta-analysis. *J Psychiatry Neurosci* 2005;30:83–90.
94. Mayberg HS, Lozano AM, Voon V, McNeely HE, Seminowicz D, Hamani C, et al. Deep brain stimulation for treatment-resistant depression. *Neuron* 2005;45:651–660.
95. Ioannides C. Pharmacokinetic interactions between herbal remedies and medicinal drugs. *Xenobiotica* 2002;32:451–478.
96. Lecrubier Y, Clerc G, Didi R, Kieser M. Efficacy of St. John's wort extract WS 5570 in major depression: a double-blind, placebo-controlled trial. *Am J Psychiatry* 2002;159:1361–1366.
97. Hypericum Depression Trial Study Group. Effect of *Hypericum perforatum* (St. John's wort) in major depressive disorder: a randomized controlled trial. *JAMA* 2002;287:1807–1814.
98. van Gurp G, Meterissian GB, Haiek LN, McCusker J, Bellavance F. St. John's wort or sertraline? Randomized controlled trial in primary care. *Can Fam Physician* 2002;48:905–912.
99. Mischoulon D, Fava M. Role of S-adenosyl-L-methionine in the treatment of depression: a review of the evidence. *Am J Clin Nutr* 2002;76:1158S–1161S.
100. CW Fetrow, JR Avila. Efficacy of the dietary supplement S-adenosyl-L-methionine. *Ann Pharmacother* 2001;35:1414–1425.
101. Saletu B, Anderer P, Di Padova C, Assandri A, Saletu-Zyhlarz GM. Electrophysiological neuroimaging of the central effects of S-adenosyl-L-methionine by mapping of electroencephalograms and event-related potentials and low-resolution brain electromagnetic tomography. *Am J Clin Nutr* 2002;76:1162S–1171S.
102. Bottiglieri T. S-Adenosyl-L-methionine (SAMe): from the bench to the bedside: molecular basis of a pleiotrophic molecule. *Am J Clin Nutr* 2002;76:1151S–1157S.
103. Pancheri P, Scapicchio P, Chiaie RD. A double-blind, randomized parallel-group, efficacy and safety study of intramuscular S-adenosyl-L-methionine 1,4-butanedisulphonate (SAMe) versus imipramine in patients with major depressive disorder. *Int J Neuropsychopharmacol* 2002;5:287–294.
104. Delle Chiaie R, Pancheri P, Scapicchio P. Efficacy and tolerability of oral and intramuscular S-adenosyl-L-methionine 1,4-butanedisulfonate (SAMe) in the treatment of major depression: comparison with imipramine in 2 multicenter studies. *Am J Clin Nutr* 2002;76:1172S–1176S.
105. Fava M, Giannelli A, Rapisarda V, Patralia A, Guaraldi GP. Rapidity of onset of the antidepressant effect of parenteral S-adenosyl-L-methionine. *Psychiatry Res* 1995;56:295–297.
106. Brottiglieri T. Homocysteine and folate metabolism in depression. *Prog Neuropsychopharmacol Biol Psychiatry* 2005;29:1103–1112.
107. Penninx BW, Guralnik JM, Ferrucci L, Fried LP, Allen RH, Stabler SP. Vitamin B(12) deficiency and depression in physically disabled older women: epidemiologic evidence from the Women's Health and Aging Study. *Am J Psychiatry* 2000;157:715–721.
108. Fafouti M, Paparrigopoulos T, Liappas J, Mantouvalos V, Typaldou R, Christodoulou G. Mood disorder with mixed features due to vitamin B(12) and folate deficiency. *Gen Hosp Psychiatry* 2002;24:106–109.
109. Bell IR, Edman JS, Morrow FD, Marby DW, Mirages S, Perrone G, et al. B complex vitamin patterns in geriatric and young adult inpatients with major depression. *J Am Geriatr Soc* 1991;39:252–257.
110. Tiemeier H, Hofman A, Kiliaan Aj, Meijer J, Breteler MM. Vitamin E and depressive symptoms are not related. The Rotterdam Study. *J Affect Disord* 2002;72:79–83.

111. Bloch M, Schmidt PJ, Danaceau MA, Adams LF, Rubinow DR. Dehydroepiandrosterone treatment of midlife dysthymia. *Biol Psychiatry* 1999;45:1531–1532.
112. Almeida OP, Barclay L. Sex hormones and their impact on dementia and depression: a clinical perspective. *Expert Opin Pharmacother* 2001;2:527–535.
113. Margolese HC. The male menopause and mood: testosterone decline and depression in the aging male: is there a link? *J Geriatr Psychiatry Neurol* 2000;13:93–101.
114. Keller MB. Issues in treatment resistant depression. *J Clin Psychiatry* 2005;66(Suppl 8):5–12.
115. Berman RM, Narasimhan M, Charney DS. Treatment-refractory depression: definitions and characteristics (review). *Depress Anxiety* 1997;5:154–164.
116. Cadieux RJ. Practical management of treatment resistant depression. *Am Fam Physician* 1998;58:2059–2068.
117. Hirschfeld RM, Montgomery SA, Aguglia E, Amore M, Delgado PL, Gastpar M, et al. Partial response and nonresponse to antidepressant therapy: current approaches and treatment options. *J Clin Psychiatry* 2002;63:826–837.
118. Posternak MA, Zimmerman M. Switching versus augmentation: a prospective, naturalistic comparison in depressed, treatment-resistant patients. *J Clin Psychiatry* 2001;62:135–142.
119. Cowen PJ. New drugs old problems, revisiting pharmacological management of treatment resistant depression. *Adv Psychiatr Treat* 2005;11:19–27.
120. Morley JE. Anorexia and weight loss in older persons. *J Gerontol A Biol Sci Med Sci* 2003;58:131–137.
121. Sullivan DH. What do the serum proteins tell us about our elderly patients? *J Gerontol Med Sci* 2001;56A:M71–M74.
122. Reynolds R. Comparative efficacy of dronabinol and megestrol acetate. *J Clin Oncol* 2002;20:2912–2913.
123. Yuh S, Wu SY, Levin DM, Parker TS, Olson JS, Stevens MR, et al. Quality of life and stimulation of weight gain after treatment with megestrol acetate: correlation between cytokine levels and nutritional status, appetite in geriatric patients with wasting syndrome. *J Nutr Health Aging* 2000;4:246–251.

23 Nutrition and Behavior

John E. Morley, M.B., B.Ch.

CONTENTS

Memory is a passion no less powerful or pervasive than love.

—Elie Wiesel, *All Rivers Run to the Sea*

23.1 NUTRITION AND BEHAVIOR

The concept that nutrition status can modulate behavior is well established. Severe isolated nutrient deficiencies such as niacin can lead to the dementia associated with pellagra, and thiamine deficiency results in Wernicke's encephalopathy. The nutrient alcohol can have devastating acute effects on behavior and the central nervous system when ingested in excess. Long-term use of alcohol may result in the memory disturbances and confabulation associated with Korsakoff's syndrome. Minamata disease occurred in persons ingesting fish that came from a bay in which excess inorganic mercury compounds had been transformed by methanogenetic bacteria into methylmercury. Minamata disease is characterized by delirium, memory problems, irritability, headaches, tremors, dysarthria, and an ataxic diet. The role of nutrients in chronic diseases of the central nervous system is less clear. For example, while high cholesterol levels are associated with atherothrombotic strokes, low cholesterol levels are associated with hemorrhagic strokes. In older persons, nutrition deficits rarely present with clear-cut changes, but rather often occur as borderline deficiency states that may be associated with subtle behavioral alterations. This chapter briefly reviews some of the recognized effects of altered nutrient status in older persons.

23.2 PROTEIN-ENERGY UNDERNUTRITION

Goodwin et al.[1] found that older persons with poor protein, ascorbate, thiamine, riboflavin, pyridoxine, niacin, or folate intake had poorer performance on the Wechsler Memory Test than those with excellent intakes. The best studies of the behavioral effects of poor nutrient intake in adults were those conducted at the University of Minnesota during World War II.[2] Caloric intakes were reduced from 3500 kcal daily to 1570 kcal daily for 6 months. The major psychological findings of this study were that decreased caloric intake resulted in a decrease in social initiative; apathy; a feeling of tiredness; decreased mental alertness, libido, motivation, and self-discipline; and increased moodiness and irritability. Cognitive performance did not show a significant deterioration. There was an increased interest in food and its preparation, with the subjects lingering longer over meals. Evidence that food may play a role in memory function comes from anecdotal descriptions of marked deterioration in functional status in Alzheimer patients when they lose weight and improved functioning with refeeding.

Food can either have direct effects on the brain after absorption from the gastrointestinal tract or produce effects by releasing hormones from the gastrointestinal tract, and then can either stimulate ascending fibers of the vagus or cross the blood–brain barrier and produce direct effects on the brain.

It is now well established that if animals are fed following learning a task, they have a better ability to recall the task.[3] We showed that cholecystokinin (CCK) enhances acquisition and memory by activating the ascending fibers of the vagus. We trace the pathway for this memory-enhancing effect from the duodenum–vagus to the nucleus tractus solitaries to amygdale to the hippocampus.[2,4] Feeding releases CCK. A CCK antagonist inhibits the ability of food to improve memory, providing evidence that this is a physiologic effect.[5] Other duodenal peptides that are released during feeding, e.g., glucagons-like peptide I and gastrin-releasing peptide, also improve memory.

Ghrelin is a peptide hormone that is released from the fundus of the stomach and increases food intake and growth hormone release. Ghrelin receptors are present in the hippocampus.[6] Ghrelin enhances recall of memories in rodents and improves long-term potentiation, an electrical measurement of activation of memory circuits.

Logically, this gut–brain axis makes sense. The ability of food to enhance acquisition would allow the animal to remember the details of a successful hunt or where it hid the leftovers from the meal. When hungry, the elevated ghrelin levels would allow the animal to recall where the food was stored or what were the essential elements to the success of the previous foraging expedition.

23.3 FAT–BRAIN AXIS

Adipose tissue produces a peptide hormone called leptin. Leptin has been demonstrated to enhance memory.[7] On the other hand, high triglycerides in obese animals and humans are associated with a decline in cognition. Central administration of triglycerides impaired retention of a learned task and also decreased long-term potentiation. Lowering triglyceride levels in rodents and humans with a PPAR-alpha agent, gemfibrozil, improved cognitive capacity and cerebral blood flow.[8] Hypertriglyceridemia blocks the ability of leptin to cross the blood–brain barrier, explaining, in part, the failure of increased leptin levels in obese humans to enhance memory.

Adipose tissue also produces cytokines such as tumor necrosis factor (TNF)-alpha and interleukin-1. These cytokines cross the blood–brain barrier and impair memory.[9] Elevated levels of the soluble TNF receptors have been shown to be highly related to a decline in cognition and function. We have shown that a caloric supplement with the prebiotic oligofructosaccharide can attenuate the production of μRNA for interleukin-6 and TNF, thus potentially improving cognition.

23.4 GLUCOSE AND MEMORY

In a large human cohort the presence of diabetes for 6 years led to a two-fold increase in cognitive impairment.[10] Diabetes is associated with a decrease in reading, gardening, telephoning, writing letters, and going out socially.[11] Two studies have shown that in older persons, lowering glucose improves memory.[12,13] In addition, metabolic control improved psychomotor speed and concentration.[14]

The effects of glucose on memory display a classic bell-shaped curve, i.e., high and very low doses showing toxicity, with doses from normal to mildly increased enhancing memory. Hypoglycemia produces delirium. Glucose levels greater than 200 ml/dl are associated with poor memory. Long-term diabetes leads to vascular dementia.

The causes of memory impairment in diabetes are multifactorial (Table 23.1). Insulin is degraded by insulin-degrading enzymes, which also degrade beta-amyloid. Thus, high levels of insulin can lead to a marked increase in beta-amyloid and a cognitive deficit. Insulin can also lead to phosphorylation of Tau protein. These effects are in concert with the findings that insulin can alter memory function and that type II diabetes is associated with an increased prevalence of Alzheimer's disease.

TABLE 23.1
Causes of Memory Impairment in Diabetes

1. Hyperglycemia
2. Oxidative stress
3. Small hippocampal volumes
4. Hypertriglyceridemia
5. Elevated homocysteine
6. Increased ACE activity
7. Elevated cytokines
8. Altered amylin levels
9. Hyperinsulinemia in type II diabetics
10. Hypogonadism
11. Vascular dementia and possibly Alzheimer's disease

23.5 ALZHEIMER'S DISEASE AND OXIDATIVE DAMAGE

Alzheimer's disease is associated with oxidative damage. Protein oxidation by amyloid beta (1-42)-protein leads to abnormalities of the cytoskeleton, protein folding, neuronal communication, energy metabolism, proteasome function, and cell signaling. All of these are responsible for the neuronal degeneration that is a hallmark of Alzheimer's disease.

Studies with vitamin E have failed to demonstrate improved memory in patients with Alzheimer's disease.[15] This has led to the search for other antioxidants that may be more effective. Two of these are alpha-lipoic acid and N-acetyl cysteine. The dextro form of alpha-lipoic acid, R(+)-lipoic acid, is transformed into dihydrolipoic acid in mitochondria by private dehydrogenase. This decreases mitochondrial superoxide and increases methionine sulfoxide reductase, whose effects are beneficial in preventing oxidative damage and enhancing cell repair. While the (–)-lipoic acid may also have positive effects, it reduced glutathione synthase, thus potentially increasing oxidative damage in some cells. Alpha-lipoic acid binds Fe, preventing the Fenton reaction and thus further protecting neural tissue. Alpha-lipoic acid has been shown to decrease oxidative damage in diabetic animals and in humans to improve diabetic peripheral neuropathy.

In a rodent model of Alzheimer's disease, the SAMP8 mouse, both alpha-lipoic acid and N-acetyl cysteine improved memory. Alpha-lipoic acid restored protein carbonyl levels, thiobarbituric acid, and oxidative changes in the synatosomal membrane proteins to normal.[16] Preliminary data suggest that alpha-lipoic acid may increase the life span in SAMP8 mice.

Overall, limitation of oxidative damage would appear to be a reasonable approach to attempting to prevent Alzheimer's disease.

23.6 DIETARY FACTORS AND ALZHEIMER'S DISEASE

Numerous studies have suggested that high intake of fish and omega-3 polyunsaturated fatty acids are associated with a reduced risk of cognitive impairment.[17] These benefits are stronger in persons without the APOE episolon-4 gene.[18] In rodent models, docosahexaenoic acid improves memory in young and old animals as well as in a variety of Alzheimer's disease rodent models.[19] In an Alzheimer model, docosahexanoic acid decreased amyloid burden.[20]

High cholesterol and saturated fats were associated with poor memory, but so is low cholesterol.

Blueberry extracts reversed the deleterious effects of aging on motor behavior and neuronal signaling and prevented memory deficits in rodents transgenic for the Alzheimer gene.[21] Blueberry extracts modulate oxidative stress in cells and block the toxic effects of amyloid beta-peptide.[22] These findings are in concert with epidemiological studies that suggest that high-fruit diets may be associated with a lower prevalence of Alzheimer's disease.[23]

The curry spice curcumin has antioxidant, anti-inflammatory, and antiamyloid activity.[24] In an Alzheimer transgenic mouse, curcumin lowered oxidative proteins, interleukin-1 beta, the astrocyte marker GFAP, and amyloid beta-peptide and the plaque burden.[25] There was also a decrease in microgliosis.

Moderate alcohol intake is associated with better cognitive scores.[26] This appears to be true not only of red wine, which contains resveratol, but of all alcohol. Resveratol acts on the melatonin-3 binding site (quinine reductase 2) to reduce oxidative damage in the brain.[27]

23.7 NEUROTRANSMITTER PRECURSORS AND BEHAVIOR

Numerous studies have suggested that neurotransmitter levels in the central nervous system may be modulated by circulating levels of their nutrient precursors. Choline and acetyl coenzyme A (CoA) are transformed by choline acetyltransferase into the neurotransmitter acetylcholine. Intake of foods with high concentrations of choline or lecithin (phosphatidyl choline), e.g., eggs, liver, fish, and peanuts, leads to increases in plasma choline levels. Choline readily crosses the blood–brain barrier, and as choline acetyltransferase is normally unsaturated, ingestion of choline results in increased synthesis of acetylcholine and enhanced release of acetylcholine with stimulation of cholinergic nerves.

Certain diseases, such as tardive dyskinesia, Huntington's disease, and Alzheimer's disease, are, in part, due to a deficit in cholinergic function. In each of these diseases, both choline and lecithin have been demonstrated to ameliorate symptoms in some but not all studies.[28–30] The cholinergic hypothesis of Alzheimer's disease has been extremely well studied. Despite this, the majority of studies have found minimal or no improvement in memory function when these neurotransmitter precursors are given to patients with Alzheimer's disease.[31,32] However, there are continuing attempts to administer choline or lecithin together with agents that inhibit the breakdown of acetylcholine (e.g., tacrine) to improve memory function in this disease. Rodent studies have suggested that administration of oral ceridene-5[1]-monophosphate increases the synthesis of cytidine diphosphatidye choline, the immediate precursor of phosphatidyl choline, and that this enhances memory.[33,34]

Serotonin is synthesized when the amino acid tryptophan is taken up from the blood into the brain. Tryptophan is one of a number of large neutral amino acids that share the same transport system across the blood–brain barrier. High-protein meals decrease tryptophan transport into the brain, as the other large neutral amino acids compete with tryptophan for entry into the brain. High-carbohydrate meals stimulate insulin release, which reduces the plasma levels of all the large neutral amino acids except for tryptophan. Thus, high-carbohydrate meals result in greater amounts of tryptophan entering the central nervous system. Tryptophan has been demonstrated to increase sleep duration and frequency of awakenings.[35] An uncontrolled trial has demonstrated similar effects in older persons.[36] The potential utility of L-tryptophan in the management of insomnia has been limited by the development of eosinophilia-myalgia syndrome in persons taking L-tryptophan. This syndrome consists of myalgias, edema, indurated skin, and dyspnea.[37] Whether this was due to the high doses of L-tryptophan ingested (~1.5 g/day), a contaminant in the L-trypotophan, or a genetic defect in tryptophan in certain susceptible individuals is uncertain.

23.8 VITAMINS

Thiamine deficiency can lead to sixth nerve palsies, nystagmus, ataxia, anorexia, and delirium. Prolonged thiamine deficiency may lead to Korsakoff's syndrome, which is characterized by difficulty in forming new memories, hallucinations, and confabulation. Brains from persons with thiamine deficiency show atrophy of the mamillary bodies and thalamus. Thiamine deficiency is associated with a decrease in acetylcholine turnover and loss of glutamate and -aminobutyric acid nerve terminals. In older Irish women, thiamine supplementation was demonstrated to increase activity, appetite, and general well-being, improve sleep patterns, and decrease fatigue.[38]

Pyridoxine deficiency can lead to headache, sleepiness, dysarthria, convulsions, depression, and paranoia. Pyridoxine is important for the synthesis of -aminobutyric acid, dopamine, serotonin, and dopamine. Pyridoxine supplementation in older persons enhanced long-term memory.[39]

Vitamin B_{12} deficiency can lead to cognition disturbances in the absence of anemia. Vitamin B_{12} deficiency is also associated with autonomic dysfunction, which can lead to postural hypotension and incontinence. Elevated serum or urine methylmalonic acid levels can facilitate the diagnosis of vitamin B_{12} deficiency in the presence of borderline serum vitamin B_{12} levels. Epidemiological studies have shown that elevated homocysteine and decreased folate are independent predictors of the development of dementia.[40] However, a randomized control trial was conducted of a daily supplement containing folate (1000 μg) and vitamins B_{12} (500 μg) and B_6 (10 mg) for 2 years of treatment. During the course, concentration showed no significant differences between the vitamin and placebo groups in the scores on tests of cognition.[41]

Chome et al.[42] reported that healthy older subjects with marginal thiamine, riboflavin, vitamin B_{12}, or vitamin C levels were more likely to be fatigued and dysphoric and have short-term memory impairment. Vitamin supplementation for 1 week improved mood in healthy young males who had suboptimal vitamin status.

23.9 ALUMINUM

Dementia occurs in 5% of persons over the age of 65 years. In the U.S. the majority of persons with dementia have Alzheimer's disease. Aluminum produces an encephalopathy in cats, dogs, and rabbits that is characterized by degeneration of cerebral neurons, brain stem demyelination, and neurofibrillary degeneration. Patients undergoing dialysis developed marked behavioral changes, cognitive decline, loss of muscle coordination, and seizures. This appears to be due to high levels of aluminum in the dialysis water, and symptoms can be reduced by utilizing deionized water.[43,44] However, persons with dialysis dementia do not develop neurofibrillary tangles, as has been reported in some animals exposed to excess aluminum.[45] It has been suggested that patients with dialysis dementia have an increase in amyloid beta protein, which is a hallmark of Alzheimer's disease and is associated with memory disturbances.[46] Memory problems and visuospatial coordination problems have been associated with high serum aluminum concentrations in normal elderly.[47,48] Aluminum is strongly associated with the development of intraneuronal neurofibrillatory tangles in Alzheimer's disease,[49] and aluminum complexing enhances amyloid beta-protein penetration of the blood–brain barrier.[50]

High concentrations of aluminum in the water supply have been correlated with a high prevalence of Alzheimer's disease in some epidemiologic studies.[51] Elevations of aluminum concentrations have been reported in the neurofibrillary tangles of persons with Alzheimer's disease.[52] Nevertheless, the overall findings do not confirm a primary role for aluminum in Alzheimer's disease, but rather that it may play a secondary role in the disease due to altered brain metabolism.[53,54]

23.10 CARBOHYDRATE METABOLISM

The hyperglycemia associated with diabetes mellitus produces cognitive disturbances.[55] These memory disturbances associated with hyperglycemia interfere with the ability of the diabetic to comply with medical advice.[56] In animals, a single injection of insulin, which normalizes glucose levels, also returns memory retention to normal.[57] Two studies have shown that normalizing glucose levels in older type II diabetics improves memory function.[12,13]

Elevations of glucose levels are associated with an increased perception of pain.[58] This appears to be secondary to glucose inhibiting the binding of beta-endorphin to its opiate receptors.

Food intake (especially carbohydrates) in older persons can produce a marked decrease in blood pressure, which can decrease cerebral perfusion, leading to the "sundown" syndrome.[59]

23.11 LIPIDS

Lowering cholesterol levels in rats resulted in decreased memory retention by altering brain membrane fluidity.[60] The senescent-accelerated mice develop premature memory dysfunction, and this is associated with lower cholesterol levels than in the control strain. Menhaden oil (a mixture of eicosopentanoic and docosahexanoic acid) improved memory retention in mice.[61] In identical twins, the twin with a lower cholesterol level shows greater cognitive impairment with aging.[62] There is epidemiological evidence that at mid-life high cholesterol levels are associated with subsequent development of Alzheimer's disease.[63] Statins (cholesterol-lowering drugs) may attenuate this risk. Simvastatin lowers beta-amyloid levels in the cerebrospinal fluid.[64] However, in nondemented persons statins have failed to improve cognition,[65] and a small study suggested minimal improvement in patients with Alzheimer's disease treated with atovastatin.[66] In contrast, hypertriglyceridemia also results in memory dysfunction.[67]

Low cholesterol levels have been demonstrated to be associated with a greater prevalence of depression in older persons.[68] Whether this was secondary to depression producing weight loss and hypoglycemia or the low cholesterol levels played a role in the development of depression could not be determined in this study.

REFERENCES

1. Goodwin, J.S., Goodwin, J.M., and Garry, P.J., Association between nutritional status and cognitive functioning in a healthy elderly population, *JAMA*, 249, 2917, 1983.
2. Keys, A., Brozek, J., Henschel, A., et al., *The Biology of Human Starvation*, Vols. 1 and 2, University of Minnesota Press, Minneapolis, 1950.
3. Flood, J.F., Smith, G.E., and Morley, J.E., Modulation of memory processing by cholecystokinin: dependence on the vagus nerve, *Science*, 236, 832, 1987.
4. Flood, J.F. and Morley, J.E., Cholecystokinin receptors mediate enhanced memory retention by feeding and gastrointestinal peptides, *Peptides*, 10, 809, 1989.
5. Flood, J.F., Garland, G.E., and Morley, J.E., Evidence that cholecystokinin-enhanced retention is mediated by changes in opioid activity in the amygdala, *Brain Res.*, 585, 94, 1992.
6. Diano, S., Farr, S.A., Benoit, S.C., et al., Ghrelin controls hippcampal spine synapse density and memory performance, *Natl. Neurosci.*, 9, 381, 2006.
7. Farr, S.A., Banks, W.A., and Morley, J.E., Effect of leptin on memory processing, *Peptides*, 24, 1420, 2006.
8. Rogers, R.L., Meyer, J.S., McDlintic, K., et al., Reducing hypertriglyceridemia in elderly patients with cerebrovascular disease stabilizes or improves cognition and cerebral perfusion, *Angiology*, 40, 260, 1969.
9. Banks, W.A., Farr, S.A., and Morley, J.E., Entry of blood-borne cytokines into the central nervous system: effects on cognitive process, *Neuroimmunomodulation*, 10, 319, 2003.
10. Gregg, E.W., Yaffe, K., Cauley, J.A., et al., Is diabetes associated with cognitive impairment and cognitive decline among older women: Study of Osteoporotic Fractures Research Group, *Arch. Intern. Med.*, 160, 174, 2000.
11. Sinclair, A.J., Diabetes in the elderly: a perspective from the United Kingdom, *Clin. Geriatr. Med.*, 15, 225, 1999.
12. Meneilly, G.S., Cheung, E., Tessier, D., et al., The effect of improved glycemic control on cognitive functions in the elderly patient with diabetes, *J. Gerontol.*, 48, M117, 1993.
13. Gradman, T.J., Laws, A., Thompson, L.W., et al., Verbal learning and/or memory improves with glycemic control in older subjects with non-insulin-dependent diabetes mellitus, *J. Am. Geriatr. Soc.*, 41, 1305, 1993.
14. Naor, M., Steingraber, H.J., Westhoff, K., et al., Cognitive function in elderly non-insulin-dependent diabetic patients before and after inpatient treatment for metabolic control, *J. Diabetes Complications*, 11, 40, 1997.
15. Blacker, D., Mild cognitive impairment: no benefit from vitamin E, little from donepezil, *N. Engl. J. Med.*, 352, 2439, 2005.
16. Poon, H.F., Farr, S.A., Thonboonkerd, V., et al., Proteomic analysis of specific brain proteins in aged SAMP8 mice treated with alpha-lipoic acid: implications for aging and age-related neurodegenerative disorders, *Neurochem. Int.*, 45, 156, 2005.
17. Morris, M.C., Evans, D.A., Bienias, J.L., et al., Consumption of fish and n-3 fatty acids and risk of incident Alzheimer disease, *Arch. Neurol.*, 60, 940, 2003.
18. Huang, T.L., Zandi, P.P., Tucker, K.L., et al., Benefits of fatty fish on dementia risk are stronger for those without APOE epsilon4, *Neurology*, 65, 1409, 2005.
19. Hashimoto, M., Tassabe, Y., Faja, Y., et al., Chronic administration of docosahexaenoic acid ameliorates the impairment of spatial cognitive learning ability in amyloid beta-infused rats, *J. Nutr.*, 135, 549, 2005.

20. Hashimoto, M., Hassain, S., and Agdul, H., Cocosahexaenoic acid-induced amelioration on impairment of memory learning in amyloid beta-infused rats relates to the decreases of amyloid beta and cholesterol levels in detergent-insoluble fractions, *Biochem. Biophys. Acta*, 1738, 91, 2005.
21. Joseph, J.A., Fisher, D.R., and Carey, A.N., Fruit extracts antagonize Abeta- or DA-induced deficits in Ca2+ flux in M1-transfected COS-7 cells, *J. Alzheimers Dis.*, 6, 403, 2004.
22. Joseph, J.A., Denisova, N.A., Arendash G., et al., Blueberry supplementation enhances signaling and prevents behavioral deficits in an Alzheimer disease model, *Nutr. Neurosci.*, 6, 153, 2003.
23. Dai, Q., Borenstein, W.R., Wu Y, et al., Fruit and vegetable juices and Alzheimer's disease: the KAME project, *Am. J. Med.*, 119, 751, 2006.
24. Ringman, J.M., Frautschy, S.A., Cole, G.M., et al., A potential role of the curry spice curcumin in Alzheimer's disease, *Curr. Alzheimer Res.*, 2, 131, 2005.
25. Lim, G.P., Chu, T., Yang, F., et al., The curry spice curcumin reduces oxidative damage and amyloid pathology in an Alzheimer transgenic mouse, *J. Neurosci.*, 21, 8370, 2001.
26. Sherman, F.T. The case for alcohol in the primary prevention of dementia: abstinence may be bad for your health! *Geriatrics*, 61, 10, 2006.
27. Vella, F., Ferry, G., Delagrange, P., et al., NRH:quinone reductase 2: an enzyme of surprises and mysteries, *Biochem. Pharmacol.*, 71, 1, 2005.
28. Growdon, J.H., Hirsch, M.J., Wurtman, R.J., et al., Oral choline administration to patients with tardive dyskinesia, *N. Engl. J. Med.*, 297, 524, 1977.
29. Gelenberg, A.J., Wojcik, J., Falk, W.E., et al., CDP-choline for the treatment of tardive dyskinesia: a small negative series, *Compr. Psychiatry*, 30, 1, 1989.
30. Aquilonius, S. and Eckernas, S., Choline therapy in Huntington's chorea, *Neurology*, 27, 887, 1977.
31. Growden, J.H., Neurotransmitter precursors in the diet: their use in the treatment of brain diseases, in *Nutrition and the Brain*, Vol. 3, Wurtman, R.J. and Wurtman J.J., Eds., Raven Press, New York, 1983, p. 117.
32. Ereshefsky, L., Rospond, R., and Jann, M., Organic brain syndromes, in *Pharmacotherapy: A Pathophysiological Approach*, DiPiro, J.T., Ed., Elsevier, New York, 1989, p. 678.
33. Cansev, M., Watkins, C.J., van der Beek, E.M., et al., Oral uridine-5'-monophosphate (UMP) increases brain CDP-choline levels in gerbils, *Brain Res.*, 1058, 101, 2005.
34. Teather, L.A. and Wurtman, R.J., Dietary cytidine (5')-diphosphocholine supplementation protects against development of memory deficits in aging rats, *Prog. Neuro-psychopharmacol. Biol. Psychiatry*, 27, 711, 2003.
35. Wyatt, R.J., Engelman, K., Kupfer, D.J., et al., Effects of L-tryptophan (a nature sedative) on human sleep, *Lancet*, 2, 842, 1970.
36. Fitten, L.J., Profita, J., and Bidder, T.G., L-Tryptophan as a hypnotic in special patients, *J. Am Geriatr. Soc.*, 33, 294, 1985.
37. Medsger, T.A., Jr., Tryptophan-induced eosinophilia-myalgia syndrome, *N. Engl. J. Med.*, 322, 926, 1990.
38. Smidt, L.J., Cremin, F.M., Grivetti, L.E., et al., Influence of thiamin supplementation on the health and general well-being of an elderly Irish population with marginal thiamin deficiency, *J. Gerontol.*, 46, M16, 1991.
39. Deijen, J.B., van der Beek, E.J., Orlebeke, J.F., et al., Vitamin B-6 supplementation in elderly men: effects on mood, memory, performance and mental effort, *Psychopharmacology*, 109, 489, 1992.

40. Ravaglia, G., Forti, P., Maioli, F., et al., Homocysteine and folate as risk factors for dementia and Alzheimer disease, *Am. J. Clin. Nutr.*, 82, 636, 2005.
41. McMahon, J.A., Green, T.J., Skeaff, C.M., et al., A controlled trial of homocysteine lowering and cognitive performance, *N. Engl. J. Med.*, 354, 2817, 2006.
42. Chome, J., Paul, T., Pudel, V., et al., Effects of suboptimal vitamin status on behavior, *Bibl. Nutr. Diet.*, 38, 94, 1986.
43. Alfrey, A.C., LeGendre, G.R., and Kaehny, W.D., The dialysis encephalopathy syndrome. Possible aluminum intoxication, *N. Engl. J. Med.*, 294, 184, 1976.
44. McDermott, J.R., Smith, A.I., Ward, M.K., et al., Brain-aluminum concentration in dialysis encephalopathy, *Lancet*, 1, 901, 1978.
45. Markesberry, W.R., and Ehmann, W.D., Trace elements in dementing disorders, in *Nutritional Modulation of Neural Function*, Morley, J.E., Sterman, M.B., and Walsh, J.H., Eds., Academic Press, New York, 1988, p. 170.
46. Flood, J.F., Robert, E., Sherman, M.A., et al., Topography of a binding site for small amnestic peptides deduced from structure-activity studies. Relation to amnestic effect on amyloid B-protein, *Proc. Natl. Acad. Sci. U.S.A.*, 91, 380, 1994.
47. Bowdler, N.C., Beasley, D.S., Fritze, E.C., et al., Behavioral effects of aluminum ingestion on animal and human subjects, *Pharmacol. Biochem. Behav.*, 10, 505, 1979.
48. Yokel, R.A., Aluminum produces age related behavioral toxicity in the rabbit, *Neurotoxicol. Teratol.*, 11, 237, 1989.
49. Walton, J.R., Aluminum in hippocampal neurons from humans with Alzheimer's disease, *Neurotoxicology*, 27, 385, 2006.
50. Banks, W.A., Niehoff, M.L., Drago, D., et al., Aluminum complexing enhances amyloid beta protein penetration of blood-brain barrier, *Brain Res.*, 28, 215–221, 2006.
51. Edwardson, J.A., Alzheimer's disease and brain mineral metabolism, in *Nutrition of the Elderly*, Munro, H. and Schlierf, G., Eds., Raven Press, New York, 1992, p. 193.
52. Crapper, D.R., Krishnan, S.S., and Quittkat, S., Aluminum, neurofibrillary degeneration and Alzheimer's disease, *Brain*, 99, 67, 1976.
53. Crapper-McLachlan, D.R. and DeBoni, U., Aluminum in human brain disease: an overview, *Neurotoxicology*, 1, 3, 1980.
54. Savory, J., Exley, C., Forbes, W.F., et al., Can the controversy of the role of aluminum in Alzheimer's disease be resolved? What are the suggested approaches to this controversy and methodological issues to be considered? *Toxicol. Environ. Health*, 48, 615, 1996.
55. Morley, J.E. and Flood, J.F., Psychosocial aspects of diabetes mellitus in older persons, *J. Am. Geriatr. Soc.*, 38, 604, 1990.
56. Mooradian, A.D., Perryman, K., Fitten, L.J., et al., Cortical function in elderly non-insulin dependent diabetic patients. Behavioral and electrophysiological studies, *Arch. Intern. Med.*, 148, 2369, 1988.
57. Flood, J.F., Mooradian, A.D., and Morley, J.E., Characteristics of learning and memory in streptozocin-induced diabetic mice, *Diabetes*, 39, 1391, 1990.
58. Morley, G.K., Mooradian, A.D., Levine, A.S., et al., Mechanism of pain in diabetic peripheral neuropathy. Effect of glucose on pain perception in humans, *Am. J. Med.*, 77, 79, 1984.
59. Morley, J.E., The ultimate "Big Mac" attack, *Nurs. Home Med.*, 1, 3, 1993.
60. Kessler, A.R., Kessler, B., and Yehuda, S., *In vivo* modulation of brain cholesterol level and learning performance by a novel plant lipid: indications for interactions between hippocampal-cortical cholesterol and learning, *Life Sci.*, 38, 1185, 1986.
61. Flood, J.F., Hernandez, E.N., and Morley, J.E., Memory enhancement in mice with chronic menhaden oil administration, in *Geriatric Nutrition*, Morley, J.E., Glick, Z., and Rubenstein, L.Z., Eds., Raven Press, New York, 1990, p. 435.

62. Swan, G.E., LaRue, A., Carmelli, D., et al., Decline in cognitive performance in aging twins. Heritability and biobehavioral predictors from the National Heart, Lung, and Blood Institute Twin Study, *Arch. Neurol.*, 49, 476, 1992.
63. Sjogren, M., Mielke, M., Gustafson, D., et al., Cholesterol and Alzheimer's disease: is there a relation? *Mech. Ageing Dev.*, 127, 138, 2006.
64. Sjogren, M., Gustafsson, K., Syversen, S., et al., Treatment with simvastatin in patients with Alzheimer's disease lowers both alpha- and beta-cleaved amyloid precursor protein, *Dement. Geriatr. Cogn. Disord.*, 16, 25, 2003.
65. Xiong, G.L., Benson, A., and Doraiswamy, P.M., Statins and cognition: what can we learn from existing randomized trials? *CNS Spectr.*, 10, 867, 2005.
66. Sparks, D.L., Connor, D.J., Sabbagh, M.N., et al., Circulating cholesterol levels, apolipoprotein E genotype and dementia severity influence the benefit of atovastatin treatment in Alzheimer's disease: results of the Alzheimer's Disease Cholesterol-Lowering Treatment (ADCLT) trial, *Acta Neurol. Scand. Suppl.*, 185, 3, 2006.
67. Perlmuter, L.C., Nathan, D.M., Goldfinger, S.H., et al., Triglyceride levels affect cognitive function in noninsulin-dependent diabetics, *J. Diabet. Complications*, 2, 210, 1988.
68. Morgan, R.E., Palinkas, L.A., Barrett-Connor, E.L., et al., Plasma cholesterol and depressive symptoms in older men, *Lancet*, 341, 75, 1993.

24 Nutritional Management of Hypertension

Ramzi R. Hajjar, M.D.

CONTENTS

24.1 INTRODUCTION

Hypertension is a common condition in older persons with potentially devastating consequences if left untreated. It is a major risk factor for atherosclerotic vascular disease and may affect up to 70% of individuals over the age of 65.[1,2] In the elderly, as in younger adults, essential hypertension, that is, high blood pressure without an identifiable cause, is by far the most common type of hypertension. To some extent, hypertension is an affliction of modern society. Until recent history, humans employed the hunter–gatherer lifestyle for survival. Such "primitive" peoples experienced vigorous daily physical activity and a diet rich in potassium and fiber and low in fat and sodium. Patterns of nature led to periods of diminished food intake, and obesity and high blood pressure were virtually unheard of in those communities. Modern-day populations who enjoy relatively low incidences of hypertension tend to practice daily routines that mimic the primitive lifestyle of old, particularly in relation to nutrition and physical activity. Furthermore, blood pressure does not rise with age in these populations, suggesting that this condition is not an inevitable consequence of aging.[1,3] The blood pressure profiles of immigrants from such regions, however, may change over the course of a few generations to resemble that of the host community. The overabundance of foods rich in sodium, calories, and fat in Westernized societies without doubt contributes to the epidemic of hypertension. Data from the third

National Health and Nutrition Examination Survey (NHANES III) indicate that dietary intake of potassium, calcium, and magnesium is below the Recommended Daily Allowances (RDAs) for adults over the age of 50, whereas intake of sodium and fat (saturated and total) exceeds the RDAs.[4] Despite the multiple anatomical and physiological age-associated changes responsible for the increasing prevalence of hypertension with age, much can be done by way of lifestyle modification to retard, if not arrest, the progression of hypertension. With the abundance of effective medications available for treatment of hypertension, nonpharmacologic strategies have received far less attention than they deserve at the clinical level. This is, in part, due to the burden and high rate of discontinuation of lifestyle modification.

Nonpharmacological interventions have been shown to lower blood pressure by a few mmHg at best. It is important to note at this point that from an epidemiological standpoint, small declines in blood pressure can result in significant reduction in mortality and morbidity from cardiovascular disease.[5,6] For example, reduction of systolic blood pressure (SBP) by only 3 mmHg will decrease stroke and cardiac mortality by 8 and 5%, respectively. A reduction in SBP by 5 mmHg will increase the decline in stroke and cardiac mortality by 14 and 9%, respectively.[1] These blood pressure changes can easily be achieved with dietary interventions, and patients should be encouraged to adhere to lifestyle modifications, particularly in the absence of a discernable decline in their blood pressure. Additional incentives are the health benefits of dietary interventions independent of blood pressure.

Several dietary components, such as sodium and alcohol, have a well-known influence on blood pressure regulation and have been studied extensively. The roles of others, such as calcium, potassium, magnesium, and folate, are less established, and study results are inconsistent. Nutritional research on single dietary factors involves a host of challenging problems inherent to the study design.[7] These include:

- Many observational and prospective trials utilize food frequency recall questionnaires, which may be unreliable and do not reflect nutritional intake during the duration of the trial.[8]
- When measuring small blood pressure changes in response to nutritional factors, it is difficult to control for normal short-term blood pressure fluctuations and for the multiple compounding factors that may affect blood pressure.
- The effect of an individual nutrient may be too small to be detected in an underpowered trial, yet be significant from a public health standpoint.
- Nutrients present in foods simultaneously may have a synergistic effect on blood pressure.
- Nutrients supplied as supplements may have different physiological effects than when obtained in their natural form.
- Manipulation of a single nutrient under isocaloric conditions will invariably change the intake of other nutrients.

For these reasons, most clinically relevant trials are designed to study the influence of comprehensive dietary modifications on blood pressure, while controlling for multiple nutritional factors simultaneously. This chapter will briefly review data supporting the role of individual nutrients on blood pressure, and dietary patterns that have been proven effective in controlling blood pressure. Few trials have investigated disease outcome as an endpoint, rather than blood pressure per se. These will also be discussed when available.

24.2 WEIGHT LOSS

The single most effective nonpharmacological intervention for lowering blood pressure is weight loss, particularly in obese persons.[9–13] In the Trial of Nonpharmacologic Intervention in the Elderly (TONE), the hazard ratio of developing hypertension requiring treatment or developing a cardiovascular event at 30 months follow-up in older obese subjects randomized to the weight loss group was 0.64 (95% confidence interval (CI), 0.49 to 0.85; $p = 0.002$) relative to usual care.[14] Weight loss not only reduces blood pressure in the immediate follow-up period, but has also been shown to decrease the progression and development of hypertension in the future, even though the long-term weight loss may not be sustained.[11,14] A 5% or greater loss of body weight is likely to reduce the need of antihypertensive medications in many elderly.[15] Despite encouraging results, weight loss in the elderly must be recommended with caution, and perhaps only for those ≥10% above their ideal body weight. The elderly are at high risk for continued weight loss and malnutrition, and micronutrient deficiencies must be screened for.

24.3 INDIVIDUAL DIETARY COMPONENTS AFFECTING BLOOD PRESSURE

24.3.1 Sodium

A large number of observational studies[16–19] and interventional trials[20–22] support the relationship between sodium intake and hypertension. Reduced sodium intake has been shown to lower blood pressure in subjects with hypertension and prehypertension. Prehypertension is defined by the seventh report of the Joint National Committee on Detection, Evaluation, and Treatment of High Blood Pressure (JNC 7) as a systolic blood pressure (SBP) of 120 to 139 mmHg or diastolic blood pressure (DBP) of 80 to 89 mmHg.[23] Salt restriction furthermore prevented the recurrence of hypertension in subjects previously controlled on antihypertensive medications.[24] In a meta-analysis of 32 randomized controlled trials, Cutler and colleagues estimated the overall impact of moderate sodium reduction to be a decline in blood pressure of 4.8/2.5 mmHg in hypertensive subjects and 1.9/1.1 mmHg for normotensive subjects.[21] Similar findings were documented by He and MacGregor in a meta-analysis of 28 trials.[25] A reduction of sodium intake of 78 meq/day for 4 or more weeks resulted in a reduction in blood pressure of 5.0/2.7 mmHg in hypertensive subjects. In normotensive subjects, the blood pressure reduction was 2.0/1.0 mmHg when sodium intake was reduced by 74 meq/day. In the International Study of Salt and Blood Pressure (INTERSALT),[16] and in the reanalysis of the original data,[17] salt intake was positively associated with blood pressure. INTERSALT included over 10,000 subjects from 52 centers around the world. The 24-hour urinary sodium excretion was used as an indicator of salt intake.

A 100 mmol/day (2.3 g sodium) increase in urinary sodium excretion was associated with a 3 to 6 mmHg increase in SBP.[17]

Blood pressure in older patients tends to be more salt-sensitive than in younger ones. A sodium load is excreted less rapidly and less completely as renal function declines with age. African Americans have a steeper age-related decline in creatinine clearance and are particularly sensitive to salt intake. Decreased vascular compliance further limits the ability of the vascular system to adjust to intravascular volume changes.[1] Sodium reduction may therefore be particularly effective in managing blood pressure in the elderly. In older nonhypertensive subjects, a greater blood pressure response to salt restriction was found than in younger nonhypertensives.[26,27] Finally, salt restriction has been found to prevent the development of overt hypertension in elderly with normal blood pressure or prehypertension.

Salt restriction in the elderly is not without risk. Data on the potential ill-effects of salt restrictions are incomplete and continue to be debated. Salt restriction, along with fat and sugar restriction, renders food less palatable for older persons who may already be suffering from loss of taste. Therapeutic diets should be recommended with caution in nonobese elderly, as they have been shown to contribute to weight loss and malnutrition. Up to 34% of older patients with salt restrictions reported excessive fatigue compared to 16% of subjects with normal salt intake.[28] In a meta-analysis of 56 randomized trials, extreme sodium reduction was associated with a 10% increase in total and low-density lipoprotein (LDL) cholesterol levels, possibly due to hemoconcentration effect of volume depletion.[29] With moderate salt restriction (80 to 100 meq/day), no such effect was noted.[30]

Although the effect of sodium intake on blood pressure is clearly established in the elderly, very few trials have investigated the effect of salt restriction on clinical outcome. Intuitively, one would expect the risk of cardiovascular disease to decrease with salt restriction due to mitigation of hypertension, a major risk factor. This does not bear out in the few imperfect trials that have addressed this issue. Analysis of NHANES I suggested that low sodium intake may be associated with increased mortality.[31] In a multiple regression analysis, an inverse relationship was noted between sodium intake and all-cause mortality ($p = 0.007$) as well as cardiovascular mortality ($p = 0.006$) over nearly two decades. In another analysis of the same data in which subjects consuming a low-salt diet at baseline were excluded, a statistically significant positive association between salt intake and all-cause mortality (including stroke and cardiac mortality) was noted only in subjects who were overweight. No similar association was shown for subjects who were not overweight.[32] Several study limitations and design flaws prevent these results from being interpreted with any degree of authority.

The NHANES III data indicate that the average American continues to consume sodium in amounts that exceed the recommendations for blood pressure control.[4] Current sodium intake in the elderly is approximately 2500 to 3100 mg/day, whereas the recommendation of the World Health Organization and other groups is for 2300 mg/day or less[4,23,33,34]; 2.3 g of sodium is approximately 100 meq sodium and 6.0 g of salt. Approximately 80% of ingested salt in a Western diet is derived from processed foods.[35] The most effective way of reducing sodium intake population-wide is to consume natural foods and to decrease the amount of salt involved in food processing and preservation.[36]

24.3.2 Potassium

An inverse relationship between potassium intake and blood pressure has been documented in observational studies[16,37–39] as well as interventional trials,[40–43] but the strength of the association varies widely. Increased potassium has also been associated with decreased stroke-related mortality.[38] Several investigators have indicated that potassium has a greater antihypertensive effect in subjects with salt-sensitive hypertension, and the mechanism appears to be related to natriuresis.[7,43,44] In the Nurses' Health Study II, Sacks and colleagues supplemented potassium, calcium, magnesium, all three, or placebo in women with low habitual intake of these minerals.[42] After 4 months, only the potassium supplement group showed a modest but significant drop in blood pressure. This trial, however, did not include older subjects (mean age, 39 years). A smaller crossover trial was conducted on 22 subjects with mild hypertension age 60 years or older.[43] Participants were administered isocaloric controlled diets and supplemented with placebo or 120 mmol potassium.[43] In just 8 days, blood pressure decreased in the treatment group by an impressive 8.6/4.0 mmHg. Urinary sodium excretion averaged 192 mmol/day after placebo and 221 after potassium treatment ($p < 0.02$). The authors postulate that the antihypertensive effect of sodium may be the result of potassium-induced natriuresis. Other proposed mechanisms include an effect of potassium on aldosterone secretion, the renin/angiotensin system, the renal kallikrein system, eicosanoids, and the atrial natriuretic peptide, but none of these mechanisms have been proven. Potassium may additionally have a direct effect on vascular smooth muscles.

The elderly consume less potassium than recommended by the JNC 7 for non-pharmacological management of blood pressure. Potassium intake does not significantly change with age, but total body potassium declines with age in both sexes, in part due to age-related sarcopenia, which starts as early as age 30,[45–47] and the consequent decline in lean body mass. Nonetheless, potassium intake should be balanced against the risk of hyperkalemia, which occurs not infrequently in the elderly. The risk is enhanced by certain pharmaceutical agents, such as angiotensin-converting enzyme (ACE) inhibitors and potassium-sparring diuretics, particularly in the face of declining renal function. Some commercial herbal blends intended to replace table salt may be rich in potassium. Careful monitoring of serum potassium is essential when changes in medications or eating habits are made. Current recommendations are to obtain sufficient potassium from potassium-rich fruits and vegetables. Potassium supplements are reserved for those with low serum levels and play no role in the management of hypertension.

24.3.3 Calcium

Over the past two decades, there has been considerable interest in the use of calcium for the management of blood pressure. There is general consensus on a modest inverse association between calcium intake and blood pressure, though not all trials have consistently shown this relationship. Several observational studies have indicated a small association between lower blood pressure and consumption of greater amounts of calcium,[48–51] although the 24-hour calcium recall method and daily variations in dietary intake and blood pressure may have obscured these findings. Interventional trials and meta-analysis of these trials have similarly shown a modest relationship between calcium and blood pressure.[52–59] A few trials demonstrated a drop in the SBP of up to 10 mmHg in some subjects supplemented with 1000 mg calcium daily,[60,61] but most showed a small or nonsignificant drop in blood pressure.[53,62]

These inconsistent findings have led investigators to wonder if some individuals are "calcium responders" and if criteria could be identified to determine calcium-sensitive individuals,[63] somewhat analogous to salt sensitivity in older African Americans. Calcium responders appear to be older than nonresponders and have higher mean arterial blood pressure and parathyroid hormone levels and lower plasma renin activity. Calcium supplementation appears to limit the salt-induced rise in blood pressure in salt-sensitive persons, possibly by enhancing renal sodium excretion.[57] Calcium responders also have lower serum calcium levels at baseline. There appears to be a threshold of approximately 500 mg/day of dietary calcium intake, below which the risk of hypertension increases significantly, and above which the effect of increasing calcium intake on blood pressure is modest.[7] Existing data do not warrant public health recommendations to increase calcium intake specifically for blood pressure control,[7] but adequate calcium intake should be encouraged in the elderly for other health benefits.

24.3.4 Alcohol

The benefit of alcohol consumption in small amounts on cardiovascular health has received much attention lately.[64,65] In larger amounts alcohol increases blood pressure and the cardioprotective effect may be erased. While the mechanism behind alcohol's influence on blood pressure is not fully understood, ample clinical evidence supporting the existence of such a link has accumulated.[66–69] Over 20 years ago, Potter and Beevers demonstrated that a reduction in alcohol consumption decreased SBP as well as DBP, and when alcohol was reintroduced, blood pressure increased once again.[68] In a meta-analysis of 15 controlled trials of 2234 mostly younger subjects, Xin and colleagues found that reduced alcohol intake was associated with a significant reduction in SBP of 3.3 mmHg and DBP of 2.0 mmHg.[70] In an observational study, reducing alcohol intake over a period of 20 years resulted in less age-associated rise in blood pressure than in those who continued to consume alcohol.[69] The type of alcohol consumed does not appear to determine risk as much as the amount consumed, and habitual users are more at risk than recent or binge drinkers.[71] The cutoff point for increased blood pressure risk is not firmly established, but men who consume three or five drinks or more per day[71] and women who consume two or three drinks per day[72] may be at particularly high risk. A drink is often defined as 2 ounces of alcohol, which is roughly equivalent to 12 ounces of beer, 5 ounces of wine, or 15 ounces of 80-proof whiskey. Current recommendations are to limit alcohol consumption to two drinks or less per day.

24.4 COMPREHENSIVE DIETARY MODIFICATION TRIALS

Dietary modification for the management of high blood pressure and other conditions seldom involves single dietary components. The Dietary Approach to Stop Hypertension (DASH) eating plan was born from an initiative of the National Heart, Lung, and Blood Institute (NHLBI) and combines dietary factors known to influence blood pressure at that time. The DASH diet emphasizes fruits, vegetables, and low-fat dairy products, and is rich in potassium, calcium, and magnesium. Components of the DASH diet include:

- Vegetables: 4 to 5 servings a day
- Fruits: 4 to 5 servings a day
- Low-fat dairy products: 2 to 3 servings a day
- Grain and grain products: 7 to 8 servings a day
- Nuts and seeds: 4 to 5 servings a week
- Meat, poultry, and fish: 2 or fewer servings a day
- Fats and oils: 2 to 3 servings a day
- Sweets: 5 servings a week

Components of the DASH diet are naturally low in sodium. The low-sodium DASH plan further encourages sodium restriction to ≤2400 mg, or ≤1500 mg for those with established hypertension. Recipes adhering to the DASH principles are readily available at local bookstores or on the Internet.

Many trials have been conducted using the DASH eating plan, but surprisingly few have included older subjects. In the Treatment of Mild Hypertension Study (TOMHS), over 900 participants with diastolic blood pressure of 90 to 100 mmHg were started on a nutritional-hygienic program consisting of reduced weight, salt intake, and alcohol intake and increased physical activity.[73] Participants were than randomly allocated to a placebo group or one of five active treatment groups. As might be anticipated, the treatment groups had a greater drop in blood pressure than the placebo group, but at 4 years follow-up, the placebo group had an average drop in blood pressure of 8.6/8.6 mmHg. Furthermore, 59% of participants assigned to the placebo group and 72% of those given drug treatment remained on their initial medication as monotherapy. One might conclude, therefore, that dietary modification might avert or delay the need for antihypertensive medications in over half the patients with mild hypertension. Improvement in the serum lipid profile is an added benefit. The oldest subject in this trial was 69 years of age, and the study limitations include the relatively small number of subjects in each group.

The Trial of Nonpharmacologic Intervention in the Elderly (TONE) investigated 975 hypertensive subjects between the ages of 60 and 80 years.[14] Interventions included reduced sodium intake, weight loss, both, or "usual care." During follow-up, the reduction in blood pressure was 2.6/1.1 mmHg with sodium restriction, 3.2/0.3 mmHg with weight loss, and 4.5/2.6 mmHg with combined interventions. All three treatment groups had statistically significant lower odds of remaining free of high blood pressure, antihypertensive medications, or cardiovascular events at 30 months follow-up compared with usual care. Even a modest 40 meq/day reduction in salt intake and a 4.7-kg weight loss in obese patients was accompanied by a 30% reduction in hypertension or the need to reinstitute antihypertensive therapy at 30 months.

Many other trials conducted in younger subjects using the DASH or other dietary plans have demonstrated impressive results.[74–81] There is no reason to believe that these findings will not extend to the elderly population based on the limited data already available, but outcome trials are still necessary.

24.5 CONCLUSION

Although dietary means of controlling blood pressure have been shown to be effective, long-term adherence to nonpharmacologic interventions remains a challenge to health care providers and patients alike. Health care providers must personalize the treatment plan and choose interventions best suited for each case based on the patient's eating and drinking habits, nutritional status, body habitus, and likelihood of compliance. Older patients should be offered the range of treatment modalities available and encouraged to adhere to the treatment plan. Frequent contact and counseling from health care professionals may favor adherence. The possibility of delaying, averting, or discontinuing a blood pressure medication may add incentive. It is estimated that up to 30% of the elderly on antihypertensive medications will experience an untoward effect.

REFERENCES

1. Hajjar, R.R. Hypertension. In *Principles and Practice of Geriatric Medicine*, 4th ed., Pathy, M.S.J., Sinclair, A.J., and Morley, J.E., Eds. Wiley, Chichester, England, 2006, chap. 48.
2. Burt, V.L. et al. Prevalence of hypertension in the US adult population: results from the third national health and nutrition examination survey, 1988–1998. *Hypertension*, 25, 305, 1995.
3. James, G.D. and Baker, P.T. Human population biology and hypertension. Evolutionary and ecological aspects of blood pressure. In *Hypertension: Pahtophysiology, Diagnosis and Management*, Laragh, J.H. and Brenner, B.M., Eds. Raven, New York, 1990, p. 137.
4. Alaimo, K. et al. *Dietary Intake of Vitamins, Minerals, and Fiber of Persons Ages 2 Months and Over in the United States: Third National Health and Nutrition Examination Survey, Phase 1, 1988–1991*. U.S. Department of Health and Human Services, Centers for Disease Control and Prevention, National Center for Health Statistics, Hyattsville, MD, 1994, pp. 1–28.
5. Cutler, J. et al. Public health issues in hypertension control: what has been learned from clinical trials. In *Hypertension: Pathophysiology, Diagnosis, and Management*, Laragh, J. and Brenner, B., Eds. Raven, New York, 1995, pp. 253–270.
6. Cook, N.R. et al. Implications of small reductions in diastolic blood pressure for primary prevention. *Arch Intern Med*, 155, 701, 1995.
7. Lin, P.H., McCullough, M., and Svetkey, L.P. Nutritional management of hypertension in the elderly. In *Handbook of Clinical Nutrition and Aging*, Bales, C.W. and Ritchie, C.S., Eds. Humana Press, Totowa, NJ, 2003, chap. 16.

8. Ferro-Luzzi, A. Individual Food Intake Survey Methods. Paper presented at the International Scientific Symposium, Food and Agriculture Organization of the United Nations, Rome, June 26–28, 2002. Accessed at http://www.fivims.net/EN/ISS.htm.
9. Stamler, J. Epidemiologic findings on weight and blood pressure in adults. *Ann Epidemiol*, 1, 347, 1991.
10. Stamler, R. et al. Primary prevention of hypertension by nutritional-hygienic means. Final report of a randomized, controlled trial. *JAMA*, 262, 1801, 1989.
11. He, J. et al. Long-term effects of weight loss and dietary sodium reduction on incidence of hypertension. *Hypertension*, 35, 544, 2000.
12. Okosun, I.S., Prewitt, T.E., and Cooper, R.S. Abdominal obesity in the United States: prevalence and attributable risk of hypertension. *J Hum Hypertens*, 13, 425, 1999.
13. The Trial of Hypertension Prevention Collaborative Research Group. The effects of nonpharmacologic interventions on blood pressure of persons with high normal levels. Results of the Trial of Hypertension, phase I. *JAMA*, 267, 1213, 1999.
14. Whelton, P.K. et al. Sodium reduction and weight loss in the treatment of hypertension in older persons. A randomized controlled trial of nonpharmacologic interventions in the elderly (TONE). *JAMA*, 279, 839, 1998.
15. Dustan, H.P. and Weinsier, R.L. Treatment of obesity-associated hypertension. *Ann Epidemiol*, 1, 371, 1991.
16. Intersalt Cooperative Research Group. Intersalt: an international study of electrolyte excretion and blood pressure: result for 24-hour urinary sodium and potassium excretion. *BMJ*, 297, 319, 1988.
17. Stamler, J. The INTERSALT study: background, methods, findings and implications. *Am J Clin Nutr*, 65 (Suppl.), 626S, 1997.
18. Elliott, P. Observational studies of salt and blood pressure. *Hypertension*, 17 (Suppl.), I-3, 1991.
19. Law, M.R., Frost, C.D., and Wald, N.J. By how much does dietary salt restriction lower blood pressure? I. An analysis of observational data among populations. *BMJ*, 302, 811, 1991.
20. Law, M.R., Frost, C.D., and Wald, N.J. By how much does dietary salt restriction lower blood pressure? III. Analysis of data from trials of salt reduction. *BMJ*, 302, 819, 1991.
21. Cutler, J.A., Follmann, D., and Allender, P.S. Randomized trials of sodium reduction: an overview. *Am J Clin Nutr*, 65, 643S, 1997.
22. Midgley, J.P. et al. Effect of reduced dietary sodium on blood pressure. *JAMA*, 275, 1590, 1996.
23. Chobanian, A.V. et al. Seventh report of the Joint National Committee on Prevention, Detection, Evaluation, and Treatment of High Blood Pressure. *Hypertension*, 42, 1206, 2003.
24. Appel, L.J. et al. Effects of reduced sodium intake on hypertension control in older individuals. *Arch Intern Med*, 161, 685, 2001.
25. He, F. and MacGregor, G. Effect of long-term modest salt reduction on blood pressure. *Cochrane Database Syst Rev*, 3, CD004937, 2004.
26. Myers, J. and To, M. Effect of alteration in sodium chloride intake on blood pressure of normotensive subjects. *J Cardiovasc Pharmacol*, 6, s204, 1984.
27. Wassertheil-Smoller, S. et al. Effect of antihypertensives on sexual function and quality of life: the TAIM study. *Ann Intern Med*, 114, 613, 1991.
28. Nestel, P. et al. Enhanced blood pressure response to dietary salt in elderly women, especially those with small waist:hip ratio. *J Hypertens*, 11, 1387, 1993.

29. Graudal, N.A., Galloe, A.M., and Garred, P. Effects of sodium restriction on blood pressure, renin, aldosterone, catecholamines, cholesterols, and triglycerides. A meta-analysis. *JAMA*, 279, 1383, 1998.
30. deWardener, H.E. and Kaplan, N.M. On the assertion that a moderate sodium restriction of sodium intake may have adverse health effects. *Am J Hypertens*, 6, 810, 1993.
31. Alderman, M.H., Cohen, H., and Madhavan, S. Dietary sodium intake and mortality: the National Health and Nutrition Examination Survey (NHANES I). *Lancet*, 251, 781, 1998.
32. He, J. et al. Dietary sodium intake and subsequent risk of cardiovascular disease in overweight adults. *JAMA*, 282, 2027, 1999.
33. 1999 World Health Organization. International Society of Hypertension guidelines for the management of hypertension. Guidelines subcommittee. *J Hypertens*, 17, 151, 1999.
34. Sacks, F.M. et al. Effects on blood pressure of reduced dietary sodium and the dietary approaches to stop hypertension (DASH) diet. *N Engl J Med*, 344, 3, 2001.
35. Engstrom, A., Tobelmann, R.C., and Albertson, A.M. Sodium intake trends and food choices. *Am J Clin Nutr*, 65, 704S, 1997.
36. Rogers, A. and Neals, B. Less salt does not necessarily mean less taste. *Lancet*, 353, 1332, 1999.
37. Ophir, O. et al. Low blood pressure in vegetarians: the possible role of potassium. *Am J Clin Nutr*, 37, 755, 1983.
38. Khaw, K.T. and Barrett-Connor, E. Dietary potassium and stroke-associated mortality. A 12-year prospective population study. *N Engl J Med*, 316, 235, 1987.
39. Langford, H.G. Dietary potassium and hypertension: epidemiologic data. *Ann Intern Med*, 98 (Part2), 770, 1983.
40. Whelton, P.K. et al. Effects of oral potassium on blood pressure. Meta-analysis of randomized controlled clinical trials. *JAMA*, 277, 1624, 1997.
41. Cappuccio, F.P. and MacGregor, G.A. Does potassium supplementation lower blood pressure? A meta-analysis of published trials. *J Hypertens*, 9, 465, 1991.
42. Sacks, F.M. et al. Effect on blood pressure of potassium, calcium, and magnesium in women with low habitual intake. *Hypertension*, 31, 131, 1998.
43. Smith, S., Klotman, P., and Svetkey, L. Potassium chloride lowers blood pressure and causes natriuresis in older patients with hypertension. *J Am Soc Nephrol*, 2, 1302, 1992.
44. MacGregor, G.A. et al. Moderate potassium supplementation in essential hypertension. *Lancet*, 2, 567, 1982.
45. Flynn, M.A. et al. Total body potassium in aging humans: a longitudinal study. *Am J Clin Nutr*, 50, 713, 1989.
46. Larsson, I. et al. Potassium per kilogram fat-free mass and total body potassium: predictions from sex, age and anthropometry. *Am J Physiol Endocrinol Metab*, 284, E416, 2003.
47. Kehayias, J.J. et al. Total body potassium and body fat: relevance to aging. *Am J Clin Nutr* 66, 904, 1997.
48. McCarron, D.A. Calcium metabolism and hypertension. *Kidney Int* 35, 717, 1989.
49. Brikett, N.J. Comments on a meta-analysis of the relation between dietary calcium intake and blood pressure. *Am J Epidemiol*, 148, 223, 1998.
50. Cutler, J.A. and Brittain, E. Calcium and blood pressure. An epidemiologic perspective. *Am J Hypertens*, 3, 137S, 1990.
51. Cappuccio, F.P. et al. Epidemiologic association between dietary calcium intake and blood pressure: a meta-analysis of published data. *Am J Epidemiol*, 142, 935, 1995.

52. Cappuccio, F.P., Siani, A., and Strazzullo, P. Oral calcium supplementation and blood pressure: an overview of randomized controlled trials. *J Hypertens*, 7, 941, 1989.
53. Bucher, H.C. et al. Effect of dietary calcium supplementation on blood pressure. *JAMA*, 275, 1016, 1986.
54. Allender, P.S. et al. Dietary calcium and blood pressure: a meta-analysis of randomized clinical trials. *Ann Intern Med*, 124, 825, 1996.
55. Griffith, L.E. et al. The influence of dietary and nondietary calcium supplementation on blood pressure. An updated meta-analysis of randomized controlled trials. *Am J Hypertens*, 12, 84, 1999.
56. Kynast-Gales, S.A. and Massey, L.K. Effect of dietary calcium from dairy products on ambulatory blood pressure in hypertensive men. *J Am Diet Assoc*, 92, 1497, 1992.
57. Sowers, J.R. et al. Calcium metabolism and dietary calcium in salt sensitive hypertension. *Am J Hypertens*, 4, 557, 1991.
58. Saito, K. et al. Effect of oral calcium on blood pressure response in salt-loaded borderline hypertensive patients. *Hypertension*, 13, 219, 1989.
59. Rich, G.M. et al. Blood pressure and renal blood flow responses to dietary calcium and sodium intake in humans. *Am J Hypertens*, 4, 642S, 1987.
60. McCarron, D.A. and Morris, C.D. Blood pressure response to oral calcium in persons with mild to moderate hypertension. A randomized, double-blind, placebo-controlled, crossover trial. *Ann Intern Med*, 103, 825, 1985.
61. Nowson, C. and Morgan T. Effect of calcium carbonate on blood pressure. *J Hypertens*, 4, 5673, 1986.
62. Nowson, C. and Morgan, T. Effect of calcium carbonate on blood pressure in normotensive and hypertensive people. *Hypertension*, 13, 630, 1989.
63. Lyle, R.M., Melby, C.L., and Hyner, G.C. Metabolic differences between subjects whose blood pressure did or did not respond to oral calcium supplementation. *Am J Clin Nutr*, 47, 1030, 1988.
64. Beilin, L.J. Alcohol, hypertension, and vascular disease. *J Hypertens*, 13, 939, 1995.
65. Rimm, E.B. et al. A prospective study of alcohol consumption and the risk of coronary disease in men. *Lancet*, 338, 464, 1991.
66. Cushman, W.C. Alcohol consumption and hypertension. *J Clin Hypertens*, 3, 166, 2001.
67. Saunders, J.B., Beevers, D.G., and Paton, A. Alcohol induced hypertension. *Lancet*, 2, 653, 1981.
68. Potter, J.F., Beevers, D.G. Pressor effect of alcohol in hypertension. *Lancet*, 1, 119, 1984.
69. Gordon, T. and Doyle, J.T. Alcohol consumption and its relationship to smoking, weight, blood pressure, and blood lipids. *Arch Intern Med*, 146, 262, 1986.
70. Xin, X. et al. Effects of alcohol reduction on blood pressure. *Hypertension*, 38, 1112, 2001.
71. Klatsky, A.L., Friedman, G.D., and Armstrong, M.A. The relationship between alcoholic beverage use and other traits to blood pressure: a new Kaiser-Permanente study. *Circulation*, 73, 628, 1986.
72. Witteman, J.C. et al. Relation of moderate alcohol consumption and risk of systemic hypertension in women. *Am J Cardiol*, 65, 633, 1990.
73. Neaton, J.D. et al. Treatment of Mild Hypertension Study: final results. *JAMA*, 270, 713, 1993.
74. Stamler, R. et al. Nutritional therapy for high blood pressure. Final report of a four-year randomized controlled trial: the Hypertension Control Program. *JAMA*, 257, 1484, 1987.

75. Nicolson, D.J. et al. Lifestyle interventions or drugs for patients with essential hypertension: a systematic review. *J Hypertens*, 22, 2043, 2004.
76. Stamler, R. et al. Primary prevention of hypertension by nutritional-hygienic means. Final report of a randomized, controlled trial. *JAMA*, 262, 1801, 1989.
77. The Trials of Hypertension Prevention Collaborative Research Group. The effects of nonpharmacologic interventions on blood pressure of persons with high-normal levels. Results of the Trials of Hypertension Prevention, Phase 1. *JAMA*, 267, 1213, 1992.
78. Appel, L.J. et al. A clinical trial of the effects of dietary patterns on blood pressure. *N Engl J Med*, 336, 1117, 1997.
79. Appel, L.J. et al. Effects of comprehensive lifestyle modification on blood pressure control: main results of the PREMIER clinical trial. *JAMA*, 289, 2083, 2003.
80. The Trials of Hypertension Prevention Collaborative Research Group. Effect of weight loss and sodium reduction intervention on blood pressure and hypertension incidence in overweight people with high-normal blood pressure. The Trials of Hypertension Prevention, Phase II. *Arch Intern Med*, 157, 657, 1997.
81. Elmer, P.J. et al. Effects of comprehensive lifestyle modification on diet, weight, physical fitness, and blood pressure control: 18-month results of a randomized trial. *Ann Intern Med*, 144, 485, 2006.

25 Nutrition and Cancer: Some Practical Approaches to Management

Heidi McKean, M.D.
Aminah Jatoi, M.D.

CONTENTS

Much has been written about nutrition and cancer, and much has been written about cancer in the elderly. However, the overlap of all three of these subjects—nutrition, cancer, and the elderly—yields a dearth of publications. In considering this convergence of subjects, three points become apparent. First, malnutrition and its association with poor outcomes is a foregone conclusion among older cancer patients, as it is among their younger counterparts. For example, Fukuse and others described postoperative complications in a cohort of 120 thoracic surgery patients, many of whom had had lung cancer.[1] Evidence of malnutrition was associated with a sevenfold increase in air leaks ($p = 0.045$), which were presumably a consequence of healing impairments related to nutritional compromise. Although this study provided no comparative data from a younger cohort, it nonetheless makes the point that older cancer patients do definitely suffer morbidity in the setting of malnutrition, and that focusing upon and understanding the implications of malnutrition even among older cancer patients is a worthwhile pursuit.

Second, although few studies seem to focus intentionally on malnutrition in elderly cancer patients, shifting geriatric demographics are inevitably putting the focus of future studies squarely on the shoulders of older cancer patients. In 2000, 12.7% of the U.S. population was ≥65 years old, but projections suggest that by 2030, this percentage will increase to 19.9% and by 2050 to 20.3%.[2] Because cancer is often regarded as a disease of the elderly, it is inevitable that epidemiological and therapeutic studies will eventually—although not necessarily intentionally—shift focus to the elderly.

Third, for the time and in the absence of clear-cut data on malnutrition in elderly cancer patients, it is perhaps reasonable to consider that the use of judicious nutritional interventions that provide benefits to younger cancer patients may well provide similar benefits to older cancer patients. Analogously, previous studies have suggested that the benefits of cancer therapy are derived to a similar extent by both young and old cancer patients. For example, the North Central Cancer Treatment Group, a major cancer cooperative group in the U.S., recently published a reanalysis of one of its therapeutic trials in patients with locally advanced non-small-cell lung cancer.[3] Separate analyses based on an age cutoff of 70 years led these investigators to conclude that elderly patients benefit from chemotherapy and radiation for lung cancer therapy to the same extent as younger patients with roughly equivalent survival rates. Admittedly, nutrition support and palliative practices represent a very different discipline than the administration of cancer therapy, but in view of these data, one must assume that perhaps nutritional interventions are likely to bring about the same favorable benefits to older cancer patients as they do to younger ones.

In short, much of what follows is derived from a younger population of cancer patients, but the paucity of data on nutrition, cancer, and the elderly suggests that making assumptions on relevance of age-unspecified studies to older patients is pragmatic and justified. Thus, this manuscript focuses on malnutrition and cancer with a heavy emphasis on the age-unspecified literature.

25.1 DEFINITIONS OF MALNUTRITION

Weight loss is often viewed as a simple but telling indicator of malnutrition. The prognostic effect of weight loss has been well validated. In a seminal study from the Eastern Cooperative Oncology group, DeWys and others observed that among 3047 cancer patients, patient-reported weight loss of greater than 5% in the preceding 6 months predicted a shorter median survival.[4] Even after a multivariate survival analysis that adjusted for tumor stage, histology, and patient performance status, weight loss continued to emerge as a powerful marker of poor outcome. Utilizing this tool to its fullest extent, many have come to define a 10% or greater loss of weight, a commonly used and validated threshold, as an indicator of severe malnutrition.[4,5]

It is true that several other parameters or tools are sometimes utilized to assess nutritional status, but from the oncologist's perspective, patient-reported or health-care-provider-documented weight loss is perhaps the best. Because prescribing chemotherapy often requires body surface area calculations that include weight, obtaining periodic weight measurements on cancer patients is a routine practice in nearly all medical oncology clinics. In contrast, other assessment tools, such as the Patient-Generated Subjective Global Assessment of Nutritional Status, carry great value,[6] but they might be viewed as more challenging to implement because they are more cumbersome. Particularly from the standpoint of the medical oncologist, who, on a daily basis, participates in time-consuming discussions on prognosis, symptom control, quality of life, and end of life, a more detailed assessment of nutritional status may create an unachievable effort of time and commitment. The simplicity of weight alone, its validation, and its availability make it an ideal parameter for assessing nutritional status.

25.2 WHEN AND HOW TO INTERVENE

In the setting of weight loss or other evidence of malnutrition, a variety of interventions can be considered, but three stand out as commonly used: (1) nutritional counseling, (2) nutritional support, and (3) pharmacological therapy to promote appetite.

25.2.1 Nutritional Counseling

Nutritional counseling is a valuable intervention, but not all studies have been consistent in documenting it efficacy. Two recently published studies show positive outcomes with nutritional counseling in cancer patients. First, Ravasco and others evaluated 111 colorectal cancer patients prior to the initiation of radiation.[7] Patients were randomly assigned to receive (1) dietary counseling on the intake of regular foods, (2) dietary counseling on the use of protein supplements, or (3) *ad libitum* intake. Patients who received dietary counseling manifested better outcomes. Patients assigned to groups 1 and 2 had higher levels of protein intake and lower rates of anorexia, nausea, vomiting, and diarrhea. Some of these favorable effects were sustained even 3 months after the completion of radiation. Utilizing validated instruments and a thoughtful design, this study concluded that nutritional counseling "positively influenced outcomes."

Along similar lines, this same group observed that nutritional counseling also helped head and neck cancer patients who were receiving radiation.[8] Seventy-five patients with this malignancy were randomly assigned to one of three groups: (1) dietary counseling on the intake of regular foods, (2) dietary counseling with the added intake of nutritional supplements, or (3) *ad libitum* intake. Again these investigators observed improved outcomes among the patients who received dietary counseling. Energy intake was greater among patients who received dietary counseling. At 3 months, favorable effects appeared sustained. Ninety percent of patients in the first group manifested improvements in anorexia, nausea, vomiting, xerostomia, and dysgeusia, whereas 67% of patients in the second group and 51% in the third group described similar benefits.

In contrast to these two studies, two others show no such benefit. Ovesen and others conducted a trial that included 105 cancer patients who were receiving chemotherapy and were randomly assigned to either dietary counseling or *ad libitum* intake.[9] The group that was provided the dietary counseling ate more and overall consumed approximately 1 MJ more calories than the other group. Despite this difference in caloric intake, however, there was no difference in tumor response rates, survival, or quality of life between the two groups. Although nutritional counseling is important, the results of this study make the point that it is difficult to gauge patient benefits with the use of traditional oncology outcome measures. Overall, even if we focus specifically on the quality of life data, it does not appear that dietary counseling provided the same favorable impact as observed in more recent studies.

In a similar negative study, Evans and others focused on 192 cancer patients with non-small-cell lung cancer and colorectal cancer.[10] All patients were newly diagnosed and about to initiate chemotherapy. These patients were randomly assigned to dietary counseling or *ad libitum* food intake. The group that had been assigned to the nutritional counseling arm manifested no evidence of favorable impact in terms of improvement in the percent of planned dose of chemotherapy administered, in lesser degree of toxicity or in lesser frequency of treatment delays. Again, it appeared that dietary counseling provided no clinical impact that could be clearly measured and referenced to justify its mandatory use in all chemotherapy-treated cancer patients.

How might we reconcile the results of these four studies, which yielded two very different sets of conclusions? First, the two earlier studies focused on radiation-treated patients, and perhaps one might argue that radiation-treated cancer patients are more likely to glean benefits from nutritional counseling than chemotherapy-treated patients. Although we agree that the study populations in these trials are quite distinct on the basis of outcome and type of cancer treatment administered, it becomes difficult to conclude at this juncture that all radiation-treated cancer patients should receive nutritional counseling. Instead, we would argue that the conclusion to draw from these trials is that more research, specifically among radiation-treated cancer patients, is appropriate and worthwhile. Second, it is important to point out that nutritional counseling entails some degree of bias. It is impossible to construct a "sham" nutritional counseling control group, and in general patients tend to tell investigators and their health care providers what they think these individuals want to hear. By virtue of simply implementing nutritional counseling—independently of whether it truly helped—patients may have reported benefits. Thus, it is possible that the investigators' anticipation of certain findings, especially if these investigators were strong advocates of dietary counseling, may well have affected the positive outcomes observed in the first two studies described above. In view of this possibility of bias, it would be important for other groups besides Ravasco and others to conduct similar research and confirm the importance findings reported in the first two trials.

Despite the foregoing, it is difficult to contest the great value of a one-on-one discussion between a cancer patient and a health care provider about eating, eating strategies, and the cancer patient's personal nutrition goals during cancer therapy. Sometimes poor food intake becomes a terrible source of guilt and personal inadequacy for cancer patients and their family members, and even interpersonal strife can occur as a result.[11] We believe that an honest and forthright discussion of these issues assuages many of these negative feelings. Moreover, the cost of nutritional counseling appears to be far less than many other medical interventions that some times entail high pharmacy costs and even higher personnel costs. Although the data may remain controversial on its utility, it remains appropriate and humane to provide nutritional counseling to cancer patients who desire it.

On a slightly more tangential note, it is also important to make the distinction between nutritional counseling among cancer patients with advanced disease and nutritional counseling among cancer patients who have completed cancer therapy with curative intent. The role of this intervention in the latter situation is gaining far greater acceptance. For example, the Women's Intervention Nutrition Study (WINS) observed that among a 2437-patient cohort of women who had received breast cancer therapy with curative intent, those patients who had been counseled to take 15% of their caloric intake from fat manifested an improved cancer-free survival (hazard ratio = 0.76, p = 0.034).[12] Again, the patients in this study had received curative cancer therapy, and thus represent a dramatic departure from the use of dietary counseling for patients who have advanced cancer and have lost the desire to eat. The results of this study underscore that under some circumstances dietary counseling does play an important role.

25.2.2 Nutritional Support

Should all cancer patients with weight loss receive supplemental calories in the form of nutritional support? The answer is no. Only under highly select circumstances does a nutritional intervention appear to favorably impact the outcome of cancer patients, and usually these circumstances center around severe malnutrition in the setting of highly treatable or curable cancers. Two circumstances where nutritional support appears to provide benefit are discussed below.

First, the use of parental nutrition in cancer patients remains highly controversial, but some data suggest that subgroups of preoperative cancer patients may derive benefit from it. One study that suggests such benefit is the Veterans Affairs Cooperative Group study that evaluated 395 malnourished cancer patients, 65% of whom had cancer.[13] In this well-designed trial, patients were randomly assigned to receive either 7 days of preoperative total parenteral nutrition along with continued therapy for a few days after surgery or no total parenteral nutrition. Patients assigned to the latter group did receive intravenous therapy, but without the same caloric value. Importantly, this study did not support the use of total parenteral nutrition overall, as outcomes based on the study arm were basically equivalent. However, an *a priori* subgroup analysis revealed that those patients with severe malnutrition (n = 24) appeared to benefit from nutritional support, as illustrated by the fact that fewer noninfectious complications arose within that cohort. A few other studies, some of which included an assessment of preoperative parenteral nutrition in patients with hepatocellular carcinoma and colorectal and gastric cancer, have served to bolster this same conclusion.[14,15] Certainly the benefits do not appear dramatic, but the use of total parenteral nutrition in the preoperative setting in severely malnourished cancer patients can be justified.

Second, the use of prophylactic parenteral nutrition appears to provide benefit to patients who are receiving high-dose antineoplastic therapy followed by blood or marrow transplantation, especially when it appears that the risk for malnutrition is high. In a seminal study to focus on and test this approach, Weisdorf and others randomly assigned 137 cancer patients to one of two arms:[16] (1) parenteral nutrition or (2) intravenous fluids. The nutrition therapy or fluids were initiated very early on, during cytoreductive therapy, in anticipation of the transplant. This study allowed a crossover of the total parenteral nutrition, but despite the possibility of crossing over, the patients who were originally assigned to receive total parenteral nutrition did better. Compared to patients who received intravenous fluids alone, those who received the total parenteral nutrition manifested improvements in cancer-free survival as well as in overall survival. Other studies have observed similar favorable outcomes,[17,18] although nuances of administration, such as whether to include glutamine,[19,20] remain controversial. Although the study by Weisdorf and others was completed over 20 years ago, and although many of the subsequent studies are also not recent, their findings continue to resonate in cancer centers throughout the U.S., and these data continue to appear to be relied upon in clinical decision making.

Despite the compelling nature of the two studies discussed and referenced above, an inevitable question centers around all the other clinical scenarios where the role of nutritional support in the form of either parenteral or enteral has not been tested. What should be recommended to patients in the absence of data? Based on the data we do have available, it appears reasonable, in our opinion, to gauge the use of nutrition support on the likelihood of making a favorable impact on the patient's cancer status. In other words, if it appears likely that the patient will acquire a marked improvement in survival or a cure from the standpoint of the cancer, and if it also appears that risk of severe malnutrition is high from the cancer treatment, it makes sense to start some type of nutritional support either prophylactically or upon the onset of weight loss. Nutritionists and oncologists may have different views on this subject, but the above represents an approach often utilized by us and that has served us well to date.

It should be noted that the American College of Physicians recommends against the use of parenteral nutrition in most cancer patients who are receiving chemotherapy.[21] This well-respected group sites complications associated with the use of total parenteral nutrition in the setting where this is little chance that cancer treatment will provide a notable and favorable clinical impact. It becomes important once again to point out that decisions on when to utilize nutrition support must be made hand-in-hand with decisions on cancer therapy, and that the clinical goals of each should be in complete alignment.

The vast majority of oncologists accept the rule as outlined by the American College of Physicians, but very occasionally a need to deviate from this approach arises. Indeed, a small but notable literature, comprised of case reports and small series, suggests that occasionally even a cancer patient with incurable metastatic disease may benefit from parenteral nutrition or a more aggressive approach to nutrition support. The Mayo Clinic reviewed its 20-year experience on the use of parenteral nutrition in patients with metastatic incurable cancer and confirmed that deviating from this rule appears on occasion to be justified.[22] The Mayo Clinic experience included 52 incurable cancer patients who had been prescribed home parenteral nutritional. This small cohort represents only a fraction of all the cancer patients treated at this institution, and in fact, it represents only 15% of the clinic's total number of patients who were receiving home parenteral nutrition during this interval. In effect, it appears that breaking the rules in this manner constitutes a rare event, and one that certainly does not define standard of care.

Several aspects of this Mayo Clinic study caution against implementing total parenteral nutrition in a wide variety of cancer patients with advanced, incurable disease. First, this Mayo Clinic retrospective study focused on cancer patients with a relatively unusual mix of tumor types. For example, a large proportion of patients with carcinoid and islet cell tumors were included. This finding in particular cautions against extrapolating the observations from this study to all other cancer patients. Second, this paper describes how the philosophy of utilizing home total parenteral nutrition among advanced cancer patients is quite conservative, so at the outset it appears that a tremendous selection bias occurred in choosing patients who would receive nutrition support. Nonetheless, it is important to describe the study's findings. Some patients lived a relatively long time. The median time from initiation of total parenteral nutrition to death was 5 months (range = 1 to 154 months); remarkably, 16 patients lived for over a year. Parenteral nutrition was well tolerated with few complications.

In attempting to define factors to allow accurate prediction of outcomes with total parenteral nutrition, the investigators were not successful. Tumor grade, interval between diagnosis of metastatic cancer and initiation of total parenteral nutrition, the presence of prominent cancer symptoms, and the administration of cancer therapy after the initiation of total parenteral nutrition failed to predict long-term survival, defined in this study as 1 year or longer. In short, these investigators concluded that on rare occasion cancer patients with metastatic disease do appear to benefit from parenteral nutrition, that it is difficult to predict who will benefit, and that a very deliberate patient-by-patient assessment that carries a strong emphasis on multidisciplinary, clinical judgment must be employed when considering the possibility of starting parenteral nutrition.

Another very specific situation in which oncologists sometimes face the prospect of considering total parenteral nutrition occurs in patients with a malignancy-associated bowel obstruction. These patients sometimes have no surgical option because of the multifocal nature of the obstruction or because of their severe debility. Attempting to explore whether there is a role for total parenteral nutrition in this group, Brard and others recently reported a retrospective study of 55 patients with "terminal bowel obstruction," or an inoperable bowel obstruction.[23] All these patients had previously treated ovarian cancer. Twenty-eight received total parenteral nutrition and 21 did not. Patients who received nutritional support lived 72 days (range = 16 to 485 days), and those who did not lived 41 days (range = 4 to 133 days). This modest survival advantage becomes all the less clinically significant when one acknowledges that in a retrospective study such as this selection bias alone may account for improved outcomes. Nonetheless, this study also suggests that the role of total parental nutrition in this cancer setting does not constitute the standard of care, but that it might potentially benefit highly select cancer patients.

Although the foregoing applies primarily to total parenteral nutrition, the same conclusions pertain to the use of enteral nutrition. The widely taught adage "If the gut works, use it" is useful in deciding whether to implement enteral vs. parenteral nutrition, but otherwise the rules for when to implement nutritional support apply to either therapeutic modality. Recently, the European Society of Parenteral and Enteral Nutrition provided evidence-based guidelines on the use of enteral nutrition in cancer patients.[24] Their recommendations, as relevant to indications for their use, describe strong evidence in implementing nutritional support in severely malnourished patients in the perioperative setting and in patients who are at risk for nutritional decline during aggressive cancer treatment. Again, the routine use of enteral nutrition during chemotherapy is not considered useful, and these guidelines do not specifically address the use of enteral nutrition in older cancer patients.

25.2.3 Pharmacological Therapy to Promote Appetite

As alluded to above, a sizable number of solid-tumor cancer patients do not carry a promise of long-term survival by the time they manifest evidence of nutritional compromise, particularly in the setting of an incurable cancer. Many of these patients live only a few months, and the majority describe anorexia, or loss of appetite, as a particularly troubling end-of-life symptom. In fact, various series describe how over 60% of solid-tumor cancer patients with metastatic disease suffer from anorexia and describe it as among their top five most troubling end-of-life symptoms.[25]

What approach should be utilized in these patients, and is there any role for even thinking about the topics of nutrition and cancer together in this setting? Four points should be raised in order to answer these questions. First, in these patients, when overall life expectancy is considered short, total parenteral nutrition or aggressive enteral feeding should not be considered for the reasons discussed above. Second, discussion of options at this juncture is often most informative if a dietitian is involved and provides patients with guidance. Often frequent small meals, avoidance of food smells immediately prior to eating, and a more liberal approach to trying a variety of food types seem helpful to patients. Third, at this juncture, it appears appropriate, as discussed earlier, to attempt to assuage any sense of guilt on the part of the patient and family members about poor eating. This is a time to emphasize to patients and family members that poor caloric intake is not their fault, but rather the fault of the disease. Fourth, for some cancer patients, this is a time when pharmacological therapy aimed at appetite stimulation is welcomed.

With regard to the latter, a large number of placebo-controlled trials point to two different hormonal agents as effective appetite stimulants in cancer patients with advanced metastatic disease: corticosteroids and progestational agents. Multiple placebo-controlled trials justify the use of these agents as appetite stimulants in the setting of anorexia in patients with advanced cancer. In the first placebo-controlled trial ever performed for purposes of palliating anorexia in patients with advanced cancer, Moertel and others proved that dexamethasone is effective in this regard.[26] Published in 1974, this paper, "Corticosteroid Therapy of Preterminal Gastrointestinal Cancer," put in place the groundwork for future symptom control clinical trials that focused on anorexia. Similarly, the first reported double-blind, placebo-controlled trial to test megestrol acetate proved that this progestational agent also carries positive effects on appetite stimulation. This multi-institutional study was conducted by the North Central Cancer Treatment Group and observed that 70% of advanced cancer patients who received megestrol acetate at a dose of 800 mg/day described an improvement in appetite.[27] Weight gain also occurred: 16% of megestrol acetate-treated patients gained 15 pounds or more in contrast to only 2% of placebo-exposed patients who manifested this degree of weight gain ($p = 0.003$). After the publication of these two important studies, over a dozen others followed and have established these two classes of drugs as the mainstay of palliation for cancer-associated anorexia.

Which works better, corticosteroids or progestational agents? A North Central Cancer Treatment Group study that compared these two classes of agents found that they basically tied with regard to efficacy: 66% of megestrol acetate-treated patients and 70% of dexamethasone-treated patients improved their appetite.[28] It is hard to know for sure whether this equivalent efficacy reflects nothing more than equivalent effects based on dose, or whether the maximally tolerated doses of each might have yielded relative differences in symptom improvement. Based on what we know and based on the findings of this study and others, reasonable palliative doses are as follows: a dose of dexamethasone between 2 and 4 mg/day and a dose of megestrol acetate of between 600 and 800 mg/day appear to carry reasonable and relatively equivalent appetite stimulatory effects. In view of the fact that patients often suffer from gastrointestinal upset and proximal muscle weakness over several weeks, it appears best to use corticosteroids if patients are anticipated to have limited life expectancy, in large part to minimize its more long-term side effect profile. If it is anticipated that a patient will live longer than a few weeks, a progestational agent might provide a better option. Side effects of the latter include thrombophlebitis, impotence, and vaginal bleeding upon withdrawal. It is important to point out that with either class of agents, abrupt discontinuation can lead to adrenal insufficiency, and the empiric initiation of corticosteroids may be necessary under such circumstances.

In our own practice, relatively few cancer patients opt for receiving an appetite stimulant, in large part because these agents appear to have only limited benefits. These limitations are two-fold in nature. First, although cancer patients with loss of appetite and weight die sooner than those who maintain their appetite and weight, these agents do not reverse this prognostic effect. This point is well made in a large, multi-institutional study that randomly assigned 243 extensive-stage small-cell lung cancer patients who were about to receive chemotherapy to either megestrol acetate or an identical placebo.[29] The median survival within the former group was 8.2 months, and in the placebo-exposed group 10 months (p = 0.49). Although these agents may augment appetite and weight, they do not impact the negative prognostic effect observed with this symptom and sign. At best, they remain only palliative agents that lessen the severity of anorexia in a subgroup of cancer patients with advanced disease.

Second, these two classes of agents do not appear to provide a positive impact on global quality of life.[30] It is rare to observe a patient with advanced incurable cancer return after the initiation of corticosteroids or a progestational agent and report, "I feel 100% better than I did before starting this drug." When patients do report such an improvement, it is usually a result of either these agents providing some antineoplastic effects in their own right or being combined with other chemotherapy agents that are conferring such antineoplastic effects. The global benefits of megestrol acetate are in fact quite modest. Nonetheless, it is important to point out that appetite improvement is an important goal to strive for. For this reason, prescribing an appetite stimulant appears to be a reasonable option for some patients.

As stated earlier, data tend to be sparse among elderly patients with regard to any of the interventions discussed above. Thus, noteworthy is a study from Yeh and others on the role of megestrol acetate in older patients.[31] This study did not evaluate cancer patients but did focus on geriatric nursing home patients who had either lost weight or appeared to be at least 20% below their ideal body weight. These patients were randomly assigned to receive either megestrol acetate 800 mg/day orally for 12 weeks or placebo. At the end of the 12-week treatment period, patients who had been assigned to megestrol acetate reported improved appetite and sense of well-being. Again, this study did not necessarily include cancer patients, but its focus on geriatric patients suggests the plausibility of improved outcomes with this agent in older cancer populations as well.

25.3 CONCLUSIONS

There remains no question that malnutrition is common and problematic in all cancer patients, including geriatric cancer patients. Evidence of weight loss and loss of appetite portends a less successful outcome than in patients without this sign and symptom. At the same time, however, a multitude of studies have shown that improving prognosis with nutritional interventions occurs, at best, in only a few subgroups of patients. The initiation of nutritional support appears justified in the setting of severe malnutrition, particularly if cancer therapy offers a chance of favorably impacting the patient's outcome. Dietary counseling remains an important option. For many cancer patients, especially if the cancer is unlikely to be positively impacted from cancer therapy, the utilization of appetite stimulants might help patients.

REFERENCES

1. Fukuse T, Satoda N, Hijiya K, Fujinaga T. Importance of a comprehensive geriatric assessment in prediction of complications following thoracic surgery in elderly patients. *Chest* 127:886–891, 2005.
2. Edwards BK, Howe HL, Ries LA, et al. Annual report to the nation on the status of cancer, 1973–1999, featuring implications of age and aging on US cancer burden. *Cancer* 94:2766–2892, 2002.
3. Schild SE, Stella PJ, Geyer SM, et al. The outcome of combined-modality therapy for stage III non-small cell lung cancer in the elderly. *J Clin Oncol* 21:3201–3206, 2003.
4. Dewys WD, Begg C, Lavin PT, et al. Prognostic effect of weight loss prior to chemotherapy in cancer patients. Eastern Cooperative Oncology Group. *Am J Med* 69:491–497, 1980.
5. Genton L, van Gemert WG, Dejong CH, et al. When does malnutrition become a risk? *Nestle Nutr Workshop Ser Clin Perform Programme* 10:73–84, 2005.
6. Ottery FD. Definition of standardized nutritional assessment and interventional pathways in oncology. *Nutrition* 12 (Suppl.):S15–S19, 1996.
7. Ravasco O, Monteiro-Grillo I, Vidal PM, Camilo ME. Dietary counseling improves patient outcomes: a prospective, randomized, controlled trial in colorectal cancer patients undergoing chemotherapy. *J Clin Oncol* 23:1348–1349, 2005.
8. Ravasco P, Monteiro-Grillo I, Marques Vidal P, Camilo ME. Impact of nutrition on outcome: a prospective randomized controlled trial in patients with head and neck cancer undergoing radiotherapy. *Head Neck* 27:659–668, 2005.

9. Ovesen L, Allingstrup L, Hannibal J, et al. Effect of dietary counseling on food intake, body weight, response rate, survival, and quality of life in cancer patients undergoing chemotherapy: a prospective, randomized study. *J Clin Oncol* 11:2043–2049, 1993.
10. Evans WK, Nixon DW, Daly JM, et al. A randomized study of oral nutritional support versus *ad lib* nutritional intake during chemotherapy for advanced colorectal and non-small cell lung cancer. *J Clin Oncol* 5:113–124, 1987.
11. McClement SE, Degner LF, Harlos M. Family responses to declining intake in a terminally ill relative. *J Palliat Care* 20:93–100, 2004.
12. Chlebowski RT, Blackburn GL, Elashoff RE, et al. Dietary fat reduction in postmenopausal women with primary breast cancer: phase III Women's Intervention Nutrition Study (WINS). *ASCO Annu Meet Proc* 23:10, 2005.
13. No authors. Perioperative total parenteral nutrition in surgical patients. The Veterans Affairs Total Parenteral Nutrition Cooperative Study Group. *N Engl J Med* 325:525–532, 1991.
14. Fan ST, Lo CM, Lai EC, et al. Perioperative nutritional support in patients undergoing hepatectomy for hepatocellular carcinoma. *N Engl J Med* 331:1547–1552, 1994.
15. Bozzetti F, Gavazzi C, Miceli R, et al. Perioperative total parenteral nutrition in malnourished, gastrointestinal cancer patients: a randomized, clinical trial. *J Parenter Enteral Nutr* 24:7–14, 2000.
16. Weisdorf SA, Lysne J, Wind D, et al. Positive effect of prophylactic total parenteral nutrition on long-term outcome of bone marrow transplantation. *Transplantation* 43:833–838, 1987.
17. Hays DM, Russell JM, White L, et al. Effect of total parenteral nutrition on marrow recovery during induction therapy for acute nonlymphocytic leukemia in childhood. *Med Pediatr Oncol* 11:134–140, 1983.
18. Muscaritoli M, Grieco G, Capria S, et al. Nutritional and metabolic support in patients undergoing bone marrow transplantation. *Am J Clin Nutr* 75:183–190, 2002.
19. Ziegler TR, Young LS, Benfell K, et al. Clinical and metabolic efficacy of glutamine-supplemented parenteral nutrition after bone marrow transplantation. A randomized, double-blind, controlled study. *Ann Intern Med* 116:821–828, 1992.
20. Schloerb PR, Amare M. Total parenteral nutrition with glutamine in bone marrow transplantation and other clinical applications. *J Parenter Enteral Nutr* 17:407–413, 1993.
21. No authors listed. Parenteral nutrition in patients receiving cancer chemotherapy. American College of Physicians. *Ann Intern Med* 110:734–736, 1989.
22. Hoda D, Jatoi A, Burnes J, et al. Should patients with advanced, incurable cancers ever be sent home with total parenteral nutrition? A single institution's 20-year experience. *Cancer* 103:863–868, 2005.
23. Brard L, Weitzen S, Strubel-Lagan SL, et al. The effect of total parenteral nutrition on the survival of terminally ill ovarian cancer patients. *Gynecol Oncol* 103(1):176–180, 2006.
24. Arends J, Bodoky G, Bozzetti F, et al. ESPEN guidelines on enteral nutrition: non-surgical oncology. *Clin Nutr* 25:245–259, 2006.
25. Sarhill N, Mahmoud F, Walsh D, et al. Evaluation of nutritional status in advanced metastatic cancer. *Support Care Cancer* 11:652–659, 2003.
26. Moertel CG, Schutt AJ, Reitemeier RJ, Hahn RG. Corticosteroid therapy of preterminal gastrointestinal cancer. *Cancer* 33:1607–1609, 1974.
27. Loprinzi CL, Ellison NM, Schaid DJ, et al. Controlled trial of megestrol acetate for the treatment of cancer anorexia and cachexia. *J Natl Cancer Inst* 82:1127–1132, 1990.

28. Loprinzi CL, Kugler JW, Sloan JA, et al. Randomized comparison of megestrol acetate versus dexamethasone versus fluoxymesterone for the treatment of cancer anorexia/cachexia. *J Clin Oncol* 17:3299–3306, 1999.
29. Rowland KM, Loprinzi CL, Shaw EG, et al. Randomized double-blind placebo-controlled trial of cisplatin and etoposide plus megestrol acetate/placebo in extensive-stage small cell lung cancer: a North Central Cancer Treatment Group study. *J Clin Oncol* 14:135–141, 1996.
30. Jatoi A, Kumar S, Sloan JA, Nguyen PL. On appetite and its loss. *J Clin Oncol* 21:79–81, 2003.
31. Yeh SS, Wu SY, Lee TP, et al. Improvement in quality of life measures and stimulation of weight gain after treatment with megestrol acetate oral suspension in geriatric cachexia: results of a double-blind, placebo-controlled study. *J Am Geriatr Soc* 48:485–492, 2000.

26 Nutrition and Type 2 Diabetes Mellitus in the Geriatric Patient

Angela Mazza, D.O.

CONTENTS

Diabetes mellitus has become one of the most common as well as complex of the chronic diseases that affect most races and generations. Twenty million individuals have diabetes, and an additional 26% of the U.S. population has an impaired fasting glucose, making this epidemic in proportions.[1] On the basis of increases in morbidity, mortality, and cost, it poses a significant health burden, a fact that has been proven without doubt.[2] The objective of the third National Health and Nutrition Examination Survey, 1988–1994 (NHANES III) was to examine the prevalence and time trends for diagnosed and undiagnosed diabetes according to age, sex, race, or ethnic groups in the U.S. population and show that the prevalence significantly increases with age, in addition to being higher among certain racial minority populations. The health care use, including office and inpatient visits, attributed to diabetes in an older population was also shown to be substantial.[3,4] NHANES 1999-2000 proceeded to show that an inability to control risk factors, such as blood pressure and cholesterol, in conjunction with a rise in the prevalence of type 2 diabetes at an earlier age leads to time-dependent vascular complications, which in turn increase as the population ages and the general life span increases. Further studies went on to demonstrate that although individuals with diabetes are at increased risk for vascular disease, including macrovascular (coronary artery disease (CAD) and stroke) and microvascular (retinopathy, neuropathy, and nephropathy), improved glycemic control definitely and positively impacts these complications.[5,6]

Approximately 20% of patients over 65 years of age suffer from diabetes.[1] Although age is a common denominator in this population, these patients are a diverse group. Some have developed diabetes early in life and possess years of complications. Others are recently diagnosed and may have had years of ongoing undiagnosed complications. Some have a multitude of other chronic comorbidities, not to mention limitations in physical or cognitive function, polypharmacy, risk of falls, persistent pain, depression, and urinary incontinence. For example, there is an association between diabetes and periodontal disease in that oral health problems tend to complicate overall diabetes management and worsen glycemic control.[7] These factors, among many others, make this population challenging to treat, and considering the fact that there are minimal long-term studies, if any, to consult, we must draw from what knowledge we have of both general diabetes management and geriatric care in order to individualize treatment on a case-by-case basis.

26.1 METABOLIC SYNDROME

Diabetes in its very essence is a metabolic disorder. Type 1 diabetes is thought to be autoimmune in nature, characterized by decreased or lack of insulin secretion, and usually seen in young people. Type 2 diabetes is associated with age and obesity, but the vast majority of patients seem to have a genetic risk as well that unveils an existing defect in insulin secretion.[8] The development of type 2 diabetes generally occurs over time, involving a period of insulin resistance with a compensatory hyperinsulinemia, in an attempt to maintain euglycemia and resulting in impaired glucose levels. Metabolic syndrome is this insulin resistance along with dyslipidemia, hypertension, and visceral adiposity, which may eventually lead to overt diabetes. There are additional environmental factors that interact with genetic susceptibility in the pathogenesis of type 2 diabetes. These factors are mainly associated with a preexisting obesity, including an elevation in free fatty acids, increased release of tumor necrosis factor-alpha (TNFa), increased synthesis of interleukin-1-beta (IL-β) by the beta cell, and a deficiency of adiponectin, in addition to a multitude of other factors in the milleu.[9,10]

26.2 MEDICAL NUTRITION THERAPY

Medical nutrition therapy (MNT) is an integral part of not only preventing diabetes but also managing diagnosed diabetes. It is crucial in preventing associated complications or slowing the progression of others.[11] Tailoring MNT to the individual patient by considering aspects such as the patient's tastes and ethnic or cultural backgrounds through a coordinated team approach, including the patient and a supportive system of care, is vital to achieving this goal.[12] Older patients require additional considerations as well. Since the general population with diabetes, mainly type 2, is obese and insulin resistant, moderate weight loss is encouraged. However, elderly patients may be malnourished already, and any strict dietary restriction could further decrease their quality of life. Weight loss and low body mass index (BMI) are associated with frailty, micronutrient deficiencies, and accelerated morbidity and mortality rates.[13]

Additionally, elderly patients may fail to respond to a monotonous diet with cravings for different foods.[14] This low dietary variety may lead to inadequate intake of energy and micronutrients, which could be ameliorated with dietary education and counseling.[15,16] There is no evidence that the prescription of "no added sugar or concentrated sweets" is beneficial to elderly patients in long-term facilities.

26.3 PROTEIN

In patients with diabetes, the general recommendation for protein intake is 15 to 20% of total daily energy intake, or approximately 0.8 g/kg body weight, and as long as renal function is not impaired, there is no need for modification.[12] Furthermore, protein restriction intended for the prevention or delay of renal damage is not advocated. Protein nutrition is a major factor for the geriatric population in general because of various changes in body metabolism, composition, and daily activities.[17,18] The apparent protein requirement is metabolic demand divided by efficiency of utilization. Healthy older persons with similar protein intakes have been shown to have lower metabolic demands and efficiency of protein utilization than controls, but patients with chronic illness actually require higher levels of protein.[19,20] Unfortunately, few studies exist that specifically focus on protein requirements in older diabetic patients.

26.4 FAT

The American Heart Association (AHA) currently recommends that the average diet contain a maximum of 30% total fat, with less than 10% in the form of saturated fat. Most studies on dietary fat and risk factors for diabetes, the older population included, are short term, but there are certain beliefs that are generally accepted.

Saturated fats tend to increase low-density lipoprotein (LDL) as well as total cholesterol. However, there are fats that have probable beneficial effects.

Polyunsaturated fats decrease LDL, while monounsaturated fats may be neutral. Some studies have shown a decrease in LDL with the addition of olive oil to the diet. It is important to note that decreasing the fat in any diet will probably also result in a decline in high-density lipoprotein (HDL) and any potential benefit associated with a higher HDL.[21] The general consensus of the American Diabetes Association (ADA) is to remain flexible in the amount of fat and to individualize the diet to the tastes of the patient.[12]

26.5 FIBER

Dietary fiber has many health benefits, particularly considering the health needs and complications of diabetic patients. Fiber has positive effects on LDL and triglycerides and has been shown to be beneficial in the control of weight and blood pressure. Of most interest in diabetes, dietary fiber has been shown to decrease postprandial serum glucose values.[22,23] A fiber intake of 25 to 50 g/day is currently recommended in diabetic individuals.[12] Water-soluble fiber, in the form of whole grains, legumes, vegetables, and fruit, is preferred over nonsoluble forms, like bran. Dietary fiber is not recommended for all elderly diabetic patients. Patients who are ambulatory may benefit from a moderate increase in fiber intake; however, since part of the benefit of fiber on lipid and carbohydrate metabolism is derived from retarding food digestion and nutrient absorption,[24] older patients who are less mobile or bed-bound may suffer bowel impaction.

26.6 CALCIUM AND VITAMIN D

Calcium and vitamin D are important factors in bone metabolism, and deficiencies of either are major risk factors for fractures. Aging in itself is associated with loss of bone and can be aggravated by multiple other influences, some modifiable and others not, such as smoking and alcohol vs. race and sex. Residents of nursing homes and people over the age of 65 have been found to have a prevalence of hypovitaminosis D of up to 50%.[25,26] Since 1,25-dihydroxyvitamin D (calcitriol) is the major regulator of intestinal calcium absorption, lower calcium absorption in the elderly may be due to lower levels of calcitriol, among other factors that may affect absorption. The relationship between diabetes and osteoporosis is poorly understood, but older diabetic populations have a definite increased risk of clinical fractures. Patients with type 1 diabetes are considered to have high rates of bone resorption and subsequent low bone mineral density. However, patients with type 2 diabetes have been found to have bone mass that is greater, lesser, or equal to controls without diabetes.[27] A recent study suggests that diabetic adults with a bone mineral density similar to that of nondiabetic adults have a greater than 60% higher risk of fracture at sites, including the hip, radius/ulna, spine, and foot.[28] The higher risk of fractures in older diabetic adults may be due to associated underlying factors, including obesity, medications, and motor or neurologic impairments.[29] Considering the increased mortality associated with hip fractures, it is important to ensure strategies not only to prevent falls, but also to maintain bone density. This includes maintaining an adequate calcium intake of at least 1.0 to 1.5 g of elemental calcium and 400 international units (iu) of vitamin D every day.

26.7 OTHER MICRONUTRIENTS OF INTEREST: ZINC AND CHROMIUM

26.7.1 Zinc

Zinc is an essential nutrient and acts as a catalyst for many enzymes and a cofactor for other proteins and enzymes, as well as being important in gene expression. It also plays a structural role in cell membranes, and any deficiency may lead to oxidative changes and free radical damage of the membrane. Clinically, zinc deficiency in the general population may lead to growth retardation, hypogonadism, immune dysfunction, and alterations in taste and may manifest similarly in the diabetic and geriatric population.

The estimated average requirements for zinc are 9.4 mg/day for elderly men and 6.8 mg/day for elderly women. A study using the data of the NHANES III to calculate usual dietary intakes for adults greater than 60 years of age found that up to 45% of elderly adults had inadequate dietary zinc intakes and up to 25% had inadequate combined dietary and supplement intakes.[30] Zinc supplementation has been shown to aid in the healing of leg ulcers in zinc-deficient geriatric patients.[31] Diabetic patients have been found to have alterations in zinc metabolism and have also been shown to possess elevated urine levels of zinc, a factor that may play a part in impaired immune function.[32] The exact role of zinc supplementation in older diabetic individuals is unclear but may be beneficial in those that are found deficient in this nutrient.

26.7.2 Chromium

An important nutrient required in both carbohydrate and lipid metabolism is chromium, and it has been reported to decrease body fat as well as improve lipid profiles, both of which tend to worsen with aging.[32] Studies evaluating chromium and its use in the setting of diabetes have been largely inconsistent, and its use is currently not recommended by the ADA due to lack of definitive randomized trials, some showing beneficial effects on both insulin sensitivity and glucose tolerance and others showing none. Adequate intake of chromium in adult men over 50 years of age is 30 μg/day, and for women older than 50 years of age adequate intake is >20 μg/day.[33] A recent study did, however, find that the addition of 500 μg of chromium picolinate, the most common supplemental form of this nutrient, twice daily to a regimen of sulfonylurea in patients with type 2 diabetes improved glycemic control and increased insulin sensitivity.[34]

26.8 FISH OIL SUPPLEMENTS

Omega-3 polyunsaturated fatty acids (PUFAs) are a group of polyunsaturated fats that can be found in fish sources in the form of eicosapentaenoic acid (EPA) and docosaheaenoic acid (DHA), as well as in some vegetables, oils, and nuts in the form of an alpha-linolenic acid (ALA).[35] Several studies have evaluated the beneficial impact of omega-3 PUFAs in fish oil upon secondary prevention of cardiovascular endpoints.

Additionally, daily doses of 3 to 12 g of omega-3 PUFAs have also been shown to decrease triglycerides when used in conjunction with diet in patients with elevated triglyceride levels.[36] Currently, Omacor is the only fish oil supplement approved by the FDA for the treatment of hypertriglyceridemia. Type 2 diabetes is generally associated with a dyslipidemia that is composed of low HDL, high LDL, as well as hypertriglyceridemia. Fish oil supplementation in this population has been proven statistically significant in lowering triglycerides by almost 30% without significantly increasing fasting glucose or hemoglobin A1c.[37] The elderly diabetic population may particularly benefit from this intervention. In addition to the obvious cardiovascular risks, elevated triglyceride levels are associated with poor cognitive performance by way of decreased verbal fluency and impaired memory tasks,[38] possibly further influenced by accompanied poor glycemic control and overall metabolic abnormalities.

26.9 EXERCISE

An additional component of diabetes management, along with diet and medication, is exercise. Most studies on the therapeutic benefit of exercise up until fairly recently have focused on young and middle-aged patients with type 2 diabetes and have shown the effectiveness of exercise in reducing glycolated hemoglobin independent of body weight and the association between training intensity and the amount of change in that value.[39,40] Aerobic exercise, such as walking, bicycling, or jogging, has generally been the focus of training programs for diabetic patients, but the older patients may not be able to tolerate this form of activity.[41] Increased age is associated with a decline in muscle mass along with a decline in metabolic control[42]; therefore, resistance exercise, activity that uses muscular strength to move a weight or work against a resistive load, has been shown to be an effective alternative. Two separate trials have evaluated high-intensity progressive resistance exercise in older diabetics, with a mean age of 66, and both succeeded in showing a significant decrease of more than 1% in hemoglobin A1c compared to the control subjects.[43,44]

26.10 CONCLUSION

Considering the growing rate of diabetes, especially in the elderly population, as well as the morbidity and mortality associated with complications, caring for the older diabetic patient is a challenge that is best met with an interdisciplinary approach and extrapolation of experience in both diabetes and geriatrics. MNT is crucial in diabetes management but should be flexible and individualized to the specific patient and should not be too restrictive, which can lead to micronutrient deficiency and further frailty. Protein restriction in the absence of renal insufficiency is not recommended. Calcium and vitamin D supplementation is encouraged for bone maintenance and prevention of fractures, an increased complication that is seen in type 2 diabetes. Zinc and chromium may further prove to be supplements of significance. Older patients with hypertriglyceridemia may benefit from the addition of fish oil. Finally, exercise implementation, resistance training in particular, should be considered in elderly diabetic persons who could be suitable candidates.

REFERENCES

1. American Diabetes Association, Standards of medical care in diabetes, *Diabetes Care*, 29, 59, 2006.
2. American Diabetes Association, Economic consequences of diabetes mellitus in the US in 2002, *Diabetes Care*, 26, 917, 2003.
3. Johnson, C.L., Rifkind, B.M., Sempos, C.T., et al., Declining serum total cholesterol levels among US adults: the National Health and Nutrition Examination Surveys, *JAMA*, 269, 3002, 1993.

4. Harris, M.I., Flegal, K.M., Cowie, C.C., et al., Prevalence of diabetes, impaired fasting glucose, and impaired glucose tolerance in US adults: the third National Health and Nutrition Examination Survey, 1988–1994, *Diabetes Care*, 21, 518, 1998.
5. UK Prospective Diabetes Study Group, Intensive blood-glucose control with sulphonylureas or insulin compared with conventional treatment and risk of complications in patients with type 2 diabetes (UKPDS 33), *Lancet*, 352, 837, 1998.
6. Saydah, S.H., Fradkin, J., and Crowie, C.C., Poor control of risk factors for vascular disease among adults with previously diagnosed diabetes mellitus, *JAMA*, 291, 335, 2004.
7. Martin, W., Oral health and the older diabetic, *Clin. Geriatr. Med.*, 15, 339, 1999.
8. Jackson, R.A., Mechanisms of age-related glucose intolerance, *Diabetes Care*, 13, 9, 1990.
9. Beck-Nielsen, H. and Groop, L.C., Metabolic and genetic characterization of prediabetic states. Sequence of events leading to non-insulin-dependent diabetes mellitus, *J. Clin. Invest.*, 94, 1714, 1994.
10. Stumvoll, M., Goldstein, B.J., and van Haeften, T.W., Type 2 diabetes: principles of pathogenesis and therapy, *Lancet*, 365, 1333, 2005.
11. American Diabetes Association, Evidence-based nutrition principles and recommendation for the treatment and prevention of diabetes and related complications, *Diabetes Care*, 25, 202, 2002.
12. American Diabetes Association, Nutrition recommendations and interventions for diabetes: 2006, *Diabetes Care*, 29, 2140, 2006.
13. Calle, E.E., Thun, M.J., Petrilli, J.M., et al., Body mass index and mortality in prospective cohort of US adults, *N. Engl. J. Med.*, 341, 1097, 1991.
14. Roberts, S.B., Hajkuk, C.L., Howarth, N.C., et al., Dietary variety predicts low body mass index and inadequate macronutrient and micronutrient intakes in community-dwelling older adults, *J. Gerontol. A Biol. Sci. Med. Sci.*, 60, 613, 2005.
15. Reed, R.L. and Mooradian, A.D., Nutritional status and dietary management of elderly diabetic patients, *Clin. Geriatr. Med.*, 6, 883, 1990.
16. Miller, C.K., Edwards, L., Kisslin, G., et al., Nutrition education improves metabolic outcomes among older adults with diabetes mellitus: results from a randomized controlled trial, *Prev. Med.*, 34, 252, 2002.
17. Millward, D.J., Fereday, A., Gibson, N., et al., Aging, protein requirements, and protein turnover, *Am. J. Clin. Nutr.*, 66, 774, 1997.
18. Pijls, L.T., deVries, J., van Eijk, J.T., et al., Protein restriction, glomerular filtration rate and albuminuria in patients with type 2 diabetes mellitus: a randomized trial, *Eur. J. Clin. Nutr.*, 12, 1200, 2002.
19. Morais, J.A., Gougeon, R., Pencharz, P.B., et al., Whole body protein turnover in the healthy elderly, *Am. J. Clin. Nutr.*, 66, 880, 1997.
20. Frieday, A., Protein requirements and aging: metabolic demand and efficiency of utilization, *Br. J. Nutr.*, 77, 685, 1997.
21. Howard, B.V., Dietary fat and diabetes: a consensus view, *Am. J. Med.*, 113, 38, 2002.
22. Riccardi, G. and Rivellese, A.A., Effects of dietary fiber and carbohydrate on glucose and lipoprotein metabolism in diabetic patients, *Diabetes Care*, 14, 1115, 1991.
23. Chandalia, M., Garg, A., Lutjohann, D., et al., Beneficial effects of high dietary fiber intake in patients with type 2 diabetes mellitus, *N. Engl. J. Med.*, 342, 1392, 2000.
24. Anderson, J.W., Randles, K.M., Kendall, C.W.C., et al., Carbohydrate and fiber recommendations for individuals with diabetes: a quantitative assessment and meta-analysis of the evidence, *J. Am. Coll. Nutr.*, 23, 5, 2004.

25. Kanyamu, H.K., Gallagher, J.C., Balhorn, K.E., et al., Serum vitamin D metabolites and calcium absorption in normal young and elderly free-living women and in women living in nursing homes, *Am. J. Clin. Nutr.*, 65, 790, 1997.
26. Thomas, M.K., Lloyd-Jones, D.M., Thadhani, R.I., et al., Hypovitaminosis D in medical patients, *N. Engl. J. Med.*, 338, 777, 1998.
27. Nicodemus, K.K. and Folsom, A.R., Type 1 and type 2 diabetes and incident hip fractures in postmenopausal women, *Diabetes Care*, 24, 1192, 2001.
28. Stratmeyer, E.S., Cauley, J.A., Schwartz, A.V., et al., Nontraumatic fracture risk with diabetes mellitus and impaired fasting glucose in older white and black adults, *Arch. Intern. Med.*, 165, 1612, 2005.
29. Volpato, S., Leveille, S.G., Blaum, C., et al., Risk factors of falls in older disabled women with diabetes: the Women's Health and Aging Study, *J. Gerontol. A Biol. Sci. Med. Sci.*, 60, 1539, 2005.
30. Ervin, R.B. and Kennedy-Stephenson, J., Mineral intakes of elderly adult supplement and non-supplement users in the third National Health and Nutrition Examination Survey, *J. Nutr.*, 132, 3422, 2002.
31. Hallbook, T. and Lanner, E., Serum zinc and healing of venous leg ulcer, *Lancet*, 2, 780, 1972.
32. Gilden, J.L., Nutrition and the older diabetic, *Clin. Geriatr. Med.*, 15, 371, 1999.
33. Amato, P., Morales, A.J., and Yen, S.S.C., Effects of chromium picolinate supplementation on insulin sensitivity, serum lipids, and body composition in healthy, non-obese older men and women, *J. Gerontol. A Biol. Sci. Med. Sci.*, 55, M250, 2000.
34. Martin, J., Wang, Z.Q., Zhang, X.H., et al., Chromium picolinate supplementation attenuates body weight gain and increases insulin sensitivity in subjects with type 2 diabetes, *Diabetes Care*, 29, 1826, 2006.
35. DeFillipis, A.P. and Sperling, L.S., Understanding omega-3's, *Am. Heart J.*, 151, 564, 2006.
36. Rivellese, A., Maffettone, A., Iovine, C., et al., Long-term effects of fish oil on insulin resistance and plasma lipoproteins in NIDDM patients with hypertriglyceridemia, *Diabetes Care*, 19, 1207, 1996.
37. Montori, V.M., Farmer, A., Wollan, P.C., et al., Fish oil supplementation in type 2 diabetes, *Diabetes Care*, 23, 1407, 2000.
38. Friedberg, C., Janssen, M.J., Heine, R.J., et al., Fish oil and glycemic control in diabetes, *Diabetes Care*, 21, 494, 1998.
39. Wasserman, D.H. and Zinman, B., Exercise in individuals with IDDM, *Diabetes Care*, 17, 924, 1994.
40. Sigal, R.J., Kenny, G.P., Wasserman, D.H., et al., Physical activity/exercise and type 2 diabetes, *Diabetes Care*, 27, 2518, 2004.
41. Schwartz, R.S., Exercise training in treatment of diabetes mellitus in elderly patients, *Diabetes Care*, 13, 77, 1990.
42. Silver, A.J., Morley, J.E., Guillen, R.D., et al., Effect of aging on body fat, *J. Am. Geriatr. Soc.*, 14, 211, 1993.
43. Castaneda, C., Layne, J.E., Munoz-Orians, L., et al., A randomized controlled trial of resistance exercise training to improve glycemic control in older adults with type 2 diabetes, *Diabetes Care*, 25, 2335, 2002.
44. Dunstan, D.W., Daly, R.M., Owen, N., et al., High-intensity resistance training improves glycemic control in older patients with type 2 diabetes, *Diabetes Care*, 25, 1729, 2002.

27 COPD and Undernutrition: A Complex Interaction

Oscar A. Cepeda, M.D.

CONTENTS

27.1 INTRODUCTION

Chronic obstructive pulmonary disease (COPD) is an important cause of morbidity and mortality in the U.S. As many as 16 million Americans have symptomatic COPD; it is the fourth most common cause of death in the U.S. and results in direct medical costs of $15 billion in the U.S. alone. It is the only one among the top 10 causes of death with a continuing increase in morbidity and mortality.[1] The diagnosis of chronic obstructive pulmonary disease is based on the presence of clinical symptoms such as chronic cough with sputum production and objective information measured in the lung function test to confirm the diagnosis and classify the disease.[2]

The treatment of COPD is complex and involves interventions at many levels in order to limit the decline in respiratory function over time. The routine use of inhalers such as bronchodilators and anti-inflammatory are well-established therapies to improve respiratory symptoms; regular vaccination to prevent infections and antibiotics when indicated are also part of the standard treatment for COPD. Lifestyle and environmental modifications, such a smoking cessation, exercise, physical therapy, and pulmonary rehabilitation, may improve functional status.[3]

Poor nutritional status is associated with an increased morbidity and mortality in patients with COPD. While a number of factors have been shown to produce tissue catabolism, no single mechanism has been clearly identified as a primary cause for weight loss in patients with severe COPD. The association between weight loss and COPD has been recognized since the late 19th century. Attempts to describe different COPD classifications found that body weight may be an important discriminant.[4] This observation led to the classic descriptions of the pink puffer (emphysema) and the blue bloater (bronchitic type). The pink puffing patient is characteristically thin and breathless; the blue and bloated patient may not be particularly breathless, at least when at rest, but has severe central cyanosis. In the 1960s, several studies reported that a low body weight and weight loss are negatively associated with survival in patients with COPD.[5]

Approximately 35 to 60% of patients with COPD are undernourished, and low body weight is associated with an impaired pulmonary status, reduced diaphragmatic mass, lower exercise capacity, and higher mortality rate than seen in adequately nourished individuals with this condition. Weight loss in COPD is a consequence of increased energy requirements and unbalanced dietary intake. Both metabolic and mechanical inefficiency contribute to the elevated energy expenditure. An imbalance between protein synthesis and protein breakdown may cause a disproportionate depletion of fat-free mass in some patients.[6]

Weight loss includes both fat and lean body mass, and it may occur even in the presence of an appropriate dietary intake for predicted energy requirements. Malnourished patients have worse scores on a respiratory disease-specific quality of life questionnaire than well-nourished individuals.[7]

27.2 WEIGHT LOSS AND BODY COMPOSITION IN COPD

Weight loss in patients with COPD may be a multifactorial phenomenon, resulting from a combination of various pathophysiological events. Abnormalities in energy balance, increased levels of cytokines, chronic hypoxia, exacerbations of COPD, and corticosteroid intake can all influence food intake, substrate utilization, and metabolic efficiency.[8] Weight loss and particular loss of fat mass occur if energy expenditure exceeds dietary intake. More specifically, muscle wasting is a consequence of an imbalance between protein synthesis and protein breakdown. Alterations in both parts of the energy balance have been extensively reported in COPD.

Airflow obstruction and loss of alveolar structure have been commonly pointed as the hallmarks for COPD symptoms, even though skeletal muscle dysfunction is also an important determinant of symptoms like dyspnea and impaired exercise.[9]

Muscle mass is the single largest tissue of body cell mass and can be assessed indirectly in clinically stable individuals by measurement of fat-free mass (FFM). The importance of measuring FFM, indicating loss of muscle mass, contributes significantly to peripheral muscle weakness and impaired exercise tolerance in COPD, as well as to health-related quality of life.[10] Patients with an FFM lower than normal are characterized as having a lower peak oxygen consumption, lower peak work rate, and early onset of lactic acidosis compared to individuals with normal FFM.

Body weight and composition are significantly different between patients with chronic bronchitis and the group of patients with emphysema, as shown by Engelen et al.: lean mass depletion was found in 37% of the emphysema patients compared to only 12% of the chronic bronchitis patients. Body weight, body mass index (BMI), and FFM index were lower in the emphysema group than in healthy controls, and these results were the consequence of a lower lean mass index and a lower bone mineral content.[11]

Fat mass also plays an important role in energy metabolism besides being just an energy reservoir. Fat produces the adipocyte-derived hormone leptin, the feedback mechanism to the brain for fat mass regulation, increases thermogenesis, and has a role regulating the lipid and glucose balance. Serum leptin levels are lower in COPD patients than in healthy individuals, and also correlates well with body mass index and percentage of fat.[12] Furthermore, leptin levels have been reported to be significantly lower in patients with emphysema (30%) than in patients with chronic bronchitis (11%), and a link among leptin levels, cytokines, and tumor necrosis soluble receptor (sTNF-R) levels in emphysematous patients was reported.[12] Leptin and sTNF-R55 are inversely related to dietary intake adjusted for resting energy expenditure.[13]

27.3 ABNORMALITIES IN ENERGY BALANCE

In mammals, there is a very tight connection between oxygen consumption and adenosine-5'-triphosphate (ATP) production and utilization; 90% of oxygen consumption is responsible for 90% of ATP synthesis, and 10% of ATP synthesis in our body is independent of oxygen. Under normal conditions, the rate of oxygen delivery to the cell must be precisely adjusted to avoid excessive free radical production. The mitochondrial respiratory chain is an essential element in the transduction of energy during life. Mitochondria occupy a pivotal position in aerobic ATP reduction through oxidative phosphorylation of adenosine diphosphate (ADP). All energy-producing reactions generate reducing equivalents in the form of reduced nicotinamide adenine dinucleotide (NADH) and reducing flavins, which are ultimately oxidized by oxygen through a chain of oxidoreduction reactions occurring in complexes that reside in the inner mitochondrial membrane.[14] This process of oxidative phosphorylation is pushed by the redox potential (NADH/NAD) and is limited by the phosphate potential (ATP/ADP.Pi).

Loss of fat mass is seen in undernourished patients as a result of reduced caloric intake or increased energy expenditure. Total energy expenditure can be considered the score of resting energy expenditure (REE), diet-induced thermogenesis, and energy spent during daily activities. REE comprises the sleeping metabolic rate and the energy cost of arousal, and it amounts to about 70% of total energy expenditure in sedentary persons.

Pulmonary symptoms such as shortness of breath and cough can cause loss of appetite and energy for eating. Shortness of breath may increase during the effort of eating, making this an unpleasant task. It is difficult to swallow and breathe at the same time, and the extremely dyspnoeic patient may be unable to coordinate breathing alternately with swallowing in an efficient manner.[15]

Schols et al.[13] reported an inadequate dietary intake for energy expenditure, especially in the more disabled COPD population; these authors found that sTNF-R55, a marker of inflammation, and leptin were significantly related to dietary intake in absolute terms as well as adjusted for REE. This theory has been emphasized with the studies by Creutzber et al.,[30] demonstrating a significant relationship between baseline dietary intake and soluble intracellular adhesion molecule-1. Aging, relative anorexia, and elevated systemic inflammatory markers, as assessed by circulating levels of sTNF-R55, might be associated with nonresponses to nutritional therapy.[16]

Mannix et al. found that malnourished patients with COPD tend to have lower forced expiratory volume in 1 second (FEV1) and forced vital capacity values, higher carbon dioxide partial pressure, lower arterial pH values, and elevated total energy expenditure; this may be largely because of an elevated *cost of breathing* in these patients.[31]

27.4 INFLAMMATORY MARKERS

Cytokine production and release during smoking and frequent infections may contribute to the anorexia and weight loss in COPD patients. The cytokine profile is unique, and unlike that seen in asthma patients, increased levels of tumor necrosis factor (TNF)-, interleukin (IL)-1, and interleukin-8 may induce a catabolic response in tissues, triggering muscle proteolysis with increasing protein degradation. Multiple molecules, including leukotrienes, hormones, TNF-, C-reactive protein, and lipolysaccharide, have been associated with increases in REE and weight loss in patients with COPD, even though elevated circulating levels of TNF- are strongly associated with impaired oxygen delivery in weight-losing patients.[17]

Chronic hypoxia is another potent stimulus to cytokine production, increasing the synthesis of IL-1B and TNF- in human macrophages in stable malnourished patients with COPD. In addition, inverse correlations between soluble TNF receptor levels and percentage of fat have been noted in this group of patients. The exact mechanism to explain this phenomenon is under study; however, evidence suggests that hypoxia may induce TNF- expression via induction of the NF- pathway in rats and mammalian cell cultures. Cyclic adenosine monophosphate response elements (CREs), which are responsible for inhibiting TNF- expression, are also diminished by hypoxia.[18]

Hypoxia is also thought to reduce serum insulin-like growth factor (IGF)-1 levels and cause grow impairment and tissue catabolism in chronic hypoxemic patients. IGF-1 injections have been shown to increase weight in hypoxic rats, as well as increase the serum total protein and albumin when the hypoxic exposure was terminated.[19]

27.5 PROTEIN AND MUSCLE DEGRADATION IN COPD

Depletion of FFM is a prominent finding in COPD patients. Accelerated muscle proteolysis is considered the primary cause of the loss of lean body mass, not only in COPD, but also in many other chronic diseases. The ubiquitin–proteaosome pathway is perhaps the most important during the normal turnover of most cellular proteins in catabolic states; this is a multienzymatic process of degradation that requires ATP.

The activation of the ubiquitine–proteasome system occurs in many clinical conditions involving elevated glucocorticoid levels and acidosis. Glucocorticoids together with other signals are required to increase messenger RNAs encoding ubiquitin and proteasome subunits; glucocorticoids also inhibit protein synthesis and the transport of amino acids into the muscle to promote the mobilization of amino acids for gluconeogenesis.[20]

Fiber types can be classified based on differences in immunoreactivity for antibodies specific to different myosin heavy-chain (MHC) isoforms. In human muscles, three different MHC isoforms are expressed: MHC-1, MHC-2A, and MHC-2B. In the same way, myosin light-chain (MLC) isoforms can be determined. The following MLC isoforms can be discerned: the fast and slow isoforms of regulatory MLC (MLC-2s and MLC-2f) and three isoforms of alkaline MLC (MLC-1s, MLC-1f, and MLC-3f). Satta et al.[32] studied the fiber type composition of the musculus vastus lateralis in COPD patients. They found that the proportion of the fast MHC-2B isoform was increased in patients with COPD. While diffusing capacity, vital capacity, and FEV1 were positively correlated with slow MHC isoform content, only diffusing capacity was negatively correlated with fast MHC isoform content. The coordinated expression between MHC and MLC isoforms was also altered in COPD patients, suggesting that the coordinated protein expression was lost in the skeletal muscles of COPD patients. The authors suggest that these changes can partially be explained by reduced availability of oxygen. An impaired diffusing capacity is generally considered a feature of emphysema in a COPD population, and arterial oxygen desaturation is a frequently reported finding in patients with impaired diffusing capacity.[21]

These adaptations of skeletal muscle toward a predominance of anaerobic glycolytic type 2 muscle fibers affect the aerobic capacity of the muscle and may cause the type 2 predominant muscle to be more prone to fatigue, because anaerobic fibers synthesize ATP less efficiently than aerobic metabolism, and because production of lactic acid is markedly higher.

27.6 NUTRITIONAL INTERVENTIONS IN COPD PATIENTS

The first clinical trials investigating the effectiveness of nutritional intervention consisted of nutritional supplementation by means of oral liquid supplements or enteral nutrition. Short-term studies (2 to 3 weeks)[22] showed a significant increase in body weight and respiratory muscle function. This short-term effectiveness is probably partly related to repletion of muscle water and potassium, as well as constitution of muscle protein nitrogen. Only one study addressed the immune response to short-term nutritional intervention in nine patients with advanced COPD. Refeeding and weight gain were associated with a significant increase in absolute lymphocyte count and with an increase in reactivity to skin test antigens after 21 days of refeeding.[22]

Also, for patients not responding to oral supplementation, prolonged interventions of 4 months with nocturnal enteral nutrition support via percutaneous endoscopic gastrostomy tube were provided. The treated group had nightly enteral feeding adjusted to maintain a total daily caloric intake greater than two times the measured resting metabolic rate for sustained weight gain. Despite the magnitude of the intervention, a mean weight gain of only 3.3% (0.2 kg/week) was seen in the treated group. The majority of increase in body weight was fat mass, and no significant improvement of physiologic function was observed. The limited therapeutic impact of isolated aggressive nutrition support could be related to the fact that the selected patients (weight-losing, unresponsive to oral supplements) were both hypermetabolic and hypercatabolic, or results could be attributed to the absence of a comprehensive rehabilitative strategy.[23–27]

The effect of oral nutritional supplementation during acute exacerbation of COPD has been evaluated. Thirty-three adults hospitalized for an acute exacerbation of COPD were randomly assigned to receive extra nutritional support or regular hospital care. Almost all patients were in negative nitrogen balance, indicating muscle wasting. The degree of muscle wasting was strongly correlated with the dose of corticosteroids. An additional intake of 10 kcal/kg/day was achieved in the supplemented group. After 2 weeks, the percentage of predicted forced vital capacity improved in the treatment group but declined in the control group (+8.7% vs. +3.5%, respectively, $p = 0.015$). No change in the FEV1 was seen ($p = 0.10$). There were no changes in handgrip strength or respiratory muscle strength. A trend toward more improvement in the general well-being score was seen (+11.96 vs. +10.25, $p = 0.07$). The use of corticosteroids in these patients may have contributed to muscle wasting.[24]

Use of anabolic steroids has been associated with increases in body mass index, lean body mass, and anthropometric measures of arm and thigh circumference. No significant changes in endurance exercise capacity have been demonstrated. In a prospective, randomized, controlled, double-blind study of 17 undernourished men with COPD undergoing pulmonary rehabilitation, 250 mg of testosterone was administered intramuscularly at baseline, and 12 mg of stanozolol per day was given orally for 27 weeks in the study group and compared with placebo. Weight increased in 9 of 10 persons who received anabolic steroids (mean weight gain = +1.8 kg ± 0.5 kg) compared with a loss in the control group (–0.4 kg ± 0.2 kg, $p < 0.05$). No change in the 6-minute walking distance or in maximal exercise capacity was identified in either group.[25–28]

Recombinant human growth hormone (rhGH) treatment has been studied in patients with stable COPD. Sixteen patients whose mean age was 66 years and whose weight was 77% of ideal body weight were randomly assigned to receive 0.15 IU/kg rhGH or placebo. After 21 days, body weight was similar in the two groups, but lean body mass increased by 2.3 ± 1.6 kg in the rhGH group compared with 1.1 ± 0.9 kg in the control group. By 81 days, patients in both groups had lost some of the weight gained, but the rhGH group retained more weight than the control group (1.9 ± 1.6 kg vs. 0.7 ± 2.1 kg, $p < 0.05$). The changes in maximal respiratory pressures, handgrip strength, maximal exercise capacity, and subjective well-being were similar in the two groups. Paradoxically, the 6-minute walking distance decreased in the rhGH group (−13% ± 31%) and increased in the control group (+10% ± 14%, $p < 0.01$). Despite an increase in lean body mass, administration of 0.15 IU/kg rhGH does not improve muscle strength or exercise tolerance in underweight patients with COPD.[26–29]

27.7 CONCLUSIONS

Nutritional depletion in COPD is common and has a negative impact on respiratory as well as skeletal muscle function, contributing to the morbidity and mortality of this condition. Strategies directed toward increasing energy balance in order to increase weight and FFM are very valuable.

Most COPD patients tolerate CHO loads; however, diet content and volume per meal may have to be modified for patients with severe dyspnea or hypercapnia. Although short-term studies of nutritional supplementation have reported a positive nitrogen balance, weight gain, and improved muscle function, nutritional support for >2 weeks did not show a significant effect in any of the main outcomes measured.

The poor response to anabolic steroids may be related to the effects of systemic inflammation on dietary intake and catabolism. Evidence for a relationship between metabolic changes and cytokine-induced inflammatory mediators has been reported among patients with COPD. Studies of nutritional repletion in COPD suggest that cytokine-induced inflammation may be the source of the nutritional deficiencies. If that is true, nutritional supplementation may not overcome this effect.

Alternative approaches to increasing appetite and caloric intake are to be encouraged. A more precise understanding of the pathophysiology of weight loss and the alterations in cellular metabolism will assist with identifying the nutritional approaches most likely to be successful for those with COPD.

REFERENCES

1. Thomas DR. Dietary prescription for chronic obstructive pulmonary disease. *Clin Geriatr Med* 2002;18:835–839.
2. Mannino DM, Buist AS, Petty TL, et al. Lung function and mortality in the United States: data from the First National Health and Nutrition Examination Survey follow up study. *Thorax* 2003;58:388–393.
3. Owens MW, Markewitz BA, Payne DK. Outpatient management of chronic obstructive pulmonary disease. *Am J Med Sci* 1999;318:79–83.
4. Filley GF, Beckwitt HJ, Reever JT, et al. Chronic obstructive bronchopulmonary disease. 2. Oxygen transport in two clinical types. *Am J Med* 1968;44:26–38.
5. Vandenbergh E, Woestijne vdKP, Gyselen A. Weight changes in the terminal stages of chronic obstructive pulmonary disease. *Am Rev Respir Dis* 1967;95:556–566.
6. Schols AM. Nutrition in chronic obstructive pulmonary disease. *Curr Opin Pulm Med* 2000;6:110–115.
7. Goris AHC, Schols AM, Weling-Sheeoers CAP, et al. Tissue depletion in relation to physical function and quality of life in patients with severe COPD. *Am J Respir Crit Care Med* 1997;A498.

8. Congleton J. The pulmonary cachexia syndrome: aspects of energy balance. *Proc Nutr Soc* 1999;58:321–328.
9. Statement A. Skeletal muscle dysfunction in chronic obstructive pulmonary disease. *Am J Respir Crit Care Med* 1999;159:S1–S40.
10. Shoup R, Dalsky G, Warner S, et al. Body composition and health-related quality of life in patients with obstructive airways disease. *Eur Respir J* 1997;10:1576–1580.
11. Engelen J, Schols A, Lamers R, et al. Different patterns of chronic tissue wasting among emphysema and chronic bronchitis patients. *Clin Nutr* 1999;18:275–280.
12. Takabatake N, Nakamura H, Abe S. Circulating leptin in patients with chronic obstructive pulmonary disease. *Am J Respir Crit Care Med* 1999;159:1215–1219.
13. Schols A, Creutzberg E, Buurman W, et al. Plasma leptin is related to pro-inflammatory status and dietary intake in patients with COPD. *Am J Respir Crit Care Med* 1999;160:1220–1226.
14. Wallace DC, Zheng XX, Lott MT, et al. Familial mitochondrial encephamalomyopathy (MERRF): genetic, pathophysiological and biochemical characterization of a mitochondrial DNA disease. *Cell* 1998;55:601–610.
15. Berry J, Baum C. Reversal of chronic obstructive pulmonary disease-associated weight loss. *Drugs* 2004;64:1041–1052.
16. Emiel FM, Wouters MD. Nutrition and metabolism in COPD. *Chest* 2000;17:274–280.
17. Pitsiou G, Kyriazis G, Hatrzizisi O, et al. Tumor necrosis factor-alpha serum levels, weight loss and tissue oxygenation in chronic obstructive pulmonary disease. *Respir Med* 2002;96:594–598.
18. Takabatake N, Nakamura H, Abe S. The relationship between chronic hypoxemia and activation of the tumor necrosis factor-alpha system in patients with chronic obstructive pulmonary disease. *Am J Respir Crit Care Med* 2000;161:1179–1184.
19. Ioko Y, Tatsumi K, Sugito K, et al. Effects of insulin-like growth factor on weight gain in chronic hypoxic rats. *J Cardiovasc Pharmacol* 2002;29:636–642.
20. Wing SS, Goldberg AL. Glucocorticoids activate the ATP-ubiquitin-dependent proteolytic system in skeletal muscle during fasting. *Am J Physiol* 1993;262:E668–E676.
21. Engelen M, Schols A, Does J, et al. Altered glutamate metabolism is associated with reduced muscle glutathione levels in patients with emphysema. *Am J Respir Crit Care Med* 2000;161:98–103.
22. Schols AM. Nutrition in chronic obstructive pulmonary disease. *Curr Opin Pulm Med* 2000;6:110–115.
23. Danahoe M, Mancino J, Constantino J, et al. The effect of an aggressive support regimen on body composition in patients with severe COPD and weight loss. *Am J Respir Crit Care Med* 1994;149:A313.
24. Saudny-Unterberger H, Martin JG, Gray DK. Impact of nutritional support on functional status during an acute exacerbation of chronic obstructive pulmonary disease. *Am J Respir Crit Care Med* 1997;156:794–799.
25. Ferreira IM, Verreschi IT, Nery LE, et al. The influence of 6 months of oral anabolic steroids on body mass and respiratory muscles in undernourished COPD patients. *Chest* 1998;114:19–28.
26. Burdet L, de Muralt B, Schutz Y et al. Administration of growth hormone to underweight patients with chronic obstructive pulmonary disease. A prospective randomized controlled trial. *Am J Respir Crit Care Med* 1997;156:1800–1806.
27. Ferreira I, Brooks D, Lacasse Y. Nutritional intervention in COPD: a systematic overview. *Chest* 2001;119;353–363.

28. Ferreira I, Brooks D, Lacasse Y, et al. Nutritional support for individuals with COPD: a meta-analysis. *Chest* 2000;117:672–678.
29. Romieu I, Trenga C. Diet and obstructive lung disease. *Epidemiol Rev* 2001;23:268–287.
30. Creutzberg EG, Wouters EF, Mostert R, et al. Efficacy of nutritional supplementation therapy in depleted patients with chronic obstructive pulmonary disease. *Nutrition* 2003;19:120–7.
31. Mannix ET, Manfredi F, Farber M. Elevated O^2 cost of ventilation contributes to tissue wasting in COPD. *Chest* 1999;115:708–13.
32. Satta A, Migliori GB, Spanevello A, et al. Fibre types in skeletal muscles of chronic obstructive pulmonary disease patients related to respiratory function and exercise tolerance. *Eur Respir J* 1997;10:2853–60.

28 Nutrition and Gastrointestinal Function

M. Louay Omran, M.D.
Wasseem Aneed, M.D.

CONTENTS

Despite an earlier increase in body weight, older persons experience a loss in both lean body mass and bone mass by the seventh decade. The loss of lean tissue, with the accompanied rise in the proportion of body fat, is mirrored by a decline in physical and metabolic output. The term *anorexia of aging* was coined to reflect the poor appetite and decreased appreciation of food commonly seen in older persons. Weight loss, however, can also be due to difficulties with food ingestion, intestinal absorption, or nutrient metabolism.

Gastrointestinal (GI) complaints are very common in older adults. While many changes in the function of the gastrointestinal system are considered aging related, only a few play a role in developing gastrointestinal pathology. The prevalence of gastrointestinal complaints in older persons can be attributed to chronic disease conditions rather than aging itself. Based on that, it is not surprising that many of the slowly developing conditions affecting the gastrointestinal tract are almost exclusively diseases of aging (Table 28.1).

This chapter covers the normal gastrointestinal functions with the relevant changes experienced by older persons. It will also discuss common conditions affecting the gastrointestinal system and their mutual effect on nutrition.

TABLE 28.1
Changes with Aging in Gastrointestinal Function with Resulting Morbidity and Nutritional Consequences

Change Observed with Aging	Cause	Consequence
Delayed swallowing	Incomplete relaxation of UES and LES	Increased mealtime
Increased gastroesophageal reflux (GER)	Decreased LES resting pressure with or without hiatal hernia Decreased secondary esophageal peristalsis	Esophagitis Peptic strictures Barrett's esophagus Esophageal cancer
Decreased mealtime fundic receptive relaxation	Decreased nitric oxide production?	Early satiation
Decreased acid production	Chronic atrophic gastritis Decreased number of parietal cells?	Iron, B12, folate, and calcium deficiency Bacterial overgrowth
Decreased mucosal defense	*Helicobacter pylori*, NSAIDs	Gastritis, peptic ulcers
Minor delay in SB transit time	Decreased contraction amplitude	None
Shortening of the absorptive villi	Aging	None
Lactose intolerance	Decrease in lactase production	Bloating, diarrhea
Bacterial overgrowth	Decreased gastric acid production	Bloating, diarrhea
Decreased vitamin D absorption and synthesis	Decreased SB vitamin D receptors Decreased exposure to sun	Osteoporosis
Slow colon transit	Decreased colon motility?	Constipation
Decreased rectal compliance	Fibrosis	Defecation urge
Decreased external sphincter tone	Thinning of external sphincter	Fecal incontinence
Decreased first-pass metabolism	Decreased perfusion and hepatic mass	Drug toxicity
Increased lethogenic potential	Increased cholesterol Decreased GB motility	Cholelithiasis

Note: UES = upper esophageal sphincter; LES = lower esophageal sphincter; SB = small bowel.

28.1 THE ESOPHAGUS

Between swallows, the esophagus is a 25-cm-long neuromuscular tube that is sealed at both ends by the upper esophageal and lower esophageal sphincters. This prevents both entry of air and reflux of acid into the esophagus. Once the food bolus is prepared in the oral cavity, it is consciously propelled by the tongue toward the pharynx. The entry of bolus into the pharynx triggers the swallowing reflex, which is involuntary and consists of a complex, precisely orchestrated series of neuromuscular events. The soft palate ascends to seal the nasopharynx while the vocal cords approximate to protect the larynx. The upper esophageal sphincter, formed by the cricopharyngeal muscle, relaxes to allow entry of the bolus into the esophagus in response to the strong contraction of the pharyngeal muscular walls. This contraction propagates through the esophageal body as a peristaltic wave guiding the bolus down the esophagus and into the stomach. Entry of food into the stomach is permitted by the spontaneous relaxation of the lower esophageal sphincter, which occurs at the initiation of swallowing and continues until the bolus has passed. The oropharynx and upper esophagus are composed of striated muscle, which is controlled by the central nervous system via the glossopharyngeal and vagus nerves. The distal esophagus is composed of smooth muscle, which is controlled by an intrinsic neuromuscular network necessary for normal peristalsis. Diseases affecting the central nervous system, the striated muscle, or the smooth muscle can lead to a derangement of the swallowing process.

Normal aging is associated with many changes that are observed but have unclear clinical significance. Changes include delayed swallowing,[1] incomplete relaxation of both upper and lower esophageal sphincters,[2] decreased secondary esophageal peristalsis, and possibly increased gastroesophageal reflux.[3] Increased gastroesophageal reflux is likely caused by increased prevalence of hiatal hernias rather than an age-associated decrease in the lower esophageal sphincter tone.[4] Some of these changes are bundled together and referred to as presbyesophagus, but the clinical significance of this term is questionable.[5] Many of the changes seen with aging may actually be a result of comorbid conditions affecting the esophageal function through its neurological component (stroke), muscular component (hypothyrodism), or both.[6] Overall, it appears that the physiologic function of the esophagus is preserved with aging in normal healthy individuals with the possible exception of the very old (>80 years old), in whom the amplitude of esophageal contractions is decreased.[7] Dysphagia is common in older persons with an estimated prevalence of 6.9% in a Midwestern community.[8] The prevalence of dysphagia is higher in long-term facilities, reaching 30 to 40%.[9] Dysphagia is more common in older persons because the conditions responsible for it are typically seen more frequently with aging.

Oropharyngeal dysphagia is caused by diseases that lead to disturbance in the oropharyngeal phase of swallowing and interference with food entry into the esophagus. Oropharyngeal dysphagia can result in food entry into the nasopharynx, leading to nasal regurgitation, or food entry into the larynx, leading to coughing during or right after eating, risking aspiration with possible pneumonitis. Causes of oropharyngeal dysphagia that are prevalent with aging include neurologic conditions (cerebrovascular events,[10] Parkinson's disease,[11] amyotrophic lateral sclerosis[12]), muscular disorders (myasthenia gravis,[13] dermatomyositis, polymyositis[14]), and metabolic conditions (hypothyroidism, diabetes mellitus). In tobacco users, consideration must always be given to the possibility of head and neck tumors. Despite a higher prevalence of cervical arthritis and spur formation in older persons, dysphagia secondary to compression of the esophagus is unusual.[15] Suspicion of oropharyngeal dysphagia should trigger a bedside swallowing evaluation best performed by a trained speech therapist. The diagnostic test is videofluoroscopy, which is also referred to as modified barium swallow. Oropharyngeal dysphagia is treated by attempting to improve the underlying cause. Manipulation of the diet and proper positioning of the head are commonly used strategies to decrease risk of aspiration. Although this approach is based on videofluoroscopic findings, these findings do not always correlate clinically with the development of aspiration pneumonia.[16] Trials conducted to assess the efficacy of this approach were inconclusive, and more trials need to be conducted.[17] Aggressive postprandial oral care (cleaning of teeth with an applicator of povidone iodine) was shown to be of borderline significance in preventing aspiration pneumonia in nursing home residents.[18] More research is needed before this strategy can be recommended. The use of pharmacologic agents (amantadine or cilostazol) was shown to be beneficial in small studies.[19] Problems in studies' design and the presence of significant side effects prevent these agents from gaining widespread acceptance.

Diseases that interfere with food transfer through the esophagus are said to cause esophageal dysphasia. If dysphagia is present with both solids and liquids, it usually suggests a motility disorder or a very advanced obstruction. Achalasia is the best understood esophageal motility disorder and is hallmarked by failure of the lower esophageal sphincter to relax and the absence of esophageal peristalsis.[20] Dysphagia to solids can represent a benign or malignant mechanical obstruction. Benign mechanical obstructions are seen with acid reflux disease; they are usually progressive with peptic strictures while intermittent with Schatzki's rings.[21] Malignant obstructions are suspected when significant weight loss is present. Esophageal cancer is a disease of older persons, occurring most commonly in the sixth decade. It affects more men than women and seems to be more aggressive in African Americans. Risk factors include smoking, alcohol, and drinking hot mate (a popular drink in South America) in the squamous cell type.[22] Long-standing gastroesophageal reflux and prolonged esophageal exposure to acid can lead to the development of Barrett's esophagus, which is the principal risk factor for the adenocarcinoma type. Unfortunately, avoidance of foods that can worsen reflux, such as dietary fat, coffee, chocolate, and mint, does not provide any significant protection against esophageal cancer. Routine intake of aspirin or nonsteroidal anti-inflammatory drugs (NSAIDs) is the only intervention that may be associated with a reduction in esophageal cancer risk (of both histological types) with evidence for a dose response. A meta-analysis found a lower risk of esophageal cancer among persons who reported frequent use of NSAIDs than in those who reported intermittent use.[23] Unfortunately, most studies did not collect information on the specific doses taken. The association between aspirin or NSAID use and the decreased risk of esophageal cancer should be interpreted cautiously. Use of aspirin and NSAIDs may be associated with certain behaviors that may have an influence on cancer risk, such as use of vitamin supplementation.[24] Also, it is likely that those with upper GI symptoms such as heartburn and regurgitation, which are risk factors for esophageal cancer, are less likely to be prescribed NSAIDs or aspirin.[25] Based on that, and despite their promise, NSAIDs are not yet recommended for the prevention or treatment of any cancers.[26]

Older persons are at a particularly increased risk for medication-induced esophageal injury presenting with odynophagia and chest pain. Risk factors in older persons include decreased salivary production, increased number of medications taken, and decreased mobility. Women are affected twice as much, possibly due to the prevalent use of certain offensive pills such as alendronate.[27] Diagnosis of esophageal dysphagia is accomplished by visualizing the esophageal lumen either directly by endoscopic means or indirectly by a barium swallow test. Definitive treatment is by removal of the mechanical obstruction, which is accomplished by endoscopic dilatation of the esophagus in the case of benign strictures. In cases of esophageal cancer, the treatment is by surgical resection in the early stages, which is usually preceded by chemoradiation. Obstruction in advanced inoperable cancers can be ameliorated by chemotherapy or endoscopic techniques such as laser debulking or placement of an intraluminal stent.

Gastroesophageal reflux disease (GERD) can frequently be seen in older persons, with the current estimate that 20% of persons above 65 years of age have GERD. This can be a consequence of age-related physiologic changes in the lower esophageal sphincter pressure or the presence of a hiatal hernia. Use of medications that diminish esophageal sphincter tone (e.g., theophylline, calcium antagonists) can be a cofactor. Chronic acid exposure can lead to complications such as peptic strictures and Barrett's esophagus, which is associated with a 0.5% per year chance of development of esophageal cancer.[28] Gatsric acid reflux occurs after meals or at night and can lead to significant decline in the quality of life. Lifestyle modifications carry a modest rate of healing (20 to 30%) and include elevation of the head of the bed, avoiding bed within 3 hours of eating, moderate-size meals, moderate amount of fat per meal, reduced intake of caffeine, chocolate, and alcohol, and smoking cessation. Effective treatment of GERD is achieved by using proton pump inhibitors, which are most effective during maximal acid production (mealtime).[29] Although proton pump inhibitors have a long half-life, a peak in plasma concentration appears shortly after oral administration. This suggests that the best time for their administration is 30 minutes before what is considered to be the largest daily meal.[30] The largest daily meal is usually dinner for most people living in the Western hemisphere.

28.2 THE STOMACH

The stomach plays a central role in food intake and regulation of appetite. The major function of the stomach is to receive ingested food and mix and triturate it into suspensions suitable for emptying into the duodenum. To best fulfill these functions, the stomach can be functionally divided into three regions: proximal stomach (cardia, fundus, proximal corpus), distal stomach (distal corpus, antrum), and pylorus. On initiation of a meal, the gastric fundus undergoes vagally mediated receptive relaxation, resulting in a dramatic two- to three-fold increase in gastric volume.[31] Food is then subjected to mechanical breakdown by gastric contractions and to a thorough mixing with hydrochloric acid, which is produced by the parietal cells in the gastric fundus. The food mix then moves to the antrum, where further trituration of the food occurs. Food particles have to be smaller than 2 mm to pass through the pylorus into the duodenum. Stretching of the antrum regulates appetite as it signals to the body that the stomach is full.[32] Aging appears to be associated with a decrease in fundic receptive relaxation, leading to early transfer of food to the antrum and stretching of the antrum, signaling satiation with much smaller amounts of food than in young adults.[33] This is one of the theories proposed to explain early satiation seen in older persons, possibly due to a decrease in the nitric oxide necessary for fundic relaxation.[34] Fundic activities play a very important role in liquid emptying. This is particularly true in cases of nutrient-containing liquids such as liquid nutritional supplements, since carbonation delays gastric emptying of liquids.[35] A decline in fundic activities may be responsible for the delay in gastric emptying of liquids in elderly patients, resulting in early satiation and decreased intake of solids afterwards.

Based on that, it is best to offer liquid nutritional supplements to older persons between meals (on an empty stomach) rather than with meals. Liquids swallowed on an empty stomach are quickly transported to the duodenum in a linear fashion under effects of the vagus nerve. Transport of solids is delayed as they are broken down into smaller particles, after which transport becomes linear. The rate of the transport is mediated by several duodenal mechanisms, including the "acid brake" effect. Aging results in a delay in the transfer of liquid and mixed liquid–solid meals into the duodenum. This leads to prolonged stretching of the antrum and prolonged sense of satiety. It is not clear whether solid transport is affected by aging since studies have shown mixed results.[36]

The primary role of hydrochloric acid is to dissolve the particulate matter in food. This is essential to allow the release of macro- and micronutrients from food. A decrease in hydrochloric acid is known to be associated with several nutritional deficiencies, including vitamin B12, iron, calcium, and folic acid. Aging is associated with a gradual decrease in acid production.[37] Until the discovery of *Helicobacter pylori*, this was thought to be an aging-related process. *H. pylori* is histologically associated with loss of gastric glandular pattern and intestinal metaplasia, leading to a significant decrease in acid production and a resultant increase in gastrin levels. *H. pylori* impairs duodenal mucosal integrity and increases its susceptibility to ulcer formation. Infection with *H. pylori* increases with aging and is most probably responsible for the hypochlorhydria seen with aging, much more than the aging process itself.[38] *H. pylori*-mediated gastric inflammation is referred to as chronic atrophic gastritis (or chronic gastritis type B) and can be responsible for nonulcer dyspepsia. Nonulcer dyspepsia can occasionally lead to a significant weight loss and failure to thrive necessitating treatment. *H. pylori* eradication is accomplished by administering a 2-week course of triple therapy, including two antibiotics and a proton pump inhibitor, with more than a 90% success rate.[39] Chronic gastritis type A is usually associated with a variety of autoimmune conditions and hallmarked by the presence of antibodies against the gastric parietal cells or against the intrinsic factor.[40] This condition leads to a decrease in acid production and a decrease in the ability to absorb vitamin B12 (pernicious anemia). Type A chronic gastritis is significantly less common than type B in older persons.

Peptic ulcer disease is seen more frequently in older persons with more serious ramifications due to higher rates of hospitalization and ulcer-related mortality. This is usually due to decreased mucosal defense mechanisms thought to be due to aging itself, the presence of chronic gastritis, the presence of *H. pylori*, and extrinsic factors such as NSAIDs.[41] An estimated 10 to 15% of older Americans use prescription NSAIDs daily, with over-the-counter use possibly being up to seven times greater.[42] NSAIDs alter mucosal circulation and mucosal ability to produce bicarbonate necessary for defense against mucosal insults. This can lead to acute inflammation, erosions, ulcers, and bleeding. One of these complications can be seen in more than 30% of old NSAID users.[43] Based on this information, routine use of NSAIDs in older individuals should be discouraged.

Uncomplicated peptic ulcers typically present with abdominal pain that is most common 2 to 3 hours after meals (when acid production is maximized) and nocturnally (when food is no longer protectively coating the ulcer). Other symptoms may include nausea, dyspepsia, and weight loss. Complications can occur and include bleeding, which can present as hematemesis or melena, perforation with full-thickness ulcers, gastric outlet obstruction when the ulcer is located in the pylorus and is associated with severe inflammatory reaction, and fibrosis. The diagnosis of ulcers is possible with an upper GI series, but the gold standard is endoscopic visualization, which also allows for biopsies. Treatment of peptic ulcers is accomplished by using twice-a-day proton pump inhibitors, which lead to ulcer healing in more than 90% of cases in 8 weeks. Although many ulcer patients report that certain foods (e.g., spicy foods) can worsen their symptoms, there is no evidence that diet has a causal role in peptic ulcer disease or that dietary adjustments affect the rate of healing. Continuous use of acid suppression medications is indicated in older persons with high risk for recurrence (e.g., continuous use of NSAIDs, steroids, warfarin). The presence of antral or duodenal ulcers should always trigger a workup for *H. pylori* and treatment if found. Treatment of *H. pylori* is associated with a decrease in the 1-year ulcer recurrence from 90% to less than 2%.

Like most cancers, gastric cancer is a disease of older individuals. In the U.S., the majority of patients present between the ages of 65 and 74 years.[44] Risk factors include a family history of gastric cancer, cigarette smoking, pernicious anemia, and hypertrophic gastropathy (Menetrier disease). A recent meta-analysis suggested a two-fold increase in risk of gastric cancer in persons with *H. pylori*.[45] Numerous dietary factors have been implicated as risk factors for gastric cancer, such as highly preserved foods due to rich content of salt (pickled foods, salted fish and meat, soy sauce), nitrates, and polycyclic aromatic amines.[46] Other dietary risk factors that are suspected but not proven include fatty and fried foods and high intake of red meat. On the other hand, a high intake of fresh fruits and raw vegetables has been found to provide a 40% decrease in the risk of gastric cancer due to its rich content of antioxidants that reduce reactive DNA damage induced by free radicals.[47]

28.3 THE SMALL INTESTINES

Most digestion and absorption occurs in the small intestines. Fat is digested utilizing bile salts and pancreatic lipase, while proteins are digested utilizing pancreatic proteases (trypsin, chemotrypsin, and elastase). Carbohydrate digestion requires pancreatic amylase and several disaccharide-specific mucosal proteases, of which lactase is the best known. Most macronutrients are absorbed in the proximal small bowel. With the exception of vitamin B12, which is absorbed in the terminal ileum, micronutrients are also absorbed in the proximal small bowel. About 9 l of fluids pass through the small intestines daily as a result of oral intake and intestinal secretion. Most of it gets absorbed in the small bowel, so only 1 to 2 l of fluids reach the colon, where further water absorption occurs. Progress of chyme from the duodenum to the colon is mediated by intestinal peristaltic movements that occur largely between meals. These peristalses originate in the duodenum and progress as a migratory motor complex toward the colon. After meals, another type of regional contraction occurs to allow mixing of chyme with the digestive enzymes and ensure adequate contact time with intestinal mucosa.

Studies have shown that intestinal motility remains intact with aging, and despite a possible decrease in the amplitude of contractions, the speed at which chyme progresses through the small bowels remains preserved.[48] Except for a possible shortening of the absorptive villi, no significant histologic or functional changes are seen with aging. Absorption of macronutirents remains adequate, particularly proteins and fat (in the absence of bacterial overgrowth). Carbohydrate absorption may be affected in individuals who develop lactase deficiency. These individuals typically present with bloating, abdominal discomfort, and diarrhea after consuming milk or dairy products and are known to be milk intolerant—better referred to as lactose intolerant. There is no specific treatment for this condition except for avoiding dairy products or using lactose-free dairy products. Several differences in micronutrient absorption or clearance exist between old and young individuals. Vitamin A clearance, for instance, decreases with aging, predisposing older persons to vitamin A toxicity at lower doses. On the other hand, most older persons require supplementation with vitamin D. This is usually due to decreased skin synthesis (decreased exposure to sunlight), decreased intestinal absorption (decreased intestinal receptors?), and decreased renal production of 1,25-dihydroxy-vitamin D. The decrease in vitamin D levels, in the absence of adequate supplementation, leads to a decrease in calcium absorption and an increased risk of osteoporosis. Folate absorption is impaired in older persons with atrophic gastritis due to failure to decrease duodenal pH for optimal folate absorption. This may lead to an increase in homocysteine levels, predisposing individuals to atherosclerotic complications. This is also true in the presence of vitamin B12 deficiency. Vitamin B12 has a complex absorption mechanism that requires adequate gastric acidity (to release vitamin B12 from food), normal pancreatic function (to produce enough bicarbonate to alkalinize the duodenum), and adequate intrinsic factor production by the parietal cells (to bind to ileal receptors). According to the Framingham Study, 11.3% of elderly subjects had laboratory evidence of vitamin B12 deficiency compared with 5.3% of younger adults.[49] Despite these facts, the need for universal screening in older adults remains controversial.[50]

Small bowel bacterial overgrowth is seen more commonly in older persons, likely due to hypochlorhydria and decreased ability to kill bacteria in the stomach. Bacteria colonizing the small bowels deconjugate bile salts, thus interfering with the absorption of fat and leading to diarrhea and eventual weight loss.[51] Fat malabsorption is usually associated with a decrease in the absorption of fat-soluble vitamins (A, D, E, K). Bacterial metabolism can lead to the production of various gases, causing bloating and possibly nausea. Increased folate on blood tests can be a subtle sign of bacterial overgrowth because bacteria manufacture folate in the intestines. Diagnosis is by duodenal aspiration or a sugar breath test (observing a quick rise in hydrogen due to early bacterial metabolism of the used sugar). Treatment with a course of antibiotics is usually effective and can be repeated periodically if overgrowth recurs.

Celiac sprue is far more common than once realized and continues to be one of the leading underdiagnosed diseases in the U.S. Although it is usually discovered at a young age, it is not uncommon for it to be diagnosed in older persons. Celiac sprue involves atrophy of the intestinal villi due to hypersensitivity to a protein called gluten, which is found in wheat, rye, and barley. This hypersensitivity leads to the formation of antibodies that attack intestinal villi and lead to their destruction. Although severe diarrhea, malabsorption, and weight loss represent the picture of a full-blown condition, celiac sprue rarely presents in this dramatic fashion. Celiac sprue can present with milder gastrointestinal symptoms such as nausea, dyspepsia, abdominal pain, bloating, and diarrhea. It can also present with nongastrointestinal symptoms, particularly psychiatric and neurologic symptoms such as ataxia. Screening can be done with serologic testing, but confirmation is accomplished endoscopically with a small bowel biopsy. The best serologic test is the use of tissue transglutaminase (TTG) immunoglobulin A (IgA) antibodies, which is a highly sensitive and specific test.[52] Antigliadin antibodies are less sensitive and less specific and are rarely used. Antiendomesial antibodies are not as sensitive but are very specific. Biopsy of the proximal small bowel reveals intraepithelial lymphocytic infiltrates and loss of villi. Celiac sprue is treated by following a gluten-free diet, which necessitates avoidance of wheat, barley, and rye. Despite not containing gluten, in the U.S. oats are often contaminated with gluten and should also be avoided.

28.4 THE COLON

The colon is a 3-foot-long muscular tube that measures about 7 cm in diameter. It starts with a blind pouch called the cecum and ends with the rectum. The chyme enters the colon via the ileocecal valve into the cecum. Muscular contractions generate peristaltic colonic movements that propel chyme toward the rectum. Although constipation is the most common gastrointestinal complaint among older persons, there is no concrete evidence that colonic motility decreases as part of aging. Chyme reaching the colon consists primarily of water, electrolytes, and indigestible food remains. Further water absorption occurs in the colon and seems to be proportionate to the time spent in the colon. Constipated individuals experience further water absorption and drying of stool, which turns into pellets, creating a vicious cycle, as this worsens constipation. Undigested and unabsorbed material in the colon can be the subject of further metabolism by the colonic bacteria. This is physiologically important since bacteria manufacture certain vitamins that the colon then absorbs. Vitamin K is the main vitamin produced by colonic bacteria. Prolonged use of antibiotics eradicates the natural colonic flora, predisposing the patient to vitamin K deficiency with easy bruising and prolongation of prothrombin time (PT). This is important to realize particularly in patients who are also on warfarin, as they can be at an increased risk of bleeding.

The rectum, a 12- to 15-cm tubular structure, serves as a storage cavity for stool in preparation for its exit. Compliance of rectal walls gives the rectum the ability to relax to accommodate stool. With aging, this ability to relax may diminish, leading to stool frequency or even fecal incontinence. Continence is maintained by the function of two muscles: the internal sphincter, which is a nonvoluntary smooth muscle, and the external sphincter, which is a voluntary striated muscle. The internal sphincter is contracted tonically at rest, preventing the involuntary loss of stool and gas. A mild increase in the thickness of the internal anal sphincter is noted with aging (probably connective tissue) without a clear functional significance.[53] Voluntary external anal sphincter pressures are consistent with the overall body muscle mass, and thus are generally lower in women than in men. With the loss of skeletal muscles noted with aging, a significant thinning of the external anal sphincter occurs, possibly contributing to a reduction in its pressure.[54]

Constipation is very common in older persons, as complaints of infrequency and difficulty with evacuation seem to increase with age, as does the frequency of regular laxative use. Constipation is practically endemic among nursing home residents.[55] The Rome criteria were developed to define constipation, but they not very practical for clinical use and are better suited as a research tool. Constipation is simplistically defined as having less than three bowel movements per week. Severe constipation can lead to decreased enteric motility and possibly decreased appetite and nausea, which ultimately affects nutrition. Besides ensuring that the patient received the appropriate colon cancer screening, most cases of constipation are mild and do not require an extensive workup. Excluding causes of secondary constipation requires screening for electrolyte abnormalities, hypothyroidism, and a thorough review of medications to identify anticholinergics and smooth muscle relaxants. Once this basic workup is completed, the most physiologic approach to treatment is to recommend adequate fluid and fiber intake, as there is a proportionate relation between water and fiber intake and fecal output.[56] The goal is to reach 25 g of fiber daily in a gradual fashion to avoid bloating and cramping. Cereal fibers resist digestion and retain water within their cellular structures, enhancing fecal bulking effects. Fiber found in citrus fruits and legumes stimulates the growth of colonic flora, thereby increasing fecal mass.[57] Adding raw bran (3 to 4 tablespoons with each meal) followed by a glass of water can be very effective. Among fruits, prunes are rich in fiber and can be added to daily nutrient intake. The daily target of fiber may be hard to reach solely from dietary sources, and a fiber supplement is often necessary. Psyllium is the fiber most studied and proven to increase stool frequency, but many others are avilable. Increased physical activity may be beneficial in treating constipation by increasing propulsive movements of the colon.[58] When fighting constipation, it is helpful to utilize the gastrocolic reflex by attempting defecation shortly after meals. Increased contractile activity of the colon and rectum is known to occur half an hour after consumption of a large meal (usually more than 400 cal). If simple measures are ineffective, a small dose of a daily laxative such as sorbitol or ethylene glycol is recommended. Stimulant laxatives such as senna or bisacodyl can be used judiciously on an as needed basis. Resistant cases justify further workup by a gastroenterologist. A new type of 4,5-hydroxytryptamine (5-HT4, serotonin-4) agonist, tegaserod (Zelnorm®), was recently approved for refractory cases of constipation in both men and women under age 65. No trial has specifically targeted elderly patients yet.

Colonic diverticulosis is another condition associated with aging and is related to poor nutritional habits. While diverticulosis is rarely seen before age 45 years, its prevalence increases to reach 80% by age 85 years. There is an association between diverticulosis and a Western diet high in refined carbohydrates and low in dietary fiber. Chronic constipation leads to increased intraluminal colonic pressure, with the resulting protrusion of the colonic mucosa through weak areas in the colonic muscle. Diverticuli are usually asymptomatic and are found incidentally during colonoscopy or radiographic imaging of the colon. Complications may occur in 20% of people, such as inflammation or bleeding. Prevention and treatment of uncomplicated diverticuli is accomplished by dietary changes to allow for more fibers and by preventing constipation.

Colorectal cancer (CRC) is mostly a disease of older persons. Less than 5% of cases are seen before age 45 years. Furthermore, aging results in a significantly higher chance of acquiring adenomatous polyps with high-grade dysplasia. CRC is the third most common cancer in the U.S. and the second killer among cancers. However, it is completely preventable with regular screening and removal of polyps before their malignant transformation. This underscores the significance of regular screening. Colon cancer is prevalent in urban industrialized countries with poor dietary habits and significantly less prevalent in agricultural communities. A diet high in fat and red meat and low on fiber seems to be associated with colon cancer. Fat stimulates secretion of primary bile acids, which are transformed eventually to secondary bile acids by colonic bacteria. In addition to the colonic toxicity induced by the secondary bile acid, fat itself can directly affect the colonic mucosa and increase mitogenesis. Consumption of heavily browned red meat is thought to be associated with a higher incidence of colorectal cancer, possibly due to the formation of chemicals called heterocyclic amines (HCAs), which are potent procarcinogens.[59] Current data support the notion that meat consumption more than once a week can increase the risk of CRC, particularly the left side. Fiber, on the other hand, is thought to dilute the carcinogenic secondary bile salts and decrease transit time and time of contact with the colonic mucosa. Surprisingly, intervention trials failed to show a protective effect of fiber against CRC.[60] High consumption of fresh fruits and vegetables is thought to help prevent colon cancer by providing helpful antioxidants, but results of studies have been inconsistent.[61] Higher calcium intake (>1250 mg daily) was associated with a significant 35% reduction in the risk of distal colon cancers according to the Nurses' Health Study and the Health Professionals' Follow-Up Study.[62] Another meta-analysis concluded that the risk of recurrence of colorectal adenomas was significantly lower in patients randomized to calcium.[63] This beneficial effect is believed to be due to calcium's ability to bind with intraluminal toxins, possibly by positively influencing mucosal proliferation. Folate deficiency may be associated with an increased risk of CRC since folate is an important supplier of the methyl groups necessary for gene regulation and nucleotide synthesis. The Nurses' Health Study suggested a protective effect from folic acid supplementation (400 μg/day for at least 15 years), as it reduced the chance of developing CRC (relative risk (RR) = 0.25). Vitamin B6 (pyridoxine) intake was also inversely related to colon cancer risk (RR = 0.51).[64] Physical activity was found to decrease the risk of left-sided CRC by half, probably due to induction of colonic activity and a decrease in transit time. Alcohol and smoking are both associated with an increase in the risk for CRC. A meta-analysis of cohort studies revealed that alcohol consumption in excess of 45 g/day can lead to a 40% increase in the risk of CRC (45 g/day equals four 12-ounce beers, four 4-ounce glasses of wine, or three 1.5-ounce shots of 80-proof liquor).[65] The risk may be related to alcohol interference with folate absorption and decreased folate intake. Tobacco consumption for more than 20 years was shown to increase the incidence and mortality from CRC.[66]

28.5 THE LIVER

The liver plays a significant role in maintaining normal nutrition and energy balance. Bile salts are manufactured in the liver and excreted in bile to help digest fat. The liver also plays a central role in the synthesis and degradation of important proteins such as albumin, transferrin, ceruloplasmin, and coagulation factors, among others. Depending on energy needs, the liver regulates the synthesis and breakdown of glycogen as an energy reservoir. The liver cells are also capable of enzymatically synthesizing glucose from several precursors when necessary in a process called gluconeogenesis. Mitochondrial fatty acid breakdown occurs in situations of glucose/glycogen deficiency as a source of energy, such as in the case of prolonged starvation. Triglyceride synthesis occurs in the liver in conditions of energy excess, after which they are stored in adipose tissues. Hepatic perfusion and liver mass seem to decrease with aging, mounting to a 30% decline by the eighth decade. This can lead to a decrease in first-pass drug metabolism in the liver and a prolonged half-life. Although some microsomal oxidating functions decline with aging, those responsible for drug metabolism are usually preserved. Histologic examination of the aged liver may reveal clinically insignificant increased fibrosis. Liver functions as reflected by liver enzymes and synthetic functions remain normal in the healthy aged.

Acute hepatitis of any kind is often associated with decreased appetite, nausea, and vomiting. Fasting hypoglycemia may be seen due to depleted glycogen and impaired gluconeogenesis. Luckily, the nutritional consequences of acute liver injury are minimal, as most cases are short-lived. Regardless of origin, cirrhosis is likely to cause patients to have abnormal anthropometric measurements (i.e., muscle wasting) and low levels of water- and fat-soluble vitamins. These nutritional deficiencies arise as a result of inadequate dietary intake, maldigestion, malabsorption, or defective metabolism.[67] There is no good clinical evidence supporting protein restriction in patients with acute hepatic encephalopathy, except for severe refractory cases. In chronic hepatic encephalopathy, vegetable proteins may be superior to proteins derived from fish, milk, or meat with regard to nitrogen balance.[68] Nonalcoholic steatohepatitis (NASH) is a liver condition that has a connection to dietary habits. It is associated with insulin resistance and is typically seen in overweight individuals with risk factors such as type II diabetes mellitus and dyslipidemia. NASH is usually asymptomatic, presenting with mildly elevated liver enzymes without other explanation. Ultrasound or computed tomography (CT) of the liver usually suggests presence of fat, but the gold standard diagnosis is by liver biopsy. Only 28% of patients slowly progress to significant fibrosis and cirrhosis. No specific treatment for NASH exists, but to ameliorate risk factors, one can lose weight and control diabetes and dyslipidemia. Because of the slow progression of the disease, it should not be of great concern as a new diagnosis in an older person.

28.6 THE GALL BLADDER

The main function of the gall bladder is to store and concentrate bile to be readily available for fat digestion when needed. Bile in the gall bladder consists mainly of bile acids, cholesterol, and bilirubin. A balance between these components prevents stone formation. With aging there is an increase in the lithogenic potential in the gall bladder due to an increase in cholesterol, while the bile acid pool, necessary to keep cholesterol solvent, does not change. This is particularly important in obese individuals or those with diets rich in fat. Acute weight loss can also lead to stone formation due to mobilization of lipid stores and to gall bladder stasis. Based on that, most gall bladder stones seen in older persons are cholesterol stones. Older persons are more likely to have silent and complicated gall bladder stones than younger adults. Also, cholecystectomy is among the most common abdominal surgeries performed in older individuals.

Most gall bladder stones remain asymptomatic, with only 20 to 30% presenting as colicky pain. This, however, may become recurrent, leading to food aversion and gradual weight loss. Complications of gall bladder stones, such as cholecystistis or acute pancreatitis, occur in 2% of patients. Asymptomatic gall bladder stones do not require any treatment. Those with recurrent pain attacks can be considered for elective cholecystectomy. Complicated gall bladder stones often require urgent surgical intervention. The best approach to gall bladder stones complicated by acute cholecystitis can be subject to a difference of opinion, but most agree that early surgical intervention (during the same hospitalization) in patients with low surgical risk decreases morbidity and cost.[69] Patients with high surgical risk, particularly those with advanced cardiac or pulmonary disease, should be managed conservatively. A postcholecystectomy diet should take into account the patient's inability to adequately digest a large fatty meal in the absence of preprepared stored bile. Many patients will experience an increase in the frequency of bowel movements, which improves with time and is usually manageable.

28.7 THE PANCREAS

The pancreas is a combined endocrine and exocrine gland that plays a central role in macronutrient digestion. Pancreatic lipase is responsible for fat digestion, while pancreatic trypsin, chemotrypsin, and elastase are responsible for protein digestion. Aging can lead to morphologic changes observed by specialized imaging. This includes epithelial hyperplasia and ductal fibrosis. Large ducts may become ecstatic and sometimes may be confused with chronic pancreatitis. Physiologic decline in pancreatic function is observed with aging and demonstrated by a steady decline in the amount of secreted pancreatic enzymes and bicarbonate. This, however, does not seem to be enough to cause overt clinical problems.

Chronic pancreatitis is usually alcohol related. In young individuals, long-term chronic pancreatitis can lead to exocrine insufficiency, fat malabsorption, and weight loss. Disease progression is significantly slower in the elderly; therefore, only a few if any show evidence of exocrine insufficiency. Pain is also less common in older persons.

About 90% of pancreatic adenocarcinomas arise in the head of the pancreas and are associated with obstruction of the pancreatic duct and severe exocrine pancreatic insufficiency. Fat malabsorption, cancer cachexia, and increased cytokines are the leading causes of weight loss in pancreatic cancer. Treatment should be optimized with aggressive pancreatic enzyme replacement, but prognosis is typically poor.

TABLE 28.2
Dietary Intervention for Promotion of Gastrointestinal Health and General Nutrition with Specific Gastrointestinal Ailments

Condition Affecting GI Tract	Dietary Recommendations for GI Health
Oropharyngeal dysphagia–laryngeal penetration	Thickened fluids to honey consistency
	Chin tuck
GERD	Avoiding bed within 3 hours of eating
	Moderate-size meals
	Moderate amount of fat per meal
	Reduced intake of caffeine, chocolate, and alcohol
	Smoking cessation
Early satiation	Smaller meals
	Liquid nutritional supplement between meals
Gastric cancer prevention	Avoid highly preserved foods (pickled foods, salted fish and meat, soy sauce)
	Increase fruits and vegetables
Lactose (milk) intolerance	Avoid dairy products, use lactose-free products
Small bowel aging	Vitamin D and calcium supplement
Celiac sprue	Avoid wheat, barley, rye; also avoid oat (in the U.S.)
Constipation with or without diverticulosis	Adequate water intake
	Ensure 25 g fiber daily (bran, fruits, psyllium)
Colon cancer prevention	Avoid fat, browned red meat
	Increase fruits and vegetables
	Adequate fiber (questionable)
	Calcium intake (>1250 mg/day)
	Avoid folate and vitamin B6 deficiency
NASH	Calorie restriction, weight loss
Gall bladder stone prevention	Avoid harsh dieting leading to acute weight loss
	Decrease daily cholesterol intake
	Avoid prolonged fasting
Aging pancreas/chronic pancreatitis	Avoid large fatty meals
	Consider pancreatic enzyme supplement

28.8 SUMMARY

It is very important for all clinicians caring for older persons to be familiar with the gastrointestinal function and aging-related changes affecting it. This is particularly important for those interested in nutrition and nutritional health, considering that the gastrointestinal system is the portal for all nutrients into the human body. Table 28.2 summarizes some of the dietary interactions that may promote gastrointestinal health in the presence of certain gastrointestinal ailments.

REFERENCES

1. Tracy JF, Logemann JA, Kahrilas PJ, et al. Preliminary observations on the effects of age on oropharyngeal deglutition. *Dysphagia* 1989;4:90–94.

2. Robbins J, Hamilton JW, Lof GL, et al. Oropharyngeal swallowing in normal adults of different ages. *Gastroenterology* 1992;103:823–829.
3. Shaker R, Staff D. Esophageal disorders in the elderly. *Gastroenterol Clin North Am* 2001;30:335–361.
4. Stilson WL, Sanders I, Gardiner GA, et al. Hiatal hernia and gastroesophageal reflux: a clinicoradiological analysis of more than 1,000 cases. *Radiology* 1969;93:1323–1327.
5. Shaker R, Kusano M, et al. Effect of aging on the secondary esophageal peristalsis: presbyesophagus revisited. *Am J Physiol* 1995;268(Pt. 1):G772–G779.
6. de Boer SY, Masclee AA, Lamers CB. Effect of hyperglycemia on gastrointestinal and gallbladder motility. *Scand J Gastroenterol Suppl* 1992;194:13–18.
7. Achem SR, Devault KR. Dysphagia in aging. *J Clin Gastroenterol* 2005;39:357–371.
8. Talley NJ, Weaver AL, Zinsmeister AR, et al. Onset and disappearance of gastrointestinal symptoms and functional gastrointestinal disorders. *Am J Epidemiol* 1992;136:165–177.
9. Siebens H, Trupe E, Siebens A, et al. Correlates and consequences of eating dependency in institutionalized elderly. *J Am Geriatr Soc* 1986;34:192–198.
10. Mann G, Hankey GJ, Cameron D. Swallowing disorders following acute stroke: prevalence and diagnostic accuracy. *Cerebrovasc Dis* 2000;10:380–386.
11. Logemann JA, Blonsky ER, Boshes B. Dysphagia in parkinsonism. *JAMA* 1975;231:69–70.
12. Hillel A, Dray T, Miller R, et al. Presentation of ALS to the otolaryngologist/head and neck surgeon: getting to the neurologist. *Neurology* 1999;53(Suppl):22–25.
13. Schon F, Drayson M, Thompson RA. Myasthenia gravis and elderly people. *Age Ageing* 1996;25:56–58.
14. Grunebaum M, Salinger H. Radiologic findings in polymyositis-dermatomyositis involving the pharynx and upper oesophagus. *Clin Radiol* 1971;22:97–100.
15. Saffouri MH, Ward PH. Surgical correction of dysphagia due to cervical osteophytes. *Ann Otol Rhinol Laryngol* 1974;83:65–70.
16. Perry L, Love CP. Screening for dysphagia and aspiration in acute stroke: a systematic review. *Dysphagia* 2001;16:7–18.
17. Loeb MB, Becker M, Eady A, et al. Interventions to prevent aspiration pneumonia in older adults: a systematic review. *J Am Geriatr Soc* 51:1018–1022, 2003.
18. Yoneyama T, Yoshida M, Matsui T, et al. Oral care and pneumonia. *Lancet* 1999;354:515–519.
19. Mutsuo Y, Masaru Y, Takashi O, et al. Antithrombotic therapy for prevention of pneumonia. *J Am Geriatr Soc* 2001;49:687–688.
20. Sonnenberg A, Massey BT, McCarty DJ, et al. Epidemiology of hospitalization for achalasia in the United States. *Dig Dis Sci* 1993;38:233–244.
21. Richter JE. Gastroesophageal reflux disease in the older patient: presentation, treatment, and complications. *Am J Gastroenterol* 2000;95:368–373.
22. De Stefani E, Deneo-Pellegrini H, Ronco AL, et al. Food groups and risk of squamous cell carcinoma of the oesophagus: a case-control study in Uruguay. *Br J Cancer* 2003;89:1209–1214.
23. Corley DA, Kerlikowske K, Verma R, et al. Protective association of aspirin/NSAIDs and esophageal cancer: a systematic review and meta-analysis. *Gastroenterology* 2003;124:47–56.
24. Patterson RE, Neuhouser ML, White E, Hunt JR, Kristal AR. Cancer-related behavior of vitamin supplement users. *Cancer Epidemiol Biomarkers Prev* 1998;7:79–81.
25. Mehta S, Johnson I, Rhodes M. Systematic review: the chemoprevention of oesophageal adenocarcinoma. *Aliment Pharmacol Ther* 2005;22:759–768.

26. Thun MJ. NSAIDs and esophageal cancer: ready for trials but not yet broad clinical application. *Gastroenterology* 2003;124:246.
27. Hey H, Jorgensen F, Sorensen K, et al. Oesophageal transit of six commonly used tablets and capsules. *Br Med J* 1982;285:1717–1719.
28. Collen MJ, Abdulian JD, Chen YK. Gastroesophageal reflux disease in the elderly more severe disease that requires aggressive therapy. *Am J Gastroenterol* 1995;90:1053–1057.
29. Klinkenberg-Knol EC, Nelis F, Dent J, et al. Long-Term Study Group. Long-term omeprazole treatment in resistant gastroesophageal reflux disease: efficacy, safety, and influence on gastric mucosa. *Gastroenterology* 2000;118:661–669.
30. Hatlebakk JG, Katz PO, Camacho-Lobato L, et al. Proton pump inhibitors: better acid suppression when taken before a meal than without a meal. *Aliment Pharmacol Ther* 2000;14:1267–1272.
31. Tack J, Piessevaux H, Coulie B, et al. Role of impaired gastric accommodation to a meal in functional dyspepsia. *Gastroenterology* 1998;115:1346.
32. Geliebter A, Westreich S, Gage D. Gastric distention by balloon and test-meal intake in obese and lean subjects. *Am J Clin Nutr* 1988;48:592–594.
33. Rayner CK, MacIntosh CG, Chapman IM, et al. Effects of age on proximal gastric motor and sensory function. *Scand J Gastroenterol* 2000;35:1041–1047.
34. Kuiken SD, Vergeer M, Heisterkamp SH, et al. Role of nitric oxide in gastric motor and sensory functions in healthy subjects. *Gut* 2002;51:212–218.
35. Collins PJ, Houghton LA, Read NW, et al. Role of the proximal and distal stomach in mixed solid and liquid meal emptying. *Gut* 1991;32:615–616.
36. Tougas G, Eaker EY, Abell TL, et al. Assessment of gastric emptying using a low fat meal: establishment of international control values. *Am J Gastroenterol* 2000;95:1456–1462.
37. Kinoshita Y, Kawanami C, Kishi K, et al. *Helicobacter pylori* independent chronological change in gastric acid secretion in the Japanese. *Gut* 1997;41:452–458.
38. Haruma K, Kamada T, Kawaguchi H, et al. Effect of age and *Helicobacter pylori* infection on gastric acid secretion. *J Gastroenterol Hepatol* 2000;15:277–283.
39. Lind T, Megraud F, Unge P, et al. The MACH2 study: role of omeprazole in eradication of *Helicobacter pylori* with 1-week triple therapies. *Gastroenterology* 1999;116:248–253.
40. Correa P. Chronic gastritis: a clinicopathological classification. *Am J Gastroenterol* 1988;83:504–506.
41. McCarthy DM. Acid peptic disease in the elderly. *Clin Geriatr Med* 1991;7:231–254.
42. Griffin MR, Piper JM, Daugherty JR, et al. Nonsteroidal anti-inflammatory drug use and increased risk for peptic ulcer disease in elderly persons. *Ann Intern Med* 1991;114:257–263.
43. Langman MJ, Weil J, Wainwright P, et al. Risk of bleeding peptic ulcer associated with individual non-steroidal anti-inflammatory drugs. *Lancet* 1994;343:1075–1078.
44. Ries L, Kosary C, Hawkey B, et al. SEE*R Cancer Statistics Review 1973–1996.* National Cancer Institute, Bethesda, MD, 1999.
45. Eslick G, Lim L, Byles J, et al. Association of *Helicobacter pylori* infection with gastric carcinoma: a meta-analysis. *Am J Gastroenterol* 1999;94:2373.
46. Ramon J, Serra L, Cerdo C, et al. Dietary factors and gastric cancer risk: a case-control study in Spain. *Cancer* 1993;71:1731.
47. Terry P, Yuen ON. Protective effect of fruits and vegetables on stomach cancer in a cohort of Swedish twins. *Int J Cancer* 1998;76:35.
48. Anuras S, Sutherland J. Small intestine manometry in healthy elderly subjects. *J Am Geriatr Soc* 1984;32:581–583.

49. Lindenbaum J, Rosenberg IH, Wilson PW, et al. Prevalence of cobalamin deficiency in the Framingham elderly population. *Am J Clin Nutr* 1994;60:2–11.
50. Stabler SP. Screening the older population for cobalamin (vitamin B_{12}) deficiency. *J Am Geriatr Soc* 1995;43:1290–1297.
51. Wanitschke R, Ammon HV. Effects of dihydroxy bile acids and hydroxy fatty acids on the absorption of oleic acid in the human jejunum. *J Clin Invest* 1978;61:178.
52. Sulkanen S, Halttunen T, Laurila K, et al. Tissue transglutaminase autoantibody enzyme-linked immunosorbent assay in detecting celiac disease. *Gastroenterology* 1998;115:1322.
53. Papachrysostomou M, Pye SD, Wild SR, et al. Significance of the thickness of the anal sphincter with age and its relevance in faecal incontinence. *Scand J Gastroenterol 1*994;29:710–714.
54. Enck P, Kuhlbusch R, Lubke H, et al. Age and sex and anorectal manometry in incontinence. *Dis Colon Rectum* 1989;32:1026–1030.
55. Robson KM, Kiely DK, Lembo T. Development of constipation in nursing home residents. *Dis Colon Rectum* 2000;43:940–944.
56. Voderholzer WA, Schatke W, Muhldorfer BE, et al. Clinical response to dietary fiber treatment of chronic constipation. *Am J Gastroenterol* 1997;92:95–98.
57. Floch MH, Wald A. Clinical evaluation and treatment of constipation. *Gastroenterologist* 1994;2:50–60.
58. De Schryver AM, Keulemans YC, Peters HP, et al. Effects of regular physical activity on defecation pattern in middle-aged patients complaining of chronic constipation. *Scand J Gastroenterol* 205;40:422–429.
59. Skog KI, Johansson MAE, Jagerstad MI. Carcinogenic heterocyclic amines in model systems and cooked foods: a review on formation, occurrence, and intake. *Food Chem Toxicol* 1998;36:879–896.
60. Park Y, Hunter DJ, Spiegelman D, et al. Dietary fiber intake and risk of colorectal cancer: a pooled analysis of prospective cohort studies. *JAMA* 2005;294:2849–2857.
61. Terry P, Giovannucci E, Michels KB, et al. Fruit, vegetables, dietary fiber, and risk of colorectal cancer. *J Natl Cancer Inst* 2001;93:525–533.
62. Wu K, Willett WC, Fuchs CS, et al. Calcium intake and risk of colon cancer in women and men. *J Natl Cancer Inst* 2002;94:437–446.
63. Shaukat A, Scouras N, Schunemann HJ. Role of supplemental calcium in the recurrence of colorectal adenomas: a metaanalysis of randomized controlled trials. *Am J Gastroenterol* 2005;100:390–394.
64. Giovannucci E, Stampfer MJ, Colditz GA, et al. Multivitamin use, folate, and colon cancer in women in the Nurses' Health Study. *Ann Intern Med* 1998;129:517–524.
65. Cho E, Smith-Warner SA, Ritz J, et al. Alcohol intake and colorectal cancer: a pooled analysis of 8 cohort studies. *Ann Intern Med* 2004;140:603–613.
66. Colangelo LA, Gapstur SM, Gann PH, et al. Cigarette smoking and colorectal carcinoma mortality in a cohort with long-term follow-up. *Cancer* 2004;100:288–293.
67. Shils ME, Olsen JA, Shikes M, Ross C. *Modern Nutrition in Health and Disease*, 9th ed. Baltimore: Lippincott Williams & Wilkins, p. 1238, 1999.
68. Bianchi GP, Marchesini G, Fabbri A, et al. Vegetable versus animal protein diet in cirrhotic patients with chronic encephalopathy. A randomized cross-over comparison. *J Intern Med* 1993;233:385–392.
69. Norrby S, Herlin P, Holmin T, et al. Early or delayed cholecystectomy for acute cholecystitis? A clinical trial. *Br J Surg* 1983;70:163–169.

29 Drug–Nutrient Interactions

David R. Thomas, M.D.

CONTENTS

29.1 INTRODUCTION

Orally administered drugs are absorbed from the gastrointestinal tract through a number of distinct mechanisms. At the same time, nutrients are absorbed through similar mechanisms. At times, this leads to a competition that alters the adsorption of either the drug or the specific nutrient, or both. A drug–nutrient interaction is defined as an alteration of the pharmacokinetics or pharmacodynamics of drug absorption, or of a nutritional element, or a compromise in nutritional status as a result of the addition of a drug.[1]

Drug–nutrient interactions result from at least four mechanisms. First, a direct interaction can take place between the drug and the nutrient before they enter the body. Examples include precipitation of the drug by an alteration of pH, binding of a nutrient by the drug, or insolubility of the drug in the nutrient medium. Often this interaction depends on the method of delivery, particularly with enteral feeding formulas. Most of these interactions can be avoided by not mixing the nutrient and drug in the same infusion device.

Second, the drug–nutrient interaction can affect absorption. Gastric pH, gastrointestinal transit time, dissolution of tablet forms, binding of the drug to the intestine, or rate of bile flow can interact to change drug bioavailability. This effect can result in either an increase or a decrease in bioavailability of the drug. Examples of the effect of gastric pH on drug absorption are shown in Table 29.1. The timing of the meal, or whether the meal contains fats, can also affect the pharmacokinetics

TABLE 29.1
Examples of Interaction of Gastric pH with Drug Absorption

Drug	Acid pH	Alkaline pH
Omeprazole	Decreased absorption	
Penicillins	Decreased absorption	
Dicloxacillin	Not affected	
Erythromycin	Decreased absorption	
Phenytoin	Decreased absorption	
Phenobarbital	Decreased absorption	
Aspirin	Decreased absorption	
Ketoconazole		Decreased absorption
Iron		Decreased absorption
Amphetamines	Increased absorption	
Tricyclic antidepressants	Increased absorption	

of the drug.[2] The transport of a drug across the intestine can be delayed by competition for a transport site or by a physical interaction with the food. The gastric and intestinal epithelial tissues contain enzymes necessary for drug metabolism. For example, cytochrome P450 (CYP) 3A4 isoenzyme in the small bowel regulates the oral bioavailability of approximately 50% of currently prescribed drugs.[3] A classic example of inhibition of intestinal cytochrome P450 3A4 by nutrients is the effect of grapefruit juice on drug metabolism. Most of these second types of interactions involving metabolism and transport cannot be avoided by separating the time of administration of the drug from the mealtime.

Third, a drug–nutrient interaction may occur after the drug is absorbed. The mechanism can be either direct or indirect. Direct interactions affect the systemic metabolism or the tissue distribution of the drug or nutrient to a specific organ. Indirect interactions affect a hormone or another cofactor necessary for drug metabolism. These types of interactions cannot be prevented, but may occasionally be overcome. For example, inhibition of folate metabolism by phenytoin or methotrexate can be overcome with supplemental folate administration. Pyridoxine deficiency caused by isoniazide can be overcome by supplemental pyridoxine.

Fourth, drug–nutrient interactions can affect the elimination or clearance of a drug or a nutrient through either renal or enterohepatic excretion. Examples include erythuria from the interaction of ranitidine and beets,[4] malodorous urine after eating asparagus, or the interaction of fava beans and monoamine oxidase inhibitors.

The interaction of drugs and nutrients is complex. There is no easily intuitive way to determine the specific influence of drug–nutrient interactions (or vice versa). A few categories of drug–nutrient interactions can be memorized; others can be covered in general guidelines. However, it is often necessary to research the specific drug prescribed for pharmacokinetic interactions with nutrients. Examples of common drug–nutrient interactions are given in Table 29.2.

TABLE 29.2
Examples of Drug–Nutrient Interactions

Drug	Effect on Nutrient
	Interaction with an Electrolyte
Amphotericin B	Decrease in potassium and magnesium
Albuterol	Decrease in potassium
Prednisone	Decrease in potassium
Furosemide, hydrochlorthiazide	Decrease in potassium, calcium, magnesium
Laxatives	Decrease in potassium and chloride
Lithium	Increase in excretion with sodium
Spironolactone	Increase in potassium
Terbutaline	Decrease in potassium
	Interaction with a Vitamin
Aspirin	Decrease in ascorbic acid
Cholestyramine	Decrease in fat-soluble vitamins, folate absorption
Colestipol	Decrease in fat-soluble vitamin absorption
Hydralazine	Decrease in pyridoxine metabolism
Phenytoin	Decrease in folate metabolism
Methotrexate	Decrease in folate metabolism
Trimethoprim	Decrease in folate metabolism
Triamterene	Decrease in folate metabolism
Warfarin	Decrease in vitamin K
	Nutrient Interaction with Drug
Levodopa	Inhibited by pyridoxine-containing foods
Isoniazide	Interaction with salmon, mackeral, or tuna; inhibits vitamin D metabolism
Monoamine oxidase inhibitors	Hypertensive crisis with tyramine
	Nutrient Interaction with Drug Absorption
Antivirals: didanosine, indinavir, zidovudine, saquinavir	Do not take within 2 hours of food
Bisphosphonates	Do not take within 2 hours of food, coffee, milk, orange juice, antacids, mineral supplements (iron or calcium)
Cancer chemotherapy drugs: estramustine, melphan, methotrexate, mercaptopurine	Do not take within 2 hours of food
Carbamazepam	Do not take within 2 hours of food or enteral feeds
Digoxin	Do not take within 2 hours of food, fiber, or antacids (calcium or magnesium)
Furosemide	Inconsistent relationship to food
Iron	Do not take within 2 hours of food, antacids, minerals; vitamin C may improve absorption
Nifedapine	Do not take within 2 hours of food

Drug–nutrient interactions can vary between serious and life-threatening (hypertensive crisis with monamine oxidase inhibitors) to clinically mild (electrolyte depletion with diurectics). Although examples of drug–nutrient interactions are given in the tables, no judgment is rendered on the clinical relevance of the interaction.

29.2 THE EFFECT OF TIMING OF MEALS

A number of drugs are not influenced by the presence of food in the stomach or gastrointestinal tract. For these drugs, no consideration need be taken in regard to mealtimes. For other drugs, improved absorption occurs in the presence of food. For example, the absorption of some lipid-lowering drugs in the presence of food is improved. Lovastatin has poor bioavailability when administered orally. Although the exact mechanism is not clear, lovastatin absorption is increased by up to 33% when administered after a meal.[5] The bioavailability of nitrofurantoin is increased in the presence of food because of delayed gastric emptying, resulting in increased absorption. The absorption of griseofulvin is improved by foods with a high fat content because the drug is lipid soluble. Some theophylline products also show increased rate of absorption when taken with high-fat meals. For example, when sustained-release theophylline is administered with a high-fat meal, almost 50% of the drug may be absorbed within 4 hours of administration.[6] This may result in toxic serum concentrations. Because of increased absorption with food, sustained-release theophylline formulations should be taken on an empty stomach. An immediate-release formulation should be selected if the medication is administered with food.

The increase in absorption of some drugs may result in higher serum concentrations of the medication, as with griesofulvin. However, increased absorption may also result in an increased incidence of side effects.

A number of other drugs exhibit a delayed absorption from the gastrointestinal tract in the presence of food. In some instances, advantage can be taken of the delayed absorption to prevent or delay gastrointestinal side effects, for example, with iron preparations. At other times, the presence of food in the stomach can decrease absorption to the extent of interfering with the pharmacological effect of the drug, for example, with certain antibiotics. Antibiotic drugs are one of the most frequently affected by the presence of food. In most, but not all, circumstances, absorption is delayed. Table 29.3 gives examples of the effect of food on antibiotic absorption.

The most common recommendation from pharmaceutical manufacturers is to administer a medication either 1 hour before a meal or 2 hours after a meal.[7] In the absence of knowledge of a specific drug–nutrient interaction, this is the most prudent strategy.

29.3 THE EFFECT OF ENTERAL FEEDING

As a general rule, enteral feeding formulas and drugs, regardless of their formulation, should not be mixed.[8] The oral absorption of warfarin, tetracycline, fluoroquinolone antibiotics, and phenytoin is decreased with concomitant enteral feeding.[9] Interaction of warfarin with enteral feeding may result from increased vitamin K for those formulas that contain vitamin K or from an interaction of warfarin with protein in the formula.[10]

TABLE 29.3
Examples of Interaction of Food with Antibiotics

Drug	Effect with Food
Erythromycin base (E-mycin, EryTabs, EYRC) and erythromycin stearate (Erythrocin)	Decreased absorption
Erythromycin estolate or erythromycin ethylsuccinate	Less decreased absorption
Fluoroquinolones: ciprofloxacin, ofloxacin, lomefloxacin	Decreased absorption (14 to 50%) with divalent cations (aluminum, calcium, magnesium, zinc); decreased absorption (90%) with antacids; decreased absorption with calcium and calcium-containing orange juice
Griseofulvin	Increased absorption with fats
Isoniazid	Decreased absorption
Ketoconazole	Decreased absorption
Nitrofurantoin	Increased absorption
Penicillin salts	Decreased absorption
Rifampin	Decreased absorption
Tetracycline and doxycycline	Decreased absorption (50%)

The classic interaction of enteral feeding formulas and a drug is observed with phenytoin. Administration of phenytoin sodium with food or different physical properties of dilantin preparations has been thought to decrease absorption, potentially leading to loss of seizure control.[11] Although food slows absorption of phenytoin, it does not appear to have an affect on the bioavailability of phenytoin. Thus, phenytoin by mouth may be taken without regard to meals.[12] However, the situation is very different in the presence of enteral feeding formulas. The absorption of phenytoin is significantly decreased, resulting in a 70 to 80% reduction in steady-state blood levels. This apparently results from phenytoin–calcium and phenytoin–protein complexes that are not absorbed through the gastrointestinal tract.[13]

Phenytoin doses should be administered at least 2 hours after a feeding, and the feeding tube should be flushed with 60 ml of water. After phenytoin administration, the feeding tube should be flushed with another 60 ml of water and the enteral feeding starting no sooner than 2 hours after dosing. Because phenytoin suspension is often administered in three to four doses per day, intermittent enteral feedings (bolus) are more desirable to deliver adequate nutrients. Serum phenytoin levels should be monitored and the dosage adjusted to achieve therapeutic concentrations. If continuous enteral feeding is necessary, intravenous phenytoin should be used.

29.4 OTHER FACTORS AFFECTING DRUG–NUTRIENT INTERACTIONS

Medications are formulated to dissolve at predictable rates, insuring a desired drug delivery. Extended-release drugs are designed to delay absorption and produce a

TABLE 29.4
Abbreviations for Long-Acting Medications

CR	Controlled release
CRT	Controlled-release tablet
LA	Long acting
SA	Sustained action
SR	Sustained release
TD	Time delay
TR	Timed release
XL	Extended release
XR	Extended release

sustained drug delivery over time. Most, but not all, extended-release products contain abbreviations affixed to their brand names. The abbreviations can be a clue that crushing these products should be avoided. Some examples of common abbreviation affixes are listed in Table 29.4.

In persons who cannot swallow, or who are fed by enteral feeding tubes, the crushing of solid medications can change their pharmacokinetic properties and may alter the delivery of the medication. Medication formulations, including sublingual or buccal, enteric-coated, and extended- or sustained-release tablets or capsules, should not be crushed for this reason.

Often, a liquid or suspension formulation of a drug is used for enteral feeding to avoid this problem. However, the pharmacokinetics of liquid forms of a drug may differ from the tablets or capsules, and dosage adjustment may be necessary when a liquid is substituted, particularly if the preferred tablet or capsule is an extended-release medication. In addition, the liquid formulations may need to be administered more frequently.

29.5 ALTERATIONS OF DRUG METABOLISM

A few nutrients have a direct effect on drug metabolism. Usually, this is mediated through a particular genetic predisposition in an individual. Fava beans have been shown to interact with the antimalarial agent primaquine and can precipitate symptoms of glucose-6-phosphorylase deficiency.[14] Watercress contains phenethyl isothiocyanate, which can inhibit CYP 2E1. Ingestion of 50 g of watercress when taken with acetaminophen, results in a reduction of the serum level of acetaminophen.[15] The classic example of the effect of a nutrient on drug metabolism is the effect of grapefruit juice on inhibition of intestinal cytochrome P450 3A4 (Table 29.5).

29.6 PHARMACOLOGIC INTERACTIONS OF MEDICATIONS WITH NUTRIENTS

Nutrient–drug interactions can interfere with the pharmacokinetics of drugs. The most common reactions include the interaction of vitamin K-rich foods and warfarin and the interaction of pyridoxine-rich foods and levodopa. Foods associated with these interactions are shown in Table 29.6 and Table 29.7.

TABLE 29.5
Potential Interaction of Grapefruit Juice with Drugs

Drug Class	Example
Antiarrhythmic	Amniodarone
Antiallergenic	Desloratadine
	Fenoxfenadine
Antibiotic	Erythromycin
Anticoagulant	Warfarin
Antidepressant	Sertraline
Antifungal	Intraconazole
Antihypertensive	Felodapine
	Nifedapine
	Nisolodapine
	Pranidapine
Antilipid	Atorvastatin
	Lovastatin
	Simvastatin
Antiretroviral	Saquinavir
	Indinivir
Antiseizure	Carbamazepine
Anxiolytic/sedative	Diazepam
	Midazolam
	Triazolam
	Buspirone
	Zaleplon
Bronchodilator	Theophylline
Chemotherapeutic agent	Cyclophosphamide
	Tammoxiphen
	Vincristine
	Vinblastine
Estrogen	Ethinyl estradiol
Immune suppressant	Cyclosporine
	Tacrolimus
	Sirolimus
Impotence	Sildenafil
	Tadalafil
Pain	Methodone

Note: Compiled from various lists. The magnitude and clinical important of the interaction may vary.

29.7 CONCLUSION

Drug–nutrient interactions result from several different mechanisms, including the absorption, metabolism, and excretion of either the drug or a nutrient. In general, it is prudent to avoid the concomitant administration of a drug with meals or enteral

TABLE 29.6
Vitamin K-Rich Foods to Limit When Taking Warfarin

Beef and pork liver	Chick peas
Green tea	Kale
Broccoli	Spinach
Brussel sprouts	Turnip greens
Cauliflower	

TABLE 29.7
Pyridoxine-Rich Foods to Avoid When Taking Levodopa

Avocado	Peas
Beans	Pork
Bacon	Sweet potatoes
Beef liver	Tuna

feeding. In certain circumstances, however, the interaction can be used to increase the absorption of a drug or to minimize the adverse effects of a drug. For known interference of a drug with a specific nutrient, strategies to overcome the interference with the nutrient must be taken.

REFERENCES

1. Chan L-N. Redefining drug-nutrient interactions. *Nutr Clin Pract* 2000;15:249–252.
2. Singh BN. Effects of food on clinical pharmacokinetics. *Clin Pharmacokinet* 1999;37:213–255.
3. Rendic S, DiCarlo FJ. Human cytochrome P450 enzymes: a status report summarizing their reactions, substrates, inducers, and inhibitors. *Drug Metab Rev* 1997;29:413–580.
4. Mitchell SC. Beeting a crimson retreat: beeturia. *Lancet* 1996;347:474–475.
5. Kirk J. Significant drug-nutrient interactions. *Am Fam Physician* 1995;51:1175–1182.
6. Edwards DJ, Zarowitz BJ, Slaughter RL. Theophylline. In *Applied Pharmacokinetics: Principles of Therapeutic Drug Monitoring*, 3rd ed., Evans WE, Schentag JJ, Jusko WJ, Eds. Applied Therapeutics, Vancouver, 1992, chap. 13.
7. Maka DA, Murphy LK. Drug-nutrient interactions: a review. *Adv Pract Acute Crit Care* 2000;11:580–589.
8. Lourenco R. Enteral feeding: drug/nutrient interaction. *Clin Nutr* 2001;20:187–193.
9. Chan LN. Drug-nutrient interaction in clinical nutrition. *Curr Opin Clin Nutr Metab Care* 2002;5:327–332.
10. Penrod LE, Allen JB, Cabacungan LR. Warfarin resistance and enteral feedings: 2 case reports and a supporting *in vitro* study. *Arch Phys Med Rehabil* 2001;82:1270–1273.
11. Wilder B, Leppik I, Hietpas TJ, Cloyd JC, Randinitis EJ, Cook J. Effect of food on absorption of Dilantin Kapseals and Mylan extended phenytoin sodium capsules. *Neurology* 2001;57:582–589.

12. Cook J, Randinitis EJ, Wilder BJ. Effect of food on the bioavailability of 100-mg Dilantin Kapseals. *Neurology* 2001;57:698–700.
13. Au Yeung SC, Ensom MHH. Phenytoin and enteral feedings: does evidence support an interaction? *Ann Pharmacother* 2000;34:896–905.
14. Cittadella R, Civitelli D, Manna I, et al. Genetic heterogeneity of glucose-6-phosphate dehydrogenase deficiency in south-east Sicily. *Ann Hum Genet* 1997;61:229–234.
15. Chen L, Mohr SN, Yang CS. Decrease of plasma and urinary oxidative metabolites of acetaminophen after consumption of watercress by human volunteers. *Clin Pharmacol Ther* 1996;60:651–660.

30 Nutrition and the Endocrine System

Neelavathi Senkottaiyan, M.D.
John E. Morley, M.B., B.Ch.

CONTENTS

Aging processes induce multiple changes in the hormonal network (hormonal pause), immune system, and nutritional state and can modulate their effectiveness in determining a response to stressors. There is increasing evidence of the coupling of immune status to the metabolic system. This communication is mediated via complex interaction of hormones, nutrients, cytokines, and neuropeptides.

Aging or frailty is a syndrome characterized by reduced functional reserve and impaired adaptive capacity that results from cumulative declines of multiple subsystems, including the endocrine system. Aging is associated with anatomic changes of the endocrine glands, as a result of programmed cell death (apoptosis), autoimmune-mediated destruction of the gland, or neoplastic transformation. Age-related changes in hormonal secretion occur secondary to physiological alterations in circadian and seasonal rhythms or in the frequency and peak of hormonal pauses.[1,2] Some of these changes are compensatory for the age-related reduction in hormonal clearance, and others are the results of changes in glandular sensitivity to secretagogues or inhibitory stimuli, altered bioactivity, altered transport of hormones to the binding sites, hormone–receptor interactions, or postreceptor changes. Aging is also associated with alterations in plasma membrane properties, intrinsic changes in cellular enzyme activity, and alterations in calcium mobilization and gene expression. Some of these changes are directly related to aging, while others are secondary to age-associated diseases and changes in nutritional state. This chapter briefly reviews the relationship of nutrition and the endocrine system in aging and some of the common endocrine disorders in the elderly population.

TABLE 30.1
Effects of Dietary Restriction and Aging on Hormones in Rodents

Hormone	Aging	Dietary Restriction
Insulin	Decrease	Decrease
Insulin receptor mRNA	Increase	Increase
Corticosterone	Increase	Increase
Insulin growth factor-1	Decrease	Decrease
Growth hormone	Decrease	Decrease
Thyroxine	Decrease	Decrease
Testosterone (males)	Decrease	Decrease
Estradiol (females)	Decrease	Decrease
Norepinephrine	Increase	No effect
25(OH) Vitamin D	Decrease	No effect
Parathyroid hormone	Increase	Decrease

Dietary restriction, which prolongs life in animals, produces many of the hormonal changes that are seen in old age.[3] This suggests that these hormonal changes may play a physiologic role in slowing the aging process.

30.1 THYROID

Several studies have pointed out that hypothyroidism occurs with increasing frequency in older populations, with a prevalence of 7 to 11% and with women being more commonly affected than men and subclinical more common than overt hypothyroidism. Virtually all cases of hypothyroidism are due to autoimmune thyroid disease with measurable titers of thyroid autoantibodies. The prevalence of hyperthyroidism is approximately 0.5 to 3% in the elderly. Thyroid nodules do occur with increasing frequency in the elderly, and well-differentiated cancers do predominate, but their course is frequently less predictable than in younger patients. Major changes in thyroid hormones occur when the person becomes ill—so-called euthyroid sick syndrome[4] (Table 30.2). Protein-energy malnutrition is a common cause of euthyroid sick syndrome in the aging population. The available evidence for age-induced changes in the hypothalamic–pituitary–thyroid axis in healthy aging humans is given in Figure 30.1.[5]

Overall, the combination of low TSH and low T3, together with normal T4 and increased reverse T3, in the elderly is interpreted as an age-induced partial central hypothyroidism, associated with an impaired activity of type I deiodinase. Sensitivity to thyroid hormones is decreased in most organs with the exception of pituitary. All these age-induced physiological changes should not lead to abnormal serum levels of thyroid hormones in the elderly. Therefore, abnormal TSH levels in the elderly have to be explained and need further investigation. In the elderly, thyroid dysfunction develops insidiously and is dominated by nonspecific symptoms and clinical findings typically related to normal aging or age-associated disease. So, case finding in combination with low threshold for biochemical control is

TABLE 30.2
Typical Changes in Thyroid Levels with Various Diseases

Hormone	Aging	Hyperthyroid	Hypothyroid	Euthyroid Sick
Thyroxine	Normal	Increase	Decrease	Normal/decrease
Triiodothyronine (T3)	Mild decrease	Increase	Normal/decrease	Decrease
T3 uptake	Normal	Increase	Decrease	Increase
Free thyroxine index	Normal	Increase	Decrease	Normal/decrease
Thyroid-stimulating hormone				
Basal	Normal	Decrease	Increase	Decrease/normal increase
Response to thyrotropin-releasing hormone	Decrease	Decrease	Increase	Decrease

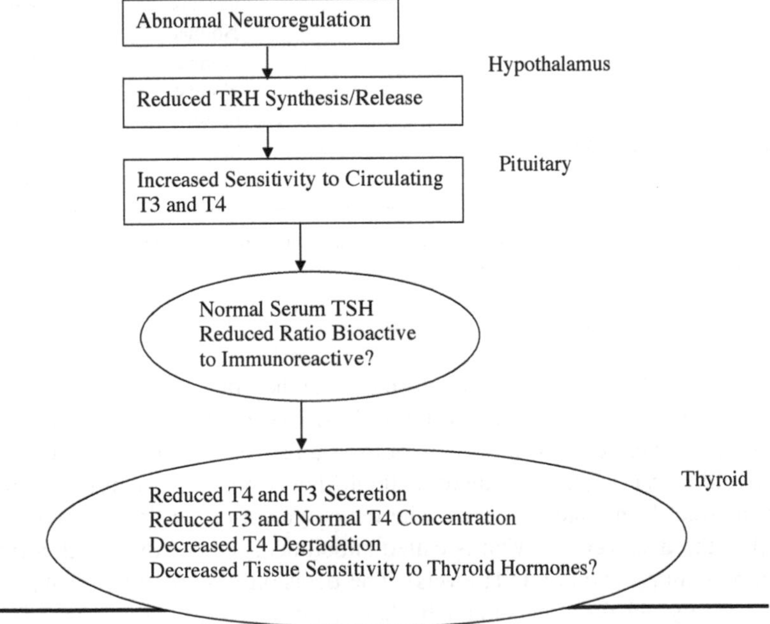

FIGURE 30.1 Changes in the hypothalamic–pituitary–thyroid axis with aging.

recommended. Additionally, the diagnosis of hyper- or hypothyroidism can be more difficult in the elderly because the symptoms may be more subtle. Hyperthyroidism may be disguised by a very apathetic presentation, myopathy, and unexplained weight loss without many of the typical adrenergic symptoms, such as tachycardia and nervousness. Some of the many ways in which hypothyroidism may present include occult congestive heart failure, severe fecal impaction, depression, or cognitive impairment.

TABLE 30.3
Effects of Thyroid Diseases on Vitamin Status

Vitamin	Hypothyroid	Hyperthyroid
Vitamin A	Increase	Decrease
Retinol-binding protein		Decrease
Thiamine		
Erythrocyte transketolase	?	Decrease[a]
In vitro thiamine pyridinylase (Thiaminase)	?	None[b]
Riboflavin	?	Increase
Erythrocyte glutathione reductase	Decrease	?
Flavine adenine nucleotide	Decrease	?
Pyridoxine		
Xanthurenic acid excretion after trytophan administration	?	Increase[c]
Vitamin B12	Decrease/normal	Decrease
Homocysteine	Increase	Normal
Folate	Normal	?
Vitamin C	Normal	Normal
25-Hydroxyvitamin D3	Normal	Normal
1,25-Hydroxyvitamin D3	Increase	Decrease
Alpha-tocopherol (vitamin E)	Increase	Decrease
Vitamin K	?	Decrease

[a] The decrease in erythrocyte transketolase suggests thiamine deficiency, but the failure of *in vitro* thiamine augmentation suggests other causes.

[b] About 5 to 10% have pernicious anemia.

[c] Suggests pyridoxine deficiency.

Because of the decrease in the plasma clearance rate and the vulnerability of elderly people to the side effects of thyroid hormones, it is recommended to start thyroid replacement at a lower dose than in younger patients (0.050 to 0.10 mg).

Thyroid extract or Armour thyroid should never be used because of wide variations in effect from batch to batch. The development of sensitive assays for TSH has led to the discovery of what is called subclinical thyroid dysfunction (isolated elevation or suppression of TSH levels). The decision to treat elderly subjects with subclinical thyroid disorder should be based on a careful assessment of risk of treatment vs. progression of the disease state. The effects of thyroid disease on vitamins are delineated in Table 30.3.

30.2 ADRENAL HORMONES

Aging in humans is accompanied by an increase in adrenal glucocorticoid secretion and a decline in adrenal androgen synthesis and secretion.[6] The intense interest in adrenal function in aging individuals in recent years is related to the potential impact of cortisol excess in the development of cognitive impairment and hippocampal neuronal loss and to the desire to provide hormone replacement and healthy aging.

During the anabolic growth period (early adulthood) the body is exposed to relatively high levels of DHEA and DHEA-S and to the relatively high levels of cortisol during infancy and the aging phase. The cortisol/DHEA-S ratio during the life span follows a U-shaped curve.

The above physiological changes in the HPA axis in aging construct the corpus of a syndrome named andrenopause, which is manifested as sarcopenia, osteopenia, atherosclerosis progression, cognitive impairment, and deterioration of the immune function.

Serum levels of norepinephrine increase and renin and aldosterone decrease in the elderly. Target organ responses to beta-adrenergic stimulation in the heart and also vascular smooth muscle decrease due to postreceptor changes contributing to hypertension and orthostatic hypotension, which characterize the elderly.

Less than 10% of patients with Addison's disease are over 60 years of age. Addison's disease, which is rare, is often missed in older patients, leading to inappropriate nursing home admissions. The classic signs and symptoms of Addison's disease include weakness, fatigue, weight loss, abdominal plain, constipation or diarrhea, salt craving, vomiting, hyponatremia, hyperkalemia, hypoglycemia, postural hypotension, hyperpigmentation, and eosinophilia. Diagnosis is made by ACTH stimulation test, demonstrating an inadequate cortisol response.

Cushing's syndrome is very rare in older persons. However, ectopic ACTH production secondary to cancer is relatively common. This is characterized by cachexia rather than obesity, proximal muscle weakness, hypokalemic alkalosis, delirium, and hyperpigmentation. The common cause of elevated corticosteroid levels in older persons is exogenous steroid administration. Glucocorticoids promote gluconeogensis, negative nitrogen balance, hyperglycemia, hyperinsulinemia, free fatty acid mobilization, hypertriglyceridemia, osteopenia, and altered vitamin D metabolism.

In older patients with severe weight loss and difficult-to-control hypertension, the possibility of pheochromocytoma should be considered.

30.3 GROWTH HORMONE

Aging is associated with a decline in the somatotroph axis.[7–10] Consequently, insulin-like growth factor (IGF)-1 levels decline progressively. This mainly reflects the impaired GH secretion, but decline in gonadal sex steroids and malnutrition also play a role. Decrease in GH secretion may partially explain the age-related changes in the metabolism, bones, muscles, cardiovascular system (CVS), central nervous system (CNS), immune system, and sense of well-being. Normal aging and GH deficiency share several clinical signs and symptoms. Owing to clinical similarities between aging and GH deficiency, the relative GH insufficiency of elderly subjects has been postulated as one important factor contributing to frailty. Hence, the assumption that hormonal therapy is a potential "fountain of youth" appears logical. However, it is currently unclear whether treatment with exogenous GH can retard or reverse age-related changes in body structure and function. Several studies showed that GH treatment was followed by an increase in lean mass, a decrease in fat mass, and an increase in bone turnover, but had no impact on physical function.

Recombinant human growth hormone (rhGH) treatment was associated with greater risk of neoplasm, hyperglycemia, and gynecomastia; hence, there is less enthusiasm for reversing the changes of somatopause with rhGH.

30.4 HYPOGONADISM

The permanent cessation of the menses (menopause) occurs at an average age of 51 years in women. Ovarian secretion of estrogens and, to lesser extent, androgens decreases, and secretion of follicle-stimulating hormone (FSH) and luteinizing hormone increases rather abruptly in about the sixth decade in women. The major metabolic effect of the lack of estrogen is rapid bone loss, which can be retarded by estrogen replacement. Estrogen therapy increases high-density lipoprotein (HDL) levels and triglycerides and decreases low-density lipoprotein (LDL) levels. But the Women's Health Initiative Study showed that estrogen replacement increases the risk of heart attack, stroke, and venous thromboembolism in high-risk individuals. So, hormone replacement therapy (HRT) is not routinely used to prevent postmenopausal bone loss.

Men have a more gradual decline in their gonadal hormones.[11] Nevertheless, by 50 years of age over half have testosterone levels below those seen in young men. Because serum sex hormone-binding globulin concentrations increase with age, older men have a greater decline in serum-free testosterone concentrations than in serum total testosterone concentrations. This decline is referred to as andropause. However, unlike menopause, where complete estrogen deficiency with known clinical consequences occurs, the decline in androgens in aging men varies from modest to severe and has unclear clinical consequences. Short-term testosterone therapy has been shown to improve muscle strength and surprisingly decrease LDL cholesterol. Low testosterone levels have been associated with minimal hip fracture in older men in nursing homes. Low testosterone levels predict mortality in older males.[12] Testosterone therapy may also decrease dehydration in older persons, increase hematocrit, produce gynecomastia, and potentially accelerate prostate growth. Sperm production is stable from soon after the completion of puberty to about age 70 years, after which it declines progressively by about 50% by age 90 years. This is accompanied by tubular fibrosis, shrinkage of testicular volume, and modest elevations of FSH.

30.5 OTHER HORMONES

Aging shifts the serum vasopressin–osmolality relationship toward increasing serum vasopressin due to altered baroreceptor input, contributing to the tendency toward hyponatremia in the elderly.[13] Paradoxically, renal responsiveness to vasopressin is reduced in older, compared with younger, subjects, making them more vulnerable to water deprivation. The vasopressin response to osmotic stimulation may or may not be increased in older subjects, whereas the vasopressin response to volume depletion, a response mediated via baroreceptors, is increased. There is a parallel decrease in thirst in response to osmotic stimulation. As a result of the decreases in thirst and renal responsiveness to vasopressin, older subjects can become more easily dehydrated, even if vasopressin secretion rises.

Aging also produces mild carbohydrate intolerance and a minimal increase in fasting serum glucose in healthy, nonobese elderly individuals, primarily due to decreasing postreceptor responsiveness to insulin (see Chapter 26).

Serum parathyroid hormone (PTH) concentrations are slightly higher in older subjects than in younger subjects. The likely cause of this increase is a fall in serum calcium concentration due to mild vitamin D deficiency and also phosphate retention caused by declining renal function. Vitamin D levels need to be maintained above 30 mg/dl in older persons. Melatonin secretion is lower in older subjects than in younger subjects, particularly the surge in melatonin secretion that occurs during sleep at night. This decrease is a possible cause of poor sleep in many older persons.

Leptin, a hormone produced by adipose tissue in proportion to body fat mass, decreases appetite.[14] Serum leptin concentrations decrease with increasing age, although some find this to be so only in women. The modest fall in serum leptin concentrations with age may contribute to increasing adiposity in older persons. Adiponectin is a protein hormone secreted by adipocytes. It reduces insulin resistance, is associated with lower risk of atherosclerosis, and has anti-inflammatory properties. Recent research shows that plasma adiponectin concentrations do not change significantly with age in women, but were higher in men over age 70 than in younger men. The higher levels of adiponectin observed in older men could reflect a longitudinal aging change or simply enhanced survival of men with more of this adipokine hormone.

REFERENCES

1. Kim, M.J. and Morley, J.E., The hormonal fountains of youth: myth or reality? *J. Endocrinol. Invest.*, 28, 5, 2005.
2. van den Beld, A.W. and Lamberts, S.W., Endocrine aspects of healthy ageing in men, *Novartis Found. Symp.*, 242, 3, 2002.
3. Morley, J.E., Aging, in *Yearbook of Endocrinology*, Bagdade, J.D., Ed., Mosby, St. Louis, 1993, p. 61.
4. De Groot, L.J., Non-thyroidal illness syndrome is a manifestation of hypothalamic-pituitary dysfunction, and in view of current evidence, should be treated with appropriate replacement therapies, *Crit. Care Clin.*, 22, 57, 2006.
5. Mooradian, A.D. and Wong, N.C., Age-related changes in thyroid hormone action, *Eur. J. Endocrinol.*, 131, 451, 1994.
6. Ferrari, M. and Mantero, F., Male aging and hormones: the adrenal cortex, *J. Endocrinol. Invest.*, 28, 92, 2005.
7. Melmed, S., Supplemental growth hormone in healthy adults: the endocrinologist's responsibility, *Natl. Clin. Pract. Endocrinol. Metab.*, 2, 119, 2006.
8. Rudman, D., Growth hormone, body composition, and aging, *J. Am. Geriatr. Soc.*, 33, 800, 1985.
9. Cohn, L., Feller, A.G., Drapper, M.W., et al., Carpal tunnel syndrome and gynaecomastia during growth hormone treatment of elderly men with low circulating IGF-I concentrations, *Clin. Endocrinol.*, 39, 417, 1986.
10. Morley, J.E., Hormones and the aging process, *J. Am. Geriatr. Soc.*, 51, S333, 2003.
11. Haren, M.T., Kim, M.J., Tariq, S.H., et al., Andropause: a quality-of-life issue in older men, *Med. Clin. North Am.*, 90, 1005, 2006.

12. Shores, M.M., Matsumoto, A.M., Sloan, K.L., et al., Low serum testosterone and mortality in male veterans, *Arch. Intern. Med.*, 166, 1660, 2006.
13. Miller, M., Hyponatremia and arginine vasopressin dysregulation: mechanisms, clinical consequences, and management, *J. Am. Geriatr. Soc.*, 54, 345, 2006.
14. Morley, J.E., The metabolic syndrome and aging, *J. Gerontol. A Biol. Sci. Med. Sci.*, 59, 139, 2004.

31 Nutritional Anemia in Older Persons

David R. Thomas, M.D.

CONTENTS

Anemia is a common disorder in the elderly population and is an independent predictor for increased morbidity and mortality over 5 years, even after adjustment for comorbid disease.[1] Older patients with anemia have a higher likelihood of physical decline, disability, hospital admission, and institutionalization.[2] Anemia has been associated with both frailty[3] and mobility impairment,[4] has been shown to lead to functional impairment,[3,4] and is a risk factor for falls in older persons.[5–7] Women with a hemoglobin concentration between 13 and 14 g/dl have better mobility and lower mortality than those with a hemoglobin concentration of less than 12 g/dl.[4] Anemia is strongly associated with an increase in myocardial infarction and poor outcomes following an infarct.[8] Prolonged anemia results in left ventricular hypertrophy.[9] Quality of life is impaired in persons with anemia[10] and produces a high level of fatigue.[11] Treatment of anemia increases hemoglobin concentration, improves quality of life, and may decrease mortality.[10–12] Patients with congestive heart failure and an ejection fraction of less than 40% who received treatment for anemia had a 42% improvement in a New York Heart Association class, compared with the control patients, who had a decrease of 11.4%.[13] The correction of anemia also produces a decrease in left ventricular hypertrophy.[9]

Despite the growing evidence of these poor outcomes associated with anemia in older persons, the diagnosis is often overlooked and, more importantly, undertreated.

31.1 DEFINITION AND PREVALENCE

The World Health Organization defines anemia as a hemoglobin concentration of less than 13 g/dl in men and less than 12 g/dl in women.[14] Hemoglobin and hematocrit values differ little between the healthy elderly population and the younger population. Thus, anemia is not a normal finding in older persons, and hemoglobin concentration should not be adjusted downward in older persons.[15,16]

In a noninstitutionalized population assessed in the third National Health and Nutrition Examination Survey (1988 to 1994), 11% of men and 10.2% of women 65 years and older were anemic by World Health Organization standards. Anemia prevalence increased to greater than 20% at age 85 and older. In the established population database, 9% of men and women age 71 to 74 years were anemic. The proportion of anemic persons increased differentially with age, reaching 41% for men and 21% for women age 90 years or older, respectively.[17,18] In this population, nutrient deficiency accounted for a third of anemia; either chronic kidney disease, anemia of chronic disease, or both accounted for an additional third,; and one third was unexplained.[19]

A marked sex difference in the frequency of anemia is observed. The corrected annual incidence of anemia was higher in men older than 65 years (90.3 per 1000 subjects) than in women older than 65 years (69.1 per 1000 subjects) in a population-based study.[20] Sex differences in hemoglobin concentration may result from differences in testosterone concentration. Hypogonadism in older males (andropause) is commonly associated with approximately a 1 g/dl fall in hemoglobin concentration.[21] Furthermore, men who have functional hypogonadism from pituitary adenomas are anemic,[22] and men with prostate cancer who are undergoing therapy with total androgen blockade are anemic.[23]

31.2 CAUSES OF NUTRITIONAL ANEMIA

The manufacture of blood proceeds in the bone marrow in a complex, regulated process. The causes of anemia can be grouped into failure of the bone marrow to manufacture adequate blood components, gradual or rapid blood loss from hemorrhage, or a rapid breakdown of blood components (hemolysis) in the marrow or peripherally. The bone marrow may fail to produce adequate blood components because of inadequate nutrients (vitamin B12, folate, pyridoxine, or iron) necessary for blood production, altered maturation of blood cells (myelodysplastic syndromes), or primary impairment of hemoglobin synthesis (hemoglobinopathy) (Table 31.1).

This review focuses on the nutrient-related causes of anemia.

31.3 IRON DEFICIENCY ANEMIA

Iron deficiency anemia occurs in 3% of children age 1 to 2 years, 2% of adolescent girls, 1% of adolescent boys and men, and 5% of women of childbearing age. Seven percent of persons older than 50 years have iron deficiency anemia.[24] Although iron deficiency, due to low iron intake or low bioavailability of dietary iron, is a main cause of anemia in younger populations, it appears to be less important in old age.

TABLE 31.1
Causes of Anemia

Causes of Anemia
Bone marrow failure
Inadequate nutrients
Inadequate erythropoiesis
Genetic
Hemorrhage
Hemolysis

The most common cause of iron deficiency in older persons is a result of acute or chronic loss through the gastrointestinal tract.[25] A dietary deficiency of iron is rare in older populations.

Since gastrointestinal (GI) blood loss accounts for most causes of iron deficiency anemia in older adults, patients should undergo both upper and lower endoscopy procedures. Upper GI endoscopy can be expected to reveal a cause in between 30 and 50% of patients. All patients should undergo examination of the lower GI tract because a second, separate disease occurs in 10 to 15% of patients. In those subjects who cannot tolerate endoscopy, barium studies may be helpful.[26]

Ferritin values less than 15 ng/ml are considered diagnostic of iron deficiency. The cutoff point for the diagnosis of iron deficiency anemia can be varied to achieve optimum sensitivity or specificity. Serum ferritin values less than 30 ng/ml will include 92 to 98% of all anemia due to iron deficiency. Levels greater than 100 mg/dl generally exclude iron deficiency. Intermediate ferritin values (30 to 99 mg/dl) represent an area of uncertain significance in terms of iron stores.

The most difficult differential diagnostic problem is distinguishing iron deficiency anemia from anemia associated with the presence of chronic inflammatory disease. Serum iron, total iron-binding capacity, and transferrin saturation do not accurately distinguish iron deficiency anemia from anemia of chronic disease. Since ferritin concentrations are elevated in inflammatory disease states, as well as in liver disease, renal disease, cancer, and in some elderly women, soluble transferrin receptors can be of use in making the diagnosis of iron deficiency.

Circulating soluble transferrin receptors is a relatively new tool in the diagnosis of anemia. The receptor assay is elevated in iron deficiency anemia even in the presence of chronic disease, but normal or only slightly raised in anemia of chronic disease. Soluble transferrin receptor divided by the log of ferritin (<2.55) is the best method of differentiating anemia of chronic disease from iron deficiency anemia[27,28] (Table 31.2).

Chronic inflammatory disease states impair iron absorption from the gut and release iron from marrow stores. Recently, attention has focused on hepcidin, a polypeptide synthesized in the liver. Chronic inflammation is a potent stimulus for the production of hepcidin. Hepcidin has been shown to reduce the intestinal absorption of iron and to block the effective use of iron stores from the reticuloendothelial system.[29] Both digestive iron absorption by enterocytes and iron recycling by macrophages appear to be controlled by hepcidin, likely through a hormonal action.[30]

TABLE 31.2
Comparison of Anemia of Chronic Disease and Iron Deficiency Anemia

	Iron Deficiency Anemia	Anemia of Chronic Disease
Mean corpuscular volume	Normal or decreased	Decreased or normal
Serum iron	Decreased	Decreased
Total iron-binding capacity	Increased	Normal to decreased
Serum ferritin	Decreased	Increased
Soluble transferrin receptor	Increased	Decreased

This mechanism is a likely explanation for the relative poor absorption of iron in chronic kidney disease. Anemia of chronic inflammation has also been reported to be associated with a diminished response to erythropoietin and a shortened red blood cell survival.[31] Whether these effects are independent of the inflammatory process or result from the restriction of iron availability is not yet known. Some patients respond to treatment with erythropoietin, but treatment of the underlying inflammatory process is the only means of restoring normal iron balance. The role of cytokines in the pathogenesis of the anemia of chronic inflammation suggests that specific modulation of the cytokine cascade may lead to development of new therapeutic approaches to the treatment of iron utilization anemia.

31.4 VITAMIN B12 AND FOLATE

Vitamin B12 and folate are two interrelated vitamins that have interdependent roles in nucleic acid synthesis (Figure 31.1). Deficiencies of either vitamin can cause megaloblastic anemia; however, inappropriate treatment of B12 deficiency with folate can cause irreversible nerve degeneration.

Little data exist about the population prevalence of pernicious anemia. Data are largely based on surveys of subjects with florid manifestations or from retrospective analyses of previously diagnosed disease. In one population-based survey, the estimated prevalence was 2.7% in women and 1.4% in men. The frequency of pernicious anemia was higher in both black women (4.3%) and white women (4.0%).[32]

Macrocytic red cell morphology is often used to highlight suspicion of a megaloblastic anemia. However, drug therapy, followed by alcohol, liver disease, and reticulocytosis, is the most common cause of macrocytosis (mean corpuscular volume greater than 100 fl) in a sample of 300 hospitalized subjects. Megaloblastic hematopoiesis accounted for less than 10% of cases. On the other hand, a mean corpuscular volume greater than 120 fl was usually caused by B12 deficiency.[33]

The recommended daily allowance for vitamin B12 is 2.4 μg, but elderly people should obtain their vitamin B12 from either supplements or fortified foods (e.g., fortified ready-to-eat breakfast cereals) to ensure adequate absorption from the gastrointestinal tract. Absorption of crystalline vitamin B12 does not decline with advancing age. However, compared with the younger population, absorption of protein-bound vitamin B12 is decreased in the elderly, owing to a high prevalence

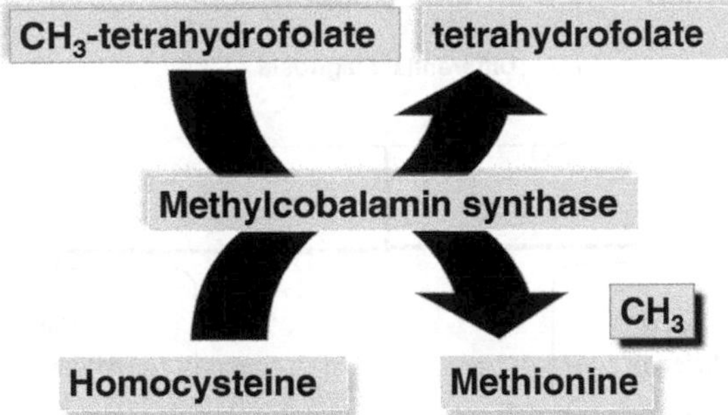

FIGURE 31.1 Metabolism of cobalamin and folate.

of atrophic gastritis in this age group. Atrophic gastritis results in a low acid–pepsin secretion by the gastric mucosa, which in turn results in a reduced release of free vitamin B12 from food proteins. In addition, hypochlorhydria in atrophic gastritis results in bacterial overgrowth of the stomach and small intestine, and these bacteria may bind vitamin B12. The ability to absorb crystalline vitamin B12 remains intact in older people with atrophic gastritis. Because the American food supply is now fortified with folic acid, concern is increasing about neurologic exacerbation in individuals with marginal vitamin B12 status and high-dose folate intake.[34]

Measurement of vitamin B12 and folate concentrations will determine these anemias in the majority of cases. However, serum cobalamin analyses have a poor sensitivity for B12 deficiency. Using a serum methylmalonic acid value of less than 0.376 μmol/l as the reference standard for B12 deficiency, a serum cobalamin assay less than 300 pmol/l had a diagnostic sensitivity of only 0.40 but a specificity of 0.98.[35]

Confirmation of vitamin B12 deficiency in those patients who have values in the lower normal range should be obtained, since about 50% of patients with subclinical disease may have normal B12 levels. A more sensitive method of screening for vitamin B12 deficiency is measurement of serum methylmalonic acid and homocysteine levels, which are increased early in vitamin B12 deficiency. A homocysteine level will be elevated in both vitamin B12 and folate deficiencies, but a methylmalonic acid level will be elevated only in vitamin B12 deficiency (Figure 31.2). Renal failure is the only other confounding cause of an elevated methylmalonic acid concentration.

Although elderly people with low vitamin B12 status frequently lack the classical signs and symptoms of vitamin B12 deficiency, e.g., megaloblastic anemia, precise evaluation and treatment in this population are important. Low folate/cobalamin levels have been linked to delirium, confusion, psychosis, depression, and dementia (Alzheimer-related dementia as well as the vascular type).[36,37] Folate/homocysteine levels have been strongly associated with cardiovascular risk. However, pharmacological interventions using folate have been disappointing.[38]

Folates are water-soluble vitamins in the vitamin B group and are found in fruit, fresh vegetables, and corn products. Insufficient food intake of folate is a common cause of low folate levels.[39] Inadequate folate nutrition during early pregnancy can cause neural tube defects in the developing fetus. In addition, folate and vitamin B12 deficiency and the compensatory increase in homocysteine are significant risk factors for cardiovascular disease.[40]

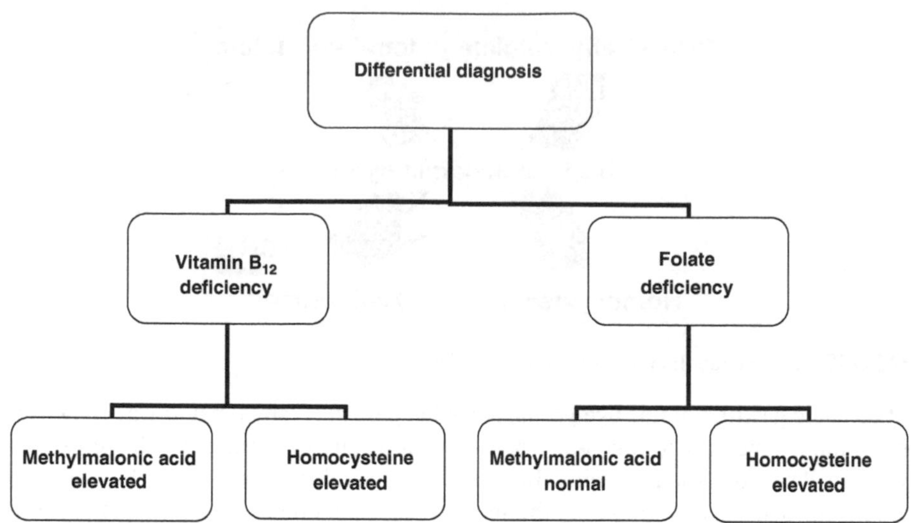

FIGURE 31.2 Differential diagnosis.

31.5 OTHER NUTRITIONAL FACTORS

Vitamins B1, B2, and B6 have been implicated in nutritional anemias. The primary cause of these anemias appears to be interference by drugs with vitamin metabolism, particularly in the case of pyridoxine. In renal dialysis patients maintained on recombinant human erythropoietin, a significant increase in erythrocyte vitamin B2 and significant decrease in erythrocyte vitamin B6 was observed. Supplementation with 20 mg/day of pyridoxine led to a significant increase in vitamin B6 at the end of the 9 months. The study suggests that erythrocyte vitamin B6 is consumed by the hemoglobin synthesis during erythropoietin therapy.[41,42]

Pyridoxine-sensitive sideroblastic anemia occurs as an X-linked genetic defect and in certain disease states such as tuberculosis and porphyuria.[43,44]

31.6 MANAGEMENT OF NUTRITIONAL ANEMIAS

In persons with iron deficiency, the recommended treatment is 325 mg ferrous sulfate three times a day,[45–47] providing 150 to 200 mg of elemental iron per day.[48] The sulfate moiety can cause gastrointestinal distress, and if this occurs, iron in the form of ferrous gluconate or fumerate may be helpful.

The duration of iron therapy may be longer when once-a-day dosing is used. Whatever the chosen dose, a reticulocyte count should be obtained 1 week after starting iron. If there is not a robust reticulocyte response, intravenous iron should be considered. Iron therapy may be discontinued when the ferritin level is normalized.

Some controversy exists about the necessary amount of iron and the frequency of dosing. Dosing iron once a day may have a similar effect to three-times-a-day dosing if absorption is normal. In a study of 90 hospitalized patients with iron deficiency anemia, subjects were randomized to receive either 15 or 50 mg of

TABLE 31.3
Iron Preparations

Iron Preparation	Tablet Size (mg)	Amount of Elemental Iron/Tablet (mg)	Approximate Number of Iron Tablets to Give 200 mg/day
Ferrous sulfate	325	65	3
Ferrous gluconate	325	38	5
Ferrous fumerate	200	66	3
Iron polysaccharide	150	150	2
Heme iron polypeptide	12	12	3–4

elemental iron as liquid ferrous gluconate or 150 mg of elemental iron as ferrous calcium citrate daily. Hemoglobin and ferritin levels were similar in each group after 60 days, but adverse effects, including abdominal discomfort, nausea, vomiting, and changes in bowel movements, were higher with the higher iron doses.[49] The time to complete resolution of the anemia was not reported. The duration of iron therapy may be longer when once-a-day dosing is used (Table 31.3).

Anemia due to vitamin B12 or folate deficiency is treated by replacement of the vitamin. Vitamin B12 can be replaced either by injections (1000 μg weekly for 1 month, then monthly thereafter), orally (1000 μg daily, which should not be given with food), or intranasally. Folate (1 mg) should be used to treat folate deficiency as well as during the first few weeks of vitamin B12 deficiency.

In 18 subjects with newly diagnosed B12 deficiency, cyanocobalamin was given either as 1 mg intramuscularly on days 1, 3, 7, 10, 14, 21, 30, 60, and 90 or as 2 mg orally daily for 120 days. There was no difference in correction of hematologic and neurologic abnormalities between the two groups. Significantly higher levels of serum cobalamin and lower serum methylmalonic acid levels were found in the oral group than in the parenteral group 4 months after treatment.[50]

31.7 SUMMARY

Nutritional anemia is easily correctable and should be aggressively sought. Anemia in older persons is a risk factor for increased mortality and decline in physical activity performance of daily living activities. The positive clinical outcomes for treating anemia, such as improved quality of life, decreased hospitalization, and decreased mortality, demand that a hemoglobin concentration of less than 12 g/dl be investigated and treated whenever possible.

REFERENCES

1. Izaks GJ, Westendorp RGJ, Knook DL. The definition of anemia in older persons. *JAMA* 1999;281:1714–1717.
2. Cohen HJ. Anemia in the elderly: clinical impact and practical diagnosis. *J Am Geriatr Soc* 2003;51(Suppl):S1–S2.

3. Kamenetz Y, Beloosesky Y, Zelter C, et al. Relationship between routine hematological parameters, serum IL-3, IL-6 and erythropoietin and mild anemia and degree of function in the elderly. *Aging Clin Exp Res* 1998;10:32–38.
4. Chaves P, Ashar T, Guralnik JM, et al. Looking at the relationship between hemoglobin concentration and previous mobility difficulty in older women: should the criteria used to define anemia in older people be changed? *J Am Geriatr Soc* 2002;50:1257–1264.
5. The prevention of falls in later life: a report of the Kellogg International Work Group on the Prevention of Falls by the Elderly. *Dan Med Bull* 1987;34(Suppl 4):1–24.
6. Baker SP, Harvey AH. Fall injuries in the elderly. *Clin Geriatr Med* 1985;1:501–512.
7. Herndon JG, Helmick CG, Sattin RW, et al. Chronic medical conditions and risk of fall injury events at home in older adults. *J Am Geriatr Soc* 1997;45:739–743.
8. Wu WC, Rathore SS, Wang Y, et al. Blood transfusion in elderly patients with acute myocardial infarction. *N Engl J Med* 2001;345:1230–1236.
9. Levin A, Singer J, Thompson CR, et al. Prevalent left ventricular hypertrophy in the predialysis population: identifying opportunities for intervention. *Am J Kidney Dis* 1996;27:347–354.
10. Valderrabano F. Quality of life benefits of early anemia treatment. *Nephrol Dialysis Transplant* 2000:15(Suppl):23–28.
11. Cella D. Factors influencing quality of life in cancer patients: anemia and fatigue. *Semin Oncol* 1998;25(Suppl 7):43–46.
12. Quirt I, Robeson C, Lau CY, Kovacs M, Burdette-Radoux S, Dolan S, Tang SC, McKenzie M, Couture F. Canadian Eprex Oncology Study Group. Epoetin alpha therapy increases hemoglobin levels and improves quality of life in patients with cancer-related anemia who are not receiving chemotherapy and patients with anemia who are receiving chemotherapy. *J Clin Oncol* 2001;19:4126–4134.
13. Silverberg OS, Wexler D, Sheps D, et al. The effect of correction of mild anemia in severe, resistant congestive heart failure using subcutaneous erythropoietin and intravenous iron: a randomized controlled study. *J Am Coll Cardiol* 2001;37:1775–1780.
14. DeMaeyer E, Adiels-Tegman M. The prevalence of anemia in the world. *World Health Stat Q Rapport Trimestriel Statistiques Sanitaires Mondiales* 1985;38:302–316.
15. Tran KH, Udden MM, Taffer GE, et al. Erythropoietin regulation of hematopoiesis is preserved in healthy elderly people. *Clin Res* 1993;41:116A.
16. Zauber NP, Zauber AG. Hematologic data of healthy very old people. *JAMA* 1987;257:2181–2184.
17. Salive ME, Cornoni-Huntley J, Guralnik JM, et al. Anemia and hemoglobin levels in older persons: relationship with age, gender, and health status. *J Am Geriatr Soc* 1992;40:489–496.
18. Hsu CY, McCulloch CE, Curhan GC. Epidemiology of anemia associated with chronic renal insufficiency among adults in the United States: results from the third National Health and Nutrition Examination Survey (NHANES III). *J Am Soc Nephrol* 2002;13:504–510.
19. Guralnik JM, Eisenstaedt RS, Ferrucci L, et al. Prevalence of anemia in persons 65 years and older in the United States: evidence for a high rate of unexplained anemia. *Blood* 2004;104:2263–2268.
20. Ania BJ, Suman VJ, Fairbanks VF, et al. Incidence of anemia in older people: an epidemiologic study in a well defined population. *J Am Geriatr Soc* 1997;45:825–831.
21. Weber JP, Walsh PC, Peters CA, Spivak JL. Effect of reversible androgen deprivation on hemoglobin and serum immunoreactive erythropoietin in men. *Am J Hematol* 1991;36:190–194.

22. Ellegala DB, Alden TD, Couture DE, et al. Anemia, testosterone, and pituitary adenoma in men. *J Neurosurg* 2003;98:974–977.
23. Bogdanos J, Karamanolakis D, Milathianakis C, et al. Combined androgen blockade-induced anemia in prostate cancer patients without bone involvement. *Anticancer Res* 2003;23:1757–1762.
24. Looker AC, Dallman PR, Carroll MD, Gunter EW, Johnson CL. Prevalence of iron deficiency in the United States. *JAMA* 1997;277:973–976.
25. Balducci L. Epidemiology of anemia in the elderly: information on diagnostic evaluation. *J Am Geriatr Soc* 2003;51:S2–S9.
26. Goddard A, McIntyre A, Scott B. Guidelines for the management of iron deficiency anaemia. *Gut* 2000;46S:1–5.
27. Malope BI, MacPhail AP, Alberts M, Hiss DC. The ratio of serum transferrin receptor and serum ferritin in the diagnosis of iron status. *Br J Haematol* 2001;115:84–89.
28. Wians FH Jr, Urban JE, Keffer JH, Kroft SH. Discriminating between iron deficiency anemia and anemia of chronic disease using traditional indices of iron status vs transferrin receptor concentration. *Am J Clin Pathol* 2001;115:112–118.
29. Roy C, Andrews, N. Anemia of inflammation: the hepcidin link. *Curr Opin Hematol* 2005;12:107–111.
30. Loreal O, Haziza-Pigeon C, Troadec MB, Detivaud L, Turlin B, Courselaud B, Ilyin G, Brissot P. Hepcidin in iron metabolism. *Curr Protein Peptide Sci* 2005;6:279–291.
31. Weiss G. Pathogenesis and treatment of anemia of chronic disease. *Blood Rev* 2002;16:87–96.
32. Carmel R. Prevalence of undiagnosed pernicious anemia in the elderly. *Arch Intern Med* 1996;156:1097–1100.
33. Savage DG, Ogundipe A, Allen RH, Stabler SP, Lindenbaum J. Etiology and diagnostic evaluation of macrocytosis. *Am J Med Sci* 2000;319:343–352.
34. Baik HW, Russell RM. Vitamin B12 deficiency in the elderly. *Annu Rev Nutr* 1999;19:357–377.
35. Holleland G, Schneede J, Ueland PM, Lund PK, Refsum H, Sandberg S. Cobalamin deficiency in general practice. Assessment of the diagnostic utility and cost-benefit analysis of methylmalonic acid determination in relation to current diagnostic strategies. *Clin Chem* 1999;45:189–198.
36. Bell IR, Erdman JS, Miller J, et al. Vitamin B12 and folate status in acute geropsychiatric inpatients: affective and cognitive characteristics of a vitamin nondeficient population. *Biol Psychiatry* 1990;2:125–133.
37. Hutto BR. Folate and cobalamin in psychiatric illness. *Comp Psychiatry* 1997;3:305–314.
38. Thomas DR. Evidence-based studies on the value of supplements and nutrients in aging. *Clin Interventions Aging*. In press.
39. Haller J. The vitamin status and its adequacy in the elderly: an international overview. *Int J Vitamin Nutr Res* 1999;69:1916–1919.
40. Klee GG. Cobalamin and folate evaluation: measurement of methylmalonic acid and homocysteine vs. vitamin B(12) and folate. *Clin Chem* 2000;46:1277–1283.
41. Mydlik M, Derzsiova K. Erythrocyte vitamins B1, B2 and B6 and erythropoietin. *Am J Nephrol* 1993;13:464–466.
42. Horl WH. Is there a role for adjuvant therapy in patients being treated with epoetin? *Nephrol Dialysis Transplant* 1999;14S:50–60.
43. May A, Bishop DF. The molecular biology and pyridoxine responsiveness of X-linked sideroblastic anaemia. *Haematologica* 1998;83:56–70.

44. Demiroglu H, Dundar S. Vitamin B6 responsive sideroblastic anaemia in a patient with tuberculosis. *Br J Clin Pract* 1997;51:51–52.
45. Provan D. Mechanisms and management of iron deficiency anaemia. *Br J Haematol* 1999;105(Suppl 1):19–26.
46. Goddard AF, McIntyre AS, Scott BB. Guidelines for the management of iron deficiency anaemia. British Society of Gastroenterology. *Gut* 2000;46(Suppl 3/4):IV1–IV5.
47. Frewin R, Henson A, Provan D. ABC of clinical haematology: iron deficiency anaemia. *BMJ* 1997;314:360–363.
48. Fairbanks VF, Beutler E. Iron deficiency. In *Williams Textbook of Hematology*, 6th ed., Beutler E, Coller BS, Lichtman MA, Kipps TJ, Eds. McGraw-Hill, New York, 2001, pp. 460–462.
49. Rimon E, Kagansky N, Kagansky M, Mechnick L, Mashiah T, Namir M, Levy S. Are we giving too much iron? Low-dose iron therapy is effective in octogenarians. *Am J Med* 2005;118:1142–1147.
50. Kuzminski AM, Del Giacco EJ, Allen RH, Stabler SP, Lindenbaum J. Effective treatment of cobalamin deficiency with oral cobalamin. *Blood* 1998;92:1191–1198.

32 The Role of Nutrition in Prevention and Management of Pressure Ulcers

David R. Thomas, M.D.

CONTENTS

32.1 INTRODUCTION AND BACKGROUND

Wound healing is intricately linked to nutrition. Severe protein-calorie undernutrition in humans alters tissue regeneration, the inflammatory reaction, and immune function.[1] Undernourished patients are more likely to have postoperative complications than well-nourished patients.[2] After vascular surgery, hypoalbuminemia and low transferrin levels have predicted wound healing complications.[3] Hospitalized patients with severe undernutrition are at a higher risk for death, sepsis, infections, and increased length of stay.[4]

Experimental studies in animal models suggest a biologically plausible relationship between undernutrition and development of pressure ulcers. When pressure was applied for 4 hours to the skin of well-nourished animals and malnourished animals, pressure ulcers occurred equally in both groups. However, the degree of ischemic skin destruction was more severe in the malnourished animals. Epithelialization of the pressure lesions occurred in normal animals at 3 days postinjury, while necrosis of the epidermis was still present in the malnourished animals.[5] These data suggest that while pressure damage may occur independently of nutritional status, malnourished animals may have impaired healing after a pressure injury.

Further indication of a relationship between nutrition and tissue damage is suggested by the finding that mitotic activity in normal epidermis is severely depressed in mice whose food intake was reduced to 70% of normal.[6] Dietary restriction to 60% of normal intake in other animal models is associated with impaired collagen cross-linking 1 week after wounding.[7] Classical studies have shown that wound dehiscence occurs more commonly in dogs with chronic protein undernutrition.[8] Nevertheless, animal studies may not accurately reflect human wound healing. For example, collagen deposition is completed in 42 days in animal wounds compared to 88 days in human wounds.[9] Hypoalbuminemia is not associated with impaired wound healing in analbuminemic rats.[10] The effects of short-term starvation are much more severe in animals than in humans.[11]

32.2 EPIDEMIOLOGICAL ASSOCIATIONS OF NUTRITION AND PRESSURE ULCERS

Nutritional status has been associated with the incidence, progression, and severity of pressure sores. Undernutrition, defined by an index of biochemical and anthropometric variables, including hemoglobin, albumin, lymphocyte count, history of weight loss, body weight, triceps skinfold thickness, and mid-arm circumference, was present in 29% of patients at hospital admission in a prospective study of high-risk patients. At 4 weeks, 17% of the undernourished patients had developed a pressure ulcer, compared to 9% of the nonundernourished patients. Thus, patients who were undernourished at hospital admission were twice as likely to subsequently develop pressure ulcers as nonundernourished patients (relative risk (RR) = 2.1, 95% confidence interval (CI) = 1.1 to 4.2).[12]

Elderly patients with decreased mobility, limited mental status, and increased skin friction and shear may have a higher risk of developing a pressure ulcer.[13]

In a study in a long-term-care setting, 59% of residents were diagnosed as undernourished on admission. Among these residents, 7.3% were classified as severely undernourished. Pressure ulcers occurred in 65% of these severely undernourished residents. No pressure ulcers developed in the mild to moderately undernourished or well-nourished groups.[14]

Dietary intake has been linked to development of pressure ulcers. In a long-term-care setting, the estimated percent intake of dietary protein, but not total caloric intake, predicted development of pressure ulcers. Patients with pressure ulcers ingested 93% of the recommended daily intake of protein compared to an intake of 119% of the recommended protein in the non-pressure ulcer group. Only dietary intake of protein was important in this study. The total dietary intake of calories or the calculated intake of vitamins A and C, iron, and zinc did not predict ulcer development.[15]

Impaired nutritional intake, defined as a persistently poor appetite, meals held due to gastrointestinal disease, or a prescribed diet less than 1100 kcal or 50 g protein/day, predicted pressure ulcer development in another long-term-care setting.[91] However, no other nutritional variable, including albumin, serum protein, hemoglobin, total lymphocyte count, body mass index, or body weight, was univariately significant.

Table 32.1 demonstrates the association of serum albumin and other nutritional variables with the development of a pressure ulcer. Pressure ulcers appear to be

TABLE 32.1
Epidemiological Association of Nutritional Markers with Development of a Pressure Ulcer

First Author	Setting	Associated with Presence of PU	Not Associated with Presence of PU
Allman[86]	AC	Albumin	Weight, hemoglobin, TLC, nutritional assessment
Gorse[87]	AC	Albumin	Nutritional assessment score
Inman[88]	AC, ICU	Albumin (measured at 3 days)	Serum protein, hemoglobin, weight
Allman[78]	AC	BMI, TLC	Albumin, TSF, arm circumference, weight loss, hemoglobin, nitrogen balance
Hargrink[50]	AC, orthopedic		Nocturnal enteral feeding
Anthony[89]	AC	Albumin < 32 g/l	
Moolten[90]	LTC	Albumin < 35 g/l	
Pinchcofsky-Devin[13]	LTC	Severe malnutrition	Mild to moderate malnutrition or normal nutrition
Berlowitz[91]	LTC	Impaired nutritional intake	Albumin, serum protein, hemoglobin, TLC, BMI/weight
Bennett[92]	LTC		Weight, BMI, weight gain
Brandeis[93]	LTC	Dependency in feeding	BMI/weight, TSF
Trumbore[94]	LTC	Albumin, cholesterol	
Breslow[95]	LTC	Albumin, hemoglobin	Serum protein, cholesterol, zinc, copper, transferrin, body weight, BMI, TLC
Bergstrom[14]	LTC	Dietary protein intake 93% of RDA vs. 119%, dietary iron	Serum protein, cholesterol, zinc, copper, transferrin, weight, BMI, TLC
Ferrell[96]	LTC		Albumin, serum protein, BMI, hematocrit
Bourdel-Marchasson[49]	LTC		Oral nutritional supplement (26 vs. 20% incidence)
Guralnik[97]	Community		Albumin, BMI, impaired nutrition, hemoglobin

Note: AC = acute care; LTC = long-term care; BMI = body mass index; TLC = total lymphocyte count; TSF = triceps skinfold thickness; ICU = intensive care unit; RDA = Recommend Daily Allowance.

associated with traditional markers of nutritional status in some, but not all, studies. However, serum albumin acts as an acute phase reactant.[16] Physiological stress (such as surgical operations), cortisol excess, and hypermetabolic states reduce serum albumin even in the presence of adequate protein intake. Decreases in serum albumin may reflect the presence of inflammatory cytokine production or comorbidity rather than nutritional status. Thus, serum albumin has not consistently been an independent predictor of pressure ulcers.

32.3 NUTRITIONAL INTERVENTIONS TO PREVENT PRESSURE ULCERS

Several attempts have been made to improve nutritional status and thus decrease the incidence of pressure ulcers (Table 32.2). Despite an epidemiological association, results of trials of nutritional intervention in prevention of pressure ulcers have been disappointing.[17] One trial of nutritional supplements has demonstrated a decrease in risk of developing pressure ulcers,[18] while others have not shown effectiveness in prevention of pressure ulcers.[19–21]

The effect of oral nutrition supplements was observed in 672 hospitalized, severely ill patients older than 65 years. Nurtritional supplements were given to 32.6% of one nonrandomized group compared to 86.9% of subjects in another hospital ward. After 15 days, the incidence of pressure ulcers (including stage 1) was 40% in the nutritional intervention group and 48% in the control group (relative risk = 0.83, 95% confidence interval (CI) = 0.70 to 0.99). There was no difference

TABLE 32.2
Nutritional Interventions in the Treatment of Pressure Ulcers

First Author	Setting	Intervention	Outcome
Breslow[18]	Long-term care	24% protein vs. 14% protein enteral feeding	–4.2 cm^2 vs. –2.1 cm^2 decrease in surface area
Chernoff[17]	Long-term care	1.8 g/kg protein vs. 1.2 g/kg protein enteral feeding	73% vs. 43% improvement in surface area
Henderson[53]	Long-term care	1.6 times basal energy expenditure,1.4 g of protein/kg/day	65% PU at onset; 61% prevalence at 3 months
Mitchell[54]	Long-term care	Enteral feeding	RR of death 1.49 (1.2–1.8) vs. RR of death 1.06 (0.8–1.4) after 2 years
Hartgrink[52]	Acute hip fracture patients	Enteral feeding	No difference in incidence
ter Riet[34]	Long-term care	Vitamin C, 10 mg vs. 1000 mg	No difference in healing rate
Taylor[32]	Acute surgical patients	Vitamin C, large dose vs. none	84% vs. 43% (control) reduction in surface area at 30 days
Norris[40]	Acute hip fracture	Zinc	No difference

Note: RR = relative risk (95% confidence intervals).

between groups in pressure ulcer prevalence at discharge (14.7% vs. 10.3%), mortality (15.6% vs. 14.2%), length of stay (17.3 days vs. 17.4 days), or nosocomial infections (26.4% vs. 19.0%).[22]

In a trial of elderly people recovering from hip fractures, the control group received a standard hospital diet and the treatment group received one oral nutrition supplement daily in addition to their hospital diet. At 6 months follow-up, there was no difference in the number of pressure ulcers among groups (relative risk = 0.79, 95% CI = 0.14 to 4.39, $p = 0.8$).[23]

Attempts to prevent development of pressure ulcers in patients with hip fracture by provision of enteral nutrition have not been successful in randomized clinical trials. The effect of overnight supplemental enteral feeding in patients with a fracture of the hip and a high-pressure-sore risk score has been evaluated. Of the 62 patients randomized for enteral feeding, only 25 tolerated their tube for more than 1 week, and only 16 tolerated their tube for 2 weeks. No differences were found for the development of a pressure ulcer, total serum protein, serum albumin, or the severity of pressure sores after 1 and 2 weeks (RR = 0.92, 95% CI = 0.64 to 1.32, $p = 0.6$). Comparison of the actually tube-fed group (n = 25 at 1 week, n = 16 at 2 weeks) and the control group showed two to three times higher protein and energy intake ($p < 0.0001$) and a significantly higher total serum protein and serum albumin after 1 and 2 weeks in the actually tube-fed group (all $p < 0.001$). However, the development of pressure ulcers and severity were not significantly influenced in the actually tube-fed group.[24]

A study of enteral tube feedings in patients with pressure ulcers in a long-term-care setting observed 49 patients for 3 months.[25] Patients received 1.6 times basal energy expenditure daily, 1.4 g of protein/kg/day, and 85% or more of their total recommended daily allowance. At the end of 3 months, there was no difference in number or healing of pressure ulcers.

In a study of survival among residents in long-term care with severe cognitive impairment, 135 residents were followed for 24 months.[26] The reasons for the placement of a feeding tube included the presence of a pressure ulcer. Having a feeding tube was not associated with increased survival; in fact, the risk of death was slightly increased (odds ratio (OR) = 1.09). There was no apparent effect on the prevalence of pressure ulcers in this group of enterally fed persons.

32.4 NUTRITIONAL INTERVENTIONS TO TREAT PRESSURE ULCERS

32.4.1 Protein

Table 32.2 summarizes the interventional trials for pressure ulcers. Greater healing of pressure ulcers has been reported with a higher protein intake irrespective of positive nitrogen balance.[27] Clinical trials have examined dietary interventions in the healing pressure ulcers. In 48 patients with stage II through IV pressure ulcers who were being fed enterally, undernutrition was defined as a serum albumin below 35 g/l or body weight more than 10% below the midpoint of the age-specific weight range. Total truncal pressure ulcer surface area showed a greater decrease (–4.2 cm^2

vs. −2.1 cm^2) in surface area in patients fed the enteral formula containing 24% protein than in patients fed a formula containing 14% protein. However, changes in body weight or biochemical parameters of nutritional status did not occur between groups. The study was limited by a small sample size (only 28 patients completed the study), nonrandom assignment to treatment groups, confounding effects of air-fluidized beds, and the use of two different feeding routes.[28]

In a small study of 12 enterally fed patients with pressure ulcers, the group who received 1.8 g/kg of protein had a 73% improvement in pressure ulcer surface area compared to a 42% improvement in surface area in the group receiving 1.2 g/kg of protein, despite the fact that the group that received the higher protein level began the study with larger-surface-area pressure ulcers (22.6 cm^2 vs. 9.1 cm^2). None of the patients in the high protein group and four patients in the very high protein group had complete healing of their ulcer, showing no difference in the relative risk of healing (0.11, 95% CI = 0.01 to 1.70).[27]

32.4.2 Amino Acids

The association of dietary protein intake with wound healing has led to investigation of the use of specific amino acids. Glutamine is essential for the immune system function, but supplemental glutamine has not been shown to have noticeable effects on wound healing.[29] Arginine enhances wound collagen deposition in healthy volunteers,[30,31] but few studies on sick, wounded patients have been done. Supplementation with 17 g of arginine did not have an effect on immune status or pressure ulcer healing compared to control in nursing homes subjects with pressure ulcers.[32] No improvement in wound healing has been demonstrated by using high supplements of branched-chain amino acid formulations.[33]

32.4.3 Vitamins

Two clinical trials have evaluated the effect of supplemental vitamin C in the treatment of pressure ulcers. In a multicenter, blinded trial, 88 patients with pressure ulcers were randomized to either 10 or 500 mg twice daily of vitamin C. The wound closure rate, relative healing rate, and wound improvement score were not different between groups.[34] An earlier trial in acute surgical patients with pressure ulcers found a mean reduction in surface area at 1 month in 84% of patients treated with 1000 mg of vitamin C compared to a reduction in surface area of 43% of the control group ($p < 0.005$).[35] Vitamin C is essential for wound healing, and impaired wound healing has been observed in clinical scurvy. However, in studies of clinically impaired wound healing, 6 months of an ascorbate-free diet is required to produce a deficient state.[36] In animals who are vitamin C deficient, wound healing is abnormal at 7 days but completely normal at 14 days.[37] Although essential, there is no evidence of acceleration of wound healing by vitamin C supplementation in patients who are not vitamin C deficient.[38,39]

The recommended daily allowance (RDA) of vitamin C is 60 mg. This RDA is easily achieved from dietary sources that include citrus fruits, green vegetables, peppers, tomatoes, and potatoes.

Vitamin A deficiency results in delayed wound healing and increased susceptibility to infection.[40] Vitamin A has been shown to be effective in counteracting delayed healing in patients on corticosteroids.[41] Vitamin E deficiency does not appear to play an active role in wound healing.[42]

Zinc was first implicated in delayed wound healing in 1967.[43] No study to date has shown improved wound healing in patients supplemented with zinc who were not zinc deficient.[44,45] Zinc levels have not been associated with development of pressure ulcers in patients with femoral neck fractures.[46] In a small study of patients (n = 10) with pressure ulcers, no effect on ulcer healing was seen at 12 weeks in zinc-supplemented vs. non-zinc-supplemented patients (weighted mean difference = 4.1 ml, 95% CI = 8.10 to 16.30, $p = 0.5$).[47]

The RDA for zinc is 12 to 15 mg, but most elderly persons intake 7 to 11 mg zinc/day,[48] chiefly from meats and cereal. Indiscriminate or long-term zinc supplementation should be avoided since high-serum zinc levels may inhibit healing, impair phagocytosis, and interfere with copper metabolism.[49–51]

Vitamins should be given only when a suspected or defined deficiency state is present.

32.5 RECOMMENDATIONS FOR GENERAL NUTRITIONAL SUPPORT FOR PERSONS WITH PRESSURE ULCERS

32.5.1 Energy

Daily caloric requirements range from 25 kcal/kg/day for sedentary adults to 40 kcal/kg/day for adults with burns, pressure ulcers, cancer, infections, and other similar conditions. In general, caloric requirements can be met at 30 to 35 kcal/kg/day for elderly patients under moderate stress. Various formulas, including the Harris–Benedict equation, can be used to predict caloric requirements, but controversy exists over accuracy in obese or severely undernourished individuals.[52] Other formulas have been adjusted for severely stressed hospitalized subjects.[53] Considerable debate exists over whether to use ideal body weight or an adjusted body weight in calculations. The best instrument for predicting nutritional requirements in older, undernourished individuals in whom ideal or usual body weight is often unknown is not clear.

The optimum dietary protein intake in patients with pressure ulcers is unknown, but may be higher than the current adult recommendation of 0.8 g/kg/day. Current recommendations for dietary intake of protein in stressed elderly patients lie between 1.2 and 1.5 g/kg/day. Yet half of chronically ill elderly persons cannot maintain nitrogen balance at this level.[54] On the other hand, increasing protein intake beyond 1.5 g/kg/day may not increase protein synthesis and may cause dehydration.[55] The optimum protein intake for these patients has not been defined, but may lie between 1.5 and 1.8 g/kg/day.

32.6 FACTORS CONTRIBUTING TO THE NUTRITIONAL PARADOX

Although correction of poor nutrition is part of total patient care and should be addressed in each patient, controversy exists about the ability of nutritional support to reduce wound complications or improve wound healing.[56,57] Despite a strong association, a causal relationship of poor nutritional status to pressure ulcers has not been established. The reported association is often confounded by lack of adjustment for comorbidity or severity of illness.[58]

Involuntary weight loss, reduced appetite, and severe undernutrition are common in the geriatric population and are often unexplained.[59] A common cause may be loss of appetite, due to dysregulation of a variety of psychological, gastrointestinal, metabolic, and nutritional factors.[60] Loss of appetite may initiate a vicious cycle of weight loss and increasing undernutrition.

The controversy may have roots in the physiological variables used to define malnutrition. There is no accepted gold standard for the diagnosis of undernutrition, and the markers for nutritional status may reflect underlying disease rather than undernutrition in older, ill persons.

Several cytokines, particularly interleukin (IL)-1, IL-1, and IL-6, have been suggested to be elevated in subjects with pressure ulcers.[61] Levels of IL-1 are elevated in persons with pressure ulcers but low in acute wound fluid.[62] Circulating serum levels of IL-6, IL-2, and IL-2R are higher in spinal cord-injured patients than in normal controls, and highest in subjects with pressure ulcers. The highest concentration of cytokines was in subjects with the slowest-healing pressure ulcers.[63] In other studies, IL-6 serum levels were increased in patients with pressure ulcers, but IL-1 and tumor necrosis factor (TNF) were not elevated.[64] In 72 male subjects admitted to a geriatric rehabilitation unit, soluble IL-2 receptor was negatively associated with albumin, prealbumin, cholesterol, transferrin, and hemoglobin.[65] This suggests that inflammation increases the incidence of hypoalbuminemia and other markers used

TABLE 32.3
Documented Relations among Cytokines, Undernutrition, and Chronic Wounds

Undernutrition
Poor wound healing
Increased risk of infection
Increased incidence of pressure ulcers
Proinflammatory Cytokines
Suppress appetite
Promote/interfere with wound healing
Chronic Wounds
Source of cytokines
Increased association with undernutrition
Increased serum levels of cytokines

for nutritional status. The use of albumin and cholesterol in these patients as nutritional markers could potentially lead to overdiagnosis of malnutrition.

A number of cytokines are also known to increase in severe undernutrition. TNF-levels are elevated in patients with severe undernutrition and congestive heart failure, but not in patients with congestive heart failure who do not have severe undernutrition.[66] IL-1 concentrations are elevated in elderly patients with severe undernutrition of unknown etiology,[67] and levels of IL-1 and IL-6 can be increased in elderly persons without evidence of infection or cancer.[68]

Existing studies are not clear on whether the elevation of cytokines is due to the presence of a pressure ulcer or to underlying severe undernutrition. Alternatively, the elevation of cytokine levels may be a common pathway for both conditions. The hypotheses are demonstrated in Figure 32.1.

Severe undernutrition occurs in both chronic infections and neoplastic disorders, suggesting that severe undernutrition develops along a common pathway and is not dependent on a specific infection or a particular neoplasm. Large reductions in body weight may indicate disease-associated cachexia rather than impaired intake alone.

Cytokines may regulate appetite directly through the central feeding drive. Significant interaction among the central feeding drive, neuropeptide Y, and IL-1 have been demonstrated in rats.[69,70] IL-1, IL-6, TNF, interferon-, leukemia inhibitory factor (D-factor), and prostaglandin E_2 have all been implicated in cancer-induced severe undernutrition.[71,72] TNF may either promote wound healing or induce cascades that interfere with inflammatory resolution and foster autoimmune reactions.[73] Leptin, a central regulator of food intake and body fat mass, increases under the stress of hip operations,[74] but is low in undernourished men.[75]

Serum albumin and weight loss may be independent markers for poor outcome regardless of nutrient intake. Poor nutritional status defined by these biochemical variables may indicate poor health rather than poor nutrient intake.

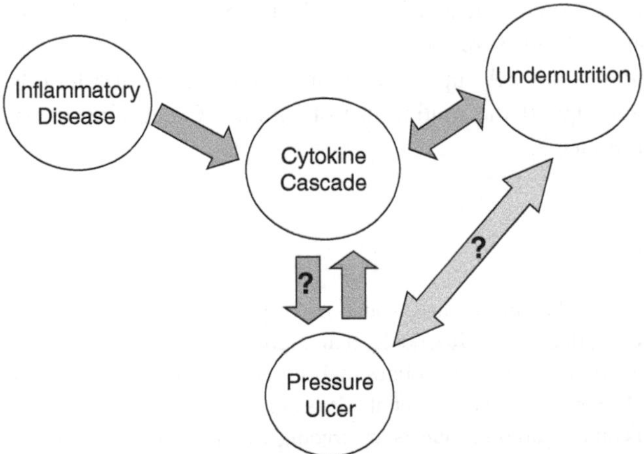

FIGURE 32.1 Interaction between proinflammatory cytokines, undernutrition, and pressure ulcers.

The lack of effect of hypercaloric feeding in pressure ulcers may reflect that the underlying pathophysiology is cytokine-induced cachexia rather than simple starvation. Starvation is amenable to hypercaloric feeding in all but the terminally undernourished patients. Cytokine-induced cachexia is remarkably resistant to hypercaloric feeding.[76,77]

Interventions to modulate cytokine activity are possible. Cytokine modulation has been postulated as a potential treatment for cachexia.[78–84] If a significant positive relationship exists between circulating cytokines and pressure ulcers, an opportunity for potential intervention to promote healing exists.

32.7 CONCLUSIONS

Wound nutrition is whole-body nutrition. Unquestionably, providing nutritional support can prevent the effects of starvation. Death is an inevitable consequence of starvation. Whether nutrition can improve the outcome of a disease remains disputable. Improvements in nutritional markers, such as serum protein concentrations, nitrogen balance, and weight gain, have not usually been accompanied by clinical benefits.[77,85]

There is no doubt that undernutrition does not have a positive effect on wound healing. However, there is no magic nutritional bullet that will accelerate wound healing. General nutritional support should be provided to persons with pressure ulcers, consistent with medical goals and patient wishes. Some evidence demonstrates that two daily supplement drinks may be able to reduce the number of older people recovering from acute illness who develop pressure ulcers.

32.8 CLINICAL RECOMMENDATIONS

1. Nutritional supplementation may prevent some pressure ulcers.
2. Optimize protein intake with a goal of 1.5 to 1.8 g/kg/day of protein in persons with pressure ulcers.
3. Consider vitamin A supplements in patients on corticosteriods.
4. No data support the routine use of vitamin C and zinc in patients with pressure ulcers.

REFERENCES

1. Young ME. Malnutrition and wound healing. *Heart Lung* 1988;17:60.
2. Detsky AS, Baker JP, O'Rourke K, et al. Predicting nutrition-associated complications for patients undergoing gastrointestinal surgery. *J Parenter Enteral Nutr* 1987;11:440.
3. Casey J, Flinn WR, Yao JST, et al. Correlation of immune and nutritional status with wound complications in patients undergoing vascular operations. *Surgery* 1983;93:822.
4. Dempsey DT, Mullen JL, Buzby GP. The link between nutritional status and clinical outcome: can nutritional intervention modify it? *Am J Clin Nutr* 1988;47(Suppl):352.
5. Takeda T, Koyama T, Izawa Y, et al. Effects of malnutrition on development of experimental pressure sores. *J Dermatol* 1992;19:602.

6. Bullough WS, Eisa EA. The effects of a graded series of restricted diets on epidermal mitotic activity in the mouse. *Br J Cancer* 1950;4:321.
7. Reiser KM. Nonenzymatic glycations and enzymatic crosslinking in a model of wound healing. *J Geriatr Dermatol* 1993;1:90.
8. Thompson W, Ravdin IS, Frank IL. The effect of hypoproteinemic on wound disruption. *Arch Surg* 1938;26:500.
9. Levenson SM. Some challenging wound healing problems for clinicians and basic scientists. In *Repair and Regeneration: The Scientific Basis for Surgical Practice*, Dunphy JE, Van Winkle W, Jr, Eds. McGraw-Hill, New York, 1969, pp. 309.
10. Felcher A, Schwartz J, Schechter C, et al. Wound healing in normal and analbuminemic rates. *J Surg Res* 1987;43:546.
11. Barbul A, Purtill WA. Nutrition in wound healing. *Clin Dermatol* 1994;12:133.
12. Thomas DR, Goode PS, Tarquine PH, Allman R. Hospital acquired pressure ulcers and risk of death. *J Am Geriatr Soc* 1996;44:1435.
13. Perneger TV, Rae AC, Gaspoz JM, Borst F, Vitek O, Heliot C. Screening for pressure ulcer risk in an acute care hospital: development of a brief bedside scale. *J Clin Epidemiol* 2002;55:498.
14. Pinchcofsky-Devin GD, Kaminski MV, Jr. Correlation of pressure sores and nutritional status. *J Am Geriatr Soc* 1986;34:435.
15. Bergstrom N, Braden B. A prospective study of pressure sore risk among institutionalized elderly. *J Am Geriatr Soc* 1992;40:747.
16. Friedman FJ, Campbell AJ, Caradoc-Davies. Hypoalbuminemia in the elderly is due to disease not malnutrition. *Clin Exp Gerontol* 1985;7:191.
17. Langer G, Schloemer G, Knerr A, Kuss O, Behrens J. Nutritional interventions for preventing and treating pressure ulcers. *Cochrane Database Syst Rev* 2004;4.
18. Bourdel-Marchasson I, Barateau M, Sourgen C, et al. Prospective audits of quality of PEM recognition and nutritional support in critically ill elderly patients. *Clin Nutr* 1999;18:233.
19. Thomas DR. The role of nutrition in prevention and healing of pressure ulcers. *Clin Geriatr Med* 1997;13:497.
20. Bergstrom N. Lack of nutrition in AHCPR prevention guideline. *Decubitus* 1993;6:4.
21. Thomas DR. Improving the outcome of pressure ulcers with nutritional intervention: a review of the evidence. *Nutrition* 2001;17:121.
22. Bourdel-Marchasson I, Barateau M, Sourgen C, et al. Prospective audits of quality of PEM recognition and nutritional support in critically ill elderly patients. *Clin Nutr* 1999;18:233.
23. Delmi M, Rapin CH, Bengoa JM, Delmas PD, Vasey H, Bonjour JP. Dietary supplementation in elderly patients with fractured neck of the femur. *Lancet* 1990;335:1013.
24. Hartgrink HH, Wille J, Konig P, et al. Pressure sores and tube feeding in patients with a fracture of the hip: a randomized clinical trial. *Clin Nutr* 1998;17:287.
25. Henderson CT, Trumbore LS, Mobarhan S, et al. Prolonged tube feeding in long-term care: nutritional status and clinical outcomes. *J Am Coll Clin Nutr* 1992;11:309.
26. Mitchell SL, Kiely DK, Lipsitz LA. The risk factors and impact on survival of feeding tube placement in nursing home residents with severe cognitive impairment. *Arch Intern Med* 1997;157:327.
27. Chernoff RS, Milton KY, Lipschitz DA. The effect of very high-protein liquid formula (Replete) on decubitus ulcer healing in long-term tube-fed institutionalized patients. Investigators Final Report 1990. *J Am Diet Assoc* 1990;90:A-130.
28. Breslow RA, Hallfrisch J, Guy DG, et al. The importance of dietary protein in healing pressure ulcers. *J Am Geriatr Soc* 1993;41:357.

29. McCauley R, Platell C, Hall J, McCulloch R. Effects of glutamine on colonic strength anastomosis in the rat. *J Parenter Enter Nutr* 1991;116:821.
30. Barbul A, Lazarous S, Efron DT, et al. Arginine enhances wound healing in humans. *Surgery* 1990;108:331.
31. Kirk SJ, Regan MC, Holt D, et al. Arginine stimulates wound healing and immune function in aged humans. *Surgery* 1993;114:155.
32. Langkamp-Henken B, Herrlinger-Garcia KA, Stechmiller JK, Nickerson-Troy JA, Lewis B, Moffatt L. Arginine supplementation is well tolerated but does not enhance mitogen-induced lymphocyte proliferation in elderly nursing home residents with pressure ulcers. *J Parenter Enteral Nutr* 2000;24:280.
33. McCauley C, Platell C, Hall J, McCullock R. Influence of branched chain amino acid solutions on wound healing. *Aust NZ J Surg* 1990;60:471.
34. ter Riet G, Kessels AG, Knipschild PG. Randomized clinical trial of ascorbic acid in the treatment of pressure ulcers. *J Clin Epidemiol* 1995;48:1453.
35. Taylor TV, Rimmer S, Day B, Butcher J, Dymock IW. Ascorbic acid supplementation in the treatment of pressure sores. *Lancet* 1974;2:544.
36. Crandon JH, Lind CC, Dill DB. Experimental human scurvy. *N Engl J Med* 1940;223:353.
37. Levenson SM, Upjohn HL, Preston JA, et al. Effect of thermal burns on wound healing. *Ann Surg* 1957;146:357.
38. Rackett SC, Rothe MJ, Grant-Kels JM. Diet and dermatology. The role of dietary manipulation in the prevention and treatment of cutaneous disorders. *J Am Acad Dermatol* 1993;29:447.
39. Vilter RW. Nutritional aspects of ascorbic acid: uses and abuses. *West J Med* 1980;133:485.
40. Hunt TK. Vitamin A and wound healing. *J Am Acad Dermatol* 1986;15:817.
41. Ehrlich HP, Hunt TK. Effects of cortisone and vitamin A on wound healing. *Ann Surg* 1968;167:324.
42. Waldorf H, Fewkes J. Wound healing. *Adv Dermatol* 1995;10:77.
43. Pories WJ, Henzel WH, Rob CG, et al. Acceleration of healing with zinc sulfate. *Ann Surg* 1967;165:423.
44. Hallbrook T, Lanner E. Serum zinc and healing of leg ulcers. *Lancet* 1972;2:780.
45. Sandstead SH, Henrikson LK, Greger JL, et al. Zinc nutriture in the elderly in relation to taste acuity, immune response, and wound healing. *Am J Clin Nutr* 1982;36(Suppl):1046.
46. Goode HF, Burns E, Walker BE. Vitamin C depletion and pressure ulcers in elderly patients with femoral neck fracture. *Br Med J* 1992:305:925.
47. Norris JR, Reynolds RE. The effect of oral zinc sulfate therapy on decubitus ulcers. *JAGS* 1971;19:793.
48. Gregger JL. Potential for trace mineral deficiencies and toxicities in the elderly. In *Mineral Homeostasis in the Elderly*, Bales CW, Ed. Marcel Dekker, New York, 1989, p. 171.
49. Goode P, Allman R. The prevention and management of pressure ulcers. *Med Clin N Am* 1989;73:1511.
50. Thomas DR. The role of nutrition in prevention and healing of pressure ulcers. *Clin Geriatr Med* 1997;13:497.
51. Reed BR, Clark RAF. Cutaneous tissue repair: practical implications of current knowledge: II. *J Am Acad Dermatol* 1985;13:919.
52. Choban PS, Burge JC, Flanobaum L. Nutrition support of obese hospitalized patients. *Nutr Clin Pract* 1997;12:149.

53. Ireton-Jones CS. Evaluation of energy expenditures in obese patients. *Nutr Clin Pract* 1989;4:127.
54. Gersovitz M, Motil K, Munro HN, Scrimshaw NS. Human protein requirements: assessment of the adequacy of the current Recommended Dietary Allowance for dietary protein in elderly men and women. *Am J Clin Nutr* 1982;35:6.
55. Long CL, Nelson KM, Akin JM, Jr, Geiger JW, Merrick HW, Blakemore WZ. A physiologic bases for the provision of fuel mixtures in normal and stressed patients. *J Trauma* 1990;30:1077.
56. Albina JE. Nutrition and wound healing. *J Parenter Enteral Nutr* 1994;18:367.
57. Thomas DR. Issues and dilemmas in managing pressure ulcers. *J Gerontol Med Sci* 2001;56:M238.
58. Finucane TE. Malnutrition, tube feeding and pressure sores: data are incomplete. *J Am Geriatr Soc* 1995;43:447.
59. Thompson MP, Merria LK. Unexplained weight loss in ambulatory elderly. *J Am Geriatr Soc* 1991;39:497.
60. Morley JE, Thomas DR. Anorexia and aging: pathophysiology. *Nutrition* 1999;15:499.
61. Matsuyama N, Takano K, Mashiko T, Jimbo S, Shimetani N, Ohtani H. The possibility of acute inflammatory reaction affects the development of pressure ulcers in bedridden elderly patients. *Jpn J Clin Pathol* 1999;47:1039.
62. Barone EJ, Yager DR, Pozez AL, Olutoye OO, Crossland MC, Diegelmann RF, Cohen IK. Interleukin-1 and collagenase activity are elevated in chronic wounds. *Plastic Reconstruct Surg* 1998;102:1023.
63. Segal JL, Gonzales E, Yousefi S, Jamshidipour L, Brunnemann SR. Circulating levels of IL-2R, ICAM-1, and IL-6 in spinal cord injuries. *Arch Physical Med Rehab* 1997;78:44.
64. Bonnefoy M, Coulon L, Bienvenu J, Boisson RC, Rys L. Implication of cytokines in the aggravation of malnutrition and hypercatabolism in elderly patients with severe pressure sores. *Age Ageing* 1995;24:37.
65. Rosenthal AJ, Sanders KM, McMurtry CT, Jacobs MA, Thompson DD, Gheorghiu D, Little KL, Adler RA. Is malnutrition overdiagnosed in older hospitalized patients? Association between the soluble interleukin-2 receptor and serum markers of malnutrition. *J Gerontol A Biol Sci Med Sci* 1998;53:M81.
66. Ikeda U, Yamamoto K, Akazawa H, et al. Plasma cytokine levels in cardiac chambers of patients with mitral stensis with congestive heart failure. *Cardiology* 1996;87:476.
67. Liso Z, Tu JH, Small CB, Schnipper SM, Rosenstreich DL. Increased urine IL-1 levels in aging. *Gerontology* 1993;39:19.
68. Cederholm T, Whetline B, Hollstrom K, et al. Enhanced generation of interleukin 1 and 6 may contribute to the cachexia of chronic disease. *Am J Clin Nutr* 1997;65:876.
69. Chasse WT, Balasubramahiam A, Dayal R, et al. Hypothalamic concentration and release of neuropeptide Y into microdialyses is reduced in anorectic tumor bearing rats. *Life Sci* 1994;54:1869.
70. Leibowitz SF. Neurochemical-neuroendocrine systems in the brain controlling macronutrient intake and metabolism. *Trends Neurosci* 1992;12:491.
71. Noguchi Y, Yoshikawa T, Marsumoto A, Svaninger G, Gelin J. Are cytokines possible mediators of cancer cachexia? *Jpn J Surg* 1996;26:467.
72. Keiler U. Pathophysiology of cancer cachexia. *Support Care Cancer* 1993;1:290.
73. Pan W, Zadina JE, Harlan RE, Weber JT, Banks WA, Kastin AJ. Tumor necrosis factor-: a neuromodulator in the CNS. *Neurosci Biobehav Rev* 1997;21:603.
74. Straton RJ, Dewit O, Crowe R, Jennings G, Viller RN, Elia M. Plasm leptin, energy intake and hunger following total hip replacement surgery. *Clin Sci* 1997;93:113.

75. Cederholm T, Arter P, Palmviad J. Low circulation leptin level in protein-energy malnourished chronically ill elderly patients. *J Intern Med* 1997;242:377.
76. Souba WW. Drug therapy: nutritional support. *N Engl J Med* 1997;336:41.
77. Atkinson S, Sieffert E, Bihari D. A prospective, randomized, double-blind, controlled clinical trial of enteral immunonutrition in the critically ill. *Crit Care Med* 1998;26:1164.
78. Bruerra E, Macmillan K, Hanson J, et al. A controlled trial of megestrol acetate on appetite, caloric intake, nutritional status, and other symptoms in patients with advance cancer. *Cancer* 1990;66:1279.
79. Allman RM, Goode PS, Patrick MM. Pressure ulcer risk factors among hospitalized patients with severe limitation. *JAMA* 1995;273:865.
80. Schmoll E, Wilke H, Thole R. Megestrol acetate in cancer cachexia. *Semin Oncol* 1991;1(Suppl):32.
81. Heckmayr M, Gatzenneier U. Treatment of cancer weight loss in patients with advance lung cancer. *Oncology* 1992;49(Suppl):32.
82. Feliu J, Gonzalez-Baron M, Berrocal A. Usefulness of megestrol acetate in cancer cachexia and anorexia. *Am J Clin Oncol* 1992;15:436.
83. Azona C, Castro L, Crespo E, et al. Megestrol acetate therapy for anorexia and weight loss in children with malignant solid tumours. *Aliment Pharmacol Ther* 1996;10:577.
84. Mantovani G, Maccio A, Bianchi A, Curreli L, Ghiani M, Santona MC, Del Giacco GS. *Megestrol Acetate in Neoplastic Anorexia/Cachexia: Clinical Evaluation and Comparison with Cytokine Levels in Patients with Head and Neck Carcinoma Treated with Neoadjuvant Chemotherapy.* Springer-Verlag, Berlin, 1995.
85. Christou NV, Meakins JL, Gordon J, et al. The delayed hypersensitivity response and host resistance in surgical patients: 20 years later. *Ann Surg* 1995;222:534.
86. Allman RM, Walker JM, Hart MK, et al. Air-fluidized beds or conventional therapy for pressure sores: a randomized trial. *Ann Intern Med* 1987;107:641.
87. Gorse GJ, Messner RL. Improved pressure sore healing with hydrocolloid dressings. *Arch Dermatol* 1987;123:766.
88. Inman KJ, Sibbald WJ, Rutledge FS. Clinical utility and cost-effectiveness of an air suspension bed in the prevention of pressure ulcers. *JAMA* 1993;269:1139.
89. Anthony D, Reynolds T, Russell L. An investigation into the use of serum albumin in pressure sore prediction. *J Adv Nurs* 2000;32:359.
90. Moolten SE. Bedsores in the chronically ill patient. *Arch Physical Med Rehab* 1972;53:430.
91. Berlowitz DR, Wilking SV. Risk factors for pressure sores: a comparison of cross-sectional and cohort-derived data. *J Am Geriatr Soc* 1989;37:1043.
92. Bennett RG, Bellantoni MF, Ouslander JG. Air-fluidized bed treatment of nursing home patients with pressure sores. *J Am Geriatr Soc* 1989;37:235.
93. Brandeis GH, Morris JN, Nash DJ, et al. Epidemiology and natural history of pressure ulcers in elderly nursing home residents. *JAMA* 1990;264:2905.
94. Trumbore LS, Miles TP, Henderson CT, et al. Hypocholesterolemia and pressure sore risk with chronic tube feeding. *Clin Res* 1990;38:760A.
95. Breslow RA, Hallfrisch J, Goldberg AP. Malnutrition in tube-fed nursing home patients with pressure sores. *J Parenter Enteral Nutr* 1991;15:663.
96. Ferrell BA, Osterweil D, Christenson P. A randomized trial of low-air-loss beds for treatment of pressure ulcers. *JAMA* 1993;269:494.
97. Guralnik JM, Harris TB, White LR, et al. Occurrence and predictors of pressure sores in the National Health and Nutrition Examination Survey follow-up. *J Am Geriatr Soc* 1988;36:807.

33 Nutrition and Fracture Risk

Kent R. Wehmeier

CONTENTS

Osteoporosis is a devastating disease that affects more than 10 million people in the U.S., with annual costs in excess of $13.5 billion.[1] According to the U.S. Surgeon General's Report, by the year 2020, 50% of all Americans older than 50 years will be at risk of an osteoporotic fragility fracture. Approximately 1.66 million hip fractures occur each year worldwide,[2] and that the incidence is set to increase four-fold by 2050 because of the increasing numbers of older people and because the age-adjusted incidence rates are many times higher in affluent developed countries than in sub-Saharan Africa and Asia.[3,4] Nearly all fractures in the elderly result from osteoporosis. The incidence of vertebral and hip fractures increases exponentially with advancing age (while that of wrist fractures plateaus after the age of 60 years).[5] Calcium and vitamin D are commonly prescribed for the prevention and treatment of osteoporosis. The paradox that hip fracture rates are higher in developed countries, where calcium intake is higher than in developing countries, clearly calls for an explanation. The report of the Joint FAO/WHO Expert Consultation on Vitamin and Mineral Requirements in Human Nutrition[6] made it clear that the recommendations for calcium intakes were based on long-term (90-day) calcium balance data for adults derived from Australia, Canada, the European Union, the U.K., and the U.S., and were not necessarily applicable to all countries worldwide. The report also acknowledged that strong evidence was emerging that the requirements for calcium might vary from culture to culture for dietary, genetic, lifestyle, and geographical reasons. Within these limitations, this chapter will attempt to review the available data for micronutrients as they apply to fracture prevention in the elderly.

Osteoporosis is characterized by low bone mass and microarchitectural deterioration of bone tissue, leading to bone fragility and a consequent increased risk of fracture. Bone is made of both organic and inorganic components. Collagen type I is the most abundant organic molecule, while crystals containing calcium and phosphorus make up most of the inorganic weight. Highly regulated at local, distant, and central levels, cells of the skeleton, the osteoclasts, which resorb bone, and the osteoblasts, which lay down new bone, are part of a process to afford the individual with adequate support for locomotion and a ready store of essential ions for homeostasis. Human bone is

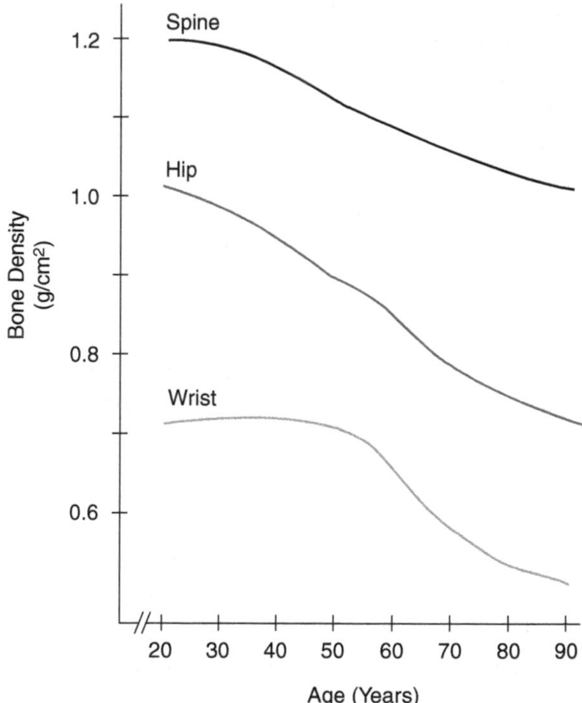

FIGURE 33.1 Areal bone mineral density of various bones as a function of advancing age.

about 60% mineralized. Variations in tissue mineral density affect function, such as the enamel of teeth having the highest tissue density of calcium. The composition and degree of collagen cross-linking also influence function.[7] The cross-links in collagen keep its three helixes fastened. The enzymes responsible for this cross-linking require trace metals for normal functioning. The skeleton's resistance to fracture is determined by geometric properties (size, shape, and connectivity of bones), the activities of the osteoclasts and osteoblasts in the tissue, and the material properties of the tissue.[8–10] The material properties of bone include the mineral content,[8] mineral composition and crystal size,[9] and matrix content and composition.[8] Bone is composed of type I collagen stiffened by crystals of hydroxyapatite (HA) [$Ca_5(PO_4)_3OH$] that may have substitutions of carbonate, acid phosphate, strontium, magnesium, or fluoride.[11] Substitutions affect the size, shape, and solubility of the crystal. HA crystal size and perfection were first suggested to contribute to the mechanical strength of bones in the early 1980s.[12] Increased bone mineral particle size is associated with increased bone fragility[12]; crystals that are too small do not reinforce the bone composite, suggesting that there also is an optimal size range for bone mineral crystals.[13] Compositional changes may be caused by alterations in crystal size (smaller crystals have more surface area to adsorb foreign ions) or may be indicative of the size changes. In osteoporosis and aging, there are reports of increased magnesium content and decreased fluoride, acid phosphate, boron, strontium, and carbonate contents. Variation in mineral content in osteoporosis is important, but other material properties beyond content alone contribute to the loss of mechanical strength in osteoporotic bones.[14–17]

To ensure adequate calcification of the bony matrix, two major hormones, parathyroid hormone (PTH) and vitamin D, are synthesized. Release of PTH is largely dependent upon signaling by the calcium-sensing receptor on parathyroid gland cells. Phosphorus, magnesium, and vitamin D levels also modulate PTH induction, processing, and release (Table 33.1). Its major focus is fostering a normal extracellular calcium and phosphorus level. Vitamin D physiology may be visualized graphically in Figure 33.2. Note that the plant source of vitamin D is called ergocalciferol (D_2) and animal vitamin D is called cholecalciferol (D_3). For reasons of clarity, vitamin D will refer to all forms of vitamin D unless otherwise stated.

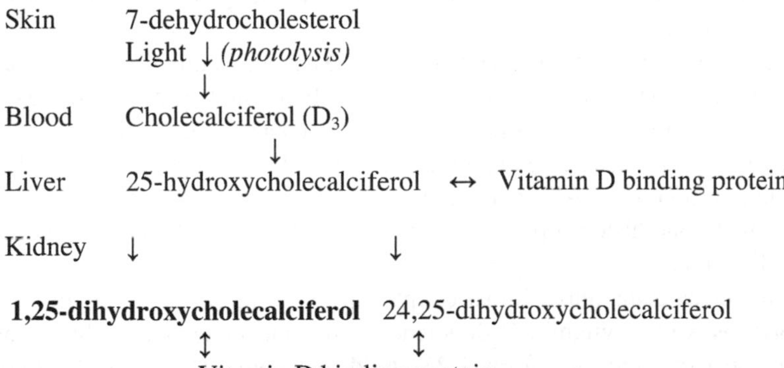

FIGURE 33.2 Synthesis of vitamin D.

Growth and strengthening of the skeleton occur due to a positive balance between bone formation and bone resorption. First, an organic matrix is laid down, or osteoid; only then can subsequent mineralization occur. Without osteoid, crystallization will not occur. During the lifetime of an individual, bone responds to increased loads by increasing bone matrix and bone mineralization as well as repairing microcracks that result from fatigue damage. Bone mineral density (BMD) is currently used as a surrogate for fracture risk, to be considered along with risk of falling when developing a treatment strategy. BMD is determined by measuring the grams of calcium content based on the absorbance of a transmitted x-ray beam, calibrated to a bone phantom, of a defined area, typically of the proximal femur and lumbar spine, and dividing that total by the area (areal BMD). A widely available instrument for BMD measurement with high reproducibility and low external radiation is the dual-energy x-ray absorptiometry machine (DXA). One of the complexities of using BMD is that widening of the bone with the same calcium content or changes in microarchitecture may lead to false assumptions that fracture risk is truly changed. Many factors contribute to changes in BMD, including age, genetic heritage, tobacco and ethanol use, performance of weight-bearing exercise, body weight, concentrations of sex steroids, and pharmacologic agents. Peak BMDs for different regions of the skeleton are attained at different ages. BMD of the hip reaches a peak in the late teens, whereas the spine may continue to accrue calcium until age 25. Similarly, loss of bone may also occur at different rates, depending on the bone and age of the individual. This discussion of micronutrients must therefore consider effects on bone formation, bone resorption, or both, when addressing mechanisms of dietary interventions. Particular problems with regard to bone density interpretation that are specific to the elderly population are the development of osteoarthritis and vascular calcification. Both of these conditions interfere with the interpretation of spinal as well as hip BMD and may be impacted by interventions such as calcium and vitamin D administration, though little data are available to answer that question. One must also consider in the evaluation of fracture studies effects on falls that are independent of changes in bone mineral density. The absorption, distribution, and excretion of micronutrients may also be altered in the geriatric patient, and this population must be evaluated before making recommendations. The issue of interaction with another micronutrient must also be considered when evaluating interventions with such minute quantities.

Based on the bone mineral density exam, one cannot readily distinguish between osteomalacia, a condition of undermineralized bone, and osteoporosis, as Fuller Allbright put it, the lack of bone in bone. The concept that osteoporosis is due primarily to calcium deficiency, particularly in the elderly, was initially put forward as a counterproposal to Albright's estrogen deficiency theory. One should note, however, that bone histomorphometry shows the absence of bone, not the absence of crystallization.

Decreased calcium intake, impaired intestinal absorption of calcium due to aging or disease, as well as vitamin D deficiency can result in secondary hyperparathyroidism. The active hormonal form, 1,25-dihydroxyvitamin D (calcitriol), is not only necessary for optimal intestinal absorption of calcium and phosphorus, but also exerts a tonic inhibitory effect on parathyroid hormone (PTH) synthesis, so that there are

TABLE 33.1
Parathyroid Hormone Regulation

Increase PTH	Lower PTH
Hypocalcemia	1,25-Dihydroxyvitamin D
Hyperphosphatemia	Hypermagnesemia

dual pathways that can lead to secondary hyperparathyroidism.[18] Vitamin D deficiency and secondary hyperparathyroidism can contribute not only to accelerated bone loss and increasing fragility, but also to neuromuscular impairment that can increase the risk of falls.[19,20] Clinical trials involving older individuals at high risk for calcium and vitamin D deficiency indicate that supplementation of both can reverse secondary hyperparathyroidism, decrease bone resorption, increase bone mass, decrease fracture rates, and even decrease the frequency of falling.[18] However, in a large recent study, calcium and vitamin D supplementation did not reduce fracture incidence significantly, perhaps because this population was less deficient in vitamin D.[21] The remainder of this chapter will discuss micronutrients in regards to osteoporosis.

33.1 RISK OF OSTEOPOROTIC FRACTURES WITH AGE

33.1.1 Calcium

Calcium is required for normal cell function. A sophisticated system of absorption, storage, release during lactation, and excretion in a manner that maintains the delicate balance between mineralization and dissolution has evolved to maintain optimal extracellular calcium concentration. The skeleton stores 99% of the body's calcium. Sustaining this depot requires adequate calcium absorption to overcome the obligatory losses of calcium through urine, feces, and sweat. This system must also regulate the highest rates of calcium accrual at a mean age of 12½ years in girls and 14 years in boys. After the rapid formation of new bone, prospective longitudinal studies in premenopausal woman have suggested that BMD falls less than 0.5%/year. During the perimenopausal period, bone resorption accelerates, causing substantial losses of bone. Fuller Albright elucidated this form of osteoporosis in 1940.[22] This form of osteoporosis was further characterized by Riggs et al.:[23] female-to-male ratio of 6:1, women between 51 and 65 years old, affects mostly trabecular bone, and is associated with decreased parathyroid function. Senile osteoporosis (type II) still affected women more than men (2:1), but occurred in men and women older than 75, affected cortical and trabecular bone, was not associated with increased bone resorption, and had mild elevations of parathyroid hormone.

Riggs et al.,[24] in cross-sectional studies evaluating women, showed a continued decline in BMD even before the onset of menopause. Efforts by some investigators to correlate changes in bone mineral density to dietary intake of calcium in otherwise normal postmenopausal women have not always been successful. Riggs et al.[25] and others[26,27] did not show a benefit with higher calcium intake on bone mineral density.

TABLE 33.2
Contributors of Reduced Bone Mineral Density

Endocrine Disorders
Hypogonadism
Hyperthyroidism
Hyperparathyroidism
Hypercortisolism
Diabetes mellitus
Medications
Glucocorticoids
Anticonvulsants
Progestins
GnRH agonists
Immunosuppressives
Nutritional Disorders
Low calcium intake
Milk intolerance
Malnutrition
Anorexia nervosa
Excess dietary protein malabsorption
Surgery
Gastric bypass
Gastrectomy
Other
Alcoholism
Tobacco use
Malignancy
Chronic kidney/liver disease
Rheumatoid arthritis
Idiopathic hypercalciuria
Immobilization

A study evaluating bone mineral density in two districts of low and high calcium intake did show an increase in BMD in the high calcium district, but differences in physical activity were not taken into account.[28] This same level of bone loss in elderly women occurs in elderly men[29] as well. As one might expect, urine calcium excretion in postmenopausal woman was inversely correlated with BMD (Table 33.2).[30,31]

This change in calcium metabolism then may make the analysis of intervention studies more challenging. In subjects on very low calcium diets (<400 mg/day), below the predicted requirement to balance obligatory losses, BMD does decline significantly in postmenopausal women.[32] In a study addressing perimenopausal bone loss,[33] large doses of total calcium intake (1700 mg/day) were associated with gains in BMD of the femoral neck and whole-body calcium by a neutron activation technique. The total-body calcium measurement is a mass measurement that has greater precision than BMD. This study was placebo controlled and double blinded for the placebo and calcium arms. In this study, a confounder was the administrator of 400 IU of vitamin D in the form of a multivitamin.

What are the calcium requirements? The classical way for this to be determined was by the use of calcium balance studies. The assumption is that healthy adults should be in balance. In a review of 212 balances,[34] the calcium requirement was calculated to be 500 to 600 mg daily. Nordin's review mentions an obligatory loss of calcium in sweat, which raises this total to nearly 800 mg daily.[35] On average, 100 to 200 mg of calcium is lost in gastrointestinal (GI) secretions daily, 50 to 300 mg/day is lost through urinary excretion, and about 100 mg is lost in sweat on a warm day.

If elderly individuals are losing bone, then calcium supplementation must overcome this deficit to maintain adequate calcium stores.

33.1.1.1 Absorption

Calcium absorption can range from 10 to 60%.[36] The highest rates occur in lactating women. This transport may occur through a vitamin D-dependent saturable transcellular means or a nonsaturable paracellular pathway. High calcium intake leads to downregulation of active transport. Two groups have evaluated calcium absorption in older subjects: Need et al.[37] and Wolf et al.[38] asked whether the efficiency of facilitated calcium absorption declines with age. In their population of 80-year-old men, Wolf et al.[38] found a significant drop in fractional calcium absorption. Other studies have documented similar findings.[39,40] Menopause represents a major loss of bone density. Heaney et al.[41] documented the changes in calcium balance with the onset of menopause.

The average adult woman over 60 years of age in the U.S. consumes 15 mol/day of calcium, whereas a man takes in 19 mmol.[42] Because a large majority of calcium is complexed, high acidity is necessary for its absorption. At the duodenum, gastric acidity is still effective in generating ionized calcium, whereas biliary and pancreatic juices neutralize the acid in the more distal portions of the intestine. 1,25-Dihydroxyvitamin D induces synthesis of the calbindins, calcium-binding proteins that are important in the transcellular transport of calcium.[43] Other dietary agents that may influence calcium absorption include a high-fat diet, forming insoluble soaps, and a high-fiber diet. Most of the ingested calcium is lost in the feces. A small amount is excreted by the kidney (4 mmol/day). Renal Ca^{2+} absorption occurs in the proximal tubules where 70% of the filtered load is reabsorbed.[44] Paracellular transport of Ca^{2+} is mediated by a transepithelial electrochemical gradient that is generated by sodium and water reabsorption. Twenty percenet of filtered calcium is absorbed at the loop of Henle, and this process requires the protein paracellin-1.[45] Fifteen percent is absorbed through an active transcellular process that is tightly regulated by parathyroid hormone (PTH), an activated form of vitamin D or 1,25-dihydroxyvitamin D {1,25(OH)$_2$D} and calcitonin. Vitamin D facilitates the diffusion of calcium for absorption by its induction of epithelial calcium channels (ECaC) at the anterolateral membrane,[46] increasing the expression of calbindins in intestinal and renal epithelial cells as well as expressing a plasma membrane Ca^{2+}-ATPase (PCMA) that actively transports calcium across the basolateral membrane.[47]

By using two separate American databases, the 1994–2004 IMS HEALTH National Disease and Therapeutic Index and the 1999–2002 National Health and Nutrition Examination Survey (NHANES), Stafford et al.[48] assessed calcium intake. Among osteoporosis patients in NHANES, 64% reported using calcium-containing supplements. Reported median calcium intake was 433 mg/day for calcium supplement nonusers and 1319 (845–1874) mg for calcium supplement users. Overall, 40% of osteoporosis patients had calcium intake exceeding 1200 mg/day.

33.1.1.2 Bone Mineral Density

Early calcium intervention trials with doses as high as 1500 mg failed to show a significant benefit on bone mineral density in postmenopausal bone loss.[49,50]

33.1.1.3 Fracture Prevention

Although this review was not exhaustive, there has been little discussion regarding the contents of placebo tablets and how they themselves may affect other micronutrients involved in bone metabolism. It is also important to recognize that mineralization of bone occurs after the matrix is produced and not before. The skeletal demands for calcium are governed by the rate of matrix synthesis rather than vice versa.[51] In addition to this consideration, calcium has effects on phosphate absorption.[52] Calcium citrate also increases the alkali load to the individual. The best evidence to support the routine use of calcium supplementation is a randomized, placebo-controlled clinical trial. In the largest trial, Chapuy et al.[53] enrolled 3270 women and showed 26% reduction in nonvertebral fractures but were confounded by vitamin D as part of the active treatment group in nursing home subjects, many of whom were vitamin D deficient. Other, smaller studies did not show a benefit with calcium administration of 800 to 1600 mg daily.[54–57]

A double-blind, placebo-controlled study enrolled 301 healthy postmenopausal women, half of whom had a usual daily calcium intake of 400 mg/day; the other half had an intake of 400 to 650 mg/day.[32] Subjects were randomized to 2 years of therapy with placebo or 500 mg/day calcium, formulated as either calcium carbonate or calcium citrate malate. Although calcium supplementation did not affect bone loss from the spine in early postmenopausal women with low calcium intake, there were small gains in BMD at the femoral neck and radius and reductions in BMD loss at the spine among women who had been postmenopausal for >6 years and who had received calcium citrate malate. Calcium carbonate maintained BMD at the femoral neck and radius, but had no effect on spine BMD.[32]

A second trial, conducted in healthy postmenopausal women who received calcium or placebo for 4 years (median intake, 640 mg/day at 4 years), found sustained, significant reductions in the rate of loss of total-body BMD in the calcium group throughout the study period.[55] Significantly fewer fractures occurred in the calcium group than in the placebo group. Combining vitamin D supplementation with calcium has been shown to reduce risk of fracture. In a 3-year double-blind study conducted in men and women age 65 years, 389 subjects were randomized to calcium (500 mg/day) plus 700 international units (IU) of vitamin D3.

Compared with placebo, combined therapy significantly increased BMD at the femoral neck and spine and over the total body. These differences were significant at 1 year; at 3 years, only total-body BMD was significantly improved by calcium/vitamin D therapy. Furthermore, the incidence of nonvertebral fracture was significantly reduced among subjects who received active therapy.[58] Reid et al., in a follow-up of their initial analysis of the longest trial of over 1400 postmenopausal women using calcium (citrate) intervention, showed a beneficial effect on BMD and markers of bone remodeling, yet failed to show a reduction in fractures.[59] Of note, the mean 25-hydroxyvitmain D {25(OH)D} levels were below 21 μg/l, the glomerular filtration rate (GFR) was 61 ml/min/1.73 m^2, and nearly a third had prevalent low trauma fractures. This suggested an excellent opportunity to see the benefit of calcium supplementation, yet a reduction in fractures was not seen in this group. This finding occurred in light of the increase in bone mineral density of the total hip. Based on previously mentioned work, the subjects may not have been able to synthesize $1,25(OH)_2D$ due to low stores of 25(OH)D, diminished GFR, and reduced ability to respond to vitamin D. Also of concern is the increased incidence of hip fractures in the calcium-treated group. Based on the intention-to-treat analysis, 5 hip fractures occurred in the placebo group and 17 in the treatment group. At other sites there was a trend favoring calcium, but it was not considered statistically significant.

The RECORD study[60] also suggested a disconnection between BMD efficacy and fracture prevention efficacy. Participants in this secondary prevention trial were randomly assigned to four equal groups and given two tablets with meals daily consisting of 800 IU vitamin D3, 1000 mg calcium (given as carbonate), 800 IU vitamin D3 combined with 1000 mg calcium, or placebo. By 2 years, compliance (defined as a participant who took >80% of tablets) was 60% of those who returned questionnaires. 25-Hydroxyvitamin D levels were measured in only a small sample (1.1% of the study population). Thus, the vitamin D status of the trial population at baseline remains largely unknown, although because the patients were younger than in other studies, ambulatory, and living in the community, they were less likely to have vitamin D deficiency. Given the latitude of the study sites, vitamin D may still be significantly deficient.

The recommended dietary intake of calcium is 1000 mg/day for men and women age <50 years. For those >50 years, the recommended intake is 1200 mg/day.[61]

The current recommended dietary intake for vitamin D (Table 33.4) is 400 IU/day for men and women age 51 to 70 years and 600 IU/day for those 71 years.[61] Women at risk for deficiency due to inadequate sunlight exposure should receive up to 800 IU/day.

Heaney et al.[62] used an isotopic method and urinary calcium load test to show that there is no significant difference between calcium carbonate when given with a light meal and calcium citrate.

33.1.1.4 Risks of Calcium Supplementation

In the Reid study,[59] 18% of subjects complained of constipation and a significant number stopped the active intervention because of it. This raises another important issue of trials using calcium: the high frequency of nonadherence due not only to constipation, but also to the need for multiple daily doses. Using data generated by the Women's Health Study, Curhan et al.[63] showed that women with the highest calcium intake had the lowest risk for symptomatic kidney stone; however, those women who took supplemental calcium were more likely to get nephrolithiasis. They also pointed out the problem of improper administration of the medication, with 67% not taking it at mealtimes or with a low oxalate meal. Similar findings of reduced stones with high calcium intake were noted in a study of men, but calcium supplements were not significantly associated with increased risk in that population.[64]

33.1.2 Vitamin D

Cholecalciferol (D_3) is the predominant form of vitamin D in fish, milk, egg yolks, and food products that are fortified with vitamin D. Bile acids bind to vitamin D in the small intestine to form micelles that are necessary for its absorption. Vitamin D is then transported into hepatocytes, where it is 25-hydroxylated. The newly formed steroid then binds to vitamin D-binding protein (DBP) or GC globulin, a globulin protein, where 99% of 25-hydroxyvitamin D is bound. The final step in the activation of vitamin D is the rate-limiting 1-hydroxylation that occurs principally in the kidney, though many tissues express the 1-alpha-hydroxylase. The expression of the enzyme is increased by low calcium, low phosphorus, and high parathyroid hormone. Vitamin D_3 may be generated endogenously by the effect of UV-B light on 7-dehydrocholesterol that is synthesized in the skin. Melanin absorbs light at the same wavelength as the light required for the formation of D_3; dark-skinned individuals synthesize less vitamin D for the same amount of light exposure. Although 1,25-dihydroxyvitamin D is considered the active compound, serum levels of total $1,25(OH)_2D$ correlate poorly with clinical disease. 25(OH)D levels are measured to assess vitamin D body stores based on a 100-times-higher concentration in serum and the now known ability of cells, including bone cells, to 1-alpha-hydroxylate 25(OH)D. The lowest plasma 25(OH)D cutoff is based on ensuring that plasma PTH will not be further reduced following a vitamin D and calcium challenge, or that seasonal variations in plasma PTH are abolished. Generally, the adverse effects of low plasma 25(OH)D begin to accumulate at levels below 50 nmol/l (20 ng/ml). This cutoff continues to be debated.[65] Center et al.[66] evaluated 25(OH)D levels and found a high correlation of fractures with serum levels below 68 nmol/l in both high-risk and low-risk elderly men. These

TABLE 33.3
Contributors to Vitamin D Deficiency in the Elderly

Inadequate dietary vitamin D intake
Inadequate sun exposure
Reduced cutaneous production
Inadequate gastrointestinal absorption
Diminished renal production of 1,25-dihydroxyvitamin D
Medication-induced metabolism of vitamin D

TABLE 33.4
Adequate Intake of Vitamin D

Age (years)	Female	Male
31–50	5	5
50–70	10	10
>70	15	15

Vitamin D (Calciferol 1 microgram = 40 IU)

findings were also corroborated by the work of Bischoff-Ferrari et al.[67] In a comprehensive study in Leeds, England, there was an almost linear fall in mean plasma 25(OH)D in females from about 50 ng/ml at age 25 to about 15 ng/ml at age 95.[68] Even in subjects over 60 there is a significant negative correlation of plasma 25(OH)D with age.[69]

As mentioned earlier, vitamin D has multiple effects on calcium metabolism. The main way that serum calcium is regulated is by the effect of activated vitamin D on absorption of calcium. The skeletal effects of vitamin D are complex and seem to be dependent upon dose and differentiation state.[70] Bone formation and mineralization are impaired in the vitamin D receptor (VDR) knockout mouse. Supplying a rescue diet returns growth to similar levels as the wild-type mouse.[71] Osteoblasts, the cells of bone formation, express receptors for vitamin D. Differentiation of preosteoblasts and expression of matrix proteins, including alkaline phosphatase, a protein required for crystal formation, are induced by vitamin D.[72] Metabolism of 1,25-dihydroxyvitamin D_3 occurs by 24-hydroxylation. Recently, though, the role of 24,25-dihydroxyvitamin D_3 has been readdressed with the finding that bone accrual increases in a rat model of osteoporosis.[73]

A number of effects occur with aging that impact on vitamin D (Table 33.3). There is less 7-dehydrocholesterol available in the skin to interact with UV-B radiation produced by the sun.[74] This reduces vitamin D synthesis. Vitamin D absorption from the duodenum may also be reduced.[40,75,76]

Evidence for resistance to the effects of vitamin D have been provided by Ebeling et al.[76] In their study they used labeled calcium with and without $1,25(OH)_2D$ administration, showing resistance to its effects, despite higher levels of baseline parathyroid hormone, due to reduced numbers of VDR in the elderly subjects based on intestinal biopsies. Manolagas et al.[77] also noted deficient synthesis of $1,25(OH)_2D$ in a population of elderly. This finding has been confirmed by others.[78,79] Data generated by Tsai and colleagues[80] suggested that the reduction in $1,25(OH)_2D$ synthesis is related to a diminished ability by PTH (using a bovine PTH(1–34) fragment) to stimulate 1-alpha-hydroxylation of vitamin D.

33.1.2.1 Vitamin D and Women

Multiple studies have shown a positive effect of calcitriol on preventing bone loss[81] and reducing the incidence of spinal fractures.[82–85]

Intervention trials with vitamin D have also given conflicting data. Lips et al.[86] gave vitamin D to a Dutch population, while Heikinheimo et al.[87] used parenteral vitamin D. The oral route did not show a significant difference, while the intramuscular vitamin D did. Cholecalciferol was administered to 213 women in Boston[58] whose mean 25-hydroxyvitamin D was 26 ng/ml with a calcium intake of 14 mmol daily. Of the 32 nonvertebral fractures that occurred, the absolute risk of fracture was not able to be calculated from the data provided, as women and men were grouped together. The results of Dawson-Hughes et al. also confirmed the findings of other groups of reduced bone remodeling by showing lower osteocalcin and pyridinoline cross-links.[88,89]

Trivedi et al.[90] examined the effects of vitamin D (100,000 IU every 4 months for 4 years) on a population of patients in Suffolk, U.K. They enrolled 2037 men and 649 women. Less than 10% of patients had assessments of vitamin 25(OH)D_3 or PTH. Compliance was recorded as 76%. Incident fractures at any site were reduced 20% for women but not for men by the addition of vitamin D in this study. Most of the effect seemed to come from wrist fractures. Effects on vertebral fractures and hip fractures were not considered significant in either gender. An open-label study[91] of over 3300 elderly female primary care clinic patients at high risk of fracture also demonstrated no benefit of 1000 mg calcium and 800 IU vitamin D_3 after 2 years. Adherence to therapy was quoted as 69%, while 25 (OH)D levels were not recorded. The latest intervention trial[92] using calcium and vitamin D was with 36,000 postmenopausal women between the ages of 50 and 79, receiving 500 mg of elemental calcium as calcium carbonate with 200 IU of vitamin D3 twice daily (for a total daily intake of 1000 mg of elemental calcium and 400 IU of vitamin D) or matching placebos for an average of 7 years. Annualized rates of hip, total, and site-specific fractures were compared between the groups. Personal use of calcium and vitamin D was permitted, as was the use of bisphosphonates or calcitonin. In addition, more than half of the participants were receiving hormone replacement therapy on entry, many as part of the active hormone replacement treatment program of the World Health Institute (WHI). Calcium with vitamin D supplementation increased total hip bone mineral density by 1% compared with placebo. According to an intention-to-treat analysis, there was no significant effect of calcium with vitamin D supplementation on any of the fracture endpoints. Calcium with vitamin D supplementation increased the risk of renal calculi by 17%. When data were excluded at the time a woman's adherence to therapy fell below 80%, the risk of hip fractures was significantly reduced (hazard ratio = 0.71, 95% confidence interval (CI) = 0.52 to 0.97).

WHI Points of Concern

Large percentage already taking vitamin D and calcium supplements
Not adequately powered to detect differences in hip fracture risk
Dose of vitamin D (10 μg) below previously published intervention trials
More than half receiving hormone therapy

In terms of data from histomorphometric analysis, Orwell et al.[95] followed a group of postmenopausal women on calcium, calcium plus vitamin D, or placebo. Interestingly, the bone biopsies suggested improved mineralization with vitamin D.

The first intervention trial of community-dwelling males did not suggest a reduction in bone loss in those that had received 25 μg of cholecalciferol. The study included individuals who were not elderly and had calcium intakes on average of over 1000 mg daily.[96] Dawson-Hughes et al.[97] used 700 IU of cholecalciferol in the elderly, showing a benefit on spinal bone mineral density over the 3-year trial. Only five fractures total occurred in the males. In a younger population, Orwell and colleagues[94] found no differences in bone density with regard to male subjects who were taking adequate oral intake of calcium.

Calcitriol or alphacalcidol (1-alpha-hydroxycholecalciferol) an activated analogue of vitamin D was used in interventions to reduce incident fractures; however, no significant difference was seen between active treatment and placebo-treated groups in these studies with a duration of up to 3 years.[95–99]

Based on previous data in women, Ebeling et al.[100] evaluated 41 men over a 2-year period that already had a baseline fracture. Administering 0.5 μg calcitriol daily did not show a benefit on spinal or femoral neck BMD when compared to 1000 mg calcium carbonate daily. A positive benefit on fractional calcium absorption was observed in the calcitriol group even though mean baseline characteristics suggested no evidence of 25-hydroxyvitamin D deficiency or elevations in parathyroid hormone.

33.1.2.2 Fall Prevention

Vitamin D has been shown to be beneficial in deficient subjects. Both calcium and phosphorus are important for muscle contraction and relaxation. Vitamin D is thought to play a role in regulating entry of these substances. Eight weeks of vitamin D3 treatment with 800 IU (20 μg) per day combined with 1200 mg calcium was reported to reduce secondary hyperparathyroidism, body sway, and number of falls after 1 year in elderly ambulatory women.[101] The number of fallers was not reduced, but the risk of falling was, by 49% (95% Cl, 14 to 71%, $p < 0.01$). Individuals with repeated falls had the greatest benefit of the treatment. However, the crude number of fallers was not reduced by the treatment. In a double-blind randomized study, 122 otherwise unselected elderly women between the ages of 63 and 99 years (mean = 85 years) in a geriatric department were treated with 800 IU (20 μg) vitamin D3 + 1200 mg calcium daily (n = 62) or 1200 mg calcium daily (n = 60) and followed for 12 weeks. Plasma 25(OH)D increased 71% ($p < 0.0001$) and plasma PTH decreased 29% ($p = 0.002$) in the group receiving vitamin D. Muscle function improved significantly in this group ($p < 0.01$). The nursing staff registered falls. An intention-to-treat analysis using a Poisson regression model to adjust for baseline covariates disclosed that calcium and vitamin D, compared with calcium alone, reduced falls. In a randomized controlled study,[102] 150 women were recruited following surgery for hip fracture and assigned to a single injection of 300,000 IU (7500 μg) D2, injection of vitamin D2 + 1000 mg Ca/day, 800 IU (20 μg) oral D3 + 1000 mg Ca/day, or no treatment and followed for 1 year. The relative risk of falling was reduced by 52% (95% Cl = 10–74, $p < 0.05$) in the groups supplemented with vitamin D compared with controls.

33.2 OTHER TRACE MINERALS OF POTENTIAL INTEREST

33.2.1 Manganese

Manganese deficiency results in abnormal skeletal development in a number of animal species. Manganese is the preferred cofactor of enzymes called glycosyltransferases, which are required for the synthesis of proteoglycans that are needed for the formation of healthy cartilage and bone.[103] In humans, demonstration of a manganese deficiency syndrome has been less clear. Young men who were fed a low-manganese diet developed decreased serum cholesterol levels and a transient skin rash.[104] Blood calcium, phosphorus, and alkaline phosphatase levels were also elevated, which may indicate increased bone remodeling as a consequence of insufficient dietary manganese. Young women fed a manganese-poor diet developed mildly abnormal glucose tolerance in response to an intravenous (IV) infusion of glucose, but changes in calcium metabolism were not noted.[105] Manganese deficiency is characterized by enlarged joints, deformed legs with thickened and shortened long bones, and lameness in pigs, ruminants, and poultry.[106] No clear syndrome of manganese deficiency has been characterized in humans. Because there was not enough information on manganese requirements to set a Recommended Dietary Allowance (RDA), the Food and Nutrition Board (FNB) of the Institute of Medicine set an Adequate Intake (AI) level, a recommended intake value based on observed or experimentally determined estimates of nutrient intake by a group of healthy people that are assumed to be adequate. Studies in the elderly are lacking. Women with osteoporosis have been found to have decreased plasma levels of manganese and an enhanced plasma response to an oral dose of manganese, suggesting they may have lower manganese status than women without osteoporosis. A study in healthy postmenopausal women found that a supplement containing manganese (5 mg/day), copper (2.5 mg/day), and zinc (15 mg/day) in combination with a calcium supplement (1000 mg/day) was more effective than the calcium supplement alone in preventing spinal bone loss over a period of 2 years.[107] However, the presence of other trace elements in the supplement makes it impossible to determine whether manganese supplementation was the beneficial agent for maintaining bone mineral density.

33.2.2 Molybdenum

Molybdenum (Mo) is a cofactor for at least three enzymes in humans: sulfite oxidase, xanthine oxidase, and aldehyde oxidase. It is considered essential because it is required for the function of these enzymes, which play a role in the catabolism of sulfur amino acids and purine and pyrimidine. Metabolism of sulfur-containing amino acids and the synthesis of sulfate used in the production of glycosaminoglycans are essential processes for bone growth.[108] Isolated sulfite oxidase deficiency has been described in which infants are born with severe brain damage. The Recommended Dietary Allowance (RDA) for molybdenum was most recently revised in January 2001.[109] It was based on the results of nutritional balance studies conducted in eight healthy young men under controlled laboratory conditions. Legumes, such as beans, lentils, and peas, are the richest sources of molybdenum. Grain products and nuts are considered good sources, while animal products, fruits, and many vegetables are generally low in molybdenum.

33.2.3 Copper

Lysyl oxidase is required for the cross-linking of collagen and elastin, which are essential for the formation of strong and flexible connective tissue. The action of lysyl oxidase helps maintain the integrity of connective tissue in the heart and blood vessels and plays a role in bone formation.[110] Abnormalities of bone development related to copper deficiency are most common in copper-deficient low-birth-weight infants and young children. Cow's milk is relatively low in copper.[110] Copper may have a significant role in bone metabolism given its role in lysyl oxidase. The RDA for copper reflects the results of depletion–repletion studies and is based on the prevention of deficiency.[111–114] Supplementation with copper prevented postmenopausal bone loss when compared to placebo.[115,116] Copper is found in a wide variety of foods and is most plentiful in organ meats, shellfish, nuts, and seeds. Wheat bran cereals and whole-grain products are also good sources of copper.

33.2.4 Phosphorus

Approximately 85% of the body's phosphorus is found in bone. Phosphorus is a major structural component of bone in the form of hydroxyapatite. Although osteoporosis is a multifactorial disease, vitamin D insufficiency can be an important contributing factor. Without sufficient vitamin D, calcium absorption cannot be maximized and the resulting elevation in PTH secretion by the parathyroid glands results in increased bone resorption, which may lead to osteoporotic fracture.[117] A prospective cohort study that followed more than 72,000 postmenopausal women in the U.S. for 18 years found that those who consumed at least 600 IU/day of vitamin D from diet and supplements had a risk of osteoporotic hip fracture that was 37% lower than women who consumed less than 140 IU/day.[118] The results of most clinical trials suggest that vitamin D supplementation can slow bone density losses or decrease the risk of osteoporotic fracture in men and women who are unlikely to be getting enough vitamin D.

Supplementation of postmenopausal women in the U.S. with 500 mg/day of calcium and either 100 or 700 IU/day of vitamin D for 2 years slowed bone density losses at the hip only in the group taking 700 IU/day.[119] Daily supplementation of elderly men and women with 500 mg/day of calcium and 700 IU/day of vitamin D for 3 years reduced bone density losses at the hip and spine and reduced the frequency of nonvertebral fractures.[58] When the calcium and vitamin D supplements were discontinued, the bone density benefits were lost within 2 years.[120] In Denmark, supplementation of elderly women with 400 IU/day of vitamin D for 2 years increased bone density at the hip.[121] An annual injection of 150,000 to 300,000 IU of vitamin D2 (ergocalciferol) for 4 years decreased the incidence of fracture in elderly Finnish women,[89] and oral supplementation with 800 IU/day of vitamin D and 1200 mg/day of calcium for 3 years decreased the incidence of hip fracture in elderly French women.[122] Oral supplementation of elderly adults in the U.K. with 100,000 IU of vitamin D once every 4 months (equivalent to about 800 IU/day) for 5 years reduced the risk of osteoporotic fracture by 33% compared to placebo.[123] However, oral supplementation with 400 IU/day of vitamin D for more than 3 years did not affect the incidence of fracture in a study of elderly Dutch men and women.[124] Overall, the evidence to date suggests that vitamin D supplements of about 800 IU/day may be helpful in reducing bone loss and fracture rates in the elderly. In order for vitamin D supplementation to be effective in preserving bone health, adequate calcium (1000 to 1200 mg/day) should also be consumed.

33.2.5 Magnesium

Magnesium is required for cell energy production, nucleic acid and protein synthesis, signaling, migration, ion transport, and a structural role in bone. Despite this, our knowledge of osteoporosis prevention is limited. Part of the problem is the measurement of an ion where only 1% is found in the blood.[125] Inadequate blood magnesium levels are known to result in low blood calcium levels, resistance to parathyroid hormone (PTH), and resistance to some of the effects of vitamin D. The active form of vitamin D (calcitriol) may increase the intestinal absorption of magnesium to a small extent. However, magnesium absorption does not seem to be calcitriol dependent, as is the absorption of calcium and phosphate. High calcium intake has not been found to affect magnesium balance in most studies. In 1997, the Food and Nutrition Board of the Institute of Medicine increased the Recommended Dietary Allowance (RDA) for magnesium, based on the results of recent, tightly controlled balance studies that utilized more accurate methods of measuring magnesium.[126] A large national survey indicated that the average magnesium intakes for men (about 320 mg/day) and women (about 230 mg/day) were significantly below the current RDA. In men and women over 70 years of age, magnesium intakes were even lower.[127] Assessments for osteoporosis prevention are lacking with this trace mineral. One epidemiologic study of magnesium intake seemed to suggest a positive relation between total BMD and magnesium; however, the effect was only seen in Caucasian populations.[128]

33.2.6 Vitamin K

Vitamin K is a fat-soluble vitamin. The *K* is derived from the German word *koagulation*, referring to the essential role of vitamin K in blood clotting. There are two naturally occurring forms of vitamin K. Plants synthesize phylloquinone, also known as vitamin K_1. Bacteria synthesize a range of vitamin K forms, using repeating five-carbon units in the side chain of the molecule. These forms of vitamin K are designated menaquinone-n (MK-n), where n stands for the number of five-carbon units. MK-n are collectively referred to as vitamin K_2.[129] MK-4 is not produced in significant amounts by bacteria, but appears to be synthesized by animals (including humans) from phylloquinone. MK-4 is found in a number of organs other than the liver at higher concentrations than phylloquinone. This fact, along with the existence of a unique pathway for its synthesis, suggests there is some unique function of MK-4 that is yet to be discovered.[130] The only known biological role of vitamin K is that of the required coenzyme for a vitamin K-dependent carboxylase that catalyzes the carboxylation of the amino acid glutamic acid, resulting in its conversion to gamma-carboxyglutamic acid (Gla).[131] Although vitamin K-dependent gamma-carboxylation occurs only on specific glutamic acid residues in a small number of proteins, it is critical to the calcium-binding function of those proteins.[132] Three vitamin K-dependent proteins have been isolated in bone. Osteocalcin is a protein synthesized by osteoblasts (bone-forming cells). The synthesis of osteocalcin by osteoblasts is regulated by vitamin D. The mineral-binding capacity of osteocalcin requires vitamin K-dependent gamma-carboxylation of three glutamic acid residues. The function of osteocalcin is unclear, but is thought to be related to bone mineralization. Matrix Gla protein (MGP) has been found in bone, cartilage, and soft tissue, including blood vessels. The results of animal studies suggest MGP prevents the calcification of soft tissue and cartilage, while facilitating normal bone growth and development. The vitamin K-dependent anticoagulant protein S is also synthesized by osteoblasts, but its role in bone metabolism is unclear. Children with inherited protein S deficiency suffer complications related to increased blood clotting as well as to decreased bone density.[133] Epidemiological studies have demonstrated a relationship between vitamin K and age-related bone loss (osteoporosis). The Nurses' Health Study followed more than 72,000 women for 10 years. Investigators found that women whose vitamin K intake was in the lowest quintile (1/5) had a 30% higher risk of hip fracture than women with vitamin K intakes in the highest four quintiles.[134] The Framingham Heart Study followed 800 elderly men and women for 7 years and found that men and women with dietary vitamin K intakes in the highest quartile (1/4) had only 35% of the risk of hip fracture experienced by those with dietary vitamin K intakes in the lowest quartile (approximately 250 µg/day vs. 50 µg/day of vitamin K). However, the investigators found no association between dietary vitamin K intake and bone mineral density (BMD) in the Framingham subjects.[135] Because the primary dietary source of vitamin K is generally green leafy vegetables, high vitamin K intake could just be a marker for a healthy diet that is high in fruits and vegetables.[136] Osteocalcin, a bone-related protein that circulates in the blood, has been shown to be a sensitive marker of bone formation. Vitamin K is required for the gamma-carboxylation of osteocalcin. Undercarboxylation of osteocalcin adversely affects its capacity to bind to bone mineral, and the degree of osteocalcin gamma-carboxylation has been found to be a sensitive indicator of vitamin K nutritional status.[137] Circulating levels of undercarboxylated osteocalcin (ucOC) were found to be higher in postmenopausal women than premenopausal women and markedly higher in women over the age of 70. In a study of 195 institutionalized elderly women, the relative risk of hip fracture was six times higher in those who had elevated ucOC levels at the beginning of the study.[138] In a much larger sample of 7500 elderly women living independently, circulating ucOC was also predictive of fracture risk.[139] Although vitamin K deficiency would seem the most likely cause of elevated blood ucOC, investigators have also documented an inverse relationship between measures of vitamin D nutritional status and ucOC levels, as well as a significant lowering of ucOC by vitamin D supplementation.[140] It is also possible that an increased ucOC level is a marker for poor vitamin D or protein nutritional status.

Certain oral anticoagulants, like warfarin, are known to be antagonists of vitamin K. A meta-analysis of the results of 11 published studies found that oral anticoagulation therapy was associated with a very modest reduction in bone density at the wrist, and no change in bone density at the hip or spine.[141] In the absence of long-term intervention studies using nutritionally optimal doses of vitamin K, evidence of a relationship between vitamin K nutritional status and bone health in adults is considered weak. Further investigation is required to determine the physiological function of vitamin K-dependent proteins in bone and the mechanisms by which vitamin K affects bone health and osteoporotic fracture risk.

33.2.7 Zinc

The biology of zinc is linked extensively to hormone metabolism. Notable examples are the zinc finger motifs of regulatory proteins required for hormonal signals to regulate gene transcription.[142] Zinc has been reported to have roles in the synthesis, transport, and peripheral action of hormones. Low dietary zinc status has been associated with low circulating concentrations of several hormones, including testosterone,[143] free T4,[144] and insulin-like growth factor (IGF)-1.[145] Previous studies of animal models have suggested a correlation between zinc deficiency and bone disease.[146] In women, a role for zinc has also been suggested.[147,148] However, no studies have directly related hormone concentrations to decreases or increases in zinc intake. In the Rancho Bernardo cohort, BMDs for the hip, spine, and distal wrist were significantly lower in men in the lowest plasma zinc quartile (11.3 mol/l) than in men with higher plasma zinc concentrations. The association between plasma zinc and BMD was cross-sectional, longitudinal, and independent of age or body mass index. However, zinc levels were not predictive of future bone loss during the 4-year trial. Most of the nutrients that were correlated with zinc intake were from animal products. The strong collinearity between zinc intake and other protein-related nutrients precludes the designation of any single nutrient, including zinc, as causally associated with osteoporosis.[149] The investigators previously reported that animal protein (correlated with zinc) is positively associated with BMD among Rancho Bernardo Study participants.[150]

33.3 CONCLUSIONS

Osteoporosis continues to claim the lives and livelihoods of many older adults. Our current view has focused on attainment of high bone mineral density as our best defense against fracture, as the reviewed studies have demonstrated that changes in bone mineral density do not always correlate with fracture reduction. Clearly, benefits from treatment with calcium supplements and vitamin D occur in those individuals with negative calcium balance and vitamin D deficiency, respectively. The recommendations to go beyond these needs do not seem to be supported by the current evidence. Fortunately, the side effects of exogenous calcium are usually low impact and self-limited. In a Westernized society, our concern is our convenience; it is usually easier to take a pill than to keep milk products available. We should continue to take extensive diet histories and counsel on lifestyle factors to attain adequate calcium intake, especially in growing adolescents, when the need is greatest. Much more research is needed to address the trace minerals in our environment that may have special applications for the elderly due to physiologic changes that occurs in these individuals. At the same time, we must be wary of those who sell various supplements for attaining better bone health, making claims that may not be supported by the available evidence. Finally, this research points to the need to better understand the matrix of bone, as this is where the crystals reside. If there is no ground substance, no castle may be built.

REFERENCES

1. U.S. Department of Health and Human Services. *Bone Health and Osteoporosis*, a report of the U.S. Surgeon General. Rockville, MD, 2004.
2. Johnell, O. The socioeconomic burden of fractures: today and in the 21st century. *Am J Med* 103, S20, 1997.
3. Royal College of Physicians. Fractured neck of femur. Prevention and management. Summary and recommendations of a report of the Royal College of Physicians. *J R Coll Physicians* 23, 8, 1989.
4. Cooper, C., Campion, G., Melton, L.J. Hip fractures in the elderly: a world-wide projection. *Osteoporos Int* 2, 285, 1992.
5. Melton, L.J., III. Epidemiology of fractures. In *Osteoporosis: Etiology, Diagnosis, and Management*, 2nd ed., Riggs, B.L., Melton, L.J., III, Eds. Lippincott-Raven, Philadelphia, 1995, p. 225.
6. World Health Organization. *Vitamin and Mineral Requirements in Human Nutrition*, Report of the Joint FAO/WHO Expert Consultation. Geneva, 2004.
7. Dalle Carbonare, L., Giannini, S. Bone microarchitecture as an important determinant of bone strength. *J Endocrinol Invest* 27, 99, 2004.
8. Roschger, P., Matsuo, K., Misof, B.M., et al. Normal mineralization and nanostructure of sclerotic bone in mice overexpressing Fra-1. *Bone* 34, 776, 1997.
9. Chatterji, S., Wall, J.C., Jeffery, J.W. Age-related changes in the orientation and particle size of the mineral phase in human femoral cortical bone. *Calcif Tissue Int* 33, 567, 1981.
10. Currey, J.D. The many adaptations of bone. *J Biomech* 36, 1487, 2003.
11. Boskey, A.L. Bone mineralization. In *Bone Biomechanics*, 3rd ed., Cowin, S.C., Ed. CRC Press, Boca Raton, FL, 2001, pp. 5.1–5.34.
12. Chatterji, S., Wall, J.C., Jeffery, J.W. Age-related changes in the orientation and particle size of the mineral phase in human femoral cortical bone. *Calcif Tissue Int* 33, 567, 1983.
13. Gao, H., Ji, B., Jager, I.L., et al. Materials become insensitive to flaws at nanoscale: lessons from nature. *Proc Natl Acad Sci USA*, 100, 5597, 2003.
14. Viguet-Carrin, S., Garnero, P., Delmas, P.D. The role of collagen in bone strength. *Osteoporos Int* 17, 319, 2006.
15. Garnero, P., Cloos, P., Sornay-Rendu, E., et al. Type I collagen racemization and isomerization and the risk of fracture in postmenopausal women: the OFELY prospective study. *J Bone Miner Res* 17, 826, 2002.
16. Bailey, A.J., Sims, T.J., Ebbesen, E.N., et al. Age related changes in the biochemical properties of human cancellous bone collagen: relationship to bone strength. *Calcif Tissue Int* 65, 203, 1999.
17. Banse, X., Sims, T.J., Bailey, A.J. Mechanical properties of adult vertebral cancellous bone: correlation with collagen intermolecular cross-links. *J Bone Miner Res* 17, 1621, 2002.

18. Lips, P. Vitamin D deficiency and secondary hyperparathyroidism in the elderly: consequences for bone loss and fractures and therapeutic implications. *Endocr Rev* 22, 477, 2001.
19. Bischoff-Ferrari, H.A., et al. Effect of vitamin D on falls: a meta-analysis. *JAMA* 291, 1999, 2004.
20. Sambrook, P.N., et al. Serum parathyroid hormone predicts time to fall independent of vitamin D status in a frail elderly population. *J Clin Endocrinol Metab* 89, 1572, 2004.
21. Grant, A.M., et al. Oral vitamin D3 and calcium for secondary prevention of low-trauma fractures in elderly people (Randomised Evaluation of Calcium or Vitamin D, RECORD): a randomized placebo-controlled trial. *Lancet* 365, 1621, 2005.
22. Albright, F., Bloomberg, E., Smith, P.H. Post-menopausal osteoporosis. *Trans Assoc Am Physicians* 55, 298, 1940.
23. Riggs, B.L., Wahner, H.W., Melton, L.J. Heterogeneity of involutional osteoporosis: evidence for two distinct osteoporosis syndromes. Clinical disorder of bone and mineral metabolism. In *Proceedings of the Frances and Anthony D'Anna Memorial Symposium*, Detroit, MI, May 9–13, 1983, pp. 337–341.
24. Riggs, B.L., Wahner, H.W., Melton, L.J., 3rd, et al. Rates of bone loss in the appendicular and axial skeletons of women. Evidence of substantial vertebral bone loss before menopause. *J Clin Invest* 77, 1487, 1986.
25. Riggs, B.L., Wahner, H.W., Melton, L.J., III, et al. Dietary calcium intake and rates of bone loss in women. *J Clin Invest* 80, 979, 1987.
26. Garn, S.M. *The Earlier Gain and the Later Loss of Cortical Bone*. C.C. Thomas, Springfield, IL, 1970.
27. Nilas, L.C., Christiansen, P., Rodbro, R. Calcium supplementation and postmenopausal bone loss. *Br Med J* 289, 1103, 1984.
28. Matkovic, V.K., Kostial, I., Simonovic, R., et al. Bone status and fracture rates in two regions of Yugoslavia. *Am J Clin Nutr* 32, 540, 1979.
29. Riggs, B.L., Wahner, H.W., Dunn, W.L., et al. Differential changes in bone mineral density of the appendicular and axial skeleton with aging: relationship to spinal osteoporosis. *J Clin Invest* 67, 328, 1981.
30. Nordin, B.E. and Polley, K.J. Metabolic consequences of the menopause. A cross-sectional, longitudinal, and intervention study on 557 normal postmenopausal women. *Calcified Tissue Int* 41, S1, 1987.
31. Reid, I.R., Ames, R., Evans, M.C., et al. Determinants of total body and regional bone mineral density in normal postmenopausal women: a key role for fat mass. *J Clin Endocrinol Metab* 75, 45, 1992.
32. Dawson-Hughes, B., Dallal, G.E., Krall, E.A., et al. A controlled trial of the effect of calcium supplementation on bone density in postmenopausal women. *N Engl J Med* 323, 878, 1990.
33. Aloia, J.F., Vaswani, A., Yeh, J.K., et al. Calcium supplementation with and without hormone replacement therapy to prevent postmenopausal bone loss. *Ann Intern Med* 120, 97, 1994.
34. Marshall, D.H., Nordin, B.E.C., Speed, R. Calcium, phosphorus and magnesium requirement. *Proc Nutr Soc* 35, 163, 1976.
35. Nordin, B.E.C. The calcium controversy. *Osteoporos Int* 7, S17, 1997.
36. Holick, M.F., Krane, S.M., Potts, J.T., Jr. Calcium, phosphorus, and bone metabolism: calcium-regulating hormones. In *Harrison's Principles of Internal Medicine*, Fauci, A.S., Braunwald, E., Isselbacher, K.J., et al., Eds. McGraw-Hill, New York, 1998, p. 2214.

37. Need, A.G., Morris, H.A., Horowitz, M., et al. Intestinal calcium absorption in men with spinal osteoporosis. *Clin Endocrinol* 48, 163, 1998.
38. Wolf, R.L., Zmuda, J.M., Charron, M., et al. Calcium absorption efficiency in older men: relationships to age and bone loss. *J Bone Miner Res* 14, A1193, 1999.
39. Gallagher, J.C., Riggs, B.L., Essman, J., et al. Intestinal calcium absorption and serum vitamin D metabolites in normal subjects and osteoporotic patients: effect of age and dietary calcium. *J Clin Invest* 64, 729, 1979.
40. Bullamore, J.R., Gallagher, J.C., Wilkinson, R., et al. Effect of age on calcium absorption. *Lancet* 2(7672), 535, 1970.
41. Heaney, R.P., Recker R.R., Saville, P.D. Menopausal changes in calcium balance performance. *J Lab Clin Med* 92, 953, 1978.
42. U.S. Department of Agriculture, Continuing Survey of Food Intake in Individuals, 1994–96. Accessible at http://www.ers.usda.gov/Briefing/dietandhealth/data/nutrients/tables.xls.
43. Buckley, M. and Bronner, F. Calcium binding protein biosynthesis in the rat: regulation by calcium and 1,25-dihydroxy vitamin D_3. *Arch Biochem Biophys* 202, 234, 1980.
44. Hoenderop, J.G., Willems, P.H., Bindels, R.J. Towards a comprehensive molecular model of active calcium reabsorption. *Am J Physiol Renal Physiol* 278, 352, 2000.
45. Simon, D.B., Lu, Y., Choate, K.A., et al. Paracellin-1, a renal tight junction protein required for paracellular Mg^{2+} absorption. *Science* 285, 103, 1999.
46. Hoenderop, J.G., van der Kemp, A.W., Hartog, A., et al. Molecular identification of the apical Ca^{2+} channel in 1,25-dihydroxyvitamin D_3 responsive epithelia. *J Biol Chem* 274, 8375, 1999.
47. Kip, S.N. and Strehler, E.E. Characterization of PCMA and their contribution to transcellular Ca^{2+} flux in MDCK cells. *Am J Physiol Renal Physiol* 284, F122, 2003.
48. Stafford, R.S., Drieling, R.L., Johns, R., Ma, J. National patterns of calcium use in osteoporosis in the United States. *J Reprod Med* 50, 885, 2005.
49. Ettinger, B., Genant, H.K., Cann, C.E. Long-term estrogen replacement therapy prevents bone loss and fractures. *Ann Intern Med* 102, 319, 1985.
50. Riis, B., Thomsen, K., Christiansen, C. Does calcium supplementation prevent postmenopausal bone loss? A double-blind, controlled clinical study. *N Engl J Med* 316,173, 1987.
51. Kanis, J.A. The use of calcium in the management of osteoporosis. *Bone* 24, 279, 1999.
52. Schiller, L.R., Santa Ana, C.A., Saheikh, M.S., et al. Effect of the time of administration of calcium acetate on phosphorus. *N Eng J Med* 1320, 1110, 1989.
53. Chapuy, M.C., Arlot, M.E., Duboeuf, F., et al. Vitamin D and calcium to prevent hip fractures in elderly women. *N Engl J Med* 327, 1637, 1992.
54. Chevaley, T., RizzolI, R., Nydegger, V., et al. Effects of calcium supplements on femoral bone mineral density and vertebral fracture rate in vitamin D replete elderly patients. *Osteoporos Int* 4, 245, 1994.
55. Reid, I.R., Ames, R.W., Evans, M.C., et al. Long-term effects of calcium supplementation on bone loss and fractures in postmenopausal women: a randomized controlled trial. *Am J Med* 98, 331, 1995.
56. Recker, R., Hinders, S., Davies, K.M., et al. Correcting calcium nutritional deficiency prevents spine fractures in elderly women. *J Bone Miner Res* 11, 1961, 1996.
57. Riggs, B.L., O'Fallon, W.M., Muhs, J., et al. Long-term effects of calcium supplementation on serum parathyroid hormone level, bone turnover, and bone loss in elderly women. *J Bone Miner Res* 13,168, 1998.

58. Dawson-Hughes, B., Harris, S.S., Krall, E.A., et al. Effect of calcium and vitamin D supplementation on bone density in men and women 65 years of age or older. *N Engl J Med* 337, 670, 1997.
59. Reid, I.R., Mason, B., Horne, A., et al. Randomized controlled trial of calcium and healthy older woman. *Am J Med* 119, 777, 2006.
60. Grant, A.M., Avenell, A., Campbell, M.K., et al. RECORD Trial Group. Oral vitamin D3 and calcium for secondary prevention of low-trauma fractures in elderly people (Randomised Evaluation of Calcium or Vitamin D, RECORD): a randomised placebo-controlled trial. *Lancet* 365, 1621, 2005.
61. National Institutes of Health, Office of Dietary Supplements. Dietary Supplement Fact Sheet. Available at http://ods.od.nih.gov/factsheets/calcium.asp. Accessed March 1, 2006.
62. Heaney, R.P., Dowell, M.S., Burger-Lux, M.J. Absorption of calcium as the carbonate and citrate salts with some observations on method. *Osteoporos Int* 9, 19, 1999.
63. Curhan, G.C., Willet, W.C., Speizer, F.E., et al. Comparison of dietary calcium with supplemental calcium and other nutrients as factors affecting the risk for kidney stones. *Ann Intern Med* 126, 497, 1997.
64. Curhan, G.C., Willet, W.C., Rimm, E.B., et al. A prospective study of dietary calcium and other nutrients and the risk of symptomatic kidney stones. *N Engl J Med* 328, 883, 1993.
65. Mosekilde, L. Vitamin D in the elderly. *Clin Endocrinol* 62, 265, 2005.
66. Center, J.R., Nguyen, T.V., Sambrook, P.N., et al. Hormonal and biochemical parameters and osteoporotic fractures in elderly men. *Jf Bone Miner Res* 15, 1405, 2000.
67. Bischoff-Ferrari, H.A., Giovannucci, E., Willett, W.C., et al. Estimation of optimal serum concentration of 25-hydroxyvitamin D for multiple health concerns. *Am J Clin Nutr* 84, 18, 2006.
68. Nordin, B.E.C., Heyburn, P.J., Peacock, M., et al. Osteoporosis and osteomalacia. *Clin Endocrinol Metab* 9, 177, 1980.
69. Hodkinson, H.M., Bryson, E., Klenerman, U., et al. Sex, sunlight, season, diet and the vitamin D status of elderly patients. *J Clin Exp Gerontol* 1, 13, 1979.
70. Aronow, M.S., Barone, L.M., Bettencourt, B., et al. Pleiotropic effects of vitamin D on osteoblasts gene expression are related to the proliferative and differentiated state of the bone cell phenotype: dependency upon basal levels of gene expression, duration of exposure, and bone matrix competency in normal osteoblast cultures. *Endocrinology* 128, 1496, 1991.
71. Amling, M., Priemel, M., Holzmann, T., et al. Rescue of the skeletal phenotype of vitamin D receptor-ablated mice in the setting of normal mineral ion homeostasis: formal histomorphometric and biomechanical analyses. *Endocrinology* 140, 4982, 1999.
72. Beresford, J.N., Gallagher, J.A., Russell, R.G. 1,25-Dihydroxy-vitamin D_3 and human bone-derived cells *in vitro*: effects on alkaline phosphatase, type I collagen and proliferation. *Endocrinology* 119, 1776, 1986.
73. Gal-Moscovici, A., Gal, M., Popovtzer, M.M. Treatment of osteoporotic ovariectomized rats with 24,25(OH)2D3. *Eur J Clin Invest* 35, 375, 2005.
74. Barragry, J.M., France, M.W., Corless, C., et al. Intestinal cholecalciferol absorption in the elderly and young adults. *Clin Sci Mol Med* 55, 213, 1978.
75. MacLaughlin, J. and Holick, M.F. Aging decreases the capacity of human skin to produce vitamin D_3. *J Clin Invest* 76, 1536, 1985.
76. Ebeling, P.R., Sandgren, M.E., DiMagno, E.P., et al. Evidence of an age-related decrease in intestinal responsiveness to vitamin D: relationship between serum 1,25-dihydroxyvitamin D3 and intestinal vitamin D receptor concentrations in normal women. *J Clin Endocrinol Metab* 75, 176, 1992.

77. Manolagas, S.C., Culler, F.L., Howard, J.E., Brickman, A.S., Deftos L.J. The cytoreceptor assay for 1,25-dihydroxyvitamin D and its application to clinical studies. *J Clin Endocrinol Metab* 56, 751, 1983.
78. Clemens, T.L., Zhou, X.Y., Myles, M., Endres, D., Lindsay, R. Serum vitamin D2 and vitamin D3 metabolite concentrations and absorption of vitamin D2 in elderly subjects. *J Clin Endocrinol Metab* 63, 656, 1986.
79. Fujisawa, Y., Kida, K., Matsuda, H. Role of change in vitamin D metabolism with age in calcium and phosphorus metabolism in normal human subjects. *J Clin Endocrinol Metab* 59, 719, 1984.
80. Tsai, K.-S., Hunter, H., III, Kumar, R., et al. Impaired vitamin D metabolism with aging in women: possible role in pathogenesis of senile osteoporosis. *J Clin Invest* 73, 1668, 1984.
81. Aloia, J.F., Vazswani, A., Yeh, J.K., et al. Calcitriol in the treatment of postmenopausal osteoporosis. *Am J Med* 84, 401, 1988.
82. Gallagher, J.C. and Goldgar, D. Treatment of postmenopausal osteoporosis with high doses of synthetic calcitriol. A randomized controlled study. *Ann Intern Med* 113, 649, 1990.
83. Gallagher, J.C., Jerphak, C.M., Jee, W.S., et al.1,25-Dihydroxyvitamin D3: short and long-term effects on bone and calcium metabolism in patients with postmenopausal osteoporosis. *Proc Natl Acad Sci USA* 79, 3325, 1982.
84. Tilyard, M.W., Spears, G.F., Thomson, J., et al. Treatment of postmenopausal osteoporosis with calcitriol or calcium. *N Engl J Med* 326, 357, 1992.
85. Gallagher, J.C., Riggs, B.L., Recker, R.R., et al. The effect of calcitriol on patients with postmenopausal osteoporosis with special reference to fracture frequency. *Proc Soc Exp Biol Med* 191, 287, 1989.
86. Lips, P., Graafmans, W.C., Ooms, M.E., et al. Vitamin D supplementation and fracture incidence in elderly persons: a randomized double blind placebo-controlled trial. *Ann Intern Med* 124, 400, 1996.
87. Heikinheimo, R.J., Inkovaara, H.A., Harju, E.J., et al. Annual injection of vitamin D and fractures of aged bones. *Calcif Tiss Int* 51, 105, 1992.
88. Delmas, P.D., Gineyts, E., Bertholin, A., et al. Immunoassay of pyridinoline crosslink excretion in normal adults and in Paget's disease. *J Bone Miner Res* 8, 643, 1993.
89. Epstein, S., Poser, J., McClintock, R., et al. Differences in serum bone GLA protein with age and sex. *Lancet* 1, 307, 1984.
90. Trivedi, D.P., Doll, R., Khaw, K.T., Effect of four monthly oral vitamin D_3 supplementation on fractures and mortality in men and women living in the community: randomized double blind controlled trial. *BMJ* 326, 469, 2003.
91. Porthouse, J., Cockayne, S., King, C., et al. Randomised controlled trial of calcium and supplementation with cholecalciferol (vitamin D3) for prevention of fractures in primary care. *BMJ* 330, 1003, 2005.
92. Jackson, R.D., LaCroix, A.Z., Gass, M., et al. Calcium plus vitamin D supplementation and the risk of fractures. *N Engl J Med* 354, 669, 2006.
93. Orwoll, E.S., McClung, M.R., Oviatt, S.K., et al. Histomorphometric effects of calcium or calcium plus 25-hydroxyvitamin D3 therapy in senile osteoporosis. *J Bone Miner Res* 4, 81, 1989.
94. Orwoll, E.S., Oviatt, S.K., McClung, M.R., et al. The rate of bone mineral loss in normal men and the effects of calcium and cholecalciferol. *Ann Intern Med* 112, 29, 1990.
95. Aloi, J.F., Vaswani, A., Yeh, J.K., et al. Calcitriol in the treatment of postmenopausal osteoporosis. *Am J Med* 84, 401, 1988.

96. Gallagher, J.C., Goldgar, D. Treatment of postmenopausal osteoporosis with high doses of synthetic calcitriol. A randomized controlled study. *Ann Intern Med* 133, 649, 1990.
97. Ott, S.M., Chestnut, C.H. Calcitriol treatment is not effective in postmenopausal osteoporosis. *Ann Intern Med* 110, 267, 1989.
98. Orimo, H., Shiraki, M., Hayashi, Y., et al. Effects of 1 alpha-hydroxyvitamin D_3 on lumbar bone mineral density and vertebral fracture in patients with postmenopausal osteoporosis. *Calcif Tissue Int* 54, 370, 1994.
99. Shiraki, M., Kushida, K., Yamakazi, K., et al. Effects of 2 years' treatment of osteoporosis with 1 alpha-hydroxyvitamin D_3 on bone mineral density and incidence of fracture: a placebo-controlled double-blind prospective study. *Endocr J* 43, 211, 1996.
100. Ebeling, P.R., Wark, J.D., Yeung, S., et al. Effects of calcitriol or calcium on bone mineral density, bone turnover, and fractures in men with primary osteoporosis: a two-year randomized, double blind, double placebo study. *J Clin Endocrinol Metab* 86, 4098, 2001.
101. Pfeifer, M., Begerow, B., Minne, H.W., et al. Effects of a short-term vitamin D and calcium supplementation on body sway and secondary hyperparathyroidism in elderly women. *J Bone Miner Res* 15, 1113, 2000.
102. Harwood, R.H., Sahota, O., Gaynor, K., et al. The Nottingham Neck of Femur (NONOF) Study. *Age Ageing* 33, 45, 2004.
103. Keen, C.L., Zidenberg-Cherr, S. Manganese. In *Present Knowledge in Nutrition*, 7th ed., Ziegler, E.E., Filer, L.J., Eds. ILSI Press, Washington, DC, 1996, p. 334.
104. Friedman, B.J., Freeland-Graves, J.H., Bales C.W., et al. Manganese balance and clinical observations in young men fed a manganese-deficient diet. *J Nutr* 117,133, 1987.
105. Johnson, P.E., Lykken, G.I. Manganese and calcium absorption and balance in young women fed diets with varying amounts of manganese and calcium. *J Trace Elem Exp Med* 4, 19, 1991.
106. Hurley, L.S., Keen, C.L. Manganese. In *Trace Elements in Human and Animal Nutrition*, 5th ed., Mertz, W., Ed., Academic Press, San Diego, 1989, p. 185.
107. Strause, L., Saltman, P., Smith, KT., et al. Spinal bone loss in postmenopausal women supplemented with calcium and trace minerals. *J Nutr* 124, 1060, 1994.
108. Rajagopalan, K.V. Molybdenum: an essential trace element in human nutrition. *Annu Rev Nutr* 8, 401, 1988.
109. Food and Nutrition Board, Institute of Medicine. Molybdenum. In *Dietary Reference Intakes for Vitamin A, Vitamin K, Boron, Chromium, Copper, Iodine, Iron, Manganese, Molybdenum, Nickel, Silicon, Vanadium, and Zinc*. National Academy Press, Washington, DC, 2001, p. 420.
110. Turnlund, J.R. Copper. In *Nutrition in Health and Disease*, 9th ed., Shils, M., Olson, J.A., Shike, M., et al., Eds. Williams & Wilkins, Baltimore, 1999, p. 241.
111. Uauy, R., Olivares, M., Gonzalez, M. Essentiality of copper in humans. *Am J Clin Nutr* 67, 952S, 1998.
112. Kelley, D.S., Daudu, P.A., Taylor, P.C., et al. Effects of low-copper diets on human immune response. *Am J Clin Nutr* 62, 412, 1995.
113. Conlan, D., Korula, R., Tallentire, D. Serum copper levels in elderly patients with femoral-neck fractures. *Age Ageing*, 19, 212, 1990.
114. Eaton-Evans, J., Mellwrath, E.M., Jackson, W.E., et al. Copper supplementation and the maintenance of bone mineral density in middle-aged women. *J Trace Elem Exp Med* 9, 87, 1996.

115. Baker, A., Harvey, L., Majask-Newman, G., et al. Effect of dietary copper intakes on biochemical markers of bone metabolism in healthy adult males. *Eur J Clin Nutr* 53, 408, 1999.
116. Eaton-Evans, J., McIlrath, E.M., Jackson, W.E., et al. Copper supplementation and the maintenance of bone mineral density in middle-aged women. *J Trace Elem Exp Med* 9, 87, 1996.
117. Lips, P. Vitamin D deficiency and secondary hyperparathyroidism in the elderly: consequences for bone loss and fractures and therapeutic implications. *Endocr Rev* 22, 477, 2001.
118. Feskanich, D., Willett, W.C., Colditz, G.A. Calcium, vitamin D, milk consumption, and hip fractures: a prospective study among postmenopausal women. *Am J Clin Nutr* 77, 504, 2003.
119. Dawson-Hughes, B., Harris, S.S., Krall, E.A., et al. Rates of bone loss in postmenopausal women randomly assigned to one of two dosages of vitamin D. *Am J Clin Nutr* 61, 1140, 1995.
120. Dawson-Hughes, B., Harris, S.S., Krall, E.A., et al. Effect of withdrawal of calcium and vitamin D supplements on bone mass in elderly men and women. *Am J Clin Nutr* 72, 745, 2000.
121. Ooms, M.E., Roos, J.C., Bezemer, P.D., van der Vijgh, W.J., et al. Prevention of bone loss by vitamin D supplementation in elderly women: a randomized double-blind trial. *J Clin Endocrinol Metab* 80, 1052, 1995.
122. Chapuy, M.C., Arlot, M.E., Delmas, P.D., et al. Effect of calcium and cholecalciferol treatment for three years on hip fractures in elderly women. *BMJ* 308, 1081, 1994.
123. Trivedi, D.P., Doll, R., Khaw, K.T. Effect of four monthly oral vitamin D3 (cholecalciferol) supplementation on fractures and mortality in men and women living in the community: randomised double blind controlled trial. *BMJ* 326, 469, 2003.
124. Lips, P., Graafmans, W.C., Ooms, M.E., et al. Vitamin D supplementation and fracture incidence in elderly persons. A randomized, placebo-controlled clinical trial. *Ann Intern Med* 124, 400, 1996.
125. Rude, R.K. Magnesium deficiency: a cause of heterogeneous disease in humans. *J Bone Miner Res* 13, 749, 1998.
126. Food and Nutrition Board, Institute of Medicine. Magnesium. In *Dietary Reference Intakes: Calcium, Phosphorus, Magnesium, Vitamin D, and Fluoride*. National Academy Press, Washington, DC, 1997, p. 190.
127. Alaimo, K., McDowell, M.A., Briefel, R.R., et al. *Dietary Intake of Vitamins, Minerals, and Fiber of Persons Ages 2 Months and Over in the United States: Third National Health and Nutrition Examination Survey, Phase I, 1988–91*, Advance data from Vital and Health Statistics 258. U.S. Department of Health and Human Services, National Center for Health Statistics, Hyattsville, MD, 1994.
128. Ryder, K.M., Shorr, R.I., Bush, A.J., et al. Magnesium intake from food and supplements is associated with bone mineral density in healthy older white subjects. *J Am Geriatr Soc* 53, 1875, 2005.
129. Shearer, M.J. Vitamin K. *Lancet* 345, 229, 1995.
130. Booth, S.L., Suttie, J.W. Dietary intake and adequacy of vitamin K. *J Nutr* 128, 785, 1998.
131. Furie, B., Bouchard, B.A., Furie, B.C. Vitamin K-dependent biosynthesis of gamma-carboxyglutamic acid. *Blood* 93, 1798, 1999.
132. Suttie, J.W. Vitamin K. In *Present Knowledge in Nutrition*, 7th ed., Ziegler, E.E., Filer, L.J., Eds. ILSI Press, Washington, DC, 1996, p. 137.

133. Shearer, M.J. The roles of vitamins D and K in bone health and osteoporosis prevention. *Proc Nutr Soc* 56, 915, 1997.
134. Booth, S.L. Skeletal functions of vitamin K-dependent proteins: not just for clotting anymore. *Nutr Rev* 55, 282, 1997.
135. Feskanich, D., Weber, P., Willett, W.C., et al. Vitamin K intake and hip fractures in women: a prospective study. *Am J Clin Nutr* 69, 74, 1999.
136. Booth, S.L., Tucker, K.L., Chen, H., et al. Dietary vitamin K intakes are associated with hip fracture but not with bone mineral density in elderly men and women. *Am J Clin Nutr* 71, 1201, 2000.
137. Booth, S.L., Mayer, J. Warfarin use and fracture risk. *Nutr Rev* 58, 20, 2000.
138. Booth, S.L., Suttie, J.W. Dietary intake and adequacy of vitamin K. *J Nutr.* 128, 785, 1998.
139. Szulc, P., Chapuy, M.C., Meunier, P.J., et al. Serum undercarboxylated osteocalcin is a marker of the risk of hip fracture in elderly women. *J Clin Invest* 91, 1769, 1993.
140. Vergnaud, P., Garnero, P., Meunier, P.J., et al. Undercarboxylated osteocalcin measured with a specific immunoassay predicts hip fracture in elderly women: the EPIDOS Study. *J Clin Endocrinol Metab* 182, 719, 1997.
141. Shearer, M.J. The roles of vitamins D and K in bone health and osteoporosis prevention. *Proc Nutr Soc* 56, 915, 1997.
142. Caraballo, P.J., Gabriel, S.E., Castro, M.R., et al. Changes in bone density after exposure to oral anticoagulants: a meta-analysis. *Osteoporos Int* 9, 441, 1999.
143. Cousins, R.J. Metal elements and gene expression. *Ann Rev Nutr* 14, 449, 1994.
144. Prasad, A.S., Mantzoros, C.S., Beck, F.W., et al. Zinc status and serum testosterone levels of healthy adults. *Nutrition* 12, 344, 1996.
145. Wada, L., King, J.C. Effect of low zinc intakes on basal metabolic rate, thyroid hormones and protein utilization in adult men. *J Nutr* 116, 1045, 1986.
146. Ninh, N.X., Thissen, J.P., Collette, L., et al. Zinc supplementation increases growth and circulating insulin-like growth factor I (IGF-I) in growth-retarded Vietnamese children. *Am J Clin Nutr* 63, 514, 1996.
147. Yamaguchi, M. Role of zinc in bone formation and bone resorption. *J Trace Elem Exp Med* 11, 119, 1998.
148. Freudenheim, J.L., Johnson, N.E., Smith, E.L. Relationships between usual nutrient intake and bone mineral content of women 35–65 years of age: longitudinal and cross-sectional analysis. *Am J Clin Nutr* 44, 863, 1986.
149. Angus, R.M., Sambrook, P.N., Pocock, N.A., Eisman, J.A. Dietary intake and bone mineral density. *Bone Miner* 4, 265, 1988.
150. Promislow, J.H.E., Goodman-Gruen, D., Slymen, D.J., et al. Protein consumption and bone mineral density in the elderly. The Rancho Bernardo Study. *Am J Epidemiol* 155, 636, 2002.

34 Multicultural Issues

Nina Tumosa, Ph.D.

CONTENTS

> Tomatoes and oregano make it Italian; wine and tarragon make it French. Sour cream makes it Russian; lemon and cinnamon make it Greek. Soy sauce makes it Chinese; garlic makes it good.
>
> **—Alice May Brock**

34.1 INTRODUCTION

The U.S. prides itself as the "melting pot of the world." This is reflected in many ways, from our fashions to our transportation choices to our food. Fast food, ranging from Southern fried anything to salad bars to stir-fried Chinese dishes, is readily available in most towns anywhere in this country with more than 10,000 residents. However, we forget how recent this phenomenon is and how much of it has been driven by the youth of the nation. A visit to the local fast food restaurant may find several elderly men drinking coffee and discussing world events, but few of them are eating food that is not some variation of steak and eggs with a side of fried potato covered with ketchup. These staples got them through years of hard work and are seldom replaced by soft drinks, flavored lattes, and rice. Although some have certainly embraced hamburgers as a more chewable substitute for steak, and some have even come to appreciate the piquante qualities of fresh salsa, most continue to enjoy good old-fashioned home cooking (even if it is done in a commercial kitchen rather than at home). Familiar food is enticing and comforting. This chapter summarizes research that shows health care providers why they should consider ethnic food preferences in diets of elderly people for whom they are making nutrition choices.

34.2 CULTURAL INFLUENCES IN FOOD PREFERENCES

Much research has shown that ethnicity plays a role in food preferences of both young[1] and old[2] humans. Gender also plays a role in food preferences for many ethnic groups.[3–6] Such results have been complemented by more cross-cultural research[7–9] on the Food Habits in Later Life (FHILL) study, in which cohorts of participants 70 years of age and older from five long-lived cultures (Swedes in Sweden, Greeks in Greece and Australia, Anglo-Celts in Australia, and Japanese in Japan) were asked about health, lifestyle, and diet. Participants were followed for 7 years. This study showed that diet is the most positive predictor of survival in these cohorts, and smoking was the most important negative predictor of survival. Nutritional variables such as a high intake and variety of plant foods (especially vegetables, legumes, and fruit) and seafood and a low intake of meat contributed to longevity across cultures.[9] The most easily recognized diet of this type is the Mediterranean diet,[10] which was the dietary pattern of people living in olive-growing areas of the Mediterranean region in the mid-20th century. Indeed, there is evidence that the overall dietary pattern of the Mediterranean diet, rather than specific food items, is what is responsible for overall survival of people over the age of 70 who are living in the Mediterranean region.[11] Another diet associated with longevity was first recognized in a study of the Okinawan food culture of the Ryukyu Island of Japan.[12] Okinawans have one of the longest life expectancies and lowest disability rates in the world. Their diet consists of large amounts of Satsamu sweet potato, plant foods such as seaweed and soy, herbaceous plants, fish and pork, and green tea and kohencha tea. Cultural food-centered festivals are thought to maintain strong ties between food and health.[12] Food and health are also strongly correlated in other cultures. Chinese philosophy holds that there must be a balance of hot and cold foods.[13] Elderly Vietnamese consume rice for both lunch and supper and 94% do not snack.[14] African Americans in Philadelphia reported specific cultural attitudes about where and with whom food is eaten.[15] African Americans in Florida reported a general perception that "eating healthfully" meant turning their back on their culture in an effort to conform.[16] Ojibway-Cree Indians in northern Ontario perceived Indian foods as healthy and white man's food as unhealthy.[17]

Culture, however, is not static. Therefore, neither is food culture static. This concept is particularly important now that the world is experiencing increased globalization, where both acculturation and ethnic mixing are becoming more common cultural phenomena.

34.2.1 First-Generation Patterns

A study of Hispanics, 60 years of age and older, in Massachusetts showed that Hispanic elders consumed significantly less saturated fats and simple sugars and more complex carbohydrates than did non-Hispanic whites. However, the more acculturated the Hispanic elders became, the fewer ethnic foods and the more foods related to a non-Hispanic-white diet they consumed.[18] Similar changes in food consumption occurred in Chinese Americans living in Pennsylvania.[19] After immigration, dietary variety increased, with consumption frequency of American food increasing and consumption frequency of traditional Chinese foods decreasing. The longer they remained in the U.S., the greater their consumption of vegetables, fats/sweets, and beverages. Similar dietary changes were observed in a study comparing food habits of ethnic Japanese living in Hiroshima with those of ethnic Japanese living in the Hawaiian Islands and in Los Angeles.[20] The Japanese Americans had increased the amount of animal fat, simple carbohydrates, and total energy intake and had decreased the complex carbohydrates in their diet,[20] compared to the Japanese. A comparison of elderly Greek immigrants in Australia with Greeks in Greece showed similar dietary changes: greater consumption of meat, legumes, protein, margarine, polyunsaturated fats, and beer and lower consumption of cereals, carbohydrates, wine, and olive oil, with corresponding increases in deteriorating health (as defined by self-reported health conditions and prescribed medications).[21] Immigrant Asian Indian families in Newfoundland self-reported that they felt that their changing eating patterns, due either to their inability to find traditional Indian foods or to the fact that they had to change methods of food preparation, carried potential health risks.[22] One study has shown that Asian American elderly in Chicago consume too little dietary calcium,[23] which puts them at risk for falls and fractures. This study also reports that many Korean elderly consume too little protein and vitamins A and C,[23] leaving them vulnerable to fatigue, vision problems, and weight loss. Finally, most Asian Americans are underweight,[23] implying that caloric intake should be a priority for this group.

34.2.2 Health Consequences of Immigration Are Not All Bad

Although immigration often causes decreased nutrition-related health of the immigrants, oftentimes the host citizenry experiences increased nutrition-related health. Australia is a prime example. Australian eating patterns have become increasingly diverse following 300 years of immigration from Europe, China, Afghanistan, Vietnam, and Southeastern Asia. Food security has increased, as has food diversity, and fresh foods have become more prevalent.[24] In Melbourne, the adoption of the Mediterranean diet for 3 years by both elderly Anglo-Celts and Greek Australians increased their survival.[25] Thus, there appears to be a compelling benefit to elderly people who adopt healthier diets than they have been accustomed to.

34.3 NOT ALL ETHNIC DIETS ARE PERFECT

Despite the plethora of research studies that have shown that specific ethnic diets improve longevity, it is also true that there is room for improvement in many ethnic diets. Several examples exist in the literature of how specific diets are correlated with increased morbidity. The amounts of sodium, potassium, and calcium ingested by South African ethnic groups differ. White South Africans have higher sodium and calcium intakes than their black and mixed-ancestry counterparts. All studied groups had potassium intakes below the recommended dietary level. These dietary differences were correlated with differences in blood pressure.[26] Risk of colon cancer in the U.S. is correlated with high refined carbohydrate and red meat consumption in Caucasians, and with frequent intake of dairy food in African Americans.[27] The risk can be mitigated somewhat in both populations with increased consumption of fruits and vegetables (particularly dark green vegetables). The role that salt plays in traditional foods in southern rural communities of African Americans, Native Americans, and Caucasians is often at odds with biomedical links to chronic disease.[28] None of the survey participants met minimum U.S. Department of Agriculture (USDA) recommendations for meats, fruits, and vegetables, and all three groups overconsumed fats, oils, sweets, and snacks.[29] A multicenter case-controlled study of African American, Caucasian, Japanese, and Chinese men in Canada and the U.S. has uncovered a link between prostate cancer and the lack of legumes and yellow-orange and cruciferous vegetables in the diet in all ethnic groups.[30]

Studies such as the ones described above have all contributed to the publication of the position paper of the American Dietetic Association that states that older Americans should have access to comprehensive food and nutrition services that are appropriate and culturally sensitive,[31] regardless of whether they live at home or in a congregate living setting. The position paper goes on to indicate that dietetics professionals can take the lead in researching and developing appropriate networks to deliver food and nutrition services across the spectrum of aging. In response to this position paper, the remainder of this chapter will discuss some of the challenges and opportunities that are faced by health care providers in accomplishing this laudable goal.

34.4 BARRIERS AND PROPOSED SOLUTIONS TO MAINTAINING NUTRITIONAL HEALTH

Good nutrition is necessary to maintain quality of life. Elderly nutrition programs (ENPs) were mandated in 1972 through Title III of the Older Americans Act. These ENPs include both pre-prepared meals and nutrition education. Some ENPs are provided to people living at home, and others are provided to elders in congregate living settings. The need for ENPs has been so great nationwide that state, local, and volunteer agencies have joined the federally financed programs in addressing the demand.

Delivery of nutritious meals is just the first step in improving the nutritional health of elderly persons. The success of these programs is also affected by how well elderly recipients perceive and utilize these meals. Several studies have addressed the various components of a successful nutrition education program, and some have addressed the role that ethnicity plays in those components.

The adoption of healthy eating habits has many influences, including the types of choices elderly persons make about their lives. European elders in Dublin identified three reasons to practice healthy eating: (1) to stay healthy, (2) to prevent disease, and (3) to promote quality of life. They also identified three barriers that prevented them from doing so: (1) self-control, (2) resistance to change, and (3) cost.[32] Knowing what needs to be done is one thing, but deciding to act, regardless of the barriers, is quite another.

Getting people to adopt healthy eating practices takes time. Perkins-Porras et al.[33] showed that people go through stages of precontemplation, contemplation, and adoption. Individuals most likely to adopt more fruits and vegetables in their diets are younger, more educated, and more likely to be female than those who are not about to change eating habits. ENPs may provide fruits and vegetables, but meal recipients may not be prepared to eat them.

Eating patterns (number and timing of meals) should also be considered when developing nutritional programs. Traditional Greek eating patterns (greater number of meals/snacks daily, two or more cooked meals daily, main meal consumed at lunchtime, consumption of alcohol with meal) were self-reported to be positively correlated with lack of obesity.[34] Such constraints may not be practical in ENPs that provide one or two meals daily, especially for elders who live in the community, but they should be considered in congregate care settings.

Some barriers to participation by ethnic populations in ENPs are due to perceptions and attitudes on the part of the people who are eligible for the service. These barriers include (1) lack of knowledge about the availability of the meal programs or misunderstanding of the eligibility rules, (2) unfamiliarity with and dislike of foods served by the ENPs, and (3) a sense of stigma attached to receiving the meals.[35] Such concerns must be addressed in education and recruitment programs associated with ENPs.

Another special aspect of ethnic meals involves the delivery of religiously appropriate meals. For example, Muslims and Mormans do not eat food prepared with alcohol. Jews require kosher food and Muslims require halal meals. The availability of these special foods is often prevented by lack of provider knowledge of special dietary laws, lack of assistance in supporting the higher cost of these meals, and difficulty in keeping up with growing demand.[36] Again, knowledge about these barriers allows the health care provider to be better prepared to address these barriers.

Delivery of nutrition education has special barriers in ethnic populations for whom English is not the primary language or for whom literacy level is low. These literacy challenges suggest that menus for healthy meals must be presented visually in a manner that is informative, engaging, appetizing, and ethnically appropriate.[37] Life is replete with examples of miscommunications about packaging. For example, care should be taken if pictures of animals are included in explanatory literature. While a picture of a goat or a cow may elucidate the origins of the entrée, mood-setting pictures of common household pets may cause misunderstanding about what is about to be eaten.

34.5 EFFECTIVENESS OF ELDERLY NUTRITION PROGRAMS (ENPS)

Because poor nutrition is associated with longer hospital stays, early entry into nursing homes, compromised immune systems, and reduced quality of life, it is important to provide nutritious meals and nutrition education through the ENPs to elders at high risk for undernutrition. Huge demands for ENPs and limited funds for such meals mandate careful allocation of resources. Therefore, it is important for programs to determine who their most vulnerable potential recipients are. People at highest nutritional risk in northern Florida are most often dwelling in urban areas, female, African American, self-reported to be in poor health, and have limited access to medical care.[38] Those at greatest risk for poor nutrition in the Texas Lower Rio Grande Valley appear to be unmarried, rural, homebound Mexican Americans.[39] The more vulnerable DeKalb County, Georgia, residents have been identified as African American women,[40] people who live alone,[41] and people who voice specific food preferences.[42] Thus, people living in the community have multiple factors that determine their degree of vulnerability to nutritional risk. Those factors differ between communities and must be reassessed periodically to determine each factor's continued applicability. Such reassessments ensure that limited resources are going to the areas of greatest need.

For nursing home residents, the maintenance of adequate nutritional intake is a special challenge. Illness, disability, and declining quality of life have already led to nursing home placement. To varying degrees, these folks require assistance with eating, from food selection to meal preparation to the actual act of eating. Dietary supplements, multivitamins, nutraceuticals, and special diets are the focus of other presentations in this book and will not be discussed here. However, one final topic of discussion for this chapter, in relation to ethnic foods, remains: the role that the ultimate ethnic food, comfort food, plays in nutritional risk.

Mealtime is an intensely social event. Shared dining experiences, most particularly those with family and friends, provide all of us with powerful memories. Whether the memories are of good food, special recipes, celebrations, special holidays, Sunday dinners, or even favorite cooking disasters, those stories add richness and pleasure to eating.[43] Comfort foods play a special role in those memories. These are foods that evoke strong memories that provide comfort and a feeling of well-being when ingested. The particular food is individualistic and often related to childhood memories of security and happiness. The identity of comfort foods differs across age, gender, and culture. In a study of 1416 individuals in North America, men were found to prefer warm, hearty comfort foods, such as steak, casserole, and soup, and reported strong positive feelings when eating these foods; women preferred foods such as chocolate and ice cream and often reported feelings of guilt when eating them; and people younger than age 55 preferred snack-related comfort foods.[44] These findings were corroborated with a different study, a Web-based survey of 275 Canadians.[45] In this study, men self-reported that they consumed comfort food when feeling positive and women reported that they consumed them because they were feeling negative. Additionally, those who were of French cultural background reported eating comfort foods when they were feeling positive, and those of English cultural background reported intense negative emotions prior to consuming comfort foods. Recent research[46] indicates that the physiological basis of eating comfort foods is stress that results in elevated glucocorticoids (GCs). The GCs, in turn, stimulate the drive to ingest comfort foods. The resulting deposition of these increased energy stores as abdominal fat appears to reduce the influence of chronic stress. While many weight-conscious individuals may not welcome this scientific explanation, it is good news for people who are planning menus for nursing home residents. The offering of comfort foods and tasty, high-calorie beverages in a social setting tends to stimulate caloric intake in people who are underweight and at risk of undernutrition.[47]

34.6 SUMMARY

Good food is an essential key to quality of life. Even as disease and disability take their toll, quality of life can be sustained if food is enjoyed and nutritional risk is minimized. The conscientious health care provider must use every arrow in the armamentarium to ensure that adequate quantity and quality of food is ingested. This provider is best aided by a more complete understanding of the psychology, as well as the physiology, of eating. Tantamount to the psychology of eating is an understanding of the role that ethnicity plays in food, its choice, its presentation, its preparation, and its ingestion. This chapter has summarized many of the studies that have contributed to that understanding. Ethnic food choices can be either good or bad for health. Adoption of the good components to maintain health is appropriate both for ethnic elders who prefer that food and for others who embrace variety in their eating choices. Limited but appropriate use of the bad components to stimulate appetite and interest in food is warranted for those ethnic elders who have lost interest in food and perhaps would benefit from increased socialization and feeling increased security, which are often associated with familiar foods. Finally, the judicious use of comfort foods, those foods that evoke feelings of security but are often of poor nutritional value, is also warranted in cases of elders who have lost interest in eating.

REFERENCES

1. Logue, A.W. and Smith, M.E., Predictors of food preferences in adult humans, *Appetite*, 7, 109, 1986.
2. Todhunter, E.N., Life style and nutrient intake in the elderly, *Curr. Concepts Nutr.*, 4, 119, 1976.
3. Bermundez, O.I. et al., Hispanic and non-Hispanic white elders from Massachusetts have different patterns of carotenoid intake and plasma concentrations, *J. Nutr.*, 135, 1496, 2005.
4. Larrieu, S. et al., Sociodemographic differences in dietary habits in a population-based sample of elderly subjects: the 3C study. *J. Nutr. Health Aging*, 8, 497, 2004.
5. Lin, W. and Lee, Y.W., Nutrition knowledge, attitudes, and dietary restriction behavior of Taiwanese elderly, *Asia Pac. J. Clin. Nutr.*, 14, 221, 2005.
6. Pareo-Tubbeh, S.L. et al., Comparison of energy and nutrient sources of elderly Hispanics and non-Hispanic whites in New Mexico, *J. Am. Diet. Assoc.*, 99, 572, 1999.
7. Darmadi-Blackberry, I. et al., Legumes: the most important dietary predictor of survival in older people of different ethnicities, *Asia Pac. J. Clin. Nutr.*, 13, 217, 2004.
8. Wahlqvist, M.L. et al., Does diet matter for survival in long-lived cultures? *Asia Pac. J. Clin. Nutr.*, 14, 2, 2005.
9. Wahlqvist, M.L., Kouris-Blazos, A., and Has-Hage, B.H., Aging, food, culture and health, *Southeast Asian J. Trop. Med. Public Health*, 28 (Suppl. 2), 100, 1997.
10. Trichopoulou, A., Mediterranean diet: the past and the present, *Nutr. Metab. Cardiovasc. Dis.*, 11 (Suppl.), 1, 2001.
11. Trichopoulou, A., et al., Diet and overall survival in elderly people, *Br. Med. J.*, 311, 1457, 1995.

12. Sho, H., History and characteristics of Okinawan longevity food, *Asia Pac. J. Clin. Nutr.*, 10, 159, 2001.
13. Chang, B., Some dietary beliefs in Chinese folk culture, *J. Am. Diet. Assoc.*, 65, 436, 1974.
14. Tong, A., Eating habits of elderly Vietnamese in the United States, *J. Nutr. Elder.*, 10, 35, 1991.
15. Airhihenbuwa, C.O. et al., Cultural aspects of African American eating patterns, *Ethn. Health*, 1, 245, 1996.
16. James, D.C., Factors influencing food choices, dietary intake, and nutrition-related attitudes among African Americans: application of a culturally sensitive model, *Ethn. Health*, 9, 349, 2004.
17. Gittelsohn, J. et al., Use of ethnographic methods for applied research on diabetes among the Ojibway-Cree in northern Ontario, *Health Educ. Q.*, 23, 365, 1996.
18. Bermudez, O.I., Falcon, L.M., and Tucher, K.L., Intake and food sources of macronutrients among older Hispanic adults: association with ethnicity, acculturation, and length of residence in the United States, *J. Am. Diet. Assoc.*, 11, 665, 2000.
19. Lv, N. and Cason, K.L., Dietary pattern change and acculturation of Chinese Americans in Pennsylvania, *J. Am. Diet. Assoc.*, 104, 771, 2004.
20. Egusa, G. et al., Westernized food habits and concentrations of serum lipids in the Japanese, *Atherosclerosis*, 100, 249, 1993.
21. Kouris-Blasos, A. et al., Health and nutritional status of elderly Greek migrants to Melbourne, Australia, *Age Ageing*, 25, 177, 1996.
22. Varghese, S. and Moore-Orr, R., Dietary acculturation and health-related issues of Indian immigrant families in Newfoundland, *Can. J. Diet. Pract. Res.*, 63, 72, 2002.
23. Kim, K.K. et al., Nutritional status of Chinese-, Korean-, and Japanese-American elderly, *J. Am. Diet. Assoc.*, 93, 1416, 1993.
24. Wahlqvist, M.L., Asian migration to Australia: food and health consequences, *Asia Pac. J. Clin. Nutr.*, 11 (Suppl. 3), S562, 2004.
25. Kouris-Blasos, A. et al., Are the advantages of the Mediterranean diet transferable to other populations? A cohort study in Melbourne, Australia, *Br. J. Nutr.*, 82, 57, 1999.
26. Charlton, K.E. et al., Diet and blood pressure in South Africa: intake of foods containing sodium, potassium, calcium, and magnesium in three ethnic groups, *Nutrition*, 21, 39, 2005.
27. Satia-Abouta, J. et al., Food groups and colon cancer risk in African-Americans and Caucasians, *Int. J. Cancer*, 109, 728, 2004.
28. Smith, S.L. et al., Aging and eating in rural, southern United States: beliefs about salt and its effect on health, *Soc. Sci. Med.*, 62, 189, 2006.
29. Vitolins, M.Z. et al., Quality of diets consumed by older rural adults, *J. Rural Health*, 18, 49, 2002.
30. Kolonel, L.N. et al., Vegetables, fruits, legumes and prostate cancer: a multiethnic case-control study, *Cancer Epidemiol. Biomarkers Prev.*, 9, 795, 2000.
31. Kuezmarski, M.F., Weddle, D.O., and American Dietetic Association, Position paper of the American Dietetic Association: nutrition across the spectrum of aging, *J. Am. Diet. Assoc.*, 105, 616, 2005.
32. de Almeida, M.D. et al., Healthy eating in European elderly: concepts, barriers and benefits, *J. Nutr. Health Aging*, 5, 217, 2001.
33. Perkins-Porras, L. et al., Does the effect of behavioral counseling on fruit and vegetable intake vary with stage of readiness to change? *Prev. Med.*, 40, 314, 2005.
34. Wahlqvist, M.L., Kouris-Blazos, A., and Wattanapenpaiboon, N., The significance of eating patterns: an elderly Greek case study, *Appetite*, 32, 23, 1999.

35. Choi, N.G. and Smith, J., Reaching out to racial/ethnic minority older persons for elderly nutrition programs, *J. Nutr. Elder.*, 24, 89, 2004.
36. Rosenzweig, L.Y., Kosher meal services in the community: need, availability, and limitation, *J. Nutr. Elder.*, 24, 73, 2005.
37. Macario, E., Factors influencing nutrition education for patients with low literacy skills, *J. Am. Diet. Assoc.*, 98, 559, 1998.
38. Weatherspoon, L.J., Worthen, H.D., and Handu, D., Nutrition risk and associated factors in congregate meal participants in northern Florida: role of elder care services (ECS), *J. Nutr. Elder.*, 24, 27, 2004.
39. Sharkey, J.R., Variation in nutritional risk among Mexican American and non-Mexican American homebound elders who receive home-delivered meals, *J. Nutr. Elder.*, 23, 1, 2004.
40. Prothro, J.W. and Rosenbloom, C.A., Description of a mixed ethnic elderly population. I. Demography, nutrient/energy intakes, and income status, *J. Gerontol. A Biol. Sci. Med. Sci.*, 54, M315, 1999.
41. Prothro, J.W. and Rosenbloom, C.A., Description of a mixed ethnic elderly population. II. Food group behavior and related nonfood characteristics, *J. Gerontol. A Biol. Sci. Med. Sci.*, 54, M325, 1999.
42. Prothro, J.W. and Rosenbloom, C.A., Description of a mixed ethnic elderly population. III. Special diets, food preferences, and medicinal intakes, *J. Gerontol. A Biol. Sci. Med. Sci.*, 54, M329, 1999.
43. Evans, B.C., Crogan, N.L., and Shultz, J.A., The meaning of mealtimes: connection to the social world of the nursing home, *J. Gerontol. Nurs.*, 31, 11, 2005.
44. Wansink, B., Cheney, M.M., and Chan, N., Exploring comfort food preferences across age and gender, *Physiol. Behavior.*, 79, 739, 2003.
45. Dube, L., LeBel, J.L., and Lu, J., Affect asymmetry and comfort food consumption, *Physiol. Behav.*, 86, 559, 2005.
46. Dallman, M.F., Pecoraro, N.C., and le Fleur, S.E., Chronic stress and comfort foods: self-medication and abdominal obesity, *Brain Behav. Immun.*, 19, 275, 2005.
47. Wood, P. and Vogen, B.D., Feeding the anorectic client: comfort food and happy hour, *Geriatr. Nurs.*, 19, 192, 1998.

35 Choice and Nutritionals: Ethical Issues

Rafi Kevorkian, M.D.

CONTENTS

Enteral and parenteral nutrition may provide sustenance to patients unable to eat or absorb food. Patients require this form of nutrition for a multitude of reasons that has led to a decline in their health, leading to death. Malnutrition is known to increase infection risk, lead to poor wound healing, prolong hospital stays, lead to multiorgan dysfunction, increase postoperative complications, and increase mortality. As in all aspects of medical decision making, one has to ask whether the benefit of a treatment outweighs its risks. The aim of providing hydration and nutrition is the perceived benefit. Yet the decision to start enteral nutrition and whether it will change mortality or improve quality of life is complex and is intertwined with much social, religious, and psychological conflict. Misperceptions remain among physicians, patients, and family members in regard to clinical tolerance to poor intake of nutrition and hydration in terminally ill patients, the risks and benefits of long-term tube feeding, and the ethical issues related to these treatments. The act of eating is of symbolic importance for patients and families. Family members associate food with health, and helping someone eat can be an important nurturing act. Thus, losing the ability to eat is felt to lead to starvation.[1] The legal system over the last several decades has developed a framework of laws to help solve some of the nutritional choices that we have. This chapter will review and analyze these issues to aid in decision making for enteral nutrition.

35.1 CONSIDERATIONS FOR ARTIFICIAL NUTRITION

Consideration for nutritional support must always take into account what the patient desires and, to a lesser degree, the family's wishes, especially if the patient is cognitively impaired (delirium, dementia) or is incapacitated (persistent vegetative state) to make a decision on the benefits or risk of nutritional support. Advance directives, if available, must be respected. There are considerations that one must consider before starting nutritional support (Table 35.1). A multitude of patients with chronic illnesses commonly receive enteral feeds. In one study by Johnson et al.,[2] 8.2% of 190,769 patients with a cancer diagnosis were receiving enteral feeding. In a group of demented patients (n = 1386), 9.7% were receiving enteral feeding.[3] Starting enteral nutrition requires informed consent. The process must be explained to the patient and its risks and benefits discussed.

The prognosis and outcome of the patient's illness and the effect of nutritional support on prognosis should also be discussed. Patient and surrogates should understand that the potential benefit of enteral nutrition or lack of benefit will require on their part a burden of undergoing a procedure as well as the risks from that procedure. The psychological and religious burden may also be discussed. The potential benefits discussed revolve around whether enteral feeding improves survival, improves quality of life, provides comfort, and corrects metabolic abnormalities that may have an impact on outcome of medical care. This beneficence is required prior to the patient giving consent. A physician is free to propose therapy, but not necessarily use such therapy. A physician who cannot explain or will not explain the unbiased risks and benefits should remove himself and find an alternate provider to obtain consent. Since many patients rely on their physician for support in decision making, the physician is also free to render an opinion or advise the patient. Self-determination must be respected, and intrusion by family or physician must be avoided. If the value of nutritional support is unclear or undefined, a limited trial may be considered and goals of care and outcome evaluated. Nutritional support is not mandatory when it is burdensome or of no proven medical value.[4] Issues of perceived improvement in quality of life and improvement in outcome must regard the underlying disease process, because unrealistic or impractical goals may cause confusion among patients and their families. There are noted appropriate indications for a percutaneous endoscopic gastrostomy (PEG) (Table 35.2).

TABLE 35.1
Nutritional Support Considerations

a) Potential benefit of therapy
b) Potential risk of therapy
c) Patient's life expectancy
d) Patient's quality of life
e) Patient's wishes for feeding tubes
f) Family's wishes if patient's wishes are unknown or unobtainable
g) Patient's prognosis

TABLE 35.2
Appropriate Indications for PEG

a) Dysphagia secondary to reversible disease
b) Incurable disease with survival potential
c) Loss of the ability to eat
d) Primary neurological disorders with likelihood of prolonged survival and improved quality of life
e) Severe upper gastrointestinal motility disorders (for decompression)
f) Growth failure in children

Several strategies exist than can be used to assess the appropriate use of feeding tubes. The feeding tube can be used as the sole source of nutrition. If oral intake is insufficient to meet nutritional requirements, it can be used in a transitory or permanent way, and as an adjuvant to parenteral nutrition if it fails to meet the nutritional needs of the patient. The percutaneous gastrostomy (PEG) tube is the most common, and it is the preferred route when enteral feeding is expected to last for more than 4 weeks, as recommended by the American Gastroenterological Association.[5] Nasogastric tube feeding carries a higher risk of self-extubation, aspiration, and patient discomfort. Gastrostomy tubes can be inserted endoscopically, surgically, or radiologically. Tube feeding is physiologically more advantageous, has fewer complications, and is less costly than parenteral nutrition.[6] Physicians, patients, and families perceive tube feeding as less invasive. Gastric rather than jejunal feeding should be used when possible. An infusion pump is not required for gastric feeding. Jejunal feeding should be considered for patients with tube feeding aspiration, clinically important gastrointestinal motility disorders, or insufficient stomach from previous resection; children gastroesophageal with reflux; and those who require feeding distal to an obstruction. Jejunal feeding requires a continuous infusion pump, and medication administration may be compromised due to certain medications being activated in the stomach or absorbed more proximally. Complications such as bleeding, infection, and peritonitis have been reported to be about 1 to 3% of patients receiving a PEG. The Veterans Administration PEG study showed serious complications to be at 3.9% at 30 days.[7] Although aspiration risk was low initially, long-term follow-up over 11 months showed that the rate of complication, including aspiration pneumonia, was 15%.[7] PEG tubes are placed successfully 98% of the time.[8] Tube feeding can be initiated as early as 4 hours after placement.

35.2 PREVALENCE OF TUBE FEEDING

PEG tube placement was introduced in 1980 and has become the method of choice for providing long-term nutrition.[9] Approximately 61,000 PEG tubes were placed in 1988, and 121,000 were placed in 1995.[10] These numbers reflect PEG tubes placed in hospitalized patients and do not include tubes placed in outpatients or in HMO–Medicare beneficiaries. The above estimates include tubes placed by all methods. Nationwide, 18% of nursing home residents who were cognitively impaired had a feeding tube in 1999, based on the National Repository of the Minimum Data

Set among 385,741 nursing home residents.[11] Resident characteristics associated with greater likelihood of feeding tube use included younger age, nonwhite race, male sex, divorced marital status, lack of an advance directive, recent decline in functional status, and no diagnosis of Alzheimer's disease. Residents who lived in facilities that were for profit, were located in an urban area, had more than 100 beds, and lacked a special dementia care unit had a higher chance of having a feeding tube.[12] The frequency of usage of enteral tube feeding varies from state to state but is not due to variability in state laws.[13] Overall, 18.1% of patients with severe dementia received a feeding tube after initial evaluation; yet, there was significant state-to-state variation, from as low as 3.8% of dementia patients in Nebraska receiving enteral feeds to as high as 41.8% of patients in the District of Columbia.[14] A European multicenter survey[15] showed differences among European centers in their usage of home enteral feeding. It showed that enteral feeding is predominantly used in patients with dysphagia from neurological disorders or cancer. The rate of usage in Europe is two to three times lower than in the U.S.[15] Differences exist between countries in regard to the age and underlying disease of those offered enteral feeding.[15] In the U.K., from 1996 to 1999, only 146 patients with head and neck cancer were on enteral feeds, compared with 5037 with cerebrovascular disease.[16] In Italy, during the period of 1992 to 1999, 1900 patients who suffered from head and neck cancer and 1647 from cerebrovascular disease received enteral feeding.[17] Intercountry differences appear to be due to recognized differences in medical practice.

35.3 IS ENTERAL NUTRITION AND ENTERAL TUBE FEEDING BENEFICIAL?

Identifying persons at risk for undernutrition is important so that prognosis can be improved as well as quality of life. Without adequate nutrition, death will occur. However, quality of life has subjective and objective meanings, and its definition varies from person to person. It is difficult to assess quality of life in a person without interference from one's own bias. Many sick patients want to eat but are unable to because of anorexia, nausea, dysphagia, depression, and altered sense of smell or taste. Anorexia, which often accompanies illness, is mediated by cytokines. In the elderly, anorexia related to illness may be superimposed with what is termed the anorexia of aging. Conflict may arise when the patient's underlying medical condition is unlikely to improve. As such, a care plan without enteral feeding can be considered. The complication rate for enteral feeding is high. Several large-scale studies have demonstrated persistent complications as well as high mortality rates (Table 35.3). No prospective, controlled, randomized studies have been conducted to examine the efficacy of PEG placement due to ethical reasons.

Enteral feedings have also not shown any benefits in existing wound healing or with protection from new pressure sores.[27,28] In an observational study, prevalence of pressure ulcers was not affected by enteral feeding.[28] Stratton et al.[30] conducted a meta-analysis on the effect of oral and enteral nutrition on wounds. They found a trend toward improved wound healing, but a fair number of the studies had small numbers of patients, historical controls, and lacked statistical power. Rimon et al.[31]

TABLE 35.3
Enteral Feeding Outcomes

Reference	Number of Patients	Mortality
1) Oyoga et al.[18]	100	41% (1 month), 4% from procedure
2) Abuksis et al.[19]	Admitted from NH	39.5% (1 month)
3) Grant et al.[10]	81,105 (retrospective)	23.9% (1 month), 63% (1 year), 81.3% (3 year)
4) James et al.[20]	126 (with CVA and dysphagia)	28% (died in hospital)
5) Kaminski et al.[21]	102 (N = 37 <65 years/old, N = 65 >65years/old)	3% <65 years/old, 35% >65 years/old
6) Loser et al.[22]	210 (followed for 4 years)	34% (1 year)
7) Nicholson et al.[23]	168 (NH)	34% (2 years)
8) Cataldi-Betcher et al.[24]	70 (NH)	46% (6 months)
9) Campos et al.[25]	70 (NH)	46% (6 months)
10) Mitchell et al.[3]	1386 dementia (NH)	No difference in 2 years between tube-fed and not
11) Finucane et al.[11]	Dementia	Survival not prolonged (wounds and ADLs not improved)
12) Dennis[26]	Stroke patients	No improvement in clinical outcome

Note: NH = nursing home; ADL = activity of daily living

TABLE 35.4
Survival after PEG Using Cox Regression

	Number of Patients	Hazard Ratio	Confidence Interval	*p* Values
Male	365	1.22	1.00–1.47	<0.05
Feeding difficulty	280	1.22	1.00–1.47	<0.05
Referral from hospital	244	1.44	1.19–1.74	<0.001
Diabetes mellitus	98	1.40	1.09–1.80	<0.01
Age >80 years	365	1.39	1.15–1.68	<0.001

looked at 674 patients in a prospective study who were severely demented and noted higher mortality in males, those with feeding difficulty, those who were diabetic, those over 80 years old, and those referred from the hospital (Table 35.4). The most serious pulmonary complication of tube feedings is aspiration of gastric contents. As many as 40% of deaths associated with tube feedings result directly from aspiration pneumonia.[32,33] Callahan et al.[34] examined 150 patients who received a PEG tube. They were monitored in a community setting. The patient groups in the above study included stroke (42%), neurodegenerative disorders (35%), and cancer (13%). Mortality at 30 days was 22 and 50% at 1 year. Nutritional as well as functional and laboratory measures were followed. Although no control group was available,

TABLE 35.5
Factors Associated with High Complications after PEG

1) Age >80
2) Dementia
3) BMI <16.5
4) Recent bronchopulmonary infection
5) Albuminemia <30 g/l

no significant improvement was seen in body mass index, triceps skinfold thickness (nutritional), activities of daily living, upper and lower body functions (functional), and albumin and total cholesterol levels (laboratory). Stratton et al.[35] looked at dialysis patients in a meta-analysis in which oral supplements or enteral nutrition was given. There was an improvement in albumin and an increase in caloric intake, but no improvement in outcome or survival was noted. Several factors have been associated with high risk of complications and early mortality after a PEG[36] (Table 35.5). Several exceptions have been found that suggest tube feedings benefit elderly patients. A study by Mazzini et al.[37] showed that patients with amyotrophic lateral sclerosis with bulbar involvement improved survival and enhanced quality of life. Kaminski et al.[21] looked at a cohort of ICU patients who were very sick and required enteral feedings. There was some benefit in comatose patients. No benefit was seen in patients who had chronic obstructive pulmonary disease, multiple-organ system failure, and end-stage renal disease. In a meta-analysis by Simpson et al.,[38] enterally fed patients performed poorly compared to parenterally fed patients in an ICU setting even though there was a higher risk of systemic infection in parenterally fed patients. Studies suggest that nutritional support may be helpful for severely malnourished patients with cancer in certain perioperative settings, those receiving chemotherapy in the setting of hematopoietic stem cell transplantation, and patients with head and neck cancer.[39,40] Thus, enteral feeding has not shown benefits in demented patients who are unable to eat; it does not improve pressure sore outcomes and has not been shown to reduce infection. Functional status has not been improved, and demented patients are not made more comfortable. Furthermore, multiple side effects have been reported.[41]

35.4 THE ETHICS OF ENTERAL FEEDING

Beauchamp[43] described four principles (Table 35.6) that are involved in the ethical decision-making process between the physician, family, and patient when discussing enteral nutrition. They are (1) autonomy (self-determination), (2) beneficence, (3) nonmaleficence, and (4) justice. Autonomy necessitates that informed and educated consent be given in order for care to be received by the patient. The physician cannot decide what is good for the patient without respect to his or her autonomy. Beneficence is the perceived benefit of a medical intervention (enteral feeding) that will provide a net positive effect on health or outcome. Nonmaleficence entails avoiding a procedure or treatment that would bring harm to the patient. Justice refers to the

TABLE 35.6
The Ethical Principles

Principle	Approach
1) Autonomy	The obligation to provide benefits and balance benefits against rights
2) Beneficence	The obligation to avoid harm
3) Nonmaleficence	The obligation to respect the decision-making capacities of autonomous persons
4) Justice	Obligations of fairness in distribution of benefits and risk

quality of care being fair and involves the just allocation of medical resources across a community. One can also consider futility, which involves the concept that an intervention has no effect or would not provide benefit to the patient if it had an effect. Precedence is given to autonomy over beneficence. If informed consent is obtained, then the presumption is that enteral feeding will provide net benefit to the patient and will not cause harm, the benefits outweigh the risk of the procedure itself, and placement would be offered regardless of socioeconomic status and financial circumstances.

Several landmark cases have shaped the laws and ethics that have influenced the decision making for enteral feeding. In the 1970s, there was a prevailing attitude that argued for providing nutritional support regardless of the disease process, clinical prognosis, or patient population.[44] Paternalism was felt to be an integral part of the decision making, in which the doctor decided what was good for the patient. Provision of nutrition and hydration was seen as ordinary care. Providing nutrition was considered a basic nonaiverable responsibility on the part of the physician. Withdrawal of nutrition and hydration was felt to result in a prolonged and painful death.[44] In the last 25 years, four landmark cases have had judgments by the Supreme Court that have led to changes in how we approach enteral feeding. The Karen Quinlan case[45] in 1976 involved a young woman who was in a vegetative state from a drug overdose for 12 months. Her parents chose to withdraw mechanical ventilation, which they viewed as extraordinary care. Her enteral feedings were continued because they were viewed as ordinary care. She went on to live 9 more years. The New Jersey Supreme Court allowed the withdrawal of mechanical ventilation, yet it did not define whether certain categories of care could be stopped or continued, and whether withdrawal of therapy was limited to incompetent patients or patients suffering from terminal conditions.[44] It confirmed that a competent person has the right to refuse unwanted life-sustaining treatments and that this right is not lost if the person becomes incompetent.

The Barber[44] case in 1983 involved a man who suffered a severe anoxic brain injury as a result of cardiopulmonary arrest after surgery. The patient's spouse requested cessation of intravenous fluids and enteral feedings because her husband had specifically indicated he never wanted to be another Karen Quinlan. The patient soon died after withdrawal of therapy. The physician and surgeon involved in the case were indicted for murder but later had charges dropped because of the wife's assertion that her husband did not want to be in that state. This case highlighted the lack of a living will, power of attorney, or written statement by the patient regarding his wishes. The Elizabeth Bouvia case in 1986[46] involved a 28-year-old woman with severe cerebral palsy, who was completely bedridden, immobile, and in constant pain from contractures and arthritis. She was totally competent, however. Her oral intake was insufficient to sustain her nutritional needs. As her weight dropped to 65 pounds, a feeding tube was placed against her wishes. After placement, the patient petitioned to have her tube removed. The lower court refused the petition on grounds that this was a form of suicide. The appellate court upheld the patient's decision for the fact that a competent patient has a fundamental right to refuse medical support. The court indicated that a nonterminally ill patient has as much right to refuse medical care as someone who is terminally ill. The tube was removed and the patient subsequently died. The Nancy Beth Cruzan case[47] in 1990 involved a young woman with severe anoxic brain injury sustained in a motor vehicle accident 7 years earlier. She was receiving hydration and enteral feeding through a PEG tube. The parents requested withdrawal of the PEG tube because they believed their daughter would never regain consciousness. She had developed contractures and had continuous drooling. A lower court upheld the parents' decision. After an appeal by the nursing home, the Missouri State Supreme Court reversed the decision on the grounds that the parents did not have proof that their daughter would not have wanted such treatment. The case went to the U.S. Supreme Court, which upheld the Missouri State Supreme Court decision. Subsequent events, in which the facility physicians reversed their position, allowed the family to repetition the Missouri lower court, which granted the withdrawal of enteral feeds. Half of the staff at the hospital refused to provide care for the patient, and 12 days later the patient died.[44]

The courts in the U.S. have determined that artificial nutrition and hydration are indistinguishable from other life-sustaining therapy (such as mechanical ventilation), and their provision should not be thought of as different from any other medical therapy. Providing artificial nutritional support is not essential, and health care providers are not obligated to provide it. All of these therapies, ranging from hydration and nutrition to provision of antibiotics, oxygen therapy, or pressure support, are all bodily functions that the patient cannot provide on his or her own. Providing artificial nutritional support is no more basic than dialysis or oxygen delivery. Health care providers should assume that patients want therapy until proven otherwise or unless evidence is found to the contrary. The decision to withdraw or withhold nutritional therapy is no different than the decision to start provision. Thus, once nutritional therapy is started, health care professionals are not bound to continue feeding. Incompetent patients who do not have an advance directive must have "clear and convincing evidence" in a written manner that they wish not to have enteral nutrition.[48] The concepts of patient autonomy and self-determination indicate that patients have a right to decide for themselves whether to receive medical therapy. The right to consent to medical treatment is meaningless without the right to refuse medical treatment. Providing unwanted care contradicts established ethical principles and diminishes patient dignity. Criminal liability has been eliminated from the ethical dilemma of forgoing nutritional therapy. It is the underlying disease process that results in the patient's death and not the cessation of nutritional therapy.[44] In the Terri Schiavo case, a persistent vegetative state was concluded, and that there was "clear and convincing evidence" that she did not want prolonged enteral feedings. As previously established, an individual has the right to withhold life-sustaining therapy. When "Terri's Law" was passed by the Florida legislature and signed by Governor Jed Bush, a violation occurred in the separation of powers. The legislative body felt that the patient was being discriminated against due to her state of disability, and as such her alienable right for life had to be protected. The Florida Supreme Court unanimously ruled that this law violated that state's constitution because of its "encroachment on the power that has been reserved for the independent judiciary."[49] Living wills and health care proxies are available to help in the decision process and, as shown above, can lead to ethical and legal dilemmas if not available.

In Australia, a study by Ashby and Mendelson[50] showed that artificial nutrition and hydration are often thought by Australian doctors to be mandated by both law and ethics for elderly persons with impaired swallowing, irrespective of the patient's prognosis or the discomfort they may cause.[51] The Medical Treatment Act of 1988[52] is the main legal guide for clinicians in Australia. Under this act, a guardian of an incompetent patient may refuse medical treatment but not palliative care. Under the Medical Treatment Act, a guardian or surrogate cannot make a decision on behalf of the patient unless a medical practitioner and another person have discussed the risks and benefits of a medical procedure. A surrogate may only refuse medical treatment on a patient's behalf if such medical treatment would cause unreasonable distress to the patient or there are reasonable grounds to believe that the patient, if competent, and after giving serious consideration to her or his health and well-being, would consider the medical treatment to be unwarranted. Presumably, the guardian will use personal knowledge of the patient, and the patient's principles and convictions, if they are known, will be respected. Enteral nutrition is felt to be equivalent to artificial respiration, as in the Nancy Cruzan decision. Common law in England, as established by *Airedale NHS Trust v. Bland*[53] from 1993, gives importance to the concept of autonomy or self-determination. Thus, historical cases in several nations have given guidance for health professionals in dealing with enteral feeding.

35.5 IS WITHHOLDING ENTERAL FEEDING HARMFUL?

In certain clinical situations and patient populations clear benefits are noted from PEG tube placement. It is appropriate to place PEG tubes in patients who have a reversible disease process who likely require 4 weeks or more of enteral nutritional support. Yet, controversy exists in regard to patients with severe dementia or incurable metastatic cancer. No consistent benefit has been shown from aggressive artificial nutritional support in end-stage, incurable metastatic cancer.[54,55] Patients with terminal cancer may experience abdominal discomfort and nausea if they eat to please their families.[55] Patients who are terminally ill and do not receive artificial nutrition do not consistently sense hunger or thirst. In a study of 32 patients who were terminally ill from cancer, 63% never experienced hunger and 62% never experienced thirst.[55] Of those experiencing hunger or thirst, the symptoms were transient, occurring initially, but were easily alleviated with small amounts of food and attentive care to the mouth to keep it from being dry (ice chips, lubrication of lips). Lack of artificial nutritional support and hydration did not appear to lead to suffering in these patients. They were able to experience comfort with only minimal intake of food and fluids.[55] A survey of hospice nurses found that voluntary dehydration by patients resulted in a peaceful death that typically occurred within 2 weeks of stopping food and fluid intake.[56] Reports in humans who fast for spiritual reasons have observed preservation of mental function and alertness without suffering.[57–59]Patients with irreversible dementia may have a life expectancy of 12 to 18 months when they have reached a point where they have loss of speech, smile, and ambulation. Of the 121,000 PEG tubes placed in the U.S. in 1995, 30% were estimated to be placed in patients with dementia.[10] The global health status of the patient with dementia may impact the decision of whether to place a feeding tube. In a review of the literature, Finucane et al.[11] proposed that PEG tube placement in patients with advanced dementia was of no benefit. Although prevention of aspiration has been the leading cause for tube placement in nursing home residents with severe cognitive impairment, to date no study in patients with dementia shows that tube feeding reduces the risk of regurgitation of gastric contents.[11] Case-controlled studies have identified enteral feeding as a risk factor for aspiration pneumonia.[60–62] In a study by Canel et al.,[63] PEG tube placement reduced lower esophageal sphincter pressure and increased the incidence of gastroesophageal reflux. A study by Sullivan[64] showed that patients with advanced dementia do not suffer when oral intake declines. Urine volumes fall, and respiratory and gastrointestinal secretions decrease, lessening cough, vomiting, and diarrhea. Suffering is not aggravated in the absence of food and water, allowing caregivers to focus on comfort care. Moreover, metabolic changes that accompany withdrawal of nutritional support in dying patients actually promote comfort.[56] The majority of cognitively intact elderly patients more often declined artificial feeding when presented with clinical scenarios of advanced neurological disease such as dementia.[65] On the other hand, surrogates' views of life-sustaining treatment in settings like this correlate poorly with the patients', in whose interest they might be acting.[66] Physicians, in one survey, would order feeding tubes more often than they would for themselves were they in similar circumstances.[67] Other surveys of physicians' attitudes generally support not placing tubes when elderly patients, or those at end of life, are no longer eating; yet in reality, feeding tubes appear to be used more often than such surveys, or existing evidence already cited, would predict.[68] Avoidance of conflicts with families and fear of litigation may impact physician behavior. Practice patterns favor feeding tube placement when dying patients no longer are eating; much time and effort is required to counsel and educate patients and families about burdens and benefits, and not surprisingly, a decision for tube placement is the easiest way out in many circumstances.[69] Studies have also found that the attitude for PEG treatment in dementia patients differs between health care workers. Nurses believe feeding is a basic human requirement that should not be denied irrespective of cognitive function, whereas geriatricians are less willing to favor tube feeding in severely demented patients.[70–72] As such, withdrawal of enteral feeding in certain patients is safe and causes minimal suffering.

35.6 DO PEG TUBES IMPROVE QUALITY OF LIFE?

It is estimated that over 70% of patients with dementia on feeding tubes get restrained.[32] In a prospective study of 150 patients who were followed after PEG tube placement for a mean of 14 months (a third of which had dementia), 70% showed no improvement in functional status or overall subjective health status.[73] A study by Weaver et al.[74] looked at 100 consecutive patients placed on PEG tube feeding or surgical gastrostomy. Objective measures of quality of life were measured and no change was noted from the time the tube was placed to 4 and 8 years follow-up. Patients were divided by diagnoses of acute central system nervous disease, chronic illness, and gastrointestinal tract dysfunction. Although no control group was available for comparison, patients with chronic dementia and age over 76 years were less likely to improve than younger patients whose tubes were placed for acute cerebrovascular accident, head trauma, or abnormality of the GI tract.[74] These studies show that quality of life does not improve in demented patients, and as such, it should not be the primary reason for PEG placement. Very short survival rates are seen in demented patients with PEG placement, with 50% mortality at 1 month and 90% mortality at 1 year.[7,10,75] In the FOOD trial collaboration, a randomized controlled trial in which stroke and dysphagia were the main indications, early case fatality was reduced but at the expense of increasing the proportion surviving with poor outcome.[76] Enteral tube feeding in terminally ill cancer patients has not shown beneficial effects on outcome or quality of life.[77] It also does not reverse weight loss from cachexia or improve outcome.[78,79] However, once the PEG tube is placed, care for the patient becomes easier and more manageable, and family and caregivers often experience a lesser sense of failure. Bannerman et al.[80] looked at two cohorts of patients and assessed quality of life. The first cohort included 55 patients with PEG tubes placed 16 months earlier and the second cohort included 54 patients who had PEG tubes placed and then followed prospectively. Only 55% of patients reported an overall positive effect on their quality of life in response to the PEG tube placement.[80] In the study by Weaver et al.,[74] although objective quality of life measures did not change, 75% of the relatives of the patients claimed that the procedure benefited the patient, and 68% claimed that it improved the patient's quality of life. If it is agreed upon to start enteral feeding because of lack of consensus, one can monitor benefits and adverse events.[81] Withdrawal of a nonbeneficial or burdensome treatment, while difficult, is no different from a moral perspective than having never initiated it.[82] It is ethically and legally permissible for patients with decision-making capacity to refuse unwanted medical interventions and to ignore recommendations of the clinicians.[83] This may differ from a clinician's desire to do good and avoid harm.[84] If sufficient information in regard to risks and benefits of acceptance and refusal are given to a patient, then the clinician should respect the patient's wishes.[85]

35.7 DECIDING TO PLACE A FEEDING TUBE

Advance directives (ADs) allow persons to express their future health care goals if they lose decision-making capacity.[86] There are two types of ADs: the living will and the durable power of attorney for health care. The living will allows persons to list interventions and other actions that should or should not be taken in specific circumstances, such as PEG tube placement. The durable power of attorney for health care identifies a surrogate decision maker who can make health care decisions if the patient no longer has decision-making capacity. Persons may also identify an alternate surrogate in case the first person designated is not available. Clinicians commonly care for patients with impaired decision making who do not have an AD.[87] When caring for a patient who lacks decision-making capacity and has not completed a durable power of attorney, clinicians must identify a surrogate decision maker. The ideal surrogate is someone who best understands the patient's health care values and goals.[88] In the U.S., some states have hierarchies for surrogate decision making (e.g., spouse, next of kin), whereas others do not. In these situations, clinicians should work with the patient's family and health care team to determine the appropriate surrogate. If the situation remains unresolved, an ethics consultation and, if necessary, a court proceeding may be required to identify the most appropriate surrogate decision maker for the patient. Surrogates must be fully informed of the risks, benefits, and alternatives to a proposed procedure or treatment. Surrogates should base their decisions on the patient's previously expressed values and goals (substituted judgment). However, patients often do not discuss their health care values and goals with their surrogate. In these situations, surrogates must make decisions based on what they regard as most appropriate for the patient's clinical condition, quality of life, and best interest.[88] Laws exist in all 50 states and the District of Columbia relating to ADs, yet they vary from state to state. Several states allow surrogates to make decisions about artificial nutrition and hydration for a patient only if the patient specifically authorized the surrogate to do so. States typically restrict the authority of default surrogates. Although none of the 50 states prohibit the forgoing or withdrawal of a feeding tube, 15 states require a written advance directive to forgo insertion of a feeding tube.[89]

When discussing tube feeding placement, clinicians overestimate the efficacy of PEG feeding persons with dementia, as shown by a survey of 416 general internal medicine and family practice physicians.[68] A high percentage of physicians believed that PEG tubes reduce aspiration pneumonia (76%) and improve pressure ulcer healing (75%), survival (61%), nutritional status (94%), and functional status (27%). The physicians' decisions to place PEG tubes were influenced by the nutrition teams, speech therapists, nursing staff, and nursing home requests. In addition, one third reported that they would honor a family's request to place a feeding tube even if the patient had previously stated that his or her preference was not to have a PEG tube placed. More than half responded that PEG tube use represents a standard of care in advanced dementia, yet three fourths said they would not personally want a feeding tube if they had advanced dementia. Surrogate decision makers listed several reasons for choosing long-term tube feeding (Table 35.7).

A telephone survey of surrogate decision makers for elderly patients residing in long-term facilities found that only 57% of surrogates felt confident that the person would have wanted long-term tube feeding.[90] Most of the patients had not completed ADs, and only one patient had specifically expressed wishes to the surrogate regarding long-term tube feeding. Approximately half of surrogates believed they had received adequate support from the health care team in making the decision. Approximately

TABLE 35.7
Reasons Why Surrogate Chose Tube Feeding

1) Improve nutrition (70%)
2) Increase patient comfort (22%)
3) Prolong life (18%)
4) Increase strength (14%)
5) Help overcome acute illness (10%)

TABLE 35.8
Survival of Patients as Predicted by Physicians

Reference	Accuracy of Death Prediction	Overestimation
1) Glare et al.[73]	20%	63%
2) Lamont et al.[74]	24-day survival	75-day survival (as predicted by doctor)

one fourth of surrogates did not speak with or did not remember speaking with a physician about the decision. Most surrogates believed they understood the benefits of tube feeding, but less than half believed they understood the potential risks. Prevention of aspiration and prolongation of life were medical benefits cited most often as reasons for requesting long-term tube feeding. Accurate predictal of life expectancy by physicians tends to be overly optimistic (Table 35.8).

On certain occasion conflict arises in defining futile therapy.[91,92] Physicians may perceive therapy as futile, whereas family may view it as prolonging and improving life. If the goal of enteral nutrition is to restore good health to a patient with terminal illness, then artificial nutrition and hydration are futile, and the medical team is obligated to discuss the reasons that this treatment is futile with the patient and the surrogate. However, if the goal is to respect the patient's belief and values, provide a means to palliate symptoms, and sustain life to allow closure for the family, then treatment would not be considered futile.[93] If conflicting views persist, an ethics consult and ultimate transfer of medical care to another clinician or institution may be necessary.[94] Jonsen et al.[95] have described a four-step approach to solve ethical dilemmas. Rabeneck et al. have proposed an algorithm for PEG tube placement.[81]

Honoring a patient's request to refuse or withdraw a life-sustaining treatment is not the same as physician-assisted suicide (PAS). In PAS, a patient intentionally terminates life by a means provided by the clinician, such as a drug. In contrast, when a patient dies after a life-sustaining procedure is refused or withdrawn, the underlying disease is the cause of the death. The intent is freedom from treatments perceived as burdensome.[96,97] The U.S. Supreme Court has rules that persons have the right to refuse unwanted life-sustaining treatments, and that such refusal is not suicidal, and that death after such refusal is not suicide, but rather due to the underlying disease.[46,98] No American court has found clinicians liable for wrongful death after honoring a patient's or surrogate's request to refuse or withdraw life-sustaining treatments.[99] Clinicians must be certain that patients who refuse or request the withdrawal of life-sustaining treatments have adequate decision-making capacity and are informed of the consequences of their request.[100] It is preferable that these issues be discussed when patients are able to make decisions, and physicians should encourage these discussions with their patients. Effective communication among clinicians, patients, and surrogate decision makers may help prevent ethical dilemmas.[101] Clinicians should take time to learn about the patient and patient's values, goals, and beliefs. The patient should be provided ample time to discuss his or her concerns related to nutrition and hydration. When conveying medical information concerning benefits and risks of long-term tube feeding, clinicians should avoid using complex medical language and frequently should assess the patient's comprehension.[102] Ineffective communication among clinicians, patients, and surrogate decision makers may result in ethical dilemmas.[103] Layson et al.[104] showed that discussions about life-sustaining treatments between clinicians and patients are reportedly uncommon.

35.8 INFLUENCE OF FAITH, CULTURE, AND MORALITY OF DECISION MAKING

Many ethical dilemmas exist in modern medicine, and understanding the culture and religion of the patient, family, and clinician is imperative to know what is considered right or wrong, and acceptable or not. These factors often influence the medical decision made or not made. Many clinicians are not of the same religious persuasion as their patients, and a lack of understanding of the patient's religious conviction may cause misunderstanding, conflict, and confusion.

Artificial nutrition is a supportive medical therapy aiming to achieve predefined objectives, which should be adjusted for changing clinical situations.[105] The goal of nutritional support must be clearly defined within a global therapeutic plan. One must consider several issues in regard to enteral feedings (Table 35.9).

In the Jewish faith, persons are responsible stewards of their bodies. The physician has clear obligations to the duty of healing. The patient has a comparable obligation regarding the duty to be healed, which allows one to seek medical advice. Although illness and death are considered a natural part of life, one is duty-bound to strive to save a life. As such, collective and individual values are highly relevant. Autonomy is felt to be of secondary importance and is secondary to the patient's health and welfare as judged by clinician and cleric. Relief of suffering is as important as the duty to care for one's parents in old age. The process of dying must be respected when it is clearly occurring, is imminent, and is irreversible. Beneficence

TABLE 35.9
Perceived Goals of Enteral Nutrition

1) Will nutritional support be well tolerated by my patients?
2) Will nutritional support improve or sustain the nutritional status of my patient?
3) Will nutritional support improve or sustain the quality of life of my patient?
4) Will nutritional support improve the outcome and extend the survival of my patient?

is a major goal, as is nonmaleficence. Distributive justice is also important. If the patient is terminally ill, and enteral feeding will not reverse that, then withdrawing or not starting support is acceptable. If it will preserve or extend life (sanctity of life), then it is allowed because it will decrease suffering. Advance directives are respected since they represent the patient's wishes.

The Catholic faith directs one to behave as the steward and not simply owner of his or her body. However, bodily life is not an absolute good to be maintained at all cost. One is therefore not obliged to continue treatment if it merely prolongs dying. Although suffering may have positive meaning from a theological perspective, it is not to be sought as an end in itself. Pain management is encouraged, especially in terminal illness. Beneficence and nonmaleficence are highly regarded. Respect for life requires that one also recognize when the patient is dying and pay attention to psychological and spiritual needs. Dying is considered a time for reconciliation and forgiveness. As such, a process that prolongs and interferes with the dying process and causes suffering is allowed to be withdrawn. It is also permissible, although not obligatory, to insert a feeding tube, an act justified on the grounds of respect for sanctity of life (beneficence) and autonomy. Advance directives are to be respected. Autonomy is primary in a patient's decision making at end of life unless it interferences with beneficence or nonmaleficence.

In Islam, sanctity of life is a paramount principle. Every moment of life is precious and must be preserved. Muslims believe that all healing comes ultimately from God, yet they have a duty to seek out medical attention when ill, and have a right to receive medical care. However, Islam recognizes that death is inevitable and part of human existence. Thus, treatment does not have to be provided if it merely prolongs the final stages of a terminal illness. Autonomy is recognized in Islam, and beneficence and nonmaleficence are major, complementary goals. Distributive justice plays a minor role.

A feeding tube is allowed if it will extend life under the sanctity of life principle. Furthermore, there is a religious obligation to provide nourishment unless such an act shortens it. Nutritional support is viewed as a basic need rather than a medical necessity. Advance directives are to be respected since they represent the patient's wishes. Autonomy is also felt to be of secondary importance and is secondary to the patient's health and welfare as judged by clinician and cleric.

In other cultures, such as Japan, it is not customary to inform the patient of a terminal diagnosis, and therefore, the patient may wish to continue therapy. In a terminally ill patient who is unaware of his diagnosis, 67.5% of surveyed multispecialty Japanese physicians would provide total parenteral nutrition (TPN) for malnutrition, although only 36% of those surveyed (only 5% of Japanese American physicians) would want such therapy for themselves in a similar situation.[106] On the contrary, only 33% of Japanese American general practice and internal medicine physicians would recommend TPN to treat malnutrition in a terminal condition. Thirty-six percent of the Japanese physicians indicated they would ignore the patient's request to withdraw TPN if the physician thought it necessary, although only 6.5% of Japanese American physicians would do so. In comparison, a survey of American neurologist and medical directors showed that 89% believed that withdrawal of artificial nutrition and hydration in a patient who was in a persistent vegetative state was ethical.[107] A survey of 580 internists in the U.S. revealed similar opinions.[108]

35.9 THE LAW AND ENTERAL FEEDING

The ethical principle of autonomy maintains the right of patients to refuse or request the withdrawal of unwanted interventions. One may refuse therapy that was previously consented for. From a legal standpoint, patients in the U.S. have a constitutional right to refuse any and all forms of medical intervention, whether or not they are terminal and whether or not such refusal may lead to their death. As a result of the Nancy Cruzan case, the U.S. Supreme Court ruled that states could adopt statutes that require clear and convincing evidence to be present prior to withdrawal of long-term enteral feeding in a patient unable to speak. Several states, such as Missouri and Florida, have laws requiring clear evidence for withdrawing long-term feeding in patients unable to speak.[89] In Germany, the withdrawal of nutrition in patients suffering from terminal illness may be considered active euthanasia unless death is imminent[109] and involves the potential of civil or criminal liability.[110] Although advance directive laws are present and recognized in all states, including the District of Columbia, their absence may lead to difficulties in decision making for the care of a patient. In this situation, a physician must identify a legal authorized surrogate. States have hierarchies of surrogates, which vary from state to state. When a surrogate is not acting in the best interest of the patient, it is the physician's duty, using beneficence, to appear in court and request the appointment of another health care surrogate. In the Wanglie[111] case, the hospital attempted to withdraw ventilatory support because it was felt that Mrs. Wanglie's medical condition was terminal and further care was futile. A request for withdrawal of artificial respiration was asked for as well, replacing her husband as surrogate. The court ruled in Mr. Wanglie's favor because he was clearly following the wishes of his wife as stated in her AD. The Terri Schiavo case highlighted the divisions in society in regard to preserving life at all cost and the respect of the autonomous decisions of patients to withhold treatment. It made it more imperative that physicians and patients discuss this matter among themselves and tell family members their wishes in regard to end-of-life care, including long-term enteral feeding. Documenting conversation in the medical chart is imperative, and ensuring that patients truly understand the advance directive and reflect their wishes is of utmost importance. In many states, conscience clauses are available to prevent discrimination against health care workers who feel withdrawal of a treatment is against their moral convictions. The Missouri statute reads:

> No physician, nurse, or other individual who is a health care provider or an employee of a health care facility shall be discharged or otherwise discriminated against in his employment or employment application for refusing to honor a health care decision withholding or withdrawing life-sustaining treatment if such refusal is based upon the individual's religious beliefs, or sincerely held moral convictions.[112]

Medical futility has been addressed with variability through several cases. In the 1994 Baby K case, the court argued against the hospital that treating respiratory distress in an anencephalic baby was medically futile.[113] As in the Weigle case, the courts determined that families should judge the appropriateness of continuing or stopping treatment that physicians or ethics committees consider medically futile.

However, in the 1995 case of *Gilgunn v. Massachusetts General Hospital*, the court found that cardiopulmonary resuscitation need not be provided to a patient dying with multiple-organ system failure, even if requested by the patent's family.[114] In 1993, Lundberg suggested that physicians define medical futility and that hospitals develop guidelines for dealing with it.[115] As the debate over medical futility progressed, some institutions developed policies for dealing with this area.[115,116] In 1999, the American Medical Association Council on Ethical and Judicial Affairs published guidelines on medical futility.[94] The guidelines recommended a process-based counseling approach to futility disputes, which attempts to transfer the patient to alternate providers if disagreements cannot be resolved. At the end of this process, if no resolution can be arranged, it is ethically acceptable to halt futile treatments. The council also noted that "the legal ramifications of this course of action are uncertain."

In 1999, the Texas legislature passed a law called the Texas Advance Directive Act.[117] The law established a legally sanctioned extrajudicial process for resolving disputes about end-of-life decisions. It grants immunity from civil and criminal liability to hospitals and physicians. This form of dispute may be used in response to a surrogate, living will, or medical power of attorney request to either "do everything" or "stop all treatment" if the physician feels ethically unable to agree to either request. A "medical futility" conflict is a situation in which the physician is asked to "do everything" but feels withdrawal of treatment is most appropriate; a "right to die" conflict is a situation in which the physician is asked to stop all treatment but feels that it should be maintained. If requested by a physician, an ethics consultation is initiated. If an outside hospital is willing to accept care, then withdrawal of support is not indicated. The broadest experience has come from the Baylor University Medical Center, in which the number of consults for medical futility increased three-fold 2 years after the law's implementation. Of the six futility cases that were pursued through the dispute resolution process, three families agreed to withdrawal of support a few days after receiving the formal written report from the ethics committee. In two cases, the patients died during the 10-day waiting period without an alternate provider being found. In one case, an alternate provider was located, but the patient died while awaiting transfer.

In conclusion, the ethics of enteral nutrition and its long-term use remain controversial and many unanswered questions remain. The legal system of the U.S. and England has offered judicial advice on the placement of feeding tubes. Yet many citizens and health care workers remain unaware and uneducated on these matters. Advance directives have become the main tool to prevent undue suffering for families and patients when filled. Hospitals have set up ethics committees to help in these matters. I suggest a similar model be used in the long-term-care setting, where outside ethics consultants can help families and patients deal with these issues. It is the responsibility of health care professionals to know the laws of their state so that they can avoid legal action for procedures that may be thought of as futile or limiting suffering, yet in the end go against the wishes of the family, especially if the patient is in a persistent vegetative state. The European parliament should adopt laws to create a uniform guideline for the placement of PEG tubes. More needs to be done to educate health care workers on the religious, ethnic, and religious beliefs of patients in regard to terminal illness and enteral feeding. International consensus through dialogue can help develop guidelines using evidence-based medicine to help the legal system adopt better laws. In the end, our ultimate goal is to do no harm.

REFERENCES

1. Orrevall Y, Tishelman C, Herrington MK, Permert J. The path from oral nutrition to home parenteral nutrition: a qualitative interview study of the experiences of advanced cancer patients and their families. *Clin Nutr* 2004;23:1280–1287.
2. Johnson VM, Teno JM, Bourbonniere M, Mor V. Palliative care needs of cancer patients in U.S. nursing homes. *J Palliative Med* 2005;8:273–279.
3. Mitchell SL, Kiely DK, Lipsitz LA. The risk factors and impact on survival of feeding tube placement in nursing home residents with severe cognitive impairment. *Arch Intern Med* 1997;157:327–332.
4. Lynn J, Childress JF. Must patients always be given food and water? *Hastings Cent Rep* 1983;13:17–21.
5. Kirby DF, Delegge MH, Fleming CR. American Gastroenterological Association technical review on tube feeding for enteral nutrition. *Gastroenterology* 1995;108:1282–1301.
6. Hurley DL, Mcmahon MM. In *Clinical Nutrition: Enteral and Tube Feeding*, 4th ed., Rolandelli RH, Backhead R, Boulatta JI, Compher CW, Eds. Elsevier Saunders, Philadelphia, 2005, pp. 498–505.
7. Rabeneck L, Wray NP, Peterson NJ. Long term outcome of patients receiving percutaneous endoscopic tubes. *J Gen Intern Med* 1996;11:287–293.
8. Laasch HU, Wilbraham L, Bullen K, et al. Gastrostomy insertion: comparing the options—PEG, RIG, or PIG? *Clin Radiol* 2003;58:398–405.
9. Ponsky JL, Gauderer MW. Percutaneous endoscopic gastrostomy: a nonoperative technique for feeding gastrotomy. *Gastrointest Endosc* 1981;27:9–11.
10. Grant MD, Rudeberg MA, Brody JA. Gastrostomy placement and mortality among hospitalized Medicare beneficiaries. *JAMA* 1998;279:1973–1976.
11. Finucane TE, Christmas C, Travis K. Tube feeding in patients with advanced dementia: a review of the evidence. *JAMA* 1999;282:1365–1370.
12. Mitchell SL, Teno JM, Roy J, Kabumoto G, Mor V. Clinical and organizational factors associated with feeding tube use among nursing home residents with advanced cognitive impairment. *JAMA* 2003;290:73–80.
13. Ahronheim JC, Mulvihill M, Sieger C, Park P, Fries BE. State practice variations in the use of tube feeding for nursing home residents with severe cognitive impairment. *J Am Geriatr Soc* 2001;49:148–152.
14. Teno JM, Mor V, Sesilva D, et al. Use of feeding tubes in nursing home residents with severe cognitive impairment. *JAMA* 2002;287:3211–3212.
15. Hebuterne X, Bozetti F, Moreno Villares JM, et al. Nutrition Working Group. Home enteral nutrition in adults: a European multicentre survey. *Clin Nutr* 2003;22:261–266.
16. Elia M, Stratton RJ, Holden C, et al. Home enteral tube feeding following cerebrovascular accident. *Clin Nutr* 2001;20:27–30.
17. Gaggiotti G, Orlandoni P, Ambrosi S, Catani M. Italian home enteral nutrition register: data collections and aims. *Clin Nutr* 2001;20(Suppl 2):69–72.
18. Oyoga S, Schein M, Gardezi S, et al. Surgical feeding gastrostomy: are we overdoing it? *J Gastrointest Surg* 1999;3:152–155.
19. Abukis G, Mor M, Segal N, et al. Percutaneous endoscopic gastrostomy: high mortality rates in hospitalized patients. *Am J Gastroenterol* 2000;95:128–132.

20. James A, Kapur K, Hawthorne AB. Long-term outcome of percutaneous endoscopic gastrostomy feeding in patients with dysphagic stroke. *Age Ageing* 1998;27:671–676.
21. Kaminski MV, Nasr NJ, Freed BA, et al. The efficacy of nutritional support in the elderly. *J Am Coll Nutr* 1982;1:35.
22. Loser C, Wolters S, Folsch UR. Enteral long-term nutrition via percutaneous endoscopic gastrostomy (PEG) in 210 patients: a four-year prospective study. *Dig Dis Sci* 1998;43:2549–2557.
23. Nicholson FB, Korman MG, Richardson MA. Percutaneous gastrostomy: a review of indications, complications and outcome. *J Gastroenterol Hepatol* 2000;15:21–25.
24. Cataldi-Betcher EL, Seltzer MH, Slocum BA, et al. Complications occurring during enteral nutrition support: a prospective study. *J Parenter Enteral Nutr* 1983;7:546–552.
25. Campos ACL, Meguid MM. A critical appraisal of the usefulness of perioperative nutritional support. *Am J Clin Nutr* 1992;55:117–130.
26. Dennis M. Nutrition after stroke. British medical bulletin. *Stroke* 2000;56:466–475.
27. Berlowitz DR, Brandeis GH, Anderson J, et al. Predictors of pressure ulcer healing among long-term care residents. *J Am Geriatr* 1997;45:30–34.
28. Berlowitz DR, Ash AS, Brandeis GH, et al. Rating long-term care facilities on pressure ulcer development: importance of case-mix adjustment. *Ann Intern Med* 1996;124:557–563.
29. Henderson CT, Trumbore LS, Mobarhan S, et al. Prolonged tube feeding in long-term care: nutritional status and clinical outcomes. *J Am Coll Nutr* 1992;11:309–325.
30. Stratton RJ, Ek A, Engfer M, Moore Z, Rigby P, Wolfe R, Elia M. Enteral nutritional support in prevention and treatment of pressure ulcers: a systematic review and meta-analysis. *Ageing Res Rev* 2005;4:422–450.
31. Rimon E, Kagansky N, Levy S. Percutaneous endoscopic gastrostomy: evidence of different prognosis in various patient subgroups. *Age Ageing* 2005;34:353–357.
32. Ciocon JO, Silverstone FA, Graver LM, et al. Tube feedings in elderly patients: indications, benefits, and complications. *Arch Intern Med* 1988;148:429–433.
33. Chowdhury MA, Batey R. Complications and outcome of percutaneous endoscopic gastrostomy in different patient groups. *J Gastroenterol Hepatol* 1996;11:835–839.
34. Callahan CM, Haag KM, Weinberger M, et al. Outcomes of percutaneous endoscopic gastrostomy among older adults in a community setting. *J Am Geriatr Soc* 2000;48:1048–1054.
35. Stratton RJ, Birscher G, Fouque D, Stenvinkel P, de Mutsert R, Engfer M, Elia M. Multinutrient oral supplements and tube feeding in maintenance dialysis: a systematic review and meta-analysis. *Amer J Kidney Dis* 2005;46:387–405.
36. Hebuterne X, Schneider SM. What Are the Goals of Nutritional Support? The example of home internal nutrition, Nestlé Nutrition Workshop Series Clinical and Performance Program 2005;10:89–98: discussion 98–102. Paper presented at the Nestle Nutrition Workshop.
37. Mazzini L, Corra T, Zaccala M, et al. Percutaneous endoscopic gastrostomy and enteral nutrition in amyotrophic lateral sclerosis. *J Neurol* 1995;242:695–698.
38. Simpson F, Doig GS. Parenteral vs. enteral nutrition in the critically ill patient: a meta-analysis of trials using the intention to treat principle. *Intensive Care Med* 2005;31:12–23.
39. Lee JH, Machtay M, Unger LD, et al. Prophylactic gastrostomy tubes in patients undergoing intensive irradiation for cancer of the head and neck. *Arch Otolaryngol Head Neck Surg* 1998;124:871–875.

40. Zogbaum AT, Fitz P, Duggy VB. Tube feeding may improve adherence to radiation treatment schedule in head and neck cancer: an outcomes study. *Topics Clin Nutr* 2004;19:95–106.
41. Finucane TE, Bynum JP. Use of tube feeding to prevent aspiration pneumonia. *Lancet* 1996;348:1421–1424.
42. Cole MJ, Smith JT, Molnar C, et al. Aspiration after percutaneous gastrostomy: assessment by Tc-99m labeling of the enteral feed. *J Clin Gastroenterol* 1987;9:90–95.
43. Beauchamp T. The four principles approach. In *Principles of Health Care Ethics*, Gillon R, Ed. John Wiley & Sons, New York, 1994, pp. 3–12.
44. Mayo TW. Forgoing artificial nutrition and hydration: legal and ethical consideration. *Nutr Clin Pract* 1996;11:254–264.
45. *In re Quinlan*, 70 NJ 10, 355 A2d 647 (1976), at 663-43.
46. *Bouvia v. Superior Court*, 179 Cal. App. 3d 1127, at 1146-47, 225 Cal. Rptr. 297 (1986).
47. *Cruzan v. Director, Missouri Dept. of Health*, 497 U.S. 261 (1990).
48. Emanuel EJ. Securing patient's right to refuse medical care: in praise of the Cruzan decision. *Am J Med* 1992;92:307–312.
49. Silverman HJ. Withdrawal of feeding tubes from incompetent patients: the Terri Schiavo case raises new issues regarding who decides in end-of-life decision making. *Intensive Care Med* 2005;31:480–481.
50. Ashby M, Mendelson D. *Natural Death in 2003: Are We Slipping Backwards?* (2003) 10(3) JLM 260 at 262.
51. Steinberg MA, et al. *Percutaneous Endoscope Gastrostomy (PEG) Feeding in Residential Aged Care Facilities*. University of Queensland, Healthy Aging Unit, Department of Social and Preventive Medicine, Brisbane, April 2000.
52. Rothschild A. *Gardner; Re BWV: Resolved and Unresolved Issues at End of Life*. (2004) JLM 11:292–311.
53. In *Airedale NHS Trust v. Bland* (1993) AC 789, it needed to be determined whether a nasogastric tube could lawfully be removed from a patient in a permanent vegetative state (PVS), knowing that to do so would almost certainly condemn him to die.
54. Braunschweig CL, Levy P, Sheean PM, et al. Enteral compared with parenteral nutrition: a meta-analysis. *Am J Clin Nutr* 2001;74:534–542.
55. Mcann RM, Hall WJ, Groth-Junker A. Comfort care for terminally ill patients: the appropriate use of nutrition and hydration. *JAMA* 1994;272:1263–1266.
56. Ganzini L, Goy ER, Miller LL, Harvath TA, Jackson A, Delorit MA. Nurses' experiences with hospice patients who refuse food and fluids to hasten death. *N Engl J Med* 2003;349:359–365.
57. Stewart WK, Fleming LW. Features of a successful therapeutic fast of 382 days duration. *Postgrad Med J* 1973;49:203–209.
58. Kerndt PR, Naughton JL, Driscoll CE, Loxterkamp DA. Fasting: the history, pathophysiology and complications. *West J Med* 1982;137:379–399.
59. Saudek CD, Felig P. The metabolic events of starvation. *Am J Med* 1976;60:117–126.
60. Pick N, Mcdonald A, Bennett N, et al. Pulmonary aspiration in a long-term care setting: clinical and laboratory observations and analysis of risk factors. *J Am Geriatr Soc* 1996;44:763–768.
61. Bourdel-Marchasson I, Dumas F, Pingaud G, et al. Audit of percutaneous endoscopic gastrostomy in long-term enteral feeding in a nursing home. *Int J Qual Health Care* 1997;9:297–302.

62. Langmore Se, Terpenning MS, Schork A, et al. Predictors of aspiration pneumonia: how important is dysphagia? *Dysphagia* 1998;13:69–81.
63. Canel D, Vane B, Gotto S. Reduction of lower esophageal sphincter pressure with Stamm gastrostomy. *J Pediatr Surg* 1987;22:54–58.
64. Sullivan RJ, Jr. Accepting death without artificial nutrition or hydration. *J Gen Intern Med* 1993;8:220–224.
65. O'Brien LAA, Siegert EA, Grisso JA, et al. Tube feeding preferences among nursing home residents. *J Gen Intern Med* 1997;12:364–371.
66. Cogen R, Patterson B, Chavin S, et al. Surrogate decision-maker preferences for medical care of severely demented nursing home patients. *Arch Intern Med* 1992;152:1885–1888.
67. Carmel S. Life-sustaining treatments: what doctors do, what they want for themselves and what elderly persons want. *Soc Sci Med* 1999;49:1401–1408.
68. Shega JW, Hougham GW, Stocking CB, et al. Barriers to limiting the practice of feeding tube placement in advanced dementia. *J Palliat Med* 2003;6:885–893.
69. Callhan CM, Haag KM, Buchanan NN, et al. Decision-making for percutaneous endoscopic adults in the community setting. *J Am Geriatr Soc* 1999;47:1105–1109.
70. Hasan M, Meara RJ, Bhowmick BK, Woodhouse K. Percutaneous endoscopic gastrostomy in geriatric patients: attitudes of health care professionals. *Gerontology* 1995;41:326–331.
71. Zanetti O, Bianchetti A, Zanetti E, Magni E, Frisoni GB, Trabucchi M. Geriatric nurses' attitudes towards the use of nasogastric feeding-tubes in demented patients. *Int J Geriatr Psychiatry* 1996;11:1111–1116.
72. Watts DT, Cassel CK, Hickam DH. Nurses' and physicians' attitudes toward tube-feeding decisions in long term care. *J Am Geriatr Soc* 1986;34:607–611.
73. Callahan CM, Haag KM. Outcomes of percutaneous endoscopic gastrostomy among older adults in a community setting. *J Am Geriatr Soc* 2000;48:1048–1054.
74. Weaver JP, Odell P, Nelson C. Evaluation of the benefits of gastric tube feeding in an elderly population. *Arch Fam Med* 1993;2:953–956.
75. Murphy LM, Lipman TO. Percutaneous endoscopic gastrostomy does not prolong survival in patients with dementia. *Arch Intern Med* 2003;163:1351–1353.
76. Dennis MS, Lewis SC, Walrow C. FOOD Trial Collaboration. Effect of timing and method of enteral tube feeding for dysphagic stroke patients (FOOD): a multicentre randomized controlled trial. *Lancet* 2005;365:764–772.
77. Braga M, Giannoti L, Nespoli L, Radelli G, Di Carlo V. Nutritional approach in malnourished surgical patients: a prospective randomized study. *Arch Surg* 2002;137:173–180.
78. Kotler DP. Cachexia. *Ann Intern Med* 2000;133:622–634.
79. Betrand PC, Piquet MA, Bordier I, Monnier P, Roulet M. Preoperative nutritional support at home in head and neck cancer patients: from nutritional benefits to the prevention of the alcohol withdrawal syndrome. *Curr Opin Clin Nutr Metab Care* 2002;5:435–440.
80. Bannerman E, Pendelburg J, Phillips F, et al. A cross-sectional and longitudinal study of health related quality of life after percutaneous gastrosotomy. *Eur J Gastroenterol Hepatol* 2000;12:1101–1109.
81. Rabeneck L, McCullough LB, Wray NP. Ethically justified, clinically comprehensive guidelines for percutaneous endoscopic gastrostomy tube placement. *Lancet* 1997;349:496–498.
82. President's Commission for the Study of Ethical Problems in Medicine and Biomedical and Behavioral Research. *Deciding to Forgo Life-Sustaining Treatment, A Report on the Ethical, Medical, and Legal Issues in Treatment Decisions*. Washington, DC, 1983.

83. Mueller PS, Hook CC, Fleming KC. Ethical issues in geriatrics: a guide for clinicians. *Mayo Clini Proc* 2004;79:554–562.
84. Pellegrino ED. Decisions to withdraw life-sustaining treatment: a moral algorithm. *JAMA* 2000;283:1065–1067.
85. Snyder L, Leffler C. Ethics and Human Rights Committee, American College of Physicians. Ethics manual: fifth edition. *Ann Intern Med* 2005;142:560–582.
86. Danis M, Southerland LI, Garrett JM, et al. A prospective study of advance directives for life-sustaining care. *N Engl J Med* 1991;324:882–888.
87. Hanson LC, Rodgman E. The use of living wills at the end of life: a national study. *Arch Intern Med* 1996;156:1018–1022.
88. Hayley DC, Cassel CK, Snyder L, Rudeberg MA. Ethical and legal issues in nursing home care. *Arch Intern Med* 1996;156:249–256.
89. Gillick MR. Advance care planning. *N Engl J Med* 2004;350:7–8.
90. Mitchell SL, Lawson FM. Decision-making for long-term tube feeding in cognitively impaired elderly people. *CMAJ* 1999;160:1705–1709.
91. American Medical Association Council on Ethical and Judicial Affairs. *Code of Medical Ethics: Current Opinions with Annotations*, 2000–2001 ed. American Medical Association, Chicago, 2000.
92. Veatch RM. Why physicians cannot determine if care is futile. *J Am Geriatr Soc* 1994;42;871–874.
93. Kasman DL. When is medical treatment futile? A guide for students, residents, and physicians. *J Gen Intern Med* 2004;19:1053–1056.
94. Medical futility in end-of-life care: a report of the Council on Ethical and Judicial Affairs. *JAMA* 1999;281:937–941.
95. Jonsen AR, Siegler M, Winslade WJ. *Clinical Ethics: A Practical Approach to Ethical Decisions in Clinical Medicine*, 5th ed. Mcgraw-Hill, New York, 2002.
96. Meisel A, Snyder L, Quill T. American College of Physicians-American Society of Internal Medicine End-of-Life Care Consensus Panel. Seven legal barriers to end-of-life care: myths, realities, and grains of truth. *JAMA* 2000;284:2495–2501.
97. Winter B, Cohen S. ABCs of intensive care: withdrawal of treatment. *BMJ* 1999;319:306–308.
98. *Vacco v. Quill*, 521 U.S. 793 (1997).
99. Gostin LO. Deciding life and death in the courtroom: from Quinlan to Cruzan, Glucksberg, and Vacco: a brief history and analysis of constitutional protection of the "right to die." *JAMA* 1997;278:1523–1528.
100. Quill TE, Barold SS, Sussman BL. Discontinuing an implantable cardioverter defibrillator as a life-sustaining treatment. *Am J Cardiol* 1994;74:205–207.
101. Orr RD, Marshall PA, Osborn J. Cross-cultural considerations in clinical ethics consultation. *Arch Fam Med* 1995;4:159–164.
102. Barrier PA, Li JT-C, Jensen NM. Two words to improve physician-patient communications: what else? *Mayo Clin Proc* 2003;78:211–214.
103. Loewy EH, Carlson RW. Talking, advance directives, and medical practice (editorial). *Arch Intern Med* 1994;154:2265–2267.
104. Layson RT, Adelman HM, Wallch PM, Pfeifer MP, Johnson S, Mcnutt RA. End of Life Study Group. Discussions about the use of life-sustaining treatments: a literature review of physicians' and patients' attitudes and practice. *J Clin Ethics* 1994;5:195–203.
105. Loeser C, von Herz U, Kuchler T et al. Quality of life and nutritional state in patients on home enteral tube feeding. *Nutrition* 2003;19:605–611.

106. Asai A, Fukuhara S, Lo B. Attitudes of Japanese and Japanese-American physicians towards life-sustaining treatment. *Lancet* 1995;346:356–359.
107. Payne K, Taylor RM Stocking C, Sachs GA. Physician's attitudes about the care of patients in the persistent vegetative state: a national survey. *Ann Intern Med* 1996;125:104–110.
108. Hodges MO, Tolle SW, Stocking C, Cassel CK. Tube feeding. Internists' attitudes regarding ethical obligations. *Arch Intern Med* 1994;154:1013–1020.
109. Budersarztekammer, Richtlinien der Bundsarztekammer fur die Sterbebegleitung. *DABL* 1993;90:B1791–B1792.
110. Schmidt P, Dettmeyer R, Madea B. Withdrawal of artificial nutrition in the persistent vegetative state: a continuous controversy. *Forensic Sci Int* 2000;113:505–509.
111. *In re Helga Wanglie*, Fourth Judicial District (Dist Ct., Probate Ct. Div.) PX-91-283, Minnesota, Hennepin County (1991).
112. Revised Statutes of Missouri Section 459.040 (2003).
113. *In re Baby "K,"* 832 F3d 590 (4th Cir), *cert denied*, 513 U.S. 825 (1994).
114. *Gilgunn v. Massachusetts General Hospital*, SUCV92-4820 (Mass Supreme Ct., Suffolk Co., April 21, 1995).
115. Johnson SH, Gibbons VP, Goldner JA, Wiener RL, Eton D. Legal and institutional policy responses to medical futility. *J Health Hosp Law* 1997;30:21–36.
116. Halevy A, Brody BA. A multi-institution collaborative policy on medical futility. *JAMA* 1996;281:937–941.
117. Texas Health and Safety Code 166.046(a) (Vernon Suppl. 2002).

Index

A

B

C

D

E

F

G

H

I

N

O

P

R

S

T

U

V

W

X

Z

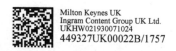

Milton Keynes UK
Ingram Content Group UK Ltd.
UKHW021930071024
449327UK00022B/1757

9 780367 389079